To Hildegard and Sophie

Sports Injuries:

Diagnosis and Management

To Hildegard and Sophie

Sports Injuries
Diagnosis and Management

Second edition

Christopher M. Norris MSc, CBA, MCSP, SRP

Director of Norris Associates, Chartered Physiotherapists, Sale, Cheshire

EDINBURGH LONDON NEW YORK OXFORD PHILADELPHIA
ST LOUIS SYDNEY TORONTO 1998

Butterworth-Heinemann
An imprint of Elsevier Science Limited
Robert Stevenson House,
1-3 Baxter's Place, Leith Walk,
Edinburgh EH1 3AF

First published 1993
Second edition 1998
Reprinted 1999, 2002

© Christopher M. Norris 1998

British Library Cataloguing in Publication Data
A catalogue record for this book is available from the British Library

Library of Congress Cataloging in Publication Data
A catalog record for this book is available from the Library of Congress

ISBN 0 7506 2873 1

your source for books,
journals and multimedia
in the health sciences
www.elsevierhealth.com

Contents

Preface

The first edition of this book has become a standard text on sports physiotherapy and sports rehabilitation courses in the UK, and feedback from countless students has shaped the second edition. The new book is expanded and brought up to date with new work from a wide area of sources. Research papers, written work, clinical practice, and taught course material have all contributed to a more detailed approach with an increased practical feel. There are new chapters on exercise therapy, sports massage, and taping. More tables and checklists have been included to guide the practitioner, and the number of line diagrams has been more than doubled to make information easier to understand 'at a glance'. The first edition of the book was designed to be 'dipped into' rather than read from cover to cover, and this intention has been maintained and expanded in the second edition. The inclusion of a new appendix on manual muscle testing is also designed with this in mind.

The chapter on physical training and injury, was the largest chapter in the first edition, demonstrating the importance given to exercise therapy in the management of the injured athlete. This importance has been firmly underlined for the second edition, with the inclusion of a separate chapter on exercise therapy in addition to that on physical training. This new chapter deals with functional rehabilitation with detailed work on muscle imbalance, posture, and proprioceptive exercise.

The chapters on sports massage, and on taping describe essentially practical material which is really best learnt through demonstration and corrected practice. It is hoped that these chapters will encourage readers to seek out courses in these areas and develop good practical skills to augment their theoretical knowledge.

It is hoped that this new edition, like the first, will be regularly used and accompany many students on their clinical placements throughout training. In addition if the book can act as a guide and 'aide-mémoire' to the experienced clinician it will have fulfilled its purpose.

C.M.N.

Preface to the first edition

Injuries relating to sport and exercise are by no means restricted to the elite athlete. The Sunday footballer, the twice-a-week aerobics devotee, and the pensioner playing badminton all deserve the same high quality of care that the professional sportsperson receives. Increases in life expectancy and changes in employment have led to an increased number of retired individuals in our society. These people are quite rightly encouraged to remain active, and exercise classes and sports centres are now being filled with older people. This trend has inevitably led to a change in the nature of those we see with sports injuries. It is now commonplace to see a fifty-year-old badminton player with an injury, and the individual with a frozen shoulder is as likely to complain that it affects their tennis serve or golf swing as much as it does the activities of everyday living. For this reason a number of complaints are included in this book which at first appear to be out of the realm of sports injuries. Conditions such as frozen shoulder, carpal tunnel syndrome and thoracic outlet syndrome are more commonly noticed when an elderly person starts exercising.

The subject area of this book is very diverse and draws on many aspects of sports science as well as sports physiotherapy. Part One deals with general aspects of injury and management, while Part Two looks at specific injuries. Part Two is arranged in individual body areas purely for convenience. Considerable overlap exists, and treatment will be far more effective when an holistic approach is taken. The book is selective in its approach, placing greater emphasis on the more commonly seen complaints. It draws on the diverse body of knowledge of sports injuries and combines this with practical experience, in an attempt to produce an academic but freely readable format. Some attention is paid to functional anatomy of the injured area, as to continue to treat well and to fully understand dysfunction we must regularly revise and update our knowledge of the normal human body. Chapter 2, which deals with the tissue response to injury, is equally important from this standpoint.

Over the years, the athletes I have treated have come from all competition levels, and the variation of sports practised by them have been countless. One central theme throughout the management of all these individuals however, has been the emphasis on active healthcare, especially by the use of therapeutic exercise in all its forms. It has always been my practice when treating injured athletes to ask the simple question, 'how can I teach this patient to help him or herself?' It is my firm belief that active therapy, by encouraging an individual to take part in his or her own treatment, places an emphasis on the patient to take a greater responsibility for their own wellbeing. I have seen countless numbers of athletes regain self-esteem and take charge of their injury, through exercise therapy. The facial expression of depression and defeat gradually gives way to confidence and the athlete becomes a 'winner' once more. In Chapter 3 we deal with the psychological consequences of injury, and the importance of changing an individual from a 'pain sufferer' to a 'pain manager'. Exercise therapy can produce this change.

It is no coincidence that Chapter 6 on physical training and injury is one of the longest in the book, and that many of the chapters include autotherapy techniques for athletes to apply themselves. Successful management of sports injuries requires an in depth knowledge of exercise therapy, and the sports physiotherapist must ensure that their standard of treatment in this area is as good as that of manual therapy or electrotherapy. Much of the material in this chapter is taught by the author on the Advanced Certificate in Sports Physiotherapy, at Alsager College, and on other postgraduate physiotherapy courses in the UK and abroad.

It is not intended that the book be read from cover to cover, but rather that it is 'dipped into', and so cross-referencing is used where appropriate. The text is written for a variety of practitioners, reflecting the multidisciplinary approach to the care of the injured athlete. It will be of particular interest to physiotherapists, at both student and postgraduate levels, and should be useful to doctors, sports scientists, coaches and athletes.

Some may say that the use of the word 'diagnosis' in the title of this book is inappropriate for physiotherapists. However, the physiotherapist dealing with the injured athlete is usually the first, and sometimes only, practitioner to see a patient. He or she must therefore take a greater responsibility for determining the nature of an injury, and be able to distinguish those conditions which are suitable for physiotherapy management from those which require referral. In this context both the therapist and medical practitioner must realize the limitations of their particular skills and recognize when a condition would be more suitably treated by each other. In Chapter 4 we look briefly at assessment techniques, and pay particular attention to the evaluation of function. This is an ongoing process, and as treatment progresses more information becomes available to the practitioner and so the exact diagnosis may change.

C.M.N.

Section I

Section I

1

Biomechanics of injury

Human tissue is governed by the laws of mechanics in the same way as other materials. While mechanics is concerned with forces, the effect of these forces on living organisms is the realm of biomechanics. The association between biological and mechanical aspects of movement has been said to give human motion its sophistication (Williams and Sperryn, 1976). For this reason, the study of biomechanics has a direct application to injury and recovery, and knowledge of this subject is essential for an understanding of the prevention, diagnosis and treatment of sports injuries (LeVeau, 1990).

Biomechanical principles

Forces

Force is a term used to describe the interaction of an object with its surroundings (Enoka, 1994). It has been defined as the physical action which tends to change the position of a body in space (Stallard, 1984). Consequently, it is an entity which will produce motion, and the study of force and motion is called kinetics. The unit of measurement of a force is the newton (N), one newton being the force which would produce an acceleration of 1 m/s^2 when acting on an object with a mass of 1 kg.

The most common forces affecting the human body are those produced by muscles, and those occurring as a result of gravity, inertia and contact. There are four important considerations when dealing with forces, the magnitude and direction of the force, and its line and point of application. The combination of magnitude and direction make force a vector quantity (Kent, 1994).

Forces can therefore be represented graphically by an arrow, the direction of which gives the direction of the force. The arrowhead represents the force's point of application, and the magnitude is given as a value in newtons, or is represented by the length of the arrow. Forces may act in the same line (in series) and are termed linear, or they may act in parallel. In addition, forces of equal magnitude may act opposite to each other to form a force couple. In this case, because the forces are aligned opposite each other no linear displacement occurs, instead a turning force is produced (Fig. 1.1).

The total force acting on a system may be calculated. For forces acting in series, this is simply a matter of subtraction or addition, but when forces act at angles to each other a parallelogram of forces can be constructed to facilitate calculation. Here, the two original or 'component' forces form the adjacent sides of the parallelogram, and the force

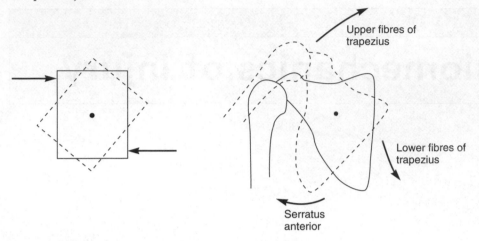

Figure 1.1 Forces of equal magnitude acting in opposite directions produce a turning effect.

which represents the two combined (the resultant) is the diagonal of the parallelogram (Fig 1.2a, b).

This principle (known as the resolution of forces) works equally well in reverse. If one force is known, its two components, acting at 90° to each other, may be determined. Thus when the heel strikes the ground (Fig 1.2c) two component forces exist causing both shear and compression.

Analysis of human motion is further simplified by using a free body diagram to help visualize the forces acting on the body. A stick figure is used to represent the body isolated from its surroundings. The diagram shows all the external forces acting on the body such as ground resistance and gravity, but not the internal forces such as muscle forces acting across a joint. The forces (input) act on the body in such a way that they produce motion (output).

In Fig. 1.3a, an athlete is running, and we want to calculate the relevant force acting on the body. First, we simplify the action by converting it to a stick figure (Fig. 1.3b), to clarify the limb position. Finally (Fig. 1.3c) we show the relevant forces imposed on the athlete's body by the surroundings. In the case of this figure these include air resistance

(Fa), the athlete's weight (Fw) and the ground reaction force (Fg).

Newton's laws of motion

Motion, defined as the continual change of relative position of an object in space (Kent, 1994), may be linear, angular or curvilinear. Linear motion occurs in a straight line (for example ice-skating). All parts of the body move the same distance in the same direction and in the same time. Angular (rotatory) motion involves movement of an object about a fixed point (the axis of rotation), so that each part of the object travels in an arc. An example is a dancer pirouetting. Curvilinear motion is the movement of all parts of an object along a curved path (for example a javelin throw). This type of motion has both linear and angular components.

The basic principles of the relationship between force and motion were set down by Newton in 1687 in his classic work *Philosophiae naturalis principia mathematica* (the mathematical principles of natural philosophy). These principles are known collectively as the 'laws of motion'.

Newton's first law of motion is the law of inertia. It states that an object remains in its

Figure 1.2 Parallelogram of forces. The two forces acting parallel to (50 N) and at right angles to (35 N) the lower leg (a) may be resolved into a single force represented by the resultant (b). (c) Components of ground reaction force in a runner.

Figure 1.3 The free body diagram. (a) An athlete sprinting from the blocks has forces imposed upon him or her from the environment. (b) A stick figure is used to simplify the action. (c) Forces due to body weight, air resistance and ground reaction are shown.

existing state of motion unless acted on by an external force. A stationary object will not begin to move unless acted on by an external unbalanced force, and a body which is moving will keep moving in the same direction and at the same velocity unless it is similarly affected by an external force. Consequently, objects have a resistance to motion change, and this property is called *inertia*.

When a ball is rolling along the ground, it will take more energy to start or stop the ball rolling than it will simply to keep it rolling at the same speed. Similarly, in a vigorous kicking action, inertia will have to be overcome to start the limb moving. If the force required to do this is large enough and rapid enough, muscle damage may occur.

A joint has a certain inertia as a result of its osteological format and the properties of the joint structures. Following immobilization the inertia is likely to be greater because the joint tissues have stiffened and the joint fluid has become more viscous. Gentle, rhythmic swinging exercises are often used to mobilize stiff joints. The continuous motion being more effective than stopping, pausing, and then starting again. In cases of severe weakness after injury, a muscle may be unable to overcome joint inertia to initiate movement. Once the movement has been started by the therapist, the patient's muscles may be strong enough to continue the action – a technique applied in sling suspension.

Heavier objects will be more difficult to start or stop than light objects travelling at the same speed, because heavier things possess more *momentum*. Momentum is the product of an object's mass and its velocity, and is an important consideration during exercise. Rapid, full range weight training exercises, for example, can be dangerous when muscle fatigue sets in. The combined momentum of the limb and weight may continue movement beyond full physiological joint range to cause tissue damage. Gleim (1984) showed momentum to be a significant factor in injuries to American football players. Taunton, McKenzie and Clement (1988) claimed that the most serious injuries in adolescent football and hockey players occur in the largest athletes, who create larger momentum forces.

Newton's second law is that of acceleration. This law states that the rate of change of momentum of a body takes place in the direction of the force and is proportional to the size of the force and the duration for which it acts.

If a hockey player hits a ball, the force (F) with which he or she hits acts for the specific time (t) that the stick is in contact with the ball. The ball has a certain mass (m), and changes its velocity from that at the start (u) to that at the finish of the action (v). We know that momentum is the product of mass and velocity, we know the velocity at the start and at the finish, so the rate of change of this momentum can be obtained by dividing the difference in velocities by time, therefore:

Rate of change of momentum

$$F = \frac{mv - mu}{t}$$

Factorizing this we are left with

$$F = \frac{m(v - u)}{t}$$

since $(v - u)/t$ is the same as change in velocity/t and this is acceleration (a), we are left with the equation $F = ma$.

The amount by which the velocity of an object is increased is dependent both on the magnitude of the force imposed on the object, and the time for which this force acts. This is an important consideration in throwing sports. A greater range of movement will allow a force to be applied on an object for longer, and as a consequence the velocity obtained will be greater. These principles are used in events such as the shot-put and discus throw, where the athlete 'winds up' and spins to apply the greatest force over the greatest time.

Newton's third law is the law of reaction, which states that action and reaction are equal in magnitude but opposite in direction. When a ball is hit with a cricket bat, the player applies a force (action force), and the ball pushes back (reaction force). From Newton's second law we know that:

$$F = \frac{m(v - u)}{t}$$

Suppose the mass of the ball (m) is 0.1 kg, the velocity at the start (u) and finish (v) is 15 m/s and 40 m/s, respectively, and the ball strikes the bat for only 0.05 s (t). Because the initial velocity and the final velocity are in opposite directions, the difference in velocity is now obtained by summing the two values.

$$F = \frac{0.1(15 - (-40))}{0.05}$$
$$= 110N$$

When a ball travelling with this force is caught, to avoid injury it is necessary to reduce its momentum. Similarly, when landing from a vertical jump, body momentum must be reduced if injury (a fractured calcaneus) is not to result. The aim in each of these cases is to extend the time taken to dissipate the reaction force (Watkins, 1983). If the cricket ball is stopped with the arms and wrists locked, injury may result from the sudden impact of the force. However, if the arms are extended to meet the ball, and flexed as the ball is brought into the body, the time taken to dissipate the ball's force (deceleration period) is extended and the injury risk reduced.

In the case of landing from a jump, the knees bend to dissipate the reaction force rather than falling directly onto the heels with straight legs.

Stress and strain

When a force acts on an object, the force, expressed per unit area, is called mechanical stress. Pushing, pulling or twisting are all examples of such forces, but three major categories of stress are important within the context of sports injury. These are tension, compression and shear (Fig. 1.4).

Tension stress is a pulling force. When the ankle is twisted by an inversion injury, the lateral ligament will stretch and tension stress is applied. Similarly, when the spine is flexed, the posterior spinal ligaments are tightened and subjected to a tension stress.

Figure 1.4 Tension, compression and shear stresses.

Compression stress is the opposite of tension. It is a pushing force, applied along the length of a tissue. In the upright posture, the menisci of the knee take weight and compression stress is applied. Another example occurs when the quadriceps contract on a bent knee, the patella is pulled against the femur and compression stress is applied to the patello-femoral joint.

Shear stress occurs when opposite forces are applied to a tissue, causing one part of the tissue to slide over another. For example, the sacro-iliac joint may encounter shearing stresses with a fall, or a finger may be subluxed by shearing forces when hit by a hard ball.

Both compression and tension stresses occur in line with the tissue fibres, a direction in which the tissues are strongest. Shearing stresses are imposed at an angle to the fibres, making this type of stress potentially the most dangerous in terms of injury. A fall onto the straight leg, for example, will cause compression stress on the joint structures, especially the cartilage and menisci of the knee. These forces will be largely absorbed, but if severe, compression fracture may occur. During the fall, tension stress will be imposed on the muscles if the joints bend. The elastic capacities of the muscles will now take some of the stress away from the joint. Falling at an angle will again cause some compression and tension, but in addition shearing will take place between the body tissues, and the foot and ground. This type of stress could cause valgus or varus strain at the joint with associated ligament damage or joint subluxation if the force is great.

The relationship between load and deformation

When a stress (load) is applied to a tissue, the tissue will deform, and the deformation is called strain. The relationship between stress and strain is shown graphically by the stress–strain curve (Fig. 1.5). Different materials will each have their own individual curves, but the general shape of the curves will be the same.

Initially, the tissue obeys Hooke's law and its deformation is proportional to the force applied to it. As the curve begins (toe region) deformation occurs with low loading. In the

case of a tendon, this initial response is due to straightening out of the 'crimp' in the fibres, which represents 2–4% elongation (Curwin, 1994). This has the effect of protecting the body as most of the movements of daily living occur within this region. As load and deformation increase, a material moves into its elastic range, which is represented by the linear portion of the curve. At any point along this part of the line, the material which is put under stress will return to its original size and shape when the stressing force is released.

When the material is stressed beyond the elastic range, it will reach a point at which deformation becomes permanent. At this point, known as the elastic limit, the object will not return to its original form when the force is released. Going past this point, further along the stress–strain curve, the material moves into the plastic range. Here, the object will permanently deform, but not rupture. The greater the force, the greater the permanent deformation. As the stress imposed on the material increases still

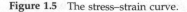

Figure 1.5 The stress–strain curve.

further, the yield point (Y) is reached. Now the material continues to deform even though the stress applied to it remains constant, a process known as creep. The stress–strain curve reaches its peak height at this point. As still greater stress is applied to the material, and we move still further along the curve, the material is failing rapidly. Little extra force is required to increase the rate of deformation which is already occurring. This is the necking region. The final load required to produce complete material failure (rupture) is the breaking strength. In the case of a tendon, this occurs when it has elongated 8–10% further than its original length (Butler et al., 1984).

Some materials (including connective tissue) demonstrate both plastic (viscous) and elastic properties, and so are termed viscoelastic. A simple mechanical model of a spring (elastic) and hydraulic cylinder (plastic) linked in series may be used to illustrate this property (Fig. 1.6).

The mechanical responses of the connective tissue are due to the complex interaction between the collagen fibres themselves and the protein matrix (ground substance) in which they are contained. The combination of these two materials gives connective tissue a biphasic nature, exhibiting both stress relaxation (a reduction in load over time) and creep (an increase in length under constant loading) (Fig. 1.7). Applying these principles to sport, repeated movement in a constant range of motion such as when jogging may lead to stress relaxation and a reduction in loading and therefore resistance to movement. Holding a stretched position (constant load) in sport or daily living will lead to creep and the consequent joint laxity may give a reduction in joint stability.

Factors influencing the stress–strain curve

The stress–strain curve may be influenced by a number of mechanical features of tissue. Of these, we will look at stiffness, creep, fatigue, resilience and toughness.

Figure 1.6 Viscoelastic tissues. (a) Schematic representation of a viscous element in material capable of permanent (plastic) deformation. (b) An elastic element in material capable of recoverable (elastic) deformation. (c) A simplified model of collagenous tissue. Connective tissue is a viscoelastic material: when stretched it behaves as if it has both viscous and elastic elements connected in series. From Sapega et al. (1981), with permission.

Structural stiffness occurs when a tissue is less elastic. In this case the initial slope of the stress–strain curve is steeper as less deformation occurs when stress increases. Scar tissue would fall into this category. Scar tissue within a ligament, for example, may be as strong or stronger than the ligament itself, but will not be as elastic and will not therefore respond to stress in the same manner.

Creep occurs when a load (usually small) is imposed on a material over a long time period, causing the material to deform very gradually. Viscoelastic materials demonstrate this property. They deform at a con-

(a)   Stress relaxation: load reduces over time

(b)   Creep: deformation increases with constant load

Figure 1.7   The biphasic nature of connective tissue.

stant rate regardless of the speed with which a force is applied to them. The degree of deformation this time is determined not just by the amount of force applied to a tissue, but also by the duration over which the force is applied. Creep is therefore time dependent. A lesser load applied over a greater time period will produce a larger amount of creep. Creep is related to the viscosity of a tissue, and elevation of temperature will cause corresponding increases in creep. This fact can be used to good effect when stretching tight connective tissue. A warmed tissue which is stretched and held being more pliable than a cold tissue stretched rapidly.

Fatigue is the characteristic of materials to fail before the yield point is reached, when a load is applied repeatedly (cyclically). The larger the load, the fewer repetitions required to produce failure, although a certain minimum load (the endurance limit) must be applied. An example of fatigue through cumulative loading is that of continually bending a wire until it breaks. Fatigue (stress) fractures occur in some athletes who place too much stress on a bone through training. Other things being equal, a heavier athlete is likely to produce fatigue more quickly than a lighter one because the heavier athlete is placing his or her tissues under greater load.

Both resilience and toughness are related to the ability of a material to absorb and release energy. Resilient materials absorb energy well in the elastic range while tough materials do the same in the plastic range. A resilient material will absorb energy and deform, returning to its original shape when the load is released. A tough material will again deform, but will not return to its original shape. Highly resilient materials tend to be bouncy. For example, a rubber ball when dropped will deform, and absorb energy. It will quickly release this stored energy and return to its original shape as it bounces back.

Tough materials will absorb a lot of energy without breaking, but when their failure point is reached, they rupture quickly. Putty is an example here. If something is dropped onto it, it will absorb energy by deforming but will not return to its original shape when released. If subjected to slow tension stress it will stretch, but when stretched quickly it will snap.

Leverage

Types of lever

A lever is simply a device for transmitting (but not creating) force. A typical lever is a rigid bar with one point (the fulcrum or pivot) about which the lever revolves. Two forces are applied to a lever, the effort which tries to move the lever, and the resistance which tries to stop movement. The product of the force, and the perpendicular distance between the line of application of the force to the fulcrum, is known as the 'moment' of the force or torque and is measured in newton-metres (Nm). Torques may be compared between agonist and antagonist muscles (torque ratio), and torque curves may be plotted to show torque generated throughout a range of motion (see Table 1.2, p. 25, Isokinetics).

The distance from the effort to the fulcrum is called the effort arm, and that from the resistance to the fulcrum, the resistance arm. The ratio between the effort arm and the resistance arm gives a value for the mechanical advantage. If the effort arm is greater than the resistance arm the mechanical advantage is greater than one. The mechanical advantage is less than one if the resistance arm is the greater of the two.

The relationship between the fulcrum, resistance and effort within a lever system determines the type or 'order' of lever. The first type, or 'first order lever', is one of balance. A typical example is a child's see-saw, in which the fulcrum lies between the force and effort. For the lever to balance, the leverage created by the effort must equal that created by the resistance.

With a simple first order lever, a resistance of 6 kg placed 3 m away from the fulcrum gives a torque of 18 Nm (6 × 3 = 18). To balance this out, the effort has to be of the same magnitude. So, the 9 kg weight has only to be placed 2 m from the fulcrum for the lever to balance (9 × 2 = 18). An example of a first-class lever in the body is the skull pivoted on the atlas. The line of gravity of the skull passes anterior to the vertebral column, and to stop the head falling forwards from its own weight, the neck extensors must exert an equivalent balancing force.

In the second order lever, the resistance lies between the fulcrum and the effort. With this type, which is commonly illustrated by a wheelbarrow, the torque produced by the effort is always greater than that produced by the resistance, so the mechanical advantage is also greater than one. The second order lever is consequently used to produce power, but is rarely found in the human body.

The third order lever is the one found most commonly in the body. Here, the resistance arm is the full length of the lever, and mechanical advantage is always less than one. The effort being applied between the fulcrum and resistance. Unlike the second order lever, this does not favour power, but rather distance and speed. With this type of lever, a contraction of a muscle (the effort) will be magnified and will cause a large movement of the resistance (the limb). In addition, as the distal end of the lever moves a greater distance than the proximal end, the speed of movement of the distal end is greater.

Leverage and injury

Increased leverage will multiply the effect of a force on body tissue, often making injury more likely (Fig. 1.8). For example, lifting a 10 kg weight is not, in itself, dangerous. However, lifting it at arm's length in a bent over position with the legs straight will place excessive leverage on the spine, increasing the effect of the weight on the lumbar spine and making injury more likely. As another example, performing a bilateral straight leg raising movement will place excessive strain on the spine, while simply bending the legs will reduce the leverage effect of the legs and so reduce the likelihood of injury.

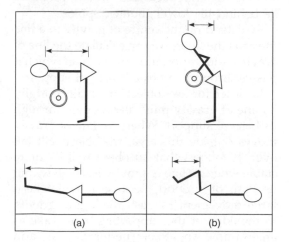

Figure 1.8 Reducing leverage can reduce the risk of injury. (a) Maximal leverage. (b) Minimal leverage.

Some types of athletic equipment may increase the risk of injury by their leverage effects. Running shoes (see p. 328) with flared heels increase the leverage effect on the ankle joints and may, under certain circumstances, predispose the athlete to injury. The face guard on an American football helmet will increase the leverage of neck extension, and a ski will increase leverage forces acting on the tibia.

Centre of gravity

The centre of gravity of an object is the point at which all the weight of the object can be considered to act. This is also the point at which the object would balance. In a symmetrical object such as a ball, the centre of gravity will be at the centre of the object. But, with asymmetrical objects, such as the human body, the centre of gravity will be nearer to the larger and heavier end.

In the human body standing in the anatomical position, the centre of gravity is at the S1/2 spinal level, but this point will vary as the body position changes. As the centre of gravity is partially determined by an object's weight, it will shift when something is carried. The centre of gravity of a hiker carrying a heavy rucksack for example, is shifted up and back and would probably lie behind his lower thoracic spine.

By extending the centre of gravity in a line towards the floor, we can calculate the line of gravity, and importantly the point at which it passes through an object's base of support.

In order for any object to remain upright, its line of gravity must always pass through its base of support. When the line of gravity moves outside this area, the object will fall over. It follows that an object will be more stable when its line of gravity lies well within its base of support, because it will take a large movement to push the line of gravity to the edge of the supporting base. Take as an example an athlete performing an arm curl exercise with a heavy barbell. In the normal standing position without the barbell his or her line of gravity will fall between the feet. However, when he or she holds the weight in front of him or her, the centre of gravity moves forwards, meaning that his or her line of gravity will now fall nearer to the toes. As the line of gravity is now closer to the edge of his or her base of support, it will take only a small movement to push it outside his or her supporting base, and cause him or her to lose balance.

Stability

During most sports and exercises, an unstable position is a dangerous one, particularly when the body becomes fatigued. An object is more stable when its centre of gravity is lower. Moreover, we say that an object is in stable equilibrium if moving it would cause its centre of gravity to rise. In Fig. 1.9c, the pyramid can either slide sideways, or it would have to be moved onto its side to raise its centre of gravity.

Unstable equilibrium exists when an object's centre of gravity would fall if it were moved (Fig. 1.9b). If the centre of gravity remains the same in all positions, as with a ball, then an object is said to be in neutral equilibrium (Fig. 1.9a).

In addition to the position of the centre of gravity, the size of an object's base of support will also affect its stability. A wide base of support is more stable than a narrow one. Take as an example an ice-skater skating a line. With only the thin blade of the skate on the ice, and the feet close together the base of support is very small. In addition the skater is standing tall, lifting the centre of gravity. The combination of these two features makes him or her quite unstable. However, a judo exponent with his or her feet wide apart has a wide base of support, the knees are bent lowering the centre of gravity and making him or her much more stable.

When moving, the base of support should be widened in the direction of movement. A pulling action such as tug-o-war is therefore safer when a wide stance is taken (increasing

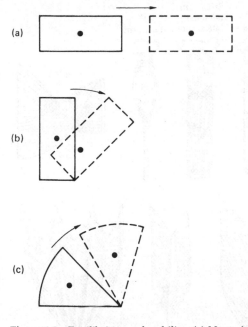

Figure 1.9 Equilibrium and stability. (a) Neutral equilibrium. The centre of gravity remains level as the object is moved. (b) Unstable equilibrium. The centre of gravity moves down as the object is moved. (c) Stable equilibrium. The centre of gravity moves up as the object is moved.

the base of support) with one foot in front of the other. Sideways actions, such as lateral flexion of the spine, become more stable and far safer with the feet astride in the frontal plane.

Biomechanics and kinesiology of muscle

Form of muscle

A great number of muscle types exist, but generally speaking muscles may be grouped according to the orientation of their fibres. The fibres may be arranged either in parallel, obliquely, or in a spiral fashion, and the arrangement will dictate the power and range of motion that the muscle can produce.

When the fibres are arranged in parallel, the muscle may be strap-like (sartorius)

where individual fibres run the whole length of the muscle. The fibres may run between adjacent tendinous intersections which divide the muscle as a whole into sections (rectus abdominis). Alternatively, the fibres may be grouped into discrete bundles producing a fusiform muscle belly which attaches to a tendon (biceps). Another fibre arrangement is the sheet attaching to a broad flat tendon or aponeurosis (internal oblique).

The oblique or 'pennate' grouping sees the muscle fibres attaching to a central tendon. Fibres joining to one side of a tendon only are termed unipennate. When the fibres bind to both sides of a central septum the muscle is bipennate, and when the muscle has several septa it is termed multipennate.

In each case, the muscle fibres can only shorten to half their original length, so the shorter fibres of a pennate muscle will produce less range of motion than the long fibres of a parallel muscle (Fig. 1.10). However, the power of a muscle is determined by the total cross-sectional area of the fibres. With a pennate muscle the total cross-sectional area is much larger than that of a parallel muscle and so the power produced is significantly greater (Fig. 1.11).

The third type of fibre arrangement is the spiralized (Fig. 1.12). Here, the muscle fibres

Figure 1.10 Muscle shortening. A muscle fibre can only shorten by half of its original length (d/2), so the range of motion is greater for a parallel arrangement of muscle fibres (a), than for a pennate arrangement (b).

Figure 1.11 Muscle power is proportional to fibre cross-sectional area (A). The total area ($A_1 + A_2$), and so the power, is greater for a pennate-shaped muscle than for a strap-shaped one.

twist as they travel between the two ends of the muscle (pectoralis major, trapezius). As the muscle contracts, the fibres tend to de-rotate and straighten out, imparting a rotation force to the bone on which they attach. In this way, a spiralized muscle not only approximates the bones of the joint over which it acts, but pulls the bones into the same plane.

Muscle attachment

The position of the muscle attachment to the bone, and the direction of the muscle will largely determine its action. As a muscle contracts, the force exerted onto its tendon may be resolved into three distinct components (Fig. 1.13a). The first component acts at 90° to the bony lever and tends to move it, causing a rotatory (swing) action at the joint. The second component acts in parallel with the bony lever and pulls it into the joint causing approximation (shunt). Finally, the offset arrangement of the muscle insertions causes the bone to rotate about its longitudinal axis (spin).

The three movements will vary tremendously between muscles and are altered by the restriction of bony configuration and soft tissue tightness. However, each of the three

Figure 1.12 Various muscle fibre arrangements. From *Grays Anatomy* (35th edn), with permission.

components is emphasized differently in various muscles. Where the muscle attachment is wrapped around the bone (Fig. 1.13d), the spin component is emphasized (pronator quadratus). The positions of the distal and proximal muscle attachments will dictate the relative amount of swing and shunt. When the distal attachment is close to the joint (brachialis) the swing component dominates (Fig. 1.13b), but when the distal attachment is placed some distance from the joint (brachioradialis) the shunt component is greater (Fig. 1.13c).

Group action of muscles

The properties of muscle contraction are often described for isolated muscle fibres in the laboratory. Functionally, however, muscles do not contract singly, but in a group.

Figure 1.13 The components of the force exerted by a muscle on its tendon (see text for details). From *Grays Anatomy* (35th edn), with permission.

The group action of muscles is an important consideration, both with injury and the process of rehabilitation.

When stimulated, a muscle fibre will develop tension tending to shorten the muscle as a whole. Whether the tension developed is sufficient to cause shortening, or indeed joint movement, will depend on a number of factors. The amount of tension developed, the resistance opposing the muscle, the mechanical leverage system, and contraction of neighbouring muscles will all have an effect.

The most effective muscle at producing a particular movement is called the prime mover (agonist). Any muscle which helps to create this same movement but is less effective at doing so is an assistant (secondary) mover. In different situations a muscle may take on both actions. Take as an example a bench-press movement in weight train-ing. If a wide grip is taken, the prime mover will be the pectoral muscles, and an assistant mover will be the triceps. If a narrow grip is taken, pulling the arms in close to the side, the pectorals are shortened and become less effective (length–tension relationship). Now, the triceps becomes the prime mover and the pectorals act as assistant movers.

The muscle which, if it contracted, would tend to oppose the action of the prime mover is the antagonist. Normally through reciprocal innervation, the contraction of the antagonist is reduced. With a co-contraction, however, both prime mover and antagonist may contract. This type of contraction can represent a lack of skill (Wells, 1966) and its reduction has been cited as one way in which strength increases are produced early on in training (Sale, 1988). In actions such as gripping, two joint muscles (see below) are acting, and there may also be a rapid alternation between opposing muscle groups or isometric action to stabilize the joint. The interaction of muscles in co-contraction is complex, and the interested reader is referred to Basmajian and Deluca (1985), and Zehr and Sale (1994) for a full review.

A muscle acts as a fixator or stabilizer when it anchors or supports a body part to supply a firm base for another muscle (usually the prime mover) to pull on. When a muscle contracts, it will tend to pull both of its ends towards each other. To produce movement at one end only, the bony attachment of one end of the muscle must be stabilized. An example is the contraction of the downwards rotators of the scapula as teres major adducts the humerus. Another situation in which a fixator can act is to resist the pull of gravity to stabilize a body segment. An example of this is a press-up action, in which the abdominal muscles contract to prevent the spine sagging into extension.

A neutralizer is a muscle which contracts to prevent an unwanted action of the prime or assistant mover. Most muscles are capable of several actions, and those not required must be counteracted by activity of a neutralizer. For example, biceps will both flex the elbow and supinate the forearm. If we wish to flex the elbow without forearm rotation, the pronators must neutralize the unwanted supinatory action of the biceps.

Ballistic and reciprocal actions

In rapid actions such as throwing or kicking, the agonist will contract powerfully, but briefly, to move the limb, allowing momentum of the moving limb to maintain the action. EMG studies of this type of action (Zehr and Sale, 1994) have shown a pre-movement silence (depression of the EMG signal) to exist just before initiation of muscle contraction. This silence may potentiate both the force and velocity of the subsequent contraction. At the end of the desired range of motion, the antagonist contracts eccentrically (to a variable degree) to decelerate the limb.

Finally, the prime mover works once more to control the final position of the limb. This triphasic muscle action (Fig. 1.14) is known as a ballistic contraction. An overlap may be present between the initial contraction of the prime mover and that of the antagonist in which case a co-contraction occurs. The ballistic action is obviously a highly skilled coordination, and when, with fatigue, the action becomes uncontrolled, injury frequently results.

When an eccentric action immediately precedes a concentric one, a reciprocal contraction occurs, giving a more powerful contraction. LaGasse (1983) demonstrated an 11.4% greater force output from the quadriceps when knee flexion was performed prior to knee extension. Reciprocal contractions occur in most functional movements such as walking and running, and form the basis of power training using plyometrics (p. 128). The stretch incurred by the elastic components of the muscle when working eccentrically is released with the concentric contraction, increasing the force output. In addition the stretch reflex is stimulated in the stretched muscle facilitating a more

Figure 1.14 Triphasic muscle action. Initially the arm is propelled forwards by the agonist muscles (AGI). As the arm reaches its target, the antagonists contract to eccentrically slow the limb (ANT). Some overlap of muscle contraction occurs (Co-cont). Finally, the agonist contracts again to finely position the limb (AG2). From McArdle et al. (1986), with permission.

powerful contraction through increased recruitment and activation of motor units.

Two-joint muscles

Most joint complexes contain two-joint or 'biarticular' muscles, and these are frequently the muscles which are torn in sport. Examples in the lower limb are the rectus femoris, hamstrings and gastrocnemius. The important characteristic of these muscles is that they are unable to permit full movement at both joints simultaneously.

When full movement is limited by passive stretch of the muscle, passive insufficiency is present. An example is passive hip extension combined with knee flexion being limited by rectus femoris. When the muscle is unable to shorten sufficiently to produce a full range movement at both joints simultaneously, active insufficiency exists. An example here is the hamstrings flexing the knee and extending the hip.

Because the muscles are not long enough to permit movement at both joints simultaneously, the tension in one muscle is transferred to the other. Using the hip as an example, as the hamstrings contract to extend the hip, tension is transmitted to the rectus femoris enabling it to extend the knee (Wells, 1966). This type of action, involving either extension or flexion at both joints at the same time, is called concurrent movement. The muscle shortens at one end but lengthens at the other, and so maintains its length and conserves tension. When the hip is flexed but the knee extended, the rectus femoris is shortened and rapidly loses tension, while the hamstrings are lengthened and rapidly gain tension, an example of countercurrent movement (Rasch, 1989).

Two-joint muscles provide three main advantages to the musculoskeletal system (Enoka, 1994). First, these muscles couple movement at both joints. For example, shoulder and elbow flexion occur together in a feeding pattern, and both actions have a contribution from biceps brachii. Second, the shortening velocity of a two-joint muscle is less than that of a single-joint muscle (van Ingen Schenau, Bobbert and van Soest 1990), contributing to more rapid limb movement. Third, two-joint muscles are said to redistribute muscle force throughout the limb (Toussaint et al., 1992). For example, if hip flexion is performed by iliopsoas, tightness in the hamstrings will tend to flex the knee. This is an appropriate action for the swing phase of gait. Hip extension will tighten rectus femoris tending to extend the knee, an action required during the propulsive gait phase.

Force–velocity relationship

When a muscle is contracting, a relationship exists between the speed of movement it creates and the force which the muscle can develop. The torque generated by the muscle decreases as the velocity of movement increases (Pipes and Wilmore, 1975; Coyle et al., 1981; Burnie and Brodie, 1986). The greatest force being produced at the slowest speeds.

One theory for the force–velocity relationship is that the myosin cross-bridges within the muscle continually move through thermal agitation. The probability of union between the actin and myosin filaments is therefore reduced at higher speeds (Bray et al., 1986), and fewer cross-bridge attachments may occur. In addition, as muscle-shortening speed increases, the rate of cross-bridge cycling increases, but the average force exerted by each cross-bridge is reduced (Enoka, 1994). The speed at which the actin and myosin cross-bridges attach is fairly uniform (a figure known as the rate constant). As force depends on the number of cross-bridges formed, greater speed of contraction means that more filaments slide past each other without binding, and therefore force is reduced. Maximal force is exerted eccentrically (muscle lengthening). As soon as the muscle begins to shorten, force reduces dramatically. When velocity increases to just 10% of maximum, force reduces by 35% (Lieber, 1992).

Length–tension relationship

A further biomechanical relationship exists between the initial length of the muscle and its force production, the so-called length–tension relationship. In the laboratory situation, an isolated muscle can exert its maximal force or tension while in a resting stretched state. If the muscle is shortened or over-stretched, less tension can be exerted.

Physiologically, this can be explained in terms of the sliding filament mechanism. In the shortened position, an overlap of the muscle filaments occurs, interfering with cross-bridge coupling. If the muscle is over-stretched, the filaments are pulled comple-tely apart, the cross-bridges will not come into contact, and no tension can be devel-oped (Fig. 1.15).

As the relaxed muscle is stretched, how-ever, a passive force due to muscle elasticity is created. This varies between muscles, for example the spinal extensors in man resist a stretching force by purely passive means. Therefore, total force developed by the mus-cle will be the sum of the active and passive forces.

The length–tension relationship can be used to advantage where two muscles work together to produce a movement as primary and secondary movers. We can emphasize the prime mover by shortening (and there-fore 'weakening') the secondary mover. For example, in a sit-up movement with the legs straight both the hip flexors and abdominal muscles are working. However, the hip flex-ors are generally strong anyway through use in everyday living, so the training effect on these muscles has to be reduced. This is accomplished by bending the knees and hips. The length–tension relationship dictates that the hip flexors will now be able to pro-duce less force.

Joint mechanics

Accessory movements

The movements of a joint are of two types, physiological and accessory. Physiological movements are those which the athlete can perform actively, for example flexion and extension of the knee. Accessory movements cannot be produced actively as individual movements, but occur automatically be-tween articulating surfaces of a joint as it moves. Three accessory movements are of particular importance when treating sports injuries, these are roll, slide and spin (Fig. 1.16).

Roll occurs when points at certain intervals on a moving surface contact points at the same intervals on the opposing surface (Hertling and Kessler, 1990). This is similar to a car tyre rolling over the road. If one point on the moving surface stays in contact with a variety of points on the opposing sur-face, slide is taking place. Spin is a pure rota-tion around a mechanical axis (Barak, Rosen and Sofer, 1990). Usually when a joint moves, both slide and roll must take place. If roll alone were the only movement, the joint would sublux before any appreciable range had been achieved. If only slide occurred, the edges of the concave aspect of the joint would impinge on the opposing convex lip.

Figure 1.15   The length–tension relationship.

Figure 1.16   Accessory joint movements. (a) Roll, (b) slide, and (c) spin.

Concave–convex motion

Synovial joints in general consist of both concave and convex surfaces created by the shapes of the bone ends within the joint and their covering cartilage. When a concave surface moves on a convex surface, roll and slide occur in the same direction, the bone sliding towards the direction of movement. When a convex surface moves on a concave surface roll and slide occur in opposite directions, the bone sliding away from the direction of movement. Take as an example knee movement. If the tibia extends on a fixed femur in a leg extension exercise (concave on convex) the joint surface of the tibia rolls and slides forwards in the direction of extension. On the other hand, if the femur extends on a stationary tibia as with standing up from a chair (convex on concave) the femoral condyles will roll forwards but slide backwards in the opposite direction to the movement. Knowledge of the direction of accessory movements is important when using joint mobilization techniques. For example, if shoulder flexion is limited, although the movement of the humerus is upward, because a convex surface is moving on a concave one, gliding of the joint should be directed downwards (caudally).

When gliding a joint, the direction of movement is altered with the angle of the joint. The glide direction chosen is called the treatment plane, and is the one in which most translatory motion is possible. In peripheral joints the joint line can be established fairly easily by palpation, and so the treatment plane is determined directly. In the spine, however, the treatment plane is determined by the joint angles of the facets, and is horizontal for C0–C1, angled at 45° between C2–T12, and almost horizontal for the lumbar area.

Close and loose pack

The two opposing surfaces of a joint do not fit together exactly; they are said to be non-congruent. But, with the joint in one particular position its surfaces will come as close together as they are able, and this is known as 'close pack'. In this position the joint capsule and ligaments twist and pull the joint surfaces together into approximation. The joint space is at a minimum and the concave surface of one bone fits tightly into the convex shape of the other. No further movement is possible in a joint which is close packed, and so this position is avoided when trying to mobilize the joint.

Loose pack position is exactly the opposite. As the joint surfaces are released from their close pack position, elastic recoil of the soft tissues surrounding the joint enables its surfaces to move apart, maximizing the joint space. The loose pack position is the resting position often taken up after injury because more joint fluid can accumulate. In loose pack positions joint play is possible. This consists of small accessory movements which give the joint its 'spring'. These are essential to the normal functioning of the joint and play a part in joint nutrition and combined movements.

Interestingly many fractures of the upper limb occur with a fall onto the outstretched arm, which is a close packed position, and many ligament sprains occur in loose packed position (Hertling and Kessler, 1990). Examples of close and loose pack positions are given in Table 1.1.

Axes and planes

The human body may for descriptive purposes be divided into three planes. The sagittal plane passes through the body from front to back, dividing it into right and left halves. The frontal plane divides the body into anterior and posterior sections, and lies at right angles to the sagittal plane. The transverse plane divides the body into upper and lower portions, and rests at right angles to the other two planes.

Each of the three body planes has an associated axis which passes perpendicularly through it (Fig. 1.17). Movement occurs *in* a plane but *about* an axis. Abduction and adduction occur in the frontal plane about the anteroposterior axis, flexion and extension occur in a sagittal plane about a transverse axis, and rotations occur in a transverse plane about a vertical axis.

In reality, movements do not occur in one plane, but several. For example, we talk of 'tri-plane motion' of the sub-taloid joint in a runner (see p. 211). This is because a complex series of movements link together to give a motion which occurs in all three planes about an oblique axis.

Figure 1.17   Axes and planes of the body.

Biomechanical analysis

Video movement analysis

Analysis of human movement is vital for the prevention and rehabilitation of sports injuries. The most basic analysis may be performed by the clinician simply observing the subject. This type of analysis may be useful, but is limited by the visual memory of the observer. The clinician is unable to follow and retain much of the important detail in even the slowest movement. Although the trained observer may extract considerably more data than the lay person, even when an action is repeated a number of times, precise analysis is not possible.

The situation is improved considerably when an action is recorded on videotape or cine film to be played back later for accurate analysis. This procedure has previously been complex and expensive, but with the steadily reducing cost and increasing standard of video equipment the task is much easier.

Table 1.1 Close packed and loose packed positions of selected joints

Joint(s)	Close packed position	Loose packed (resting) position
Facet (spine)	Extension	Midway between flexion and extension
Temporomandibular	Clenched teeth	Mouth slightly open
Gleno-humeral	Abduction and external rotation	55° abduction, 30° horizontal abduction, rotated so that the forearm is in the transverse plane
Acromioclavicular	Arm abducted to 30°	Arm resting by side, shoulder girdle in the physiological position
Sternoclavicular	Maximum shoulder elevation	Arm resting by side, shoulder girdle in the physiological position
Ulnohumeral (elbow)	Extension	70° elbow flexion, 10° forearm supination
Radiohumeral	Elbow flexed 90°, forearm supinated 5°	Full extension, full supination
Proximal radioulnar	5° supination	70° elbow flexion, 35° forearm supination
Distal radioulnar	5° supination	10° forearm supination
Radiocarpal (wrist)	Extension with ulnar deviation	Midway between flexion–extension (so that a straight line passes through the radius and third metacarpal) with slight ulnar deviation
First carpometacarpal	Full opposition	Midway between abduction-adduction and flexion-extension
Metacarpophalangeal (fingers)	Full flexion	Slight flexion
Metacarpophalangeal (thumb)	Full opposition	
Interphalangeal	Full extension	Slight flexion
Hip	Full extension, internal rotation and abduction	30° flexion, 30° abduction, and slight external rotation
Knee	Full extension and external rotation of the tibia	25° flexion
Talocrural (ankle)	Maximum dorsiflexion	10° plantarflexion, midway between maximum inversion and eversion
Subtalar	Full supination	Midway between extremes of inversion and eversion
Midtarsal	Full supination	Midway between extremes of range of movement
Tarsometatarsal	Full supination	Midway between extremes of range of movement
Metatarsophalangeal	Full extension	Neutral
Interphalangeal	Full extension	Slight flexion

From Clarkson and Gilewich (1989), with permission.

Observing and recording movement

In order to accurately record an action, the subject and environment in which he or she performs must be prepared. Subjects should be suitably dressed in shorts or bathing costume to enable accurate location of body segments and joints. Bony reference points or centres of motion are marked on the skin with adhesive tape or reflective markers. The background is cleared, where possible, to allow unobscured vision of the whole movement. The video camera is set up on a stand at a set distance from the subject. The camera should be capable of recording in poor lighting conditions (low lux number), and have a timing/counting facility. If two or more analyses are to be made, the distance between the camera and the subject must remain the same to reduce parallax error. Complex motions are better recorded with two synchronized cameras placed at 90° to each other.

Lighting must be adequate to illuminate the subject in all positions, and where this cannot be controlled (on the field) a low-light camera should be used. Reference points, such as a measuring stick placed in the field of view, can be useful to give a comparison of distance. Ideally, the whole action should be filmed without moving the camera. To do this the observer must be far enough away from the subject to get a wide field of view.

Analysing movement

The simplest way to analyse a movement is to slow the action down and use an experienced clinical eye. Where the video image is sufficiently clear and reference markers are visible this is an inexpensive and extremely useful method. The analysis may be taken further, by digitizing the image. Essentially this involves establishing X–Y coordinates of the various marked reference points. The video film is played back on a large flat screen monitor, and the freeze frame facility used to stop the action at a predetermined point. The relative positions of the various reference points are then recorded. A number of commercially available computer software programs allow the clinician to do this using a 'digitizing pen'. Alternatively, a 'mouse' is used to move the computer cursor to the selected reference point. The software package then records the position of the point in two dimensions. Gradually an image is built which may be used to create a stick figure (Fig. 1.18).

By progressing frame to frame, the limb and centres of rotation for the subject are recorded throughout the movement. Various parameters such as linear and angular displacements and accelerations of the body segments are then calculated. The overall action is reviewed by analysing the stick figure display, and the path described by individual reference points (loci) (Fig. 1.19) are studied. In addition, if sufficient joint locations are used, the body's centre of gravity may be determined.

Video analysis still has limitations, particularly with respect to joint rotation and three-dimensional images, although the use of two synchronized cameras reduces this problem. However, with the increasing availability of these systems, they are useful clinical tools for the sports physiotherapist.

Figure 1.18 Stick figure compiled by digitizing a video image.

Figure 1.19   Paths described by the hip, knee and ankle reference points. From Williams and Davis (1990), with permission.

Figure 1.20   Three force components of a force plate. a and b represent 'offset' position from centre of force plate.

Force plates

The force that an athlete exerts on a sports surface may be measured using a force plate. This is essentially a rigid plate set flush into the floor. Beneath the plate, at each corner, sit four transducers capable of recording various components of the ground reaction force (Fig. 1.20). The vertical component (F_z) is a compression force, while the horizontal components (F_y and F_x) are shearing forces. F_y is in line with the long edge of the force plate and is parallel to the direction of travel, whereas F_x is at right angles to the line of travel and parallel to the short edge of the force plate.

In addition to these three fundamental measurements, the force plate will show the moment (turning force) about the central z axis. The position of the line of action of a force is shown by measuring the distance from the force to the centre of the plate, represented by the values a and b.

Using these measurements, ground reaction forces can be plotted for vertical, anterior-posterior, and mediolateral forces (Fig. 1.21). On the time axis, zero represents the point of first contact with the platform (heel strike) and 1 shows the point of last contact (toe off). The vertical force component of running (normal heel–toe gait) has two peaks. The first (vertical impact force peak) occurs

Figure 1.21   Example for the components of the ground reaction force during running at a speed of 4 m/s (left and right foot). Adapted from Nigg (1994).

from 5 to 30 ms after ground contact and shows the first foot contact with the ground. In barefoot running the peak occurs sooner (5–10 ms), while running in a soft soled shoe on asphalt gives a slower peak (20–30 ms). In running, impact forces may be as high as four times body weight, while at take off in a jump, forces as high as twelve times body weight may be expected (Nigg, 1994). The second peak (vertical active force peak) is due to movement caused by muscle contraction. This occurs in the middle of the stance phase (100–200 ms after first ground contact). In sprint running vertical active forces may reach four times body weight (Nigg, 1994).

Isokinetic assessment

The use of isokinetic dynamometry is increasing in sports physiotherapy, and the system has both advantages and disadvantages. The system consists of a fixed axis of rotation and a lever driven either hydraulically or electrically. Both systems offer constant angular velocity. Originally hydraulic systems only offered isometric and concentric modes, but electrically powered systems now offer eccentric testing and continuous passive motion (CPM).

Advantages and disadvantages of isokinetic exercise

One of the disadvantages of isokinetics is that dynamometer velocities normally range from 1 to 500 degrees per second (°/s), a speed which is far slower than those obtained in ballistic actions in sport, which may exceed 6000°/s (Perrin, 1993). In addition, normal muscle contractions do not occur at constant velocities, as offered by a dynamometer. Concentric contractions accelerate, while eccentric actions decelerate a limb. Finally, all human movements are tri-plane in nature, consisting usually of elements of flexion/extension, abduction/adduction, and rotation. Most isokinetic

dynamometers will only allow an action in a single plane at any one time. The combination of limited speed, constant speed and single plane motion means that movements on an isokinetic dynamometer cannot be totally functional. In the clinical setting, a number of other factors must by taken into account. The expertise required to perform assessment and exercise accurately and consistently is only acquired with in-depth training. In addition, both the space taken up by the dynamometer and the purchase cost may themselves be limiting factors within a physiotherapy department specializing in sport.

The great advantage of an isokinetic system, used for measurement or training, is the objectivity and reliability that the system has brought to musculoskeletal assessment. Providing the machine is calibrated, and the joint to be measured is accurately positioned and stabilized, reliability is high (Nitschke, 1992). This is especially true when using test velocities lower than 180°/s for the knee (Wilhite, Cohen and Wilhite, 1992). From the point of view of both safety and effectiveness, isokinetic dynamometers score highly. They give continually variable resistance which will match the strength curve of the tested muscle exactly. Because of this, strength testing is not limited to the weakest point in the range of motion, and in addition, testing can accurately identify a weakness at a point within the whole range.

An isokinetic dynamometer can give a number of useful measures to assess muscle function (Table 1.2).

Muscle force

The measurement of torque during maximal concentric contraction is the most common method of isokinetic strength testing. Torque is measured for a single joint movement, the axis of the joint being aligned with that of the dynamometer. In some instances, a rapidly performed movement, such as a throwing action, may exceed the velocity limit of the dynamometer. Equally, extre-

Table 1.2   Parameters measured in isokinetic dynamometry

Torque
The turning effect produced by a force, measured in Newton metres (Nm). Peak torque (PT) is a measure of the force-generating capacity of the muscle and is represented by the highest point on a patient's torque/angle curve. Mean peak torque (MPT) averages this effect over a number of repetitions

Peak torque to weight
Torque expressed per unit of body mass. This measure makes comparisons between patients possible

Time to peak torque
Time to PT measures the ability to produce maximal torque rapidly, and is relevant for ballistic actions. Prolonged time to PT normally represents inefficient recruitment of type II muscle fibres

Torque velocity ratio
The ratio of torque (Nm) to angular velocity (rad/s). Concentric force reduces as velocity increases whereas eccentric force stays constant or may even increase

Work and power
Work is force multiplied by distance, and is represented by the area under the torque curve. Power is work per unit of time, and represents a subject's 'work rate'

Torque ratio
The ratio of agonist to antagonist peak torques expressed as a percentage, for example hamstring to quadriceps (H:Q) ratio

Endurance and fatigue
Endurance is measured as a 'fatigue index'. This gives an indication of type I fibre action. For example

$$\frac{\text{Mean torque for contractions } 47 - 50 \times 100}{\text{Mean torque for contraction} \quad 1 - 3}$$

Torque production and decay
Torque production rate (TPR) is the gradient of the ascending part of the torque curve (from start to peak torque). The torque decay rate (TDR) is the slope of the descending part of the torque curve from peak torque to the end of contraction

Adapted from Urquhart et al. (1995), with permission.

mely strong subjects, may produce movements in excess of the torque capacity of the isokinetic apparatus.

When measuring maximum torque, between two to six repetitions are usually performed before a stable measurement is achieved. The maximum torque is normally described as the highest single torque value recorded (Baltzopoulos and Brodie, 1989). However, some authors (Morris et al., 1983; Patton and Duggan, 1987) have used mean values of three or five repetitions respectively, and so the testing methods should always be defined.

The velocity of movement (degree per second or rads per second) is also recorded, and it must be remembered that torque will reduce as angular velocity increases (Fig. 1.22).

Muscle endurance

Muscular endurance can be assessed using isokinetic dynamometry by computing a fatigue index. Various methods have been used to calculate this index. Probably the most common for knee extension is that described by Thorstensson and Karlson (1976). In this

Figure 1.22   The maximum torque at different angular velocities of knee extension and flexion. From Baltzopoulos and Brodie (1989), with permission.

Figure 1.23   Torque overshoot (boxed area) during knee extension–flexion movements. From Baltzopoulos and Brodie (1989), with permission.

test, subjects perform 50 consecutive knee extensions at 180°/s. The decline in torque over the 50 repetitions is calculated as the percentage difference between the mean torque of the first and last three repetitions.

Patten et al. (1978) used time to muscular exhaustion, Barnes (1981) used the difference (as a percentage value) between the maximum torque and that obtained in the tenth maximal contraction. Norris (1987) used the time to 50% maximal torque, and Baltzopoulos, Eston and McLaren (1988) used the decline in maximum torque over time using a 30-second test period.

Effects of inertia and gravity

Chart recordings of torque from subjects working at high velocities, may show an initial high peak known as the 'impact artifact' or 'torque overshoot', followed by oscillations decreasing in amplitude (Fig. 1.23). This occurs in the time from rest, to the limb catching up with the preset speed of the dynamometer. During this phase, the limb is accelerating towards the preset speed and is therefore not exercising isokinetically.

The torque overshoot is greater during proximal joint testing due to the greater limb mass and longer distance between the

limb's centre of gravity and the axis of rotation. If the overshoot is interpreted as the peak torque, the subject's muscular capacity will be overestimated (Baltzopoulos and Brodie, 1989).

Signal damping and resistance damping may be used to reduce the effect of torque overload. Signal damping ignores the first part of the torque data, while resistance damping introduces the braking force gradually.

With sagittal and frontal plane movements the effects of gravity must be considered. With small force outputs the effect of gravity may obscure results. The dynamometer will only record the force used against its internal resistance. It would normally not show that used to overcome gravity in an upwards movement or the contribution made by gravity in a downward action. Nelson and Duncan (1983) determined the gravitational torque generated by the limb-lever system when it was allowed to fall passively at various angular positions. From this a correction factor was calculated to be added to the maximum torque registered by the dynamometer. Using this method, results will only be valid if the limb is allowed to fall against the resistance of the dynamometer with the subject's muscles relaxed.

Various computer programs have been produced which correct for gravity and inertial effects. These replace the need for manual data analysis and increase the accuracy of isokinetic dynamometry.

References

Baltzopoulos, V. and Brodie, D.A. (1989) Isokinetic dynamometry. Applications and limitations. *Sports Medicine*, **8**, (2) 101–116

Baltzopoulos, V., Eston, R.G. and McLaren, D. (1988) A comparison of power outputs on the Wingate test and on a test using an isokinetic device. *Ergonomics*, **31**, 1693–1699

Barak, T., Rosen, E.R. and Sofer, R. (1990) Basic concepts of orthopaedic manual therapy. In *Orthopaedic and Sports Physical Therapy* (ed. J.A. Gould), C.V. Mosby, St Louis, pp. 195–211

Barnes, W. (1981) Isokinetic fatigue curves at different contractile velocities. *Physical Therapy*, **60**, 1152–1158

Basmajian, J.V. and Deluca, C.J. (1985) *Muscles Alive*, Williams and Wilkins, Baltimore

Bray, J.J., Cragg, P.A., Macknight, A.D.C., Mills, R.G. and Taylor, D.W. (1986) *Lecture Notes on Human Physiology*, Blackwell Scientific, Oxford

Burnie, J. and Brodie, D.A. (1986) Isokinetics in the assessment of rehabilitation: a case report. *Clinical Biomechanics*, **1**, 140–146

Butler, D.L., Grood, E.S., Noyes, F.R., Zernicke, R.G. Barckett, K. (1984) Effects of structure and strain measurement technique on the material properties of young human tendons and fascia. *Journal of Biomechanics*, **17**, 579–596

Coyle, E.F., Feiring, D.C., Rotkis, T.C., Cote, R.U. and Roby, F.B. (1981) Specificity of power improvements through slow and fast isokinetic training. *Journal of Applied Physiology*, **51**, 1437–1442

Curwin, S.L. (1994) The aetiology and treatment of tendinitis. In *Oxford Textbook of Sports Medicine* (eds M. Harries, C. Williams, W.D. Stanish and L.J. Micheli), Oxford University Press, Oxford

Enoka, R.M. (1994) *Neuromechanical Basis of Kinesiology*, 2nd edn, Human Kinetics, Illinois

Gleim, G.W. (1984) The profiling of professional football players. *Clinics in Sports Medicine*, **3**, (1) 185–197

Hertling, D. and Kessler, R.M. (1990) *Management of Common Musculoskeletal Disorders*, J.B. Lippincott, Philadelphia

Kent, M. (1994) *The Oxford Dictionary of Sports Science and Medicine*, Oxford University Press, Oxford

LaGasse, P. (1983) Neuromuscular facilitation of muscle tension output by reciprocal muscle work. *Annals of the French-Canadian Association for the Advancement of Science*, **50**, 222

LeVeau, B.F. (1990) Basic biomechanics in sports and orthopaedic therapy. In *Orthopaedic and Sports Physical Therapy* (ed. J.A. Gould), C.V. Mosby, Philadelphia

Lieber, R.L. (1992) *Skeletal Muscle Structure and Function*, Williams and Wilkins, Baltimore

McArdle, W.D., Katch, F.I. and Katch, V.L. (1986) *Exercise Physiology. Energy, Nutrition, and Human Performance*. Lea and Febiger, Philadelphia

Morris, A., Lussier, K., Bell, G. and Dooley, J. (1983). Hamstring/quadriceps strength ratios in collegiate middle-distance and distance runners. *Physician and Sportsmedicine*, **11**, 71–77

Nelson, S. and Duncan, P. (1983) Correction of isokinetic torque recordings for the effect of gravity. *Physical Therapy*, **63**, 674–676

Nigg, B.M. (1994) Biomechanics as applied to sports. In *Oxford Textbook of Sports Medicine* (eds M. Harries, C. Williams, W.D. Stanish and L.J. Micheli), Oxford University Press, Oxford

Nitschke, J.E. (1992) Reliability of isokinetic torque measurements: a review of the literature. *Australian Journal of Physiotherapy*, **38**, 125–134

Norris, C.M. (1987) The assessment of a novel physiotherapy technique – combined vacuum and pressure. MSc thesis, University of Liverpool

Patten, W.R., Hinson, M., Arnold, B.R. and Lessard, M.A. (1978) Fatigue curves of isokinetic contractions. *Archives of Physical Medicine and Rehabilitation*, **59**, 507–509

Patton, J. and Duggan, A. (1987) An evaluation of tests of anaerobic power. *Aviation, Space and Environmental Medicine*, **3**, 237–242

Perrin, D.H. (1993) *Isokinetic Exercise and Assessment*, Human Kinetics Publishers, Leeds

Pipes, T.V. and Wilmore, J.H. (1975) Isokinetic vs isotonic strength training in adult men. *Medicine in Science and Sports*, **7**, 262–274

Rasch, P.J. (1989) *Kinesiology and Applied Anatomy*, Lea and Febiger, Philadelphia

Sale, D.G. (1988) Neural adaptation to resistance training. *Medicine and Science in Sports and Exercise*, **20**, (5) 135–145

Sapega, A.A., Quedenfel, T.C., Moyer, R.A. and Butler, R.A. (1981) Biophysical factors in range of motion exercise. *The Physican and Sportsmedicine*, **9**, (12) 57–65

Stallard, J. (1984) The mechanics of lower limb orthoses. In *Cash's Textbook of Orthopaedics and Rheumatology for Physiotherapists* (ed. P.A. Downie), Faber and Faber, London, pp. 21–42

Taunton, J.E., McKenzie, D.C. and Clement, D.B. (1988) The role of biomechanics in the epidemiology of injuries. *Sports Medicine*, **6**, 107–120

Thorstensson, A. and Karlson, J. (1976) Fatigability and fibre composition of human skeletal muscle. *Acta Physiologica Scandinavica*, **98**, 318–322

Toussaint, H.M., van Baar, C.E., van Langen, P.P., de Looze, M.P. and van Dieen, J.H. (1992) Coordination of the leg muscles in backlift and leglift. *Journal of Biomechanics*, **25**, 1279–1289

Urquhart, D.S., Garbutt, G., Cova, K., Lennox, C.M.E. and McLatchie, G.R. (1995) Isokinetics: applications in the management of knee soft-tissue injuries. *Sports Exercise and Injury*, **1**, (3) 138–147

van Ingen Schenau, G.J., Bobbert, M.F. and van Soest, A.J. (1990) The unique action of bi-articular muscles in leg extensions. In *Multiple Muscle Systems: Biomechanics and Movement Organisation* (eds J.M. Winters and S.L. Woo, Springer-Verlag, New York

Warwick, R. and Williams, P.L. (1973) *Gray's Anatomy* (35th edition) Longman, Harlow

Watkins, J. (1983) *An Introduction to Mechanics of Human Movement*, MTP Press, Lancaster

Wells, K.F. (1966) *Kinesiology*, W.B. Saunders, Philadelphia

Wilhite, M.R., Cohen, E.R. and Wilhite, S.C. (1992) Reliability of concentric and eccentric measurements of quadriceps performance using the Kin-Com dynamometer: the effect of testing order for three different speeds. *Journal of Orthopaedic and Sports Physical Therapy*, **15**, 175-182

Williams, J.G.P. and Sperryn, P.N. (1976) *Sports Medicine*, Edward Arnold, London

Williams, J.G. and Davis, M. (1990) KINEMAN: A micro-computer-based video digitising system for movement analysis. *Physiotherapy*, **76**, (6) June 436–440

Zehr, E.P. and Sale, D.G. (1994) Ballistic movement: muscle activation and neuromuscular adaptation. *Canadian Journal of Applied Physiology*, **19**, 363–378

2

Healing

The basic processes of soft tissue healing underlie all treatment techniques for sports injuries. We need to know what occurs in the body tissues at each successive stage of healing to be able to select the treatment technique which is most appropriate.

A technique aimed at reducing the formation of swelling, for example, would be inappropriate when swelling had stopped forming and adhesions were the problem. Similarly, a manual treatment designed to break up adhesions and mobilize soft tissue would not be helpful when inflammation is still forming and the tissues are highly irritable.

The stages of healing are, to a large extent, purely a convenience of description, since each stage runs into another. Traditionally, the initial tissue response has been described as inflammation, but some authors see inflammation as a response separate to the processes occurring at the time of injury. Van der Meulen (1982) described both in terms of the 'reaction phase', arguing that the classical inflammatory period is preceded by a short (10 min) period before the inflammatory mechanism is activated. The second stage of healing has been variously called repair, proliferation and regeneration. The tertiary stage has been termed remodelling (Van der Meulen, 1982; Kellett, 1986; Dyson, 1987). The terms injury, inflamma-

tion, repair and remodelling will be used in this text.

When describing the stage of healing, the terms acute, sub-acute and chronic are helpful. The acute stage (up to 48 hours following injury) is the stage of inflammation. The sub-acute stage, occurring between 14 and 21 days after injury, is the stage of repair. The chronic stage (after 21 days) is the stage of remodelling. The term chronic is also sometimes used to describe self-perpetuating inflammation, where the inflammatory process has re-started due to disruption or persistent irritation of the healing tissues. The total healing process occurs over a continuum, shown in Fig. 2.1.

Injury

This stage represents the tissue effects at the time of injury, before the inflammatory process is activated. With tissue damage, chemical and mechanical changes are seen. Local blood vessels are disrupted causing a cessation in oxygen to the cells they perfused. These cells die, and their lysosome membranes disintegrate releasing the hydrolysing enzymes the lysosomes contained. The release of these enzymes has a two-fold effect. First they begin to break down the dead cells themselves, and sec-

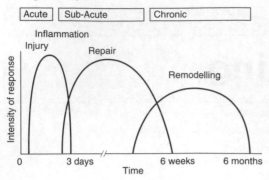

Figure 2.1 Timescale of tissue healing. From Oakes (1992).

ondly, they release histamines and kinins which have an effect on both the live cells nearby, and the local blood capillary network.

The disruption of the blood vessels which caused cell death also causes local bleeding (extravasated blood). The red blood cells break down, leaving cellular debris and free haemoglobin. The blood platelets release the enzyme thrombin which changes fibrinogen into fibrin. The fibrin in turn is deposited as a meshwork around the area (a process known as walling off). The dead cells intertwine in the meshwork forming a blood clot. This network contains the damaged area.

The changes occurring at injury are affected by age (Lachman, 1988). Intra-muscular bleeding, and therefore haemor-rhage formation, are more profuse in indivi-duals over 30 years of age. The amount of bleeding which occurs will be partially dependent on the vascularity of the injured tissues. A fitter individual is likely to have muscle tissue which is more highly vascular-ized, and therefore greater bleeding will occur with muscle injury. In addition, exer-cise itself will affect gross tissue responses. Muscle blood flow is greatly increased through dilatation of the capillary bed, and again bleeding subsequent to injury will be greater.

Inflammation

The next stage in the healing sequence is that of inflammation. This may last from 10 min to several days depending on the amount of tissue damage which has occurred. The inflammatory response to injury is the same regardless of the nature of the injuring agent or the location of the injury itself (Hettinga, 1990). Various agents can give rise to injury, and Evans (1990a) listed physical, thermal, radiational, electri-cal and chemical causes.

Inflammation is not simply a feature of soft tissue injuries. It occurs when the body is infected, in immune reactions and when infarction stops blood flowing to an area. Some of the characteristics of the inflamma-tory response have even been described as excessive (Cyriax, 1982) and better suited to dealing with infection, by preventing bac-terial spread, than healing injury (Evans, 1990a).

The cardinal signs of inflammation are heat (calor), redness (rubor), swelling (tumor) and pain (dolor). These in turn give rise to the so-called fifth sign of inflammation disturbance of function of the affected tissues (functio laesa).

Heat and redness

Heat and redness take a number of hours to develop, and are due to the opening of local blood capillaries and the resultant increased blood flow. Chemical and mechanical changes, initiated by injury, are responsible for the changes in blood flow.

Chemically, a number of substances act as mediators in the inflammatory process. The amines, including histamine and 5–hydroxytriptamine (5–HT or serotonin) are released from mast cells, red blood cells and platelets in the damaged capillaries and cause vessel dilatation and increased per-meability lasting 10–15 min (Lachman, 1988). Kinins (physiologically active poly-peptides) cause an increase in vascular permeability and stimulate the contraction of smooth muscle. They are found normally in an inactive state as kininogens. These in turn are activated by the enzyme plasmin, and degraded by kininases.

The initial vasodilatation is maintained by prostaglandins. These are one of the arachidonic acid derivatives, formed from cell membrane phospholipids when cell damage occurs, and released when the kinin system is activated. The drugs aspirin and indomethacin act to inhibit this change—hence their use as anti-inflammatory agents in sports injury treatment. The prostaglandins E1 and E2 are two of the substances responsible for pain production, and they will also promote vasodilatation, blood vessel permeability and lymph flow (Oakes, 1992).

The complement system, consisting of a number of serum proteins circulating in an inactive form, is activated and has a direct effect on the cell membrane as well as helping to maintain vasodilatation. Various complement products are involved, and these are activated in sequence.

Finally, polymorphs produce leucotrienes, which are themselves derived from arachidonic acid. These help the kinins maintain the vessel permeability.

Blood flow changes also occur through mechanical alterations initiated by injury. Normally, the blood flow in the venules in particular, is axial. The large blood proteins stay in the centre of the vessel, and the plasmatic stream, which has a lower viscosity, is on the outside in contact with the vessel walls. This configuration reduces peripheral resistance and aids blood flow.

In a damaged capillary, however, fluid is lost and so the axial flow slows. Marginalization occurs as the slower flow rate allows white blood cells to move into the plasmatic zone and adhere to the vessel walls. This, in turn, reduces the lubricating effect of this layer and slows blood flow. The walls themselves become covered with a gelatinous layer (Wilkinson and Lackie,

1979), as endothelium changes occur (Walter and Israel, 1987).

Some 4 hours after injury (Evans, 1980) diapedesis occurs as the white cells pass through the vessel walls into the damaged tissue. The endothelial cells of the vessel contract (Hettinga, 1990), pulling away from each other and leaving gaps through which fluids and blood cells can escape (Fig. 2.2). Various substances including histamine, kinins and complement factors have been shown to produce this effect (Fox, Galey and Wayland, 1980; Walter and Israel, 1987).

Swelling

The normal pressure gradients inside and outside the capillary, balance the flow of

Figure 2.2 Vascular changes which occur in inflammation. (a) Blood vessel starts to dilate. (b) Dilated vessel showing marginalization. (c) White blood cells and fluid pass into tissue. From Evans (1990a), with permission.

fluid leaving and entering the vessel (Fig. 2.3). The capillary membrane is permeable to water, and so water will be driven out into the interstitial fluid. However, because the tissue fluids usually contain a small amount of protein, and the blood contains a large amount, an osmotic pressure is created which tends to suck water back from the tissue fluid and into the capillary once more. The magnitude of this osmotic pressure is roughly 25 mmHg. At the arteriole end of the capillary the blood pressure (32 mmHg) exceeds the osmotic pressure and so tissue fluid is formed. At the venous end of the capillary the blood pressure has reduced (12 mmHg) and so, because the osmotic pressure now exceeds this value, tissue fluid is reabsorbed back into the capillary.

During inflammation the capillary bed opens and blood flow increases (heat and redness). The larger blood volume causes a parallel increase in blood pressure. Coupled with this, the tissue fluid now contains a large amount of protein, which has poured out from the more permeable blood vessels. This increased protein concentration causes a substantial rise in osmotic pressure, and this together with the larger blood pressure in the capillary, forces fluid out into the interstitium, causing swelling.

Protein exudation in mild inflammation occurs from the venules only and is probably mediated by histamine (Evans, 1990a). More severe inflammation, as a result of trauma, results in protein exudation from damaged capillaries as well.

During inflammation, lymphatic vessels open up and assist in the removal of excess fluid and protein. The lymph vessels are blind-ending capillaries which have gaps in their endothelial walls enabling protein molecules to move through easily. The lymph vessels lie within the tissue spaces, and have valves preventing the backward movement of fluid. Muscular contraction causes a pumping action on the lymph vessels and the excess tissue fluid is removed to the subclavian veins in the neck.

Pain

Pain is the result of both sensory and emotional experiences, and is associated with tissue damage or the probability that damage will occur. It serves as a warning which may cause us to withdraw from a painful stimulus and so protect an injured body part. Unfortunately, pain often continues long after it has ceased to be a useful form of protection. Associated muscle spasm, atrophy, habitual postures, guarding

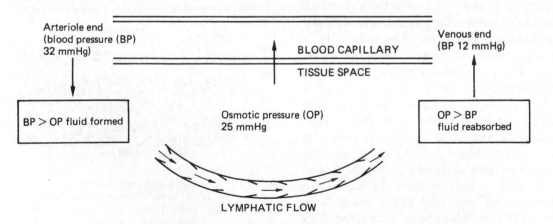

Figure 2.3 Formation and reabsorption of tissue fluid.

and psychological factors all combine to make chronic pain almost a disease entity in itself.

Types of pain

Pain may be classified as somatogenic (acute or chronic), neurogenic or psychogenic. Chronic pain may be considered as that which generally lasts for more than 6 weeks, while acute pain is that of sudden onset which lasts for less than 6 weeks (Donley and Denegar, 1990).

Musculoskeletal pain is not in general well localized, the surface site where the pain is felt rarely correlates directly to injured subcutaneous tissue. Generally, the closer an injured tissue is to the skin surface, the more accurate the athlete can be at localizing it.

Deep pain is normally an aching ill-defined sensation. It usually radiates in a characteristic fashion, and may be associated with autonomic responses such as sweating, nausea, pallor and lowered blood pressure (Lynch and Kessler, 1990). Pain referral corresponds to segmental pathways, most often dermatomes. The extent of radiation largely depends on the intensity of the stimulus, with pain normally radiating distally, and rarely crossing the midline of the body (Cyriax, 1982).

Neurogenic pain is different again. Compression of a nerve root gives rise to ill-defined tingling, especially in the distal part of the dermatome supplied by the nerve. This is a pressure reaction, which quickly disappears when the nerve root is released. Greater pressure causes the tingling to give way to numbness. Compression or tension to the dural sleeve covering the nerve root gives severe pain generally over the whole dermatome. In contrast, pressure on a nerve trunk generally causes little or no pain, but results in a shower of 'pins and needles' as the nerve compression is released. Pressure applied to a superficial nerve, distally, gives numbness and some tingling, with the edge of the affected region being well defined (Cyriax, 1982).

Irritability

Irritability may be defined as 'the vigour of activity which causes pain' (Maitland, 1991). It is determined by the degree of pain which the patient experiences, and the time this takes to subside, in relation to the intensity of activity that brought the pain on in the first place. The purpose of assessing irritability is to determine how much activity (joint mobilization, exercise, etc.) may be prescribed without exacerbating the patient's symptoms.

An assessment of irritability may be made at the second treatment session. The amount of movement which the patient was subjected to in the previous session is known, as is the discomfort that he or she feels now. These subjective feelings are then used to determine the intensity of the second treatment session. Similarly, at the beginning of each subsequent treatment session the irritability is again assessed.

Pain production

Free or 'bare' nerve endings (type IV) respond to painful stimuli and are termed nociceptors (from the Latin nocere, to damage). They are largely unresponsive to normal stimuli, but have a low threshold to mechanical and thermal injury, anoxia, and irritation from inflammatory products. Tissues vary in the intensity of pain they will produce when stimulated. The joint capsule and periosteum are the most sensitive to noxious stimuli. Subchondral bone, tendons and ligaments are the next in line in terms of sensitivity, followed by muscle and cortical bone. The synovium and cartilage being largely insensitive.

The pain receptors are supplied by a variety of different nerve fibres. Skin receptors are supplied by thinly myelinated (A delta) fibres which carry 'fast' pain and respond to strong mechanical stimuli and heat above 45°C (Low and Reed, 1990). They give the initial sharp well-localized pain feeling. The function of fast pain is to help the body avoid tissue damage and it often provokes a flexor withdrawal reflex.

Impulses from free nerve endings found in deeper body tissues are carried by non-myelinated C fibres. This is 'slow' pain, which tends to be aching and throbbing in nature, and poorly defined. Its onset is not immediate, and the sensation it produces persists after the pain stimulus has gone. The function of slow pain seems to be to enforce inactivity and allow healing to occur and it is therefore often associated with muscle spasm. The C fibres respond to many different types of stimuli and, as such, are said to be 'polymodal'. However, they are most sensitive to chemicals released as a result of tissue damage. Histamine, kinins, prostaglandins E1 and E2, and 5–HT have all been implicated in this type of pain production during inflammation (Walter and Israel, 1987; Lachman 1988).

It can be seen that the pain experienced as a result of sporting injury will usually be either mechanical or chemical in nature. Mechanical pain is the result of forces which deform, or damage the nociceptive nerve endings, and so may be caused by stretching contracted tissue or by fluid pressure. This type of pain is influenced by movement. Chemical pain, on the other hand, results from irritation of the nerve endings, and is less affected by movement or joint position, but will respond to rest.

Articular neurology

In addition to pain receptors (type IV), three other joint receptors are important. Type I receptors are located in the superficial layers of the joint capsule. They are slow adapting, low-threshold mechanoreceptors, which respond to both static and dynamic stimulation. These receptors provide information about the static position of a joint, and con-

tribute to the regulation of muscle tone and movement (kinaesthetic) sense. The type I receptors sense both the speed and direction of movement.

Type II receptors are found mainly in the deeper capsular layers, and within fat pads. These are dynamic receptors with a high threshold, and they adapt quickly. They respond to rapid changes of direction of joint movement.

The type III fibres are found in the joint ligaments, and are again high threshold dynamic mechanoreceptors, but are slow adapting. These receptors monitor the direction of movement, and have a 'braking' effect on muscle tone if the joint is moving too quickly or through too great a range of motion. The type IV receptor is the nociceptor described above. Table 2.1 provides a synopsis of the various movement categories to which the receptors respond.

Alteration in the feedback provided by joint receptors is of great importance following sports injury, and is dealt with in the section on proprioceptive training (p. 171).

Pain pathways

Three categories or 'orders' of neurone make up the pain pathways. First order neurones travel from the pain receptors to the spinal cord, second order neurones travel within the cord to the brainstem and third order

Table 2.1   Function of joint receptors

Function	Receptor
Static position	Type I
Speed of movement	Type I
Change in speed	Type II
Direction of movement	Types I and II
Postural muscle tone	Type I
Tone at initiation of movement	Type II
Tone during movement	Type II
Tone during harmful movements	Type III

Adapted from Hertling and Kessler (1990).

neurones travel from the brainstem to the higher centres of the cerebral cortex.

Seventy percent of the C fibres (slow pain) enter the spine via the dorsal root, while 30% of the fibres enter via the ventral root. The C fibres synapse with second order neurones in the substantia gelatinosa of the cord and these neurones ascend in the anterolateral funiculus on the opposite side of the cord (Fig. 2.4). From here they travel via the reticular formation to the intralaminar nuclei of the thalamus. The neurones synapse here once more and travel to the prefrontal region of the cerebral cortex.

The A delta fibres (fast pain), on the other hand, synapse in the outer part of the posterior horn of the cord and cross to ascend in the spinothalamic tract to the ventrobasal nuclei in the thalamus, and then to the postcentral gyrus of the cortex.

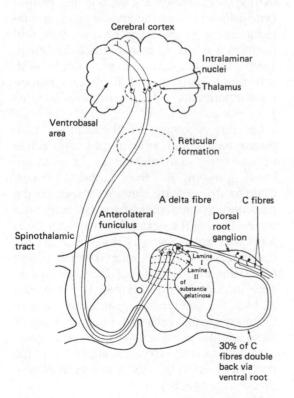

Figure 2.4 Pain pathways. From Low and Reed (1990), with permission.

Fast pain is registered in the parietal lobe and visceral pain in the insula cortex. Emotional responses to pain are generated in the limbic system and states of anxiety, fear and dread of pain are generated by the frontal lobes.

Pain relief mechanisms

Three concepts of pain control are generally used within physiotherapy. First, stimulation of ascending fibres to block pain messages (pain gate theory), second, endogenous opioid formation, and third, descending fibre stimulation within the dorsal horn of the spinal cord (descending inhibition).

The pain gate

The pain gate theory (Melzack and Wall, 1965) proposed that pain perception was regulated by a 'gate' which could be opened or closed. When stimulated, mechanoreceptors in the skin send impulses via A beta fibres to the posterior horn of the cord. Here, collateral branches are given off. These collaterals affect A delta and C pain fibres in the substantia gelatinosa (SG), reducing their excitability by presynaptic inhibition. Stimulation of A delta fibres by low intensity, high frequency transcutaneous electrical nerve stimulation (TENS) (100–200 Hz) will therefore reduce pain through this gating mechanism (Fig. 2.5).

Endogenous opioids

Interneurones within the substantia gelatinosa are able to produce endogenous (made in the body) opioid peptides, which have similar effects to opioids such as morphine, heroin, and codeine, which are some of the most powerful analgesics known. These opioids inhibit C fibre cells. Collateral branches of A delta fibres in the posterior horn connect to the interneurones and stimulate them to produce opioids.

The opioids, including enkephalins and endorphins, are produced in various areas of the central nervous system (CNS) includ-

Figure 2.5 The pain gate mechanism. Central control — effects caused by higher centre (brain), action system — pain response. SG, substantia gelatinosa. From Melzack and Wall (1965), with permission.

ing the limbic system and thalamus, the pituitary gland, the substantia gelatinosa, and nerve terminals. These substances inhibit transmission in the A delta and C fibre pathways and so block pain before it reaches sensory levels. Stimulation of the A delta fibres with high intensity low frequency TENS (2–10 Hz) will damp down C fibre activity and reduce pain through this method.

Descending inhibition
In addition, activity of the A delta fibres may provoke impulses from the periaqueductal grey matter of the midbrain. These impulses travel back down the cord to inhibit nociceptor neurones. Inhibition is by the release of serotonin and possibly noradrenaline. Stimulation at frequencies above 50 Hz may affect this system (De Domenico, 1982).

Management of inflammation

The effects of acute inflammation can be reduced by slowing the body's response represented by the cardinal signs. Redness and heat are therefore treated by trying to reduce localized bleeding by the use of cold or ice and compression. Swelling is similarly managed by the use of compression to contain local oedema, and gentle movement to assist lymphatic drainage. By reducing the chemical and mechanical effects of the three inflammatory signs above, pain is also reduced.

The amount of rest prescribed during inflammation will depend on the stage of inflammation and the amount of tissue damage.

Repair

Inflammation may continue for 5 days, but with minor trauma it is usually complete by the third day after injury (Evans, 1980). Following this, tissue repair can take place. Repair is by resolution, organization or regeneration, depending on the severity of the injury and the nature of the injured tissues.

A minor injury will result in acute inflammation as described above, and the phagocytic cells will clear the area. If there is little tissue damage, the stage of resolution will result in a return to near normal (Lachman, 1988). True resolution rarely occurs with soft tissue injuries, but is more common with inflammatory tissue reactions such as pneumonia.

On the periphery of the injured area, macrophages and polymorphs are active because they can tolerate the low oxygen levels present in the damaged tissue. Cellular division by mitosis is seen in the surrounding capillaries about 12 hours after injury. During the next 3 days capillary buds form and grow towards the lower oxygen concentration of the injured area. These capillaries form loops and blood begins to flow through them. This new capillary-rich material is known as granulation tissue. Plasma proteins, cells and fluid pour out of these highly permeable vessels. The gradually increasing oxygen supply to the previously deoxygenated area means phagocytosis can now begin.

New lymphatic vessels bud out from the existing lymphatics, linking to form a renewed lymphatic drainage system. As this process is occurring, fibroblast cells multiply and move towards the injured tissue. By the fifth day after injury they begin to lay down fibrils of collagen, a process requiring adequate amounts of vitamin C.

The individual fibrils form into parallel bundles lying in the direction of stress imposed on the tissue. If no movement occurs to stress the collagen bundles, they are laid down in a haphazard and weaker pattern (Cyriax, 1982). Controlled movement causes the fibrils to align lengthways along the line of stress of the injured structure (Burri, Helbing and Spier, 1973). Variation in longitudinal fibre alignment will determine the stress–strain response of the tissue to loading (Fig. 2.6). Where fibre alignment is parallel to the tissue body, the steep stress–strain curve (C) indicates that less deformation will occur for a given tissue loading. The tissue is therefore 'stronger'.

It becomes clear that external mechanical factors, and not the previous organization of the tissue, dictate the eventual pattern of fibril arrangement (Stearns, 1940). Total rest during this stage of healing is, therefore, contraindicated in most cases.

In some tissue regeneration occurs, damaged cells being replaced by functioning normal tissue. Fractured bone exhibits this property as do torn ligaments and peripheral nerves providing conditions are suitable (Evans, 1990b).

Figure 2.6   Relationship between fibre orientation and stress–strain response. From Oakes (1992).

Remodelling

The remodelling stage overlaps repair, and may last from 3 weeks to 12 months (Kellett, 1986). During this stage, collagen is modified to increase its functional capacity. Remodelling is characterized by a reduction in the wound size, an increase in scar strength and an alteration in the direction of the collagen fibres (Van der Meulen, 1982).

Contraction of granulation tissue will occur for as long as the elasticity of the fibres will allow (Van der Meulen, 1982). Fibroblast cells transform into myofibroblasts which then form intercellular bonds. These contain contractile proteins (actomyosin) and behave much like smooth muscle fibres.

Three weeks after injury, the quantity of collagen has stabilized (Van der Meulen, 1982) but the strength of the fibres continues to increase. Strength increases are a result of an expansion in the number of cross-bonds between the cells, and the replacement collagen cells themselves. There is a continuous turnover of collagen, a process influenced by a number of factors, including the age of the patient, the type of tissue injured, the quantity of scar tissue present, the site and direction of the scar and external forces (Van der Meulen, 1982; Frank et al., 1983).

Tissue response to injury

In this section we will look at the responses of the individual tissues to injury, and the effects these have upon subsequent rehabilitation. Aspects of tissue structure relevant to sports injury is discussed.

Synovial membrane

The synovium consists of two layers, the intima, or synovial lining, and the subsynovial (subintimal) tissue. The intimal layer is made up of specialized cells known as synoviocytes, arranged in multiple layers. Two types of synoviocytes are present, type A cells, which are phagocytic, and type B cells, which synthesize the hyaluronoprotein of the synovial fluid. The two types are not distinct however, and appear to be functional stages of the same basic cells (Hettinga, 1990).

The subsynovial tissue lies beneath the intima as a loose network of highly vascular connective tissue. Cells are interspaced with collagen fibres and fatty tissue. The subsynovial tissue itself merges with the periosteum of bone lying within the synovial membrane of the joint. Similar merging occurs with the joint cartilage through a transitional layer of fibrocartilage.

The blood vessels of the joint divide into three branches, one travelling to the epiphysis, the second to the joint capsule and the third to the synovial membrane (Paget and Bullough, 1981). From here the vessels of the subsynovium are of two types. The first is thin walled and adapted for fluid exchange, and the second thick walled and capable of gapping to allow particles, especially nutrients, to pass through.

Once free of the vessels, any material must pass through the synovial interstitium before entering the synovial fluid itself. The passage of this material is by diffusion on the whole, but by active transport for glucose molecules.

The synovium must adapt to movement with normal function of the joint. Rather than stretching, the synovium unfolds to facilitate flexion. The synovium is well lubricated by the same hyaluronate molecules found within the synovial fluid itself, and so the various layers slide over each other. Since the synovium must alter shape within the confines of the joint capsule, the process of synovial adaptation is at its best when the fluid volume of the joint is at a minimum.

Synovial fluid plays a significant role in joint stability. The negative atmospheric pressure within the joint creates a suction effect, which, aided by the surface tension of the synovial fluid, draws the bony surfaces of the joint together.

Response to injury

With minor trauma the synovium is not microscopically disturbed, but will instead suffer a vasomotor reaction (Hettinga, 1990). The synovium will dilate and fluid filtration increases. Protein leaks into the interstitium, changing the osmotic pressure and causing local oedema and joint exudation. This process constitutes a post-traumatic synovitis.

The slight hyperaemia gives way later to alterations of the intimal layer, the total number of layers increasing three-fold. If the trauma does not continue, the protein molecules which were released are cleared by the lymphatics and the osmotic pressures return to normal. If mechanical irritation persists, the intimal layer will continue to thicken. The deep synovial cells now show increased activity and protein synthesis escalates.

Alterations occur in the number of type A and type B synoviocyte cells. The number of type A cells reduces as some of these move into the synovial fluid to become macrophages. The synovial lining becomes filled with fibroblasts, which in turn change into type B cells. Neutrophil cells die, releasing proteolytic enzymes which attack the near joint structures. This process can self-perpetuate the synovitis even in the absence of further trauma, giving rise to a reactive synovitis.

Onset of symptoms following post-traumatic synovitis usually occurs between 12 and 24 hours after injury and can last for between 1 and 2 weeks. Patients complain mainly of joint tightness, with warmth, erythema and pain being encountered less often. The tightness is due to joint effusion, the increased fluid volume causing the normally negative intra-articular pressure to become positive.

The stability of the joint, no longer created by a negative intra-articular pressure, comes from joint distension instead. This places a traction force on the joint capsule and surrounding ligaments. Pressures are greatest in the effused joint in extremes of flexion and extension, and are reduced at about 30° flexion, this being the resting position taken up by the patient. Haemarthrosis is usually present if swelling occurs within 2 hours of injury, and pain is intense.

Synovial fluid

Synovial fluid is similar in many ways to blood plasma. The main differences being that synovia does not contain fibrinogen or prothrombin and so is unable to clot. The mucopolysaccharide hyaluronate (hyaluronic acid) secreted by the synoviocytes is contained within the fluid.

The amount of synovial fluid present in a joint is very little, about 0.5–4 ml within large joints such as the knee, and this is spread throughout the joint by structures such as the cartilage, menisci and fat pads.

Synovial fluid is a highly viscous fluid, which becomes more elastic as the rate of joint movement increases. As weight is taken by the joint, synovial fluid is squeezed out from between the opposing joint surfaces. This is resisted by the tenacity of the fluid itself.

As the joint moves, the synovial fluid is pulled in the direction of movement and so a layer of fluid is maintained between the joint surfaces. Any friction produced by movement will therefore occur within the synovial fluid rather than between the joint surfaces. When the joint is statically loaded, however, fluid flows away from the point of maximal load and the joint relies on the articular cartilage to provide lubrication (see below). The synovial fluid provides nutrition for about two thirds of the articular cartilage bordering the joint space.

Following injury, fluid volume may increase as much as ten or 20 times, with a decrease in hyaluronate and, with it, fluid viscosity. Pain due to the accumulation of synovial fluid is dependent not on the amount of fluid present, but on the speed with which it forms. Blau (1979) claimed that as much as 100 ml may be extracted from a joint which caused little pain because it took a long time to form while 15 ml may be exquisitely painful if formed rapidly following trauma.

With injury in which bleeding is not present, the constituents of the synovial fluid remain basically the same. In reactive synovitis, the protein concentration is slightly elevated, and the number of white blood cells increases somewhat from normal values of 100/ml to as much as 300/ml. With post-traumatic synovitis, however, the white cell count is further increased, to as much as 2000/ml.

Haemarthrosis (blood within the joint) causes rapidly developing fluid, which contains fibrinogen. If the synovial membrane is torn, fat may can enter the joint from the extrasynovial adipose tissue and will show up in the synovial fluid. The blood from haemarthrosis will mostly stay fluid, and is quickly absorbed by the phagocytic cells to ultimately disappear after several days.

Bone

Types

Bone is essentially a fibrous matrix impregnated by mineral salts (mainly calcium phosphate), and it therefore combines the properties of both elasticity and rigidity. It is a living tissue, which is continually remodelled, and subject to hormonal control.

Two types of bone are generally described, cancellous or spongy bone and compact bone, and important differences exist in both their mechanical properties and methods of healing. Cancellous bone is found at a number of sites, including the bone ends, and is arranged in a system of trabeculae aligned to resist imposed stresses. The shaft of a long bone consists of a ring of compact bone surrounding a hollow cavity. This structure in turn is surrounded by a further layer of compact bone. The bone cavity contains marrow. In infants the bone marrow is red, but this is gradually replaced by yellow bone marrow until, by puberty, only the cancellous bone cavities at the ends of the long bones contain red marrow. With age the bone marrow in these cavities too is replaced, but red bone marrow may still be found in the vertebrae, sternum, and ribs, as well as the proximal ends of the femur and humerus.

The bone is enclosed in a dense membrane called the periosteum, which is absent in the region of the articular cartilage. The periosteum is highly vascular and responsible for the nutrition of the bone cortex which underlies it. The deep layers of periosteum contain bone-forming cells (osteoblasts). These lay down successive layers of bone during growth, and so the periosteum is responsible for alterations in the bone width, in addition these cells play an important part in bone healing. In contrast, the bone cavity is lined by bone-destroying cells (osteoclasts) which erode the inner surface of the bone. A direct blow to the bone which produces bleeding beneath the periosteum will lift it, causing bone deposition by the osteoblasts. This is a common problem over the anterior tibia in footballers and hockey players.

Bone may be further classified into four major types. The long bones are found within the limbs, and consist of a shaft and two enlarged ends. Short bones have a block-like appearance such as those of the carpals, and are mainly cancellous bone. Flat bones are thinner, and consist of two layers of compact bone sandwiching a thin layer of cancellous bone, examples are the skull vaults and the ribs. Finally, irregular bones consist of a thin layer of compact bone surrounded by cancellous bone, examples are the vertebrae.

Development

Skeletal development begins with loosely arranged mesodermal cells which are mostly converted to hyaline cartilage. Between the seventh and twelfth intrauterine week a primary ossification centre appears within the shaft of the long bone, and spreads towards the bone ends. The centre of the shaft is hollowed out and filled with red bone marrow, and the whole shaft is called a diaphysis. At the end of the bone, secondary centres of ossification appear, usually after birth. Gradually the main part of the cartilage is replaced, leaving only the articular cartilage, and a cartilage plate (growth plate, or physis) between the shaft and end of the bone.

The growth plate is of great importance in paediatric sports medicine. This cartilage layer is responsible for the increase in bone length. As the cartilage grows it becomes thicker, and its upper and lower surfaces are converted to bone. Eventually the cartilage stops growing, but its ossification continues so that the cartilage becomes thinner, until it eventually disappears. At this point the diaphysis and epiphysis are united, and growth in length of the bone is no longer possible. The point at which this occurs may be influenced by a number of factors, including impact stresses (see below).

Intramembranous ossification occurs in the mandible, clavicle, and certain bones of the skull (Palastanga, Field and Soames, 1989). Here, the intermediate stage of cartilage formation is omitted and the bone ossifies directly from connective tissue.

Epiphyseal injury

Two types of epiphysis are found. Pressure epiphyses are found at the end of long bones, and are interarticular. They are subjected to compression stress with weight-bearing, and are responsible for changes in bone length. Traction epiphyses (apophyses) occur at the insertion of major muscles. They experience tension stress as the muscles contract, and alter bone shape.

The growth plate itself forms a weak link in the immature skeleton, and shearing or avulsion stresses can cause it to be dislodged. Because the epiphyses are weaker than the major joint structures, injuries, which in the adult would cause dislocation or tendon rupture, may cause epiphyseal injury in a child.

Five types of injury have been described (Salter and Harris, 1963) as shown in Fig. 2.7. The type I lesion involves horizontal displacement of the growth plate while with the type II lesion the fracture line runs through to the adjacent metaphysis. In the type III and IV fractures the joint surface is involved so the complication rate is higher (Watson, 1992). Gentle manipulation under anaesthetic is normally used to realign the epiphysis in the first fracture types. Crush injuries and those through the growth plate may cause more severe problems of growth disturbance. When a fracture crosses the growth plate, bone may fill the gap formed, giving unequal growth. Crush injuries may lead to premature closure of the plate with associated deformities of shortening and altered bony angulation.

Osteochondrosis

Osteochondrosis affects the pressure epiphyses during their growth period, and are the most common overuse injuries seen in children. There is an interference with the epiphyseal blood supply, causing an avascular necrosis to the secondary ossification centre. The bone within the epiphysis softens, dies, and is absorbed (Fig. 2.8). Because the cap of articular cartilage surrounding the epiphysis receives nutrition from the synovial fluid, it remains largely unaffected. The combination of softening bone contained within an intact articular cap leads to flattening of the epiphysis. Gradually the dead bone is replaced by new bone by a process of 'creeping substitution'. Trauma may be one factor which initiates the ischaemic process, either through direct injury or vascular occlusion as a result of traumatic synovitis (Gartland, 1987).

The osteochondroses may be categorized into four groups (Pappas, 1989). Traction osteochondroses (apophysitis) affect the attachments of major tendons, particularly to the knee and heel. Crushing osteochondroses occur in the hip, wrist, and forefoot, while articular chondral osteochondroses involve splitting of bone near an articular site, with resultant bone fragment formation. Finally, physeal injuries affect the growth plate and result in irregular growth and/or angular deformity.

Any pressure epiphysis may be affected by osteochondrosis, the condition taking the

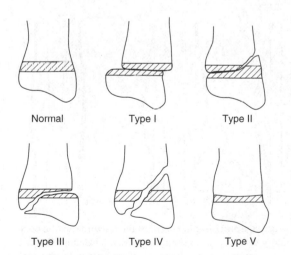

Figure 2.7 Epiphyseal injuries. After Salter and Harris (1963).

Figure 2.8 Stages of osteochondritis. (a) Normal epiphysis. (b) The bony nucleus undergoes necrosis, loses its normal texture and becomes granular. (c) The bony nucleus becomes fragmented during the process of removal of dead bone. (d) If subjected to pressure the softened epiphysis becomes flattened. (e) Re-ossification with restoration of normal bone texture but deformity may persist. The whole process takes two to three years. From Gartland (1987), with permission.

name of the person who first described it in that region. The most common conditions are shown in Table 2.2, and details of these are given in the relevant clinical chapters in Section II of this book.

Healing

Bone healing (see also 'stress fractures' p. 294) is governed by a number of factors, including the type of tissue which is damaged, the extent of the damage and posi-

tion of the bony fragments, the amount of movement present at the fracture site as healing progresses, and the blood supply. In a long bone, healing may be divided into five stages, as shown in Fig. 2.9 (Crawford-Adams, 1978; Apley and Solomon, 1988). The first stage is that of tissue destruction and haematoma formation. As local blood vessels are torn at the time of injury, blood is released forming a haematoma within and surrounding the fracture site. The bone periosteum and surrounding soft tissues contain

Table 2.2   The osteochondroses

Classification	Name	Site(s)
Non-articular traction (pulling)	Osgood–Schlatter's	Tibial tubercle
	Sinding-Larsen-Johannsson's disease	Interior pole of patella (quadriceps)
	Sever's disease	Calcaneus (gastrocnemius)
Articular subchondral (crushing)	Perthes' disease	Femoral head
	Kienböck's disease	Lunate (wrist)
	Köhler's disease	Navicular (mid-foot)
	Freiberg's disease	Second metatarsal head
Articular chondral (splitting)	Osteochondritis dissecans	Medical femoral Condyle (knee) Capitellum (elbow Talar dome (ankle)
Physeal	Scheuermann's disease	Thoracic spine
	Blount's disease	Tibia (proximal)

Figure 2.9   Stages in fracture healing. (a) Haematoma: Tissue damage and bleeding occur at the fracture site, the bone ends die back a few millimetres. (b) Inflammation: Inflammatory cells appear in the haematoma. (c) Callus: The cell population changes to osteoblasts and osteoclasts, dead bone is mopped up and woven bone appears in the fracture callus. (d) Consolidation: Woven bone is remodelled to resemble the normal struture. From Apley and Solomon (1988), with permission.

the blood, and the periosteum itself is lifted from the bone surface. The deprivation of blood to the bone surfaces immediately adjacent to the fracture line causes these surfaces to die back for up to 2 mm. Some 8 hours after fracture, inflammation and proliferation may be detected as stage two of healing. The deep periosteal cells, and those of the damaged medullary canal, proliferate, and cellular tissue begins to grow forward to meet similar material from the other side of the fracture site and bridge the area. Capillary growth into the region allows the haematoma to be slowly reabsorbed, and the congealed blood itself takes little part in the repair process.

The appearance of osteogenic and chondrogenic cells marks the beginning of the third stage of healing. New bone and, in some cases, cartilage is laid down, while osteoclastic cells remove remaining dead bone. The cellular mass which forms is called a callus, and becomes increasingly mineralized into woven bone, uniting the fracture. The callus is larger where there has been much periosteal stripping, when bone displacement is marked, and if the haematoma has been large. The woven bone is transformed into lamellar bone by osteoblasts in the fourth stage of healing.

As the fracture site is bridged by solid bone, the fifth and final stage of healing commences, that of remodelling. A combination of bone reabsorption and formation reshapes the callus, laying down thicker lamellae in areas of high stress and removing excessive bone. The medullary cavity is re-formed.

The rate of healing is dependent on a number of factors. The type of bone is important, cancellous bone healing far more quickly than cortical bone. Also, the fracture type will dictate the speed of healing, with a spiral fracture healing more quickly than a transverse type. If the blood supply has been compromised at the time of injury, or if the fracture has occurred in an area with a poor blood supply, the healing rate will be slower. The age and health of the patient are other determining factors, with fractures in children healing almost twice as fast as those in adults. In general terms, callus may be visible radiographically within 2–3 weeks of injury, with firm fracture union taking about 4–6 weeks for upper limb fractures and 8–12 weeks for those in the lower limb. Full consolidation may take as much as 8 and 16 weeks for upper and lower limb fractures, respectively.

In contrast to long bone, cancellous bone remains fairly immobile when fractured, and heals by 'direct repair' with a minimum of callus formation. The main difference occurs because there is no medullary canal in cancellous bone, and the area of contact between the two injured bone fragments is much greater. Following haematoma formation, new blood vessels and osteogenic cells penetrate the area and meet similar tissue from the opposite bone fragment. The intercellular matrix which is laid down by osteoblasts is calcified into woven bone. This type of healing also occurs when internal fixation is used.

Mechanical properties

Bone responds to mechanical stress in similar ways to other connective tissue, but at a considerably slower rate. Its ability to adapt its structure, size and shape depends on the mechanical stresses placed upon it. When stress is reduced, by prolonged bed rest for example, mineral reabsorption occurs and the bone reduces in strength. Raising stress to an optimal level, by exercise, leads to an increase in bone strength. In addition to changes in total mineral content, bone varies its strength according to the direction of the imposed stress. At bony attachment sites such as tubercles, alignment of collagen fibres is parallel to the direction of the imposed force. In the shaft of a long bone, fibre orientation is along the bone axis, indicating that this part of the bone is designed to resist tension and compression forces. In cancellous bone at the epiphysis, shear stresses are maximal and so fibre alignment is in the direction of the shearing forces.

A number of mechanisms have been proposed to explain how the bone remodels to imposed stress. Bassett (1965) argued that, in theory, mechanical stresses on bone create electrical charges (piezoelectric effect). Areas of compression were said to develop negative charges while those subjected to tensile stress are more positive. The suggestion is that bone deposition by osteoblasts occurs in negatively charged areas, while reabsorption by osteoclasts takes place in regions of positive excitation. Experiments with dogs (Bassett and Pawlick, 1964) have shown that new bone is laid down at an implanted cathode site, although other authors have described bone deposition at both negative and positive sites (Hert and Zalud, 1971) so the effects of polarity are still uncertain.

Electrical fields formed in bone as a result of imposed stresses have been shown to stimulate protein synthesis in frog osteogenic cells (Becker and Murray, 1970), and increased rate of bone formation has been shown as a result of direct current (d.c.) administered through implanted electrodes (Becker, Spadaro and Marino, 1977).

Bone trabeculae subjected to maximum stress will be strengthened by bone deposition, in the direction of the imposed force. Regions of high stress have denser trabeculae, aligned to minimize the bending effect on a bone. Where a bone is subjected to an unbalanced force, which would tend to bend it, remodelling occurs as a result of changes in surface strain (Riegger, 1990). On the convex surface of the bone, osteoclastic activity leads to bone reabsorption while on the concave surface the reverse occurs and bone deposition is seen. Bone therefore moves towards the concavity which has been induced through loading of the shaft, to minimize the bending effect, a process known as flexural drift. The stress imposed on the bone causes an increase in the calcium concentration found within the interstitial fluid, as a result of changes in bone crystal solubility.

Osteoporosis

Osteoporosis (bone mineral loss) has now reached epidemic proportions in the Western world (Carbon, 1992). The condition involves a progressive decrease in bone density, due to an imbalance between bone formation and bone reabsorption. Bone mass reaches its peak in the third and fourth decade, and loss occurs normally in both sexes with ageing, but this rate is increased markedly with osteoporosis. Normal bone loss of 3% per decade may increase to as much as 10% per decade for trabecular bone.

Osteoporosis may be either primary, governed by age and sex, or secondary as a result of disease. The most common primary types are post-menopausal osteoporosis and senile osteoporosis. The loss of mass makes the bone susceptible to fracture, particularly as a result of microtrauma. Common fracture sites include the distal radius and vertebrae for post-menopausal osteoporosis, and the proximal femur for senile osteoporosis. Fracture of the distal radius presents as a Colles' fracture, while vertebral wedging gives rise to an increased thoracic kyphosis or 'dowagers hump'.

There is a marked increase in the risk of fracture once bone density reduces below a certain level (known as the fracture threshold, Fig. 2.10). The incidence of hip and vertebral fractures rises with age (Fig. 2.11), but the rise in hip fracture incidence in men occurs some 5 years later than that of women (Wolman and Reeve, 1994), an indication of the effect of post-menopausal osteoporosis.

Three main factors are important in the development of osteoporosis: diet, oestrogen level, and physical activity.

Diet

Modern diet can fail to provide an adequate daily intake of calcium. Recommended

Figure 2.10 Change in bone density with age. From Wolman and Reeve (1994).

Figure 2.11 Incidence of common osteoporotic fractures. From Wolman and Reeve (1994).

requirements as high as 1500 mg of calcium and 400 IU of vitamin D have been made for post-menopausal women (MacKinnon, 1988), but many females may consume as little as 300 mg of calcium (McArdle, Katch and Katch, 1986), placing themselves in negative calcium balance. Excess salt or caffeine, and a large intake of meat promote calcium loss in the urine, and an excessive intake of fibre and alcohol can bind calcium in the gut preventing its absorption (Deakin and Brotherhood, 1992).

Calcium deficiency in animals has been shown to produce osteoporosis (Martin and Houston, 1987), but effects in man are less clear. Studying early post-menopausal women, Nilas, Christiansen and Rodbro (1984) gave a 500 mg calcium supplement

over a 2-year period and assessed bone density in the distal radius, while Ettinger, Genant and Cann (1987) gave a 1000 mg supplement and assessed the lumbar vertebrae. Both of these studies failed to show any significant differences between the treatment and non-treatment groups. However, in late post-menopausal women calcium supplementation may be more beneficial (MacKinnon, 1988). However, the effect of calcium supplementation on the incidence of fractures remains unproven (Evans, 1990b)

Adequate calcium is clearly necessary for health, and those individuals who show a deficiency in their calcium intake may need dietary supplementation. Others should receive advice on good diet to enable them to maintain an adequate intake of calcium and vitamin D, remembering that excessive vitamin D intake can be toxic.

Exercise

Weight-bearing exercise creates bone stress and acts as a stimulus for maintaining bone mass. Loss of bone mass has been reported both as a result of prolonged bed rest (Donaldson, Hulley and Vogel, 1970) and following weightlessness (Mazess and Whedon, 1983). Similarly, athletes have been shown to have greater bone density than non-athletes (Nilsson and Westlin, 1977), and tennis players have been shown to have a greater bone density in their dominant arm (Huddleston, Rockwell and Kuland, 1980).

A number of authors have demonstrated the beneficial effects of weight-bearing exercise in slowing bone loss. Smith, Smith and Ensign (1984) assessed the effects of exercise (45 min, 3 days per week) on bone loss in post-menopausal women and showed a 1.4% increase in bone mass during the second and third years of their study. Krolner, Toft and Nielsen (1983) studied the effects of exercise (1 hour, twice per week) on post-menopausal women. They showed a 3.5% increase in bone mineral content of the lumbar spine for the exercising group compared to 2.7% for their control.

Clearly, regular weight-bearing exercise is important for the prevention and management of osteoporosis. However, the increased risk of fracture in this group means that caution must be shown. Repeated spinal rotation or flexion should be avoided, as should high impact activities, especially where osteoporosis already exists.

Hormone replacement therapy
The use of low dosage oestrogen in hormone replacement therapy (HRT) to slow or even halt bone loss in post-menopausal women is widely recommended. HRT is used to make up for the decline in oestrogen levels seen during the menopause. Oestrogen plays an important part in calcium absorption by the body. Secreted by the ovaries and corpus luteum, oestrogen (a steroid hormone) stimulates regeneration of the endometrium, increases mucus output from the cervical glands, and promotes epiphyseal closure and growth of the bones and skeletal muscle.

HRT has been linked with an increased risk of endometrial carcinoma, although the risk is reduced when oestrogen is combined with progesterone (Hedlund and Gallagher, 1988).

Articular cartilage

Cartilage is essentially a connective tissue consisting of cells embedded in a matrix permeated by fibres. Two major types are recognized, hyaline cartilage and fibrocartilage. Hyaline cartilage is found over bone ends and is described in more detail below. Fibrocartilage may be either white or yellow. White fibrocartilage is found in areas such as the intervertebral discs and glenoid labrum. Yellow fibrocartilage is found in structures such as the ears and larynx.

Articular (hyaline) cartilage is made up of collagen fibres, a protein–polysaccharide complex, and water. Fibres of collagen are embedded in a ground substance of gel-like material. The water content of cartilage is high, between 70 and 80% of its total weight (Bullough, 1981).

Cartilage has no blood vessels, lymphatics or nerve fibres. Nutrition is supplied directly from the synovial fluid, and by diffusion of blood products from the sub-chondral bone. The tangled structure of cartilage causes it to behave in some ways like a microscopic sieve, filtering out large molecules such as plasma proteins. Fluid movement through the cartilage is by osmosis and diffusion. Movement of the joint increases the rate of diffusion, but in the mature joint there is no transfer across the bone–cartilage interface (Hettinga, 1990).

Intermittent loading creates a pumping effect, squeezing fluid from the cartilage and allowing fresh fluid to be taken up as the load is released. Prolonged loading will gradually press fluid out of the cartilage, without allowing new fluid to be taken up. As much as a 40% reduction in cartilage depth can occur by compression (Hettinga, 1990).

The cartilage is arranged in four layers (Fig. 2.12). The collagen fibres of the calcified zone bind the cartilage to the sub-chondral bone, resisting shear stresses. Within the mid-zone the fibres are randomly oriented. With joint compression, these fibres stretch and will resist the tension forces created within them (Fig. 2.13). This property of elastic deformation (spring) occurs instantly. However, the fluid within the matrix of the cartilage will be compressed. As it does so, proteoglycans within the cartilage will tend to retain water and control its movement through the cartilage matrix. The cartilage will slowly flow away from the compression force, demonstrating the property of creep. When the load is removed, the fluid lost at the time of compression is reabsorbed. These two properties of instant spring and slower creep make cartilage a viscoelastic material.

Cartilage assists joint lubrication by two processes, called boundary and weeping lubrication. Boundary lubrication occurs

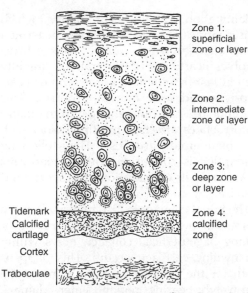

Figure 2.12 Zones in articular cartilage. From Gould (1990), with permission.

when hyaluronic acid molecules found in the joints' synovial fluid adhere momentarily to the cartilage surfaces of the joint. As the joint moves, the two molecular layers slide, a system which occurs mostly under light loads.

Weeping or fluid lubrication occurs when the cartilage is loaded and releases fluid which lies between the opposing surfaces—so-called squeeze film lubrication. The layer of fluid (the squeeze film) is under pressure and so keeps the cartilage surface apart. The fluid molecules act almost as tiny ball-bearings rolling between the opposing joint surfaces (Pascale and Grana, 1989).

Injury

Articular cartilage is to a great extent protected from injury by the elasticity of other

Figure 2.13 Effects of joint compression on articular cartilage. (a) Compressive loading of the cartilage results in (b) tension stress to the collagenous elements and compression stress to the mucopolysaccharide–water complex. (c) The total response is viscoelastic. The viscous creep with sustained loading is largely the result of a time-dependent squeezing out of fluid. From Hertling and Kessler (1990), with permission.

joint structures, and the neuromuscular reflexes. Reflex muscular contraction and soft tissue 'give' will largely dampen shock before it reaches the cartilage. However, unexpected loading (such as trauma) which occurs too rapidly to invoke reflex protection, will cause injury, but this is more frequently bony fracture rather than damage to the cartilage itself.

If cartilage injury does occur, it is most likely due to slip or shear. Three injury stages have been described (Hettinga, 1990). First, splitting of the cartilage layer at the tidemark between the calcified and uncalcified tissue. Secondly, cartilage depression into the sub-chondral bone, and, thirdly, fissuring of the cartilage and underlying bone.

Partial thickness injuries, limited to the articular cartilage alone, heal poorly. The healing which does take place is by proliferation and invasion from soft tissue, and the further away from this tissue the injured area is, the poorer the healing. Full thickness defects, extending through the sub-chondral bone heal by superficial tissue bridging the break. Blood vessels grow into the uncalcified cartilage. Osteogenic cells and granulation tissue from the base of the break invade the area resulting in the formation of fibrous tissue, bony trabeculae, and fibrocartilage. There is obvious demarcation of the region into zones, a chondrin-free ring surrounding the uninjured tissue. The healed defect appears as a slightly discoloured roughened area of fibrous tissue.

Intra-articular injection of hydrocortisone has resulted in a temporary reduction in cartilage matrix synthesis (Mankin and Conger, 1966) and destructive changes to the cartilage itself (Salter, Gross and Hall, 1967).

Arthritis

The term arthritis tends to be used to describe any chronic inflammatory reaction affecting a joint. However, the term simply means 'joint inflammation', and as such must be qualified by a description of the cause of inflammation. Acute joint injury which causes intracapsular swelling may be termed 'traumatic arthritis'. True osteoarthritis involves cartilage degeneration, initially with little inflammation, so the term osteoarthrosis would seem more appropriate. This condition must be differentiated from inflammatory states affecting multiple joints such as rheumatoid arthritis. The following description is concerned with osteoarthritis (OA) and its connection to sport and exercise.

The initial changes in OA are usually painless and show no swelling. Mild fraying or flaking of superficial collagen fibres within the hyaline cartilage occurs. This happens firstly at the periphery of the joint in the non-weight-bearing region. Later, damage (fibrillation) is to the deeper cartilage layers in the weight-bearing areas of the joint, extending down to one third of the cartilage thickness. Small cavities form (blistering) between the cartilage fibres which gradually extend to become vertical clefts. If cartilage fragments break off, they may float free in the joint fluid as loose bodies, giving rise to joint locking and sudden twinges of pain. The presence of a loose body and the by-products of cartilage destruction causes the synovium to inflame, and it is only now that many patients become aware that a problem exists.

Turnover of proteoglycan and collagen within the cartilage ground substance is increased, and the proteoglycan molecules near the fibrillated cartilage are smaller than normal. Mechanically, this altered cartilage is weaker to both compression and tension stresses, but it is still resistant to gliding, and its coefficient of friction remains low (Threlkeld and Currier, 1988). As the cartilage thins the joint space is reduced.

The sub-chondral bone beneath the fibrillated cartilage becomes shiny and smooth (eburnated). Below the eburnated region the area becomes osteoporotic and local avascular necrosis causes cyst formation where there is complete bone loss. Osteophytes covered with fibrocartilage form at the periphery of the joint, and may protrude into the joint space or more frequently into surrounding soft tissue.

The synovial membrane becomes thickened and its vascularity increases in line with an inflammatory response (see above). The joint capsule demonstrates small tears filled with fibrous tissue causing thickening. Contracture usually alters both physiological and accessory movements (see p. 18). For example, when OA affects the knee joint, flexion is often limited and mediolateral stability reduced.

Arthritis secondary to sports injury

The changes which occur in OA, if detected early enough may be reversible (Hertling and Kessler, 1990). Altered biomechanics of a joint, if corrected, can result in regrowth of fibrocartilage. However, subtle alterations in normal joint mechanics, which may remain long after an injury has 'resolved', may be largely undetectable to a patient or physician. It is not until these changes are well developed and limit physiological joint movement or cause deformity that they become readily apparent. Accessory movements when limited, are, however, detectable to a manipulative physiotherapist at a much earlier stage. It would seem logical therefore to assess and restore accessory movements after joint injury rather than simply full range physiological movement and muscle strength. In this way the onset of OA may be slowed or even avoided.

The use of biomechanical analyses after injury with apparatus such as video playback, isokinetic dynamometry and force plates is helpful to ensure that joint function has been restored.

Arthritis and exercise

Arthritis is often considered a normal ageing process. However, Panush and Brown (1987) cite a study of a population in the age range 70–79 years in which 85% had OA. Importantly, the result indicated that 15% of this age group did not suffer OA, so it seems likely that although ageing is an important factor, other considerations must exist.

Animal studies have failed to show a direct link between exercise and arthritis. Radin, Eyre and Schiller (1979) found no evidence of cartilage deterioration in sheep forced to walk for four hours daily on concrete for 12 and 30 months. Videman (1982) found that running did not affect the development of OA in rabbits. Experimentally induced OA was not increased when the animals were forced to run over 2000 m per week for 14 consecutive weeks.

Studies on runners have also failed to show any significant difference with non-runners. Puranen et al. (1975) found less hip OA in Finnish distance runners than in non-runners of a similar age. Panush et al. (1986) found no greater clinical or radiological evidence of OA in male runners of average age 55 years.

Studies have linked OA of particular joints with specific sports. In a review on the subject, Panush and Brown (1987) cited studies describing OA in the cervical spine and lower extremities of ballet dancers, the upper limb of baseball pitchers, the hands of boxers, cricketers, and downhill skiers, and the ankles and feet of soccer players. Whether these results reflect overuse of the joints involved, or altered mechanics following injury to these more frequently used body parts remains uncertain.

It would seem logical that maintaining the normal mobility and strength of a joint throughout life could help maintain the health of the joint structures and perhaps delay the onset of OA. Conversely, high impact loading of an already degenerating joint, such as may occur with running or aerobics on hard unforgiving surfaces, may exacerbate symptoms.

The advice to a patient with OA must be to reduce impact but maintain mobility and strength in a controlled fashion. Athletes must also be made aware of the danger of 'running through the pain' and training with an injury which alters the forces across a joint. Similarly, athletes must be conscious that the cessation of pain following injury does not indicate that full function has returned. Total rehabilitation has only occurred when normal joint mechanics has been restored.

The joint capsule

The joint capsule is in two parts. The outer part (stratum fibrosum) is fibrous and thickened in areas to form ligaments. The inner layer (stratum synoviale) is loose and highly vascular and blends with the synovial membrane. The capsule consists of parallel fascicles of collagen and some fibrocytes. Blood vessels enter the sub-chondral bone at the line of capsular attachment and small vessels are found between the individual cartilage fascicles. The nerve supply is very rich, with large fibres giving proprioceptive feedback and small fibres terminating in pain endings.

The capsular response to trauma is an increase in vascularity and eventually the development of fibrous tissue. Cross-linking of collagen fibres occurs, causing a palpable thickening of the capsule. Capsular shrinkage combined with fibrous adhesions will cause loss of movement and occurs particularly after immobilization.

Accumulation of joint fluid through swelling will stretch the capsule and capsular ligaments. The nerve endings situated between the collagen fascicles of the capsule will be stretched giving rise to mechanical pain. Should the fluid accumulation exceed the elastic limit of the joint capsule, rupture may result.

Joint effusion will stretch portions of the capsule which are normally lax to facilitate movement. The patient will tend to rest the joint in a position where the joint cavity is of maximum volume (loose pack, see p. 19); in addition, passive movements will be limited in characteristic 'capsular patterns' (Table 2.3).

Ligaments

When a ligament is put under stress, it responds by getting progressively stiffer before later deforming in a regular manner (Amis, 1985). There are two reasons for this. First, the collagen fibres within the ligament

Table 2.3 The capsular patterns

Shoulder — so much limitation of abduction, more than that of lateral rotation, less than that of medial rotation
Elbow — flexion usually more limited than extension, rotations full and painless except in advanced cases
Wrist — equal limitation of flexion and extension, little limitation of deviations
Trapezio-first metacarpal joint — only abduction limited
Sign of the buttock — passive hip flexion more limited and more painful than straight-leg raise
Hip — marked limitation of flexion and medial rotation, some limitation of abduction, little or no limitation of adduction and lateral rotation
Knee — gross limitation of flexion, slight limitation of extension
Ankle — more limitation of plantiflexion than of dorsiflexion
Talocalcanean joint — increasing limitations of varus until fixation in valgus
Mid-tarsal joint — limitations of adduction and internal rotation, other movements full
Big toe — gross limitation of extension, slight limitation of flexion
Cervical spine — equal limitation in all directions except for flexion which is usually full
Thoracic spine — limitation of extension, side flexion and rotations, less limitation of flexion
Lumbar spine — marked and equal limitation of side flexions, limitation of flexion and extension

From Cyriax and Cyriax (1983), with permission.

are not in line, and so the initial tensile stress is used up by pulling the fibres straight. Secondly, the fibres are not attached to a single point, but to an area of bone, and so are of slightly different lengths. When the fibres are stretched, there will be a progressive tightening of the ligament with some fibres becoming taut sooner than others.

Ligaments demonstrate viscoelastic properties. Rapid stretch has been shown to increase stiffness by as much as 20% (Woo, Gomez and Akeson, 1981), and sustained stretch to cause ligament tension to reduce significantly after 2 minutes (Viidik, 1966). The mode of failure also changes with speed, avulsion occurring at slower speeds, and ligamentous rupture at higher speeds (Noyes, DeLucas and Torvik, 1974).

Clinically, three grades of ligament injuries are recognized (Fowler, 1984). Grade I sprains involve minimal tissue damage with some local tenderness. Swelling is only slight, and function is almost normal. With the grade II sprain, more ligament fibres are injured or the ligament may become partially detached from its bony attachment. Local pain is more intense and movement more limited. Grade III injuries constitute a complete rupture. There is a rapid onset of effusion with considerable pain. The joint is unstable and loss of function is complete. Noyes et al. (1984) argued that this traditional classification, although useful, could be misleading. The grade II injury could refer equally to an injury where only a few ligament fibres are torn, or to a lesion where virtually the total ligament was affected. The grade III injury, they claimed, represented not total rupture, but total loss of function of the ligament, actual continuity of the ligament often being maintained.

With grades I and II, pain is increased by placing the ligament on stretch. With a grade II injury, some instability may be present, but with a complete rupture instability is always present. However, clinically this may be difficult to assess in instances of severe pain and muscle spasm.

Ligamentous viscosity changes with age. The collagen fibres within the ligament enlarge, reducing the water content in the ground substance. Noyes and Grood (1976) showed marked reductions in tensile strength of ligament in the 48–83 year age group when compared with the 16–26 year age group.

Noyes et al. (1984) showed three-fold decreases in maximum stress, elastic modulus and strain energy between the ligaments from donors aged 50 years compared to those aged 20 years. The older ligaments failed by bony avulsion rather than ligamentous failure as occurred in the younger tissues. They claimed that ageing produced changes in the ligament/bone systems similar to those found through disuse.

Immobility also has marked effects on ligaments. Laros, Tipton and Cooper (1971) showed strength reductions of 39% after 9 weeks' immobilization. Full strength not being regained for 30 weeks. Exercise has been shown to have a beneficial effect on ligament tensile strength (Adams, 1966; Heikkinen and Vuori, 1972; Cabaud et al., 1980). Exercise seems to act as a 'mechanical stimulant', causing increased collagen turnover within the ligament (Weisman, Pope and Johnson, 1980). This has important implications for rehabilitation following ligament injury. Wherever possible, complete immobilization should be avoided. While an injured ligament should be protected against excessive external forces which could cause further damage, gentle exercise within the pain-free range should still be encouraged.

The effect of corticosteroids on ligament failure is important, since steroid usage in sport is still popular. Decreases in maximum load of 21% and 39% have been shown 6 and 15 weeks after large dosage cortisone injection (methyl prednisolone acetate), with a load reduction remaining for one year. In addition, fibrocyte death was seen within the ligament, with delay in reappearance of new fibrocytes for 15 weeks (Noyes et al., 1984).

Muscle

The term 'strain' is generally used to imply a minor injury to any soft tissue structure. However, in this book strain will be confined to injury of muscle while the term 'sprain' will be used for injured joint structures. Strains may be subdivided into acute and chronic types. Acute strains are usually the result of a single violent stretch to a contracting muscle (Fowler, 1984; Keene, 1990), while chronic strains develop over a period of time as a result of repetitive loading.

Fowler (1984) classified strains into four grades to include complete rupture as a grade four injury, while Keene (1990) used three grades and described complete rupture as a separate entity. The diversity of opinion makes it essential when describing an injury not to use a number alone.

The grade one (mild) strain is a contusion in which there is tearing of a small number of muscle fibres with the fascia remaining intact. Bleeding is minimal, with pain and spasm being localized. Muscle function is normal, but endurance may be reduced.

Grade two (moderate) strains result from more severe trauma. A larger number of muscle fibres are injured, and injury occurs over a greater area. The fascia still remains intact so bleeding is contained within the muscle, forming an intramuscular haematoma. The contained bleeding will cause an increase in intramuscular pressure, which in turn will compress the bleeding points and stop further haemorrhage (Williams and Sperryn, 1976). A definite palpable mass is evident with this injury, and pain to palpation is considerable. Function of the muscle is impaired, with contractility and extensibility being greatly reduced.

With grade three (severe) strains, a larger area of muscle is affected. The muscle fascia is partially torn, and more than one muscle may be involved. Bleeding is more profuse, and spread over a larger area, as the haemorrhage is no longer contained by the muscle sheath. The torn fascia releases the blood to form an intermuscular haematoma (Fig. 2.14). The grade four injury is a complete rupture. The muscle ends contract and a definite gap is apparent. In some cases a snapping sound may be heard at the time of injury. Bleeding and swelling are considerable, and active contraction of the muscle is not possible.

The site of the injury is especially important with regard to the treatment regime chosen. Muscle-tendon injuries can be to the muscle belly itself, the musculotendinous (MT) junction or the teno-osseous (TO) junction. Garrett (1990) showed that both passive stretching, and stretching a pre-contracted isolated rabbit muscle consistently caused failure at the MT junction. A small (0.1–1 mm) amount of muscle tissue being left attached to the tendon.

Garrett (1990) also showed that pre-contracted muscles absorbed 100% more energy than passively stretched muscle fibre, and used these results to emphasize the importance of muscles as energy absorbers. He

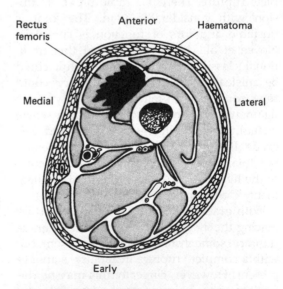

Figure 2.14 An intermuscular haematoma affecting the rectus femoris. From Fowler (1984), with permission.

argued that conditions which interfere with a muscle's contractile ability, such as fatigue or muscle weakness, might diminish the energy absorbing ability of the muscle and possibly predispose to injury.

Cyriax (1982) claimed that muscle belly injuries would respond to therapeutic exercise. Muscle contraction causes broadening of the fibres and, he claimed, would reduce intramuscular scarring. Injury at the MT or TO junctions would not respond to exercise as no muscle broadening occurs at these points. Cyriax argued that passive therapy, such as transverse frictional massage or injection, was more appropriate to these sites.

Myositis ossificans traumatica

Myositis ossificans traumatica (MOT) is soft tissue ossification of muscle resulting in the formation of non-neoplasmic bone (Booth and Westers, 1989). It usually occurs in the proximal limb muscles, and is seen most commonly following contusion of the quadriceps femoris musculature (Jackson, 1975), although other regions include the elbow flexors and hip abductors.

Several aetiological theories have been suggested (Booth and Westers, 1989). Calcification of a muscle haematoma can occur following fibrosis, or intramuscular bone formation may result from periosteal detachment. Rupture of the periosteum may lead to the proliferation of osteoblasts and their escape into the surrounding muscle. Intramuscular connective tissue may undergo metaplasia into bone, and Urist et al. (1978) demonstrated that certain skeletal muscle cells, known as inducible osteogenic precursor cells (IOPC), have the capability of differentiating into osteoblasts. Certain individuals have been shown to have a predisposition to the condition (Rothwell, 1982).

Clinically, the patient presents with severe post-traumatic pain and limitation of movement. There is local swelling and erythema, with the area being warm and tender to palpation. Tenderness usually becomes more pronounced with time, and tissue signs do not respond to conservative management. The factor which should alert the practitioner to the possibility of MOT, is a reduction in movement range over time. Normally, an increasing range would be expected as a condition resolves. Radiological evidence of ossification is usually seen within two months following injury, and other investigations including computed tomography (Vas et al., 1981), and ultrasound scanning (Kramer et al., 1979) have been used.

Management of MOT is aimed at lessening any disability rather than affecting the bone mass. Initially, the soft tissue response to trauma, especially bleeding, is limited by the use of such regimes as rest, ice, compression and elevation (RICE). Rehabilitation is slower than with a normal muscle haematoma, isometric exercises being used 7–14 days following injury, but active exercises (within the pain-free range) are not used until 2–4 weeks after injury (Booth and Westers, 1989).

Tendons

A variety of conditions may affect tendons, the most common in sport being tenosynovitis, tendinitis and tenovaginitis. Tendinitis is an inflammation and scarring of the tendon which can occur in varying degrees. Scarring may interfere with tendon function and/or cause persistent local inflammation.

Tenosynovitis is a lesion to the gliding surfaces of the outside of the tendon and the inside of its sheath, but not the sheath itself (Fowler, 1984). The lesion is usually as a result of overuse or compression (Williams and Sperryn, 1976). Pathological features are similar to those seen in rheumatoid arthritis (Williams and Sperryn, 1976), including an increase in the number of lining cells of the sheath, together with proliferation of local blood vessels, oedema and cellular changes. As the roughened surfaces of the sheath move against each other pain and crepitus occur. The same condition, occurring to tendons which do not have a true sheath, is termed peritendonitis. Here, the paratenon thickens, and shows fibrinoid degeneration and dense fibrous adhesions (Snook, 1972). Local oedema is evident, sometimes with palpable crepitus, and pain may disappear with activity (Williams and Sperryn, 1976).

Tenovaginitis occurs when the tendon sheath is chronically inflamed and thickens. It is the fibrous wall of the tendon sheath rather than the synovial lining which is affected. Common sites include the flexor sheaths of the fingers or thumb. When the sheaths of extensor pollicis brevis and abductor pollicis longus are affected, de Quervain's syndrome is present.

Skin

The initial reaction to mild skin injury is the classic triple response described by Lewis and Grant (1924). Making a firm mark across the skin with a pin, for example, causes an initial pallor, followed by a dull red line (flush) with a surrounding red area (flare). Local swelling (wheal) will occur if the skin marking was intense. This response is due mainly to the effects of histamines, and through the axon reflex.

The initial reduction in blood flow and consequent dramatic increase is the result of increases and decreases in muscle tone of the arteriole walls. The larger lumen of the vessels involved reduces peripheral resistance and a larger volume of blood enters the area. Local capillaries supplied by the affected arterioles are re-opened or dilated and the area is engorged with blood. The initial increase in blood flow will last for approximately 1 hour (Evans, 1990a), and then the blood flow gradually slows.

Blood slowing occurs by haemoconcentration, water and smaller molecules being lost through the capillary wall. The concentration of blood proteins give rise to rouleaux formation where the red cells clump together. In addition, white cells stick to the vessel walls further reducing the vessel lumen size.

Skin wounds

Skin wounds may be divided into two categories, open and closed. Closed wounds occur when there is no penetration of the epidermis, and open wounds are those where the epidermis has been pierced. Closed wounds encompass contusions, abrasions and friction burns, such as those caused by gravel. Open wounds in sport include lacerations and puncture wounds.

A contusion or bruise involves a direct blow to the skin surface. Bleeding occurs from torn blood vessels into the skin and subcutaneous tissues, forming a bruise or ecchymosis. Released blood will clot and degrade producing superficial colour changes. An abrasion or graze occurs through a glancing injury, or repeated microtrauma to the skin surface. The skin surface breaks through, but the damage is not full thickness. Extensive areas of skin may be affected, and intense pain usually occurs as raw nerve endings are exposed. Bleeding may be extensive, but healing is rapid unless infection ensues. Extensive debriding injuries involving large areas of skin loss (for example from a motor-cycle accident) may require grafting.

A laceration is a full thickness skin injury, which exposes the subcutaneous tissue. Clean lacerations may require stitching but heal well, jagged injuries involving skin tearing may leave more scarring.

Pressure or friction may cause an abrasion where the skin surface is removed, or a blister, where the epidermal surface skin layer is detached from the underlying tissue. The gap between the two layers is filled with lymph, exposing nerve endings to fluid pressure, so causing pain. When pressure or friction is applied progressively, the epidermal skin layer may adapt to form a thickened callus (Williams, 1979).

Healing of an incised wound such as a cut, where the wound edges are in apposition, occurs by first intention. If the wound edges are separated and more major skin damage has occurred (or if infection has intervened), then healing is by second intention (Evans, 1990a).

With healing by first intention, slight haemorrhage occurs and the cut is filled with a blood clot on the first day. By the second and third day the clot has become organized and epithelial cells from the two sides of the cut have joined. This single layer of covering multiplies to form stratified squamous epithelium—normal epidermis. Fibroblasts lay down collagen in the granulation tissue and a band of scar tissue is formed by two weeks after the injury.

Healing by second intention takes longer as the spread of epithelial cells over the larger area takes time. The large amount of granulation tissue results in more extensive scarring and likely contracture.

References

Adams, A. (1966) Effect of exercise upon ligament strength. *Research Quarterly*, **37**, 163–176

Amis, A.A. (1985) Biomechanics of ligaments. In *Ligament Injuries and their Treatment* (ed. D.H.R. Jenkins), Chapman and Hall, London

Apley, A.G. and Solomon, L. (1988) *Concise System of Orthopaedics and Fractures*, Butterworth-Heinemann, Oxford

Bassett, C.A.L. (1965) Electrical effects in bone. *Scientific American*, **213**(4), 18

Bassett, C.A.L. and Pawlick, R.J. (1964) Effects of electric currents on bone in vivo. *Nature*, **204**, 652

Becker, R.O. and Murray, D.G. (1970) The electrical control system regulating fracture healing in amphibians. *Clinical Orthopaedics and Related Research*, **73**, 169

Becker, R.O., Spadaro, J.A. and Marino, A.A. (1977) Clinical experience with low intensity direct current stimulation of bone growth. *Clinical Orthopaedics and Related Research*, **124**, 75–83

Blau. S.P. (1979) The synovial fluid. *The Orthopaedic Clinics of North America*, **10**, 21–35

Booth, D.W. and Westers, B.M. (1989) The management of athletes with myositis ossificans traumatica. *Canadian Journal of Sports Science*, **14**(1), 10–16

Bullough, P.G. (1981) Cartilage. In *Scientific Foundations of Orthopaedics and Traumatology* (eds R. Owen, J. Goodfellow and P. Bullough), Heinemann Medical, Oxford

Burri, C., Helbing, G. and Spier, W. (1973) Rehabilitation of knee ligament injuries. In *The Knee*, Springer, New York

Cabaud, H.E., Chatty, A., Gildengorin, V. and Feltman, R.J. (1980) Exercise effects on the strength of the anterior cruciate ligament. *American Journal of Sports Medicine*, **8**, 79–86

Carbon, R.J. (1992) The female athlete. In *Textbook of Science and Medicine in Sport* (eds J. Bloomfield, P.A. Fricker and K.D. Fitch), Blackwell Scientific Publications, Melbourne

Crawford-Adams, J. (1978) *Outline of Fractures*, Churchill Livingstone, London

Cyriax, J. (1982) *Textbook of Orthopaedic Medicine*, Vol. one (8th edn), Baillière Tindall, London

Cyriax, J.H. and Cyriax, P.J. (1983) *Illustrated Manual of Orthopaedic Medicine*, Butterworths, London

Deakin, V. and Brotherhood, J.R. (1992) Nutrition and energy sources. In *Textbook of Science and Medicine in Sport* (eds J. Bloomfield, P.A. Fricker and K. D. Fitch), Blackwell Scientific Publications, Melbourne

De Domenico, G. (1982) Pain relief with interferential therapy. *Australian Journal of Physiotherapy*, **28**(3), 14–18

Donaldson, C.L., Hulley, S.B. and Vogel, J.M (1970) Effects of prolonged bed rest on bone mineral. *Metabolism*, **19**, 1071–1084

Donley, P.B. and Denegar, C. (1990) Pain and mechanisms of pain relief. In *Therapeutic Modalities in Sports Medicine* (ed. W.E. Prentice), Times Mirror/Mosby College Publishing

Dyson, M. (1987) Mechanisms involved in therapeutic ultrasound. *Physiotherapy*, **73**(3), 116–120

Ettinger, B., Genant, H.K. and Cann, C.E. (1987) Postmenopausal bone loss is prevented by low dosage estrogen with calcium. *Annals of Internal Medicine*, **106**, 40–45

Evans, D.M.D (1990a) Inflammation and healing. In *Cash's Textbook of General Medical and Surgical Conditions for Physiotherapists* (ed. P.A. Downe), 2nd edn, Faber and Faber, London

Evans, P. (1980) The healing process at cellular level: a review. *Physiotherapy*, **66**(8), 256–259

Evans, R.A. (1990b) Calcium and osteoporosis. *Medical Journal of America*, **152**, 431–433

Fowler, J.A. (1984) Soft tissue injuries and sports injuries. In *Cash's Textbook of Orthopaedics and Rheumatology for Physiotherapists* (ed. P.A. Downie), Faber and Faber, London

Fox, J., Galey, F. and Wayland, H. (1980) Action of histamine on the mesenteric microvasculature. *Microvascular Research*, **19**, 108–126

Frank, G., Woo, S.L., Amiel, O., Harwood, F., Gomez, M. and Akeson, W. (1983) Medial collateral ligament healing. A multidisiplinary assessment in rabbits. *American Journal of Sports Medicine*, **11**, 379–389

Garrett, W.E. (1990) Muscle strain injuries: clinical and basic aspects. *Medicine and Science in Sports and Exercise*, **22**, 436–443

Gartland, J.J. (1987) *Fundamentals of Orthopaedics*, 4th edn, W.B. Saunders, Philadelphia

Gould, J.A. (ed.) (1989) *Orthopaedic and Sports Physical Therapy*. Second edition. C.V. Mosby, St Louis

Hedlund, L.R. and Gallagher, J.C. (1988) Estrogen therapy for postmenopausal osteoporosis: current considerations of the menopause. *Annals of Clinical and Laboratory Science*, **15**, 219–228

Heikkinen, E. and Vuori, I. (1972) Effect of physical activity on the metabolism of collagen in aged mice. *Acta Physiologica Scandinavica*, **84**, 543–549

Hert, J. and Zalud, J. (1971) Reaction of bone to mechanical stimuli. (VI). Bioelectrical theory of functional adaptation of bone. *Acta Chirurgicae Orthopaedicae et Traumatologicae Cechoslovaca*, **38**, 280

Hertling, D. and Kessler, R.M. (1990) *Management of Common Musculoskeletal Disorders*, J.B. Lippincott, Philadelphia

Hettinga, D.L. (1990) Inflammatory response of synovial joint structures. In *Orthopaedic and Sports Physical Therapy*, 2nd edn (ed. J.A. Gould), C.V. Mosby, St Louis, pp. 87–117

Huddleston, A.L., Rockwell, D. and Kuland, D.N. (1980) Bone mass in lifetime tennis athletes. *Journal of the American Medical Association*, **244**, 1107–1109

Jackson, D.W. (1975) Managing myositis ossificans traumatica. *Physician and Sports Medicine*, October, 56–61

Keene, J.S. (1990) Ligament and muscle tendon unit injuries. In *Orthopaedic and Sports Physical Therapy*, 2nd edn (ed. J.A. Gould), C.V. Mosby, St Louis

Kellett, J. (1986) Acute soft tissue injuries – a review of the literature. *Medicine and Science in Sports and Exercise*, **18**(5), 489–500

Kramer, F.L., Kurtz, A.B., Rubin, C. and Goldberg, B.B. (1979) Ultrasound appearance of myositis ossificans. *Skeletal Radiology*, **4**, 19–20

Krolner, B., Toft, B. and Nielsen, S. (1983) Physical exercise as a prophylaxis against involutional bone loss: a controlled trial. *Clinical Science*, **64**, 541–546

Lachman, S. (1988) *Soft Tissue Injuries in Sport*, Blackwell, Oxford

Laros, G.S, Tipton, C.M. and Cooper, R.R. (1971) Influence of physical activity on ligament insertions in the knees of dogs. *Journal of Bone and Joint Surgery*, **53A**, 275–286

Lewis, T. and Grant, R.T. (1924) Vascular reactions of the skin to injury. *Heart*, **11**, 209–265

Low, J. and Reed, A. (1990) *Electrotherapy Explained. Principles and Practice*, Butterworth-Heinemann, Oxford

Lynch, M.K. and Kessler, R.M. (1990) Pain. In *Management of Common Musculoskeletal Disorders*, 2nd edn (eds D. Hertling and R.M. Kessler), J.B. Lippincott, Philadelphia

MacKinnon, J.L. (1988) Osteoporosis. A review. *Physical Therapy*, **68**(10), 1533–1540

Maitland, G.D. (1991) *Peripheral Manipulation*, 3rd edn, Butterworth-Heinemann, Oxford

Mankin, H.J. and Conger, K.A. (1966) The acute effects of intra-articular hydrocortisone on articular cartilage in rabbits. *Journal of Bone and Joint Surgery*, **48A**, 1383–1388

Martin, A.D. and Houston, C.S. (1987) Osteoporosis, calcium and physical activity. *Canadian Medical Association Journal*, **136**, 587–593

Mazess, R.B. and Whedon, G.D. (1983). Immobilization and bone. *Calcified Tissue International*, **35**, 265–267

McArdle, W.D., Katch, F.I. and Katch, V.L. (1986) *Exercise Physiology. Energy, Nutrition, and Human Performance*, 2nd edn, Lea and Febiger, Philadelphia.

Melzack, R. and Wall, P.D. (1965) Pain mechanisms: a new theory. *Science*, **150**, 971

Nilas, L., Christiansen, C. and Rodbro, P. (1984) Calcium supplementation and post-menopausal bone loss. *British Medical Journal*, **289**, 1103–1106

Nilsson, B.E. and Westlin, N.E. (1977) Bone density in athletes. *Clinical Orthopaedics and Related Research*, **77**, 179–182

Noyes, F.R. and Grood, M.J. (1976) The strength of the anterior cruciate ligament in humans and rhesus monkeys: age-related and species-related changes. *Journal of Bone and Joint Surgery*, **58A**, 1074–1082

Noyes, F.R., DeLucas, J.L. and Torvik, P.J. (1974) Biomechanics of anterior cruciate ligament failure: an analysis of strain-rate sensitivity and mechanisms in primates. *Journal of Bone and Joint Surgery*, **56A**, 236–253

Noyes, F.R., Kelly, C.S., Grood, E.S. and Butler, D.L. (1984) Advances in the understanding of knee ligament injury, repair and rehabilitation. *Medicine and Science in Sports and Exercise*, **16**(5), 427–443

Oakes, B.W. (1992) The classification of injuries and mechanisms of injury, repair and healing. In *Textbook of Science and Medicine in Sport* (eds J. Bloomfield, P.A. Fricker and K.D. Fitch), Blackwell Scientific Publications, Melbourne

Paget, S. and Bullough, P.G. (1981) Synovium and synovial fluid. In *Scientific Foundations of Orthopaedics and Traumatology* (eds R. Owen, J. Goodfellow and P. Bullough), Heinemann Medical, Oxford

Palastanga, N., Field, D. and Soames, R. (1989) *Anatomy and Human Movement*, Heinemann Medical, Oxford

Panush, R.S. and Brown, D.G. (1987) Exercise and arthritis. *Sports Medicine*, **4**, 54–64

Panush, R.S., Schmidt, C., Caldwell, J., Edwards, N.L. and Longley, S. (1986) Is running associated with degenerative joint disease? *Journal of the American Medical Association*, **255**, 1150–1154

Pappas, A.M. (1989) Osteochondroses: diseases of growth centers. *Physician and Sports Medicine*, **17**, 51–62

Pascale, M. and Grana, W.A. (1989) Does running cause osteoarthritis? *The Physician and Sports Medicine*, **17**, (3) 157–166

Puranen, J., Ala-Ketola, L., Peltokalleo, P. and Saarela, J. (1975) Running and primary osteoarthritis of the hip. *British Medical Journal*, **1**, 424–425

Radin, E.L., Eyre, D. and Schiller, A.L. (1979) Effect of prolonged walking on concrete on the joints of sheep. Abstract. *Arthritis and Rheumatism*, **22**, 649

Reigger, C.L. (1990) Mechanical properties of bone. In *Orthopaedic and Sports Physical Therapy* 2nd edn (ed. J. A. Gould), C.V. Mosby, St Louis, pp. 3–47

Rothwell, A.G. (1982) Quadriceps haematoma. A prospective study. *Clinical Orthopaedics and Related Research*, **171**, 97–103

Salter, R.B. and Harris, W.R. (1963) Injuries involving the epiphyseal plate. *Journal of Bone and Joint Surgery*, **45A**, 587

Salter, R.B., Gross, A. and Hall, J.H. (1967) Hydrocortisone arthropathy – an experimental investigation. *Canadian Medical Association Journal*, **97**, 374–377

Smith, E.L., Smith, P.E. and Ensign, C.J. (1984) Bone involutional decrease in exercising middle-aged women. *Calcified Tissue International*, **36**, 129–138

Snook, G.A. (1972) Tenosynovitis in long distance runners. *Medicine and Science in Sports and Exercise*, **4**, 166

Sterns, M.L. (1940) Studies on development of connective tissue in transparent chambers in rabbits ear. *American Journal of Anatomy*, **67**, 55

Threlkeld, A.J. and Currier, D.P. (1988) Osteoarthritis: Effects on synovial joint tissues. *Physical Therapy*, **68** (3), 364–370

Urist, M.R., Nakagawa, M., Nakata, N. and Nogami, H. (1978) Experimental myositis ossificans: cartilage and bone formation in muscle in response to a dissufible bone matrix derived morphogen. *Archives of Pathology and Laboratory Medicine*, **102**, 312–316

Van der Meulen, J.C.H. (1982) Present state of knowledge on processes of healing in collagen structures. *International Journal of Sports Medicine*, **3**, 4–8

Vas, W., Cockshott, W.P., Martin, R.F., Pai, N.K. and Walker, I. (1981) Myositis ossificans in haemophilia. *Skeletal Radiology* **7**, 27–31

Videman, T. (1982) The effect of running on the osteoarthritic joint: an experimental matched pair study with rabbits. *Rheumatology and Rehabilitation*, **21**, 1–8

Viidik, A. (1966) Biomechanics and functional adaptation of tendons and joint ligament. In *Studies on the Anatomy and Function of Bone and Joints* (ed. F.G. Evans), Springer, Berlin

Walter, J.B. and Israel, M.S. (1987) *General Pathology*, 6th edn, Churchill Livingstone, London

Watson, A.S. (1992) Children in sport. In *Textbook of Science and Medicine in Sport* (eds J. Bloomfield, P.A. Fricker and K.D. Fitch), Blackwell Scientific Publications, Melbourne

Weisman, G., Pope, M.H. and Johnson, R.J. (1980) Cyclic loading in knee ligament injuries. *American Journal of Sports Medicine*, **8**, 24–30

Wilkinson, P.C. and Lackie, J.M. (1979) The adhesion, migration and chemotaxis of leucocytes in inflammation. *Current Topics in Pathology*, **68**, 47–88

Williams, J.G.P. (1979) *Injuries in Sport*, Bayer (UK), Haywards Heath, England

Williams, J.G.P. and Sperryn, P.N. (1976) *Sports Medicine*, Edward Arnold, London

Wolman, R.L. and Reeve, J. (1994) Exercise and the skeleton. In *Oxford Textbook of Sports Medicine* (eds M. Harries et al.), Oxford University Press, Oxford

Woo, S.L.Y., Gomez, M.A. and Akeson, W.H. (1981) The time and history-dependent viscoelastic properties of the canine medial collateral ligament. *Journal of Biomechanical Engineering*, **103**, 293–298

3

Psychological aspects of sports injury

The injury-prone athlete

A variety of psychological variables may predispose an athlete to injury. General personality make-up, trait anxiety, locus of control and self-esteem have all received attention (Kerr and Fowler, 1988). Several authors have attempted to show that specific aspects of personality make an athlete more prone to injury. Some believe that certain personality traits, which are largely genetically determined, make some athletes more likely to be injured than their peers. Others argue that temporary (transient) mood states are more liable to have a significant effect.

Jackson et al. (1978) examined footballers on the Cattell 16PF (personality factor) test, and concluded that tender-minded players were more likely to be injured. In addition, the reserved and detached players suffered more severe injuries. Reilly (1975), using the same test with professional soccer players, found a relationship between apprehensiveness and injury. Personality factors, such as being over-protective, easily distracted, or attention-seeking, may also predispose to injury.

Anxiety, and the unconscious attempt to cope with it, can cause abnormal behaviour in the athlete (Sanderson, 1981) and may increase the likelihood of injury. Coping mechanisms for tension or anxiety can in some instances create a distortion of reality. An example is the overly tense athlete who simply denies that he is anxious. This person may be emotionally vulnerable and will often lose composure easily, possibly becoming violent. Individuals of this type may harbour a sense of guilt which they try to reduce by self punishment. Injury to them may simply be a form of 'self destruction' which confirms their opinion of themselves as losers. A number of visible characteristics are displayed by the injury-prone athlete (Table 3.1), and these must be recognized by the sports injury practitioner.

Bramwell et al. (1975) investigated the effect of psychological states on injury. These authors looked at stressful life events, and measured these as the accumulation of Life Change Units (LCUs). Positive stressful life events included things like marriage, getting a better job, and passing an examination, while negative events referred to bereavement, redundancy, divorce and the like. These authors showed that injured players had amassed significantly more LCUs in both one- and two-year periods preceding injury. Categorizing athletes into low, medium and high risk depending on LCUs, it

Table 3.1   Psychological characteristics of injury-prone athletes

Counter-phobia
Athletes attempt to counter anxiety by being overtly aggressive and fearless, they repeatedly test their
  indestructibility

Sign of masculinity
Athlete uses injury as a mark of courage. Needs 'visible scars of battle' to show manhood. Continues to
  play despite injury, but exaggerates pain to seek admiration

Masochism
Punish themselves for feelings of guilt, often about failure to reach their own unrealistic targets

Injury as a weapon
Tries to punish others, for example the young athlete who is forced to play by over zealous parents

Escape
The 'training room athlete' who fears competition because of feelings of inferiority, but cannot opt out
  for fear of isolation

Psychosomatic injury
No physical injury, or slight injury made worse by emotional factors

Adapted from Sanderson (1981).

was noticeable that 73% of the high risk category experienced significant time loss through injury.

Coddington and Troxell (1980) looked at the effect of stressful life events on injuries in school children. They found that the risk of injury was five times greater when a major event such as the death of a parent, or parents separating, had occurred. Kerr and Minden (1988) showed the number of injuries in gymnasts to be four times greater and the severity to be increased by 4.5 times when athletes had experienced recent stressful life events.

There are two possible explanations for the effect of stressful life events on sports injury. First, the athlete's attention may be affected, with life events somehow hindering concentration. The method for this may be explained in terms of the psychological information processing systems used by the athlete (Kerr and Fowler, 1988).

Skilled athletes rely on two information processing systems. One is fast, allowing automatic and therefore seemingly effortless actions, the other is slower and requires more

conscious control. The slower process is used to monitor overall strategies and allows individual components of automatic actions to be pieced together (Schneider and Fisk, 1983). To perform well, an athlete must 'let go' and let these automatic actions 'flow' freely. Any attempt to control the natural rhythm of the action will hinder its automatic nature and result in a loss of efficiency. Stressful life events could lead to worry about performance which in turn may prevent an athlete from 'letting go'. Additionally, inappropriate thoughts may prevent the slower secondary system from monitoring overall performance efficiently. Several stressful life events occurring at the same time will mean an athlete has to adjust to many life changes in a short time period (Kerr and Fowler, 1988).

Kerr and Minden (1988) claimed that the majority of gymnasts in their study reported 'lack of concentration' and 'thinking of other things' as the major cause of their injuries. These statements would seem to lend support to the hypothesis that the type of information processing used may have an effect on sports injury.

Stressful life events may ultimately lead to mental fatigue and exhaustion. This may present externally as apathy and lassitude, where an athlete is 'not interested' and lacks concentration. Remedial action could involve a period of attention training, to enable the athlete to focus on a task or shift attention between different tasks rapidly. Coaches and therapists must recognize that an athlete is vulnerable to injury after a stressful life event. Training should be modified by reducing its intensity and concentrating on basic skills rather than introducing new ones.

Life stress does not have a uniform effect on all people, and individual reactions will depend on the predictability and controllability of the event, as well as the individual's psychological make-up, and 'stress resistance'. Also important is the social support available to an athlete from peers, family and sports officials.

The interplay between stress and a variety of psychosocial factors which contribute to injury has been modelled by Andersen and Williams (1988). An individual's stress response is seen as being modified by his personality, the history of stressors imposed on the athlete, the athlete's coping resources (such as social support), and any interventions (such as relaxation skills and medica-tion) used to modify the stress response (Fig. 3.1).

From this model, personality factors are seen to influence how an athlete reacts to stress, whereas coping resources and social support may attenuate the effects of life stress on injury occurrence (Yukelson and Murphy, 1993). Clearly, the more stress an athlete is under, the greater the risk of injury or illness.

Injury and rehabilitation

Reaction to injury

The psychological reaction of an athlete to a sports injury is similar to a grief response, and will often evolve through a number of definite stages (Wiess and Weiss, 1987). Initially, injury is likely to be met with denial, which quickly turns into anger. With time, as the true significance of the injury becomes apparent to the athlete, depression sets in. Finally, acceptance is seen, and the athlete takes a more constructive attitude which assists the rehabilitation process. In a study examining the reported responses of athletes to sports injury, Gordon, Milios and Grove (1991) described both positive and negative aspects (Table 3.2).

Figure 3.1 Simplified model of stress and sporting injuries.

Table 3.2   Psychological response to injury: athlete behaviour

Negative behaviour	Positive behaviour
Failure to take responsibility for own rehabilitation	Asks questions of therapist in order to understand injury
Non-acceptance of injury	Listens well to advice
Non-compliance and non-co-operation	Co-operation and compliance with therapist
Denial of seriousness or intent of injury	Receptive to restrictions placed on athlete
Displays of depression	Initiates progression of rehabilitation at home
Bargaining with therapist over treatment and time out of competition	Early acceptance of injury
Missing appointments	Does not bargain
Displays of anger	
Overdoing rehabilitation, e.g. attempting too much too early	

Adapted from Gordon, Milios and Grove (1991).

The coping mechanism that an athlete uses with respect to injury is influenced by many different factors, including personality, previous history of injury, level of competition, social support systems, and how serious the injury is perceived to be (Andersen and Williams, 1988). A history of frequent injuries is likely to lead to bitterness and frustration, demotivating the athlete and leading to apathy during rehabilitation. A severe injury may at first lead to post-trauma shock, in which the athlete is unaware of severe pain or disability, and the initial psychological effect is small. Later, however, the psychological effects of severe injury can be considerable, and personality factors are an important factor in determining the final outcome of rehabilitation.

The nature of a sport and the accepted stereotyped reaction of peers to an injured colleague is important. Severe injury in contact sports is often perceived as a sign of manhood for example, whereas a similarly severe injury in golf may be perceived as weakness. Because the latter game is not so physically demanding, to become injured is not so socially acceptable. Equally the level of competition is of importance. A top level competitor has more to lose than the weekend athlete and so his reaction to injury is likely to be more traumatic.

Certain body parts produce a greater psychological affect than others when injured. Injury to the knee and back, for example, demand a higher degree of psychological adjustment than a hamstring or groin tear (Gordon, Milios and Grove, 1991). One possible explanation for this is the perception by an athlete that any injury to the knee or spine must be 'serious', whereas muscle injuries are often dismissed as 'just a pull'.

Personality and reaction to injury

Eysenck (1957) described two major factors of personality. These were extroversion–introversion and neuroticism–stability (Fig. 3.2). The competitive sportsperson is typically extrovert, being outgoing, assertive, and optimistic. Extroverts crave excitement, and are generally less able to tolerate tasks of a mundane nature. They are more likely to find rehabilitation 'boring', and will be impatient to return to sport after injury. Extroverts are thought to have higher pain thresholds (Lynn and Eysenck, 1961).

The typical introvert is hesitant, reflective and pessimistic. Injury has greater psychological impact for him, and he or she has a lower tolerance of pain, making an injury appear more serious than it actually is. This

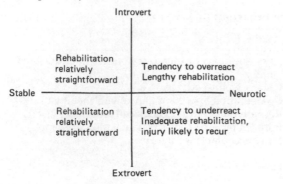

Figure 3.2 Personality factors and reaction to injury.

athlete, often only goaded into physical action by colleagues, needs strong encouragement during rehabilitation, and later when returning to sport.

Stable individuals, whether introvert or extrovert, will generally be less problematic within the sporting context, being calm, even tempered and emotionally stable. The highly neurotic athlete, on the other hand, is more difficult to deal with because he or she is nervous, anxious and moody. The neurotic-introvert is more likely to develop phobias and anxiety, and is plagued by psychological conflicts which only make his anxiety worse (Sanderson, 1977). This type of individual tends to turn his neurosis in on himself, and the psychological trauma of injury is likely to be greater for him. In addition, this athlete is likely to be more apprehensive when returning to sport and this must be considered during the final stages of rehabilitation when the aim is to restore confidence in a body part.

The extrovert generally has a strong self-esteem or self-concept, which is usually highly dependent on both physical appearance and physical function. The neurotic-extrovert will often perceive his self-esteem to be threatened by injury, and emotional problems may result. This leads to the phenomenon of 'playing through' an injury or 'working it off' in an attempt to maintain self-esteem.

Response to rehabilitation

In addition to responses to injury, the response to rehabilitation itself can be both positive and negative. Those with a positive attitude to rehabilitation tend to work hard, be cooperative with the therapist, and ask constructive questions. A negative attitude to rehabilitation is shown by such things as an unwillingness to follow a home exercise programme, failure to keep appointments, continually questioning the therapist's judgement, and a reluctance to listen.

Athletes' reactions to injury and subsequent rehabilitation differ from those of the general public (Gordon, Milios and Grove, 1991). The competitively fit athlete has already experienced greater physical discomfort during training and so may be better able to adapt to the demands of a rehabilitation programme (Sanderson, 1981). An athlete will tend to be more 'body aware' and, especially in the case of experienced athletes, more likely to act quickly to promote healing by use of measures such as RICE, for example. The general public tend to be more concerned with pain than with the consequences of injury, the reverse being true for an athlete.

The therapist is in a better position to support and influence the injured athlete than any other member of the rehabilitation team. This is because by its very nature, physiotherapy creates a close patient/carer relationship. This affinity can be helped by developing a positive and dynamic atmosphere which is professional, relaxed and cheerful.

Psychological aspects of pain

Pain perception

The sensory threshold at which a person describes actually feeling a stimulus is roughly the same for everyone. But, if the stimulus intensity is gradually increased, the point at which a subject describes this sensation as pain (pain threshold) shows a wider variation. Individual and cultural differences exist, and each is influenced by a wide variety of psychological factors. The highest intensity of pain which can be endured (pain tolerance level) varies between individuals. Personality, lifestyle, situation, accepted behaviour, cultural and religious differences may all influence pain tolerance.

Eysenck (1967) showed extroverts to have higher pain thresholds than introverts, and argued that this could be explained in terms of increased cortical inhibition. In addition, extroverts tend to express pain more freely, and are often more ready to accept the social disapproval which this can bring (Griffiths, 1980).

The situation in which the person experiences pain is also important. Injuries sustained by boxers are often not noticed until after their bout because their attention is focused elsewhere. Beecher (1959) observed that soldiers injured in battle requested less morphine than civilians with similar injuries. The social context was important here. The soldiers were grateful to be alive and looked forward to being removed from the battlefield whereas to the civilians the injury was a depressing event.

The individual's past history is also relevant. As children, we learn how to respond to a painful stimulus by observing others, and Violon and Gilurgea (1984) showed family members to respond to pain in a similar manner. Anxious subjects tend to complain of pain more, and if anxiety is reduced, pain intensity is also lowered. When a subject understands the cause of their pain, anxiety will reduce.

Patient–therapist interaction

Pain inhibition may be achieved by creating positive emotional responses, which may facilitate control of nociceptor input by descending central control. During illness the body's sensory awareness may be lowered, and positive emotions can help restore the normal pain 'body image'. In this situation the physiotherapist may act as a 'treatment modality applied directly to the mind' (Charman, 1989) and affect the intensity and meaning of the patient's pain, both positively and negatively. Body language, voice, and patient handling all give out signals which can change a patient's attitude to pain, making them a 'pain manager' rather than a 'pain victim'.

The concept of pain management by the patient was taken further by Williams (1989) with her 'school for bravery' approach. She emphasized the importance of changing from 'illness' to 'wellness' by behavioural modification. Patients were encouraged to participate in controlled exercise and recreational activities, despite being chronic pain sufferers. Combining fear reduction with confidence building she reported over 80% of patients abandoning 'illness behaviour' illustrated by such signs as lack of facial expression, excessive slow movements, altered movement patterns, use of pain gestures and attention seeking.

These concepts, although originally described in hospital in patients, have a significant overflow to sports personnel, particularly those suffering from long-term or recurring injury.

Anxiety and stress

Anxiety

Two types of anxiety are generally recognized. State anxiety, which is temporary, occurs as a result of an individual's reaction to a particular situation. Trait anxiety, on the other hand, is a more persistent feature of a person's character or personality.

Whether a situation makes a person anxious will depend very much on his or her interpretation of the events which are occurring. This is often judged in the light of past experience, and in the context of sport, an individual's ability, or perceived ability, to perform a certain task. Anticipation is a key aspect here, a person's negative expectation of an event, rather than the event itself, causing the anxiety.

One underlying cause of anxiety in many people is fear of failure. This is often associated with loss of self-esteem and prestige within their peer group, leading to humiliation. The anxiety process often leads to greater physiological responses than does a purely physical threat.

Social factors are an important factor in anxiety creation. For example, in a junior athlete, unremitting pressure from a well-meaning parent can lead to high levels of anxiety. The reverse is also true. Good social support, where a parent lets a child know it is 'OK to fail' can reduce anxiety and often lead to parallel improvements in performance.

Stress

Increased stress levels have been shown to reduce the effectiveness of the immune system, with resultant consequences on the incidence of both infection and trauma (Kennedy, Kiecolt-Glaser and Glaser, 1988). Individuals vary tremendously in their reactions to a particular situation, so the perception of stress may be a deciding factor. Stress can be described from two perspectives, the stressful agent or 'stressor' and an individual's reaction to the stress.

Stress affects the body by producing an ergotrophic response, primarily brought about by sympathetic nervous stimulation. Relaxation produces the opposite effect, through parasympathetic activity, of a trophotropic response. The ergotrophic response is basically concerned with preparing the body for physical action, and represents the classical 'fight-or-flight' response. The trophotropic response, on the other hand, is designed to reduce the metabolic rate and restore the body to its natural resting state. It embodies the 'relaxation response'. A synopsis of each response is given in Table 3.3.

In addition to physiological effects, stress can have effects on an athlete's thoughts, attitudes, feelings and emotions (Yukelson and Murphy, 1993). Fear or apprehension can lead to increases in muscle tension, fatigue and disruptions in the fluidity of movement. In turn, these changes may open an athlete to injury, providing a link between psychological and physiological processes. Increasing stress levels can lead to a narrowing of the visual field, to such an extent that vital environmental cues may be overlooked, increasing the risk of injury (Williams, Tonymon and Anderson, 1991).

In keeping with the multi-dimensional stress model (see Fig. 3.1) the key mechanism of the stress–injury relationship is an individual's responsivity and resilience to stress (Anderson and Williams, 1993). Essentially,

Table 3.3 Effects of the ergotropic and trophotropic responses

Ergotropic response	Trophotropic response
Primarily sympathetic	Primarily parasympathetic
Excitement, arousal	Relaxation
Mobilization of body	Energy conservation
↑Heart rate, blood pressure and respiration	↓Heart rate, blood pressure and respiration
↑Blood sugar	↑Gastrointestinal function
↑Muscle tension	↓Muscle tension
Pupil dilatation	Pupil constriction
↑O_2 consumption	↓O_2 consumption
↑CO_2 elimination	↓CO_2 elimination

After Hertling and Kessler (1990).

two main factors of stress are important to the development of injury. First, disruption of attention (distraction) by negative thoughts, and secondly increases in general muscle tension brought on by stress.

Stress reduction techniques

Stress management techniques fall broadly into two categories. First, there are those concerned with purely somatic (body) responses, and secondly, more mentalistic or cognitive (mind) techniques. The two categories are not distinct, but blend to form a variety of psycho-physiological responses.

A great diversity of approaches to stress management and relaxation techniques exist but the three techniques most widely used in sport are progressive relaxation, visualization and biofeedback.

With all the techniques, the reduction of initial stressors is important. Relaxation should be practised in a warm and quiet room, with low levels of lighting. The television, radio or hi-fi should be switched off, and telephones taken off the hook. The subject should ask other members of the household not to disturb them while they are relaxing. Any restrictive clothing, such as tight belts, clasps, watches and jewellery, should be removed. The body should be relaxed and supported. If the subject chooses to lie supine, the lumbar spine may be supported with a small rolled towel, and the head should rest on a small pillow or folded towel. The knees may be flexed over a pillow or roll to reduce the stretch on the popliteal structures.

Progressive relaxation

This technique was first described by Jacobsen (1929). The procedure involves repeatedly tensing particular sets of muscles, and then relaxing them. The instructions for relaxation may be recorded on tape, although a 'live performance' often gives bet-

ter results. The sequence of muscle relaxation is shown in Table 3.4.

The advantages of this technique are first, that it is easy for an athlete to practise alone, and does not involve concentrating the mind. Secondly, it teaches an athlete to recognize the difference between a tense and a relaxed muscle. This has obvious advantages in that the athlete is then able to identify when physical stress is occurring throughout the day and reduce this. The same 'tense–release' methods can be used prior to competition with the specific muscles to be used in performance.

The disadvantage of this and any other purely physical approach is that it does not occupy the mind. Subjects often complain that they were 'thinking of something else' or their 'mind was elsewhere'.

Visualization

Visualization, or mental rehearsal (practice), is used both for relaxation and performance enhancement. There are normally three components to visualization. First, the athlete

Table 3.4 Muscle sequence for progressive relaxation

Grip/straighten fingers
Flex/extend wrists
Flex/extend elbows
Rotate shoulders

Dorsiflex/plantarflex ankles
Flex (20°)/extend knees
Grip knees together
Tighten buttocks

Pull abdomen in
Arch back slightly
Brace shoulders
Shrug shoulders
Push head against floor

Grit teeth
Open mouth slightly
Frown
Raise eyebrows
Smooth forehead

must be relaxed, and often the progressive relaxation technique is used for this. Secondly, some cognitive process is used to enable the athlete to become an active participant in the healing or performance enhancing process. Thirdly, some element of self-control is introduced (such as affirmation) to replace negative thoughts with positive ones.

Once the athlete has reached a relaxed and more receptive state, various positive visual images are created by the athlete in his or her 'minds eye'. As many sensory stimuli as possible are used, sounds, feelings, pictures, smells, and tastes merging into a total vision. If the athlete wishes to see him or herself winning or achieving a particular target, he or she should try to experience feelings of elation, sensations of physical exertion and sounds of the crowd roaring.

The visualization is always positive, and may include positive statements or affirmations. Phrases such as 'I am full of energy' (positive) being used rather than 'I am not tired' (negative).

During the relaxation and visualization period, the athlete should remain alert, and in control of the images he or she uses. To facilitate this, the technique should be performed sitting rather than lying down, and the imagery should be purposeful rather than simply daydreaming. The visualization can be used either in the first person, or the third person. The athlete may imagine him or herself inside his or her own body, experiencing an ideal performance, or they may see themselves from outside, as though on video playback.

Performance enhancement can be achieved by rehearsing an ideal model of a skill. After performing well, the athlete should replay the skill and review his or her performance. Again, the positive must be emphasized, and the athlete should not replay errors, but only successful outcomes for future reference. These images may be used to rehearse a skill before competition as part of a warm-up.

Another method of enhancing performance is for the athlete to imagine not the skill itself, but the feelings of winning, or the outcome of performance. He or she may imagine him or herself as a person or animal who demonstrates a particular trait which is required, such as strength, speed, bravery, etc.

Mental practice has been shown to benefit motor skill acquisition (Vandell, Davis and Glugston, 1943; Clark, 1960; Fansler, Poff and Shepard, 1985) and strength development (Cornwall, Melinda and Barry, 1991), although this latter effect is less certain.

Biofeedback

Biofeedback is the use of instrumentation to detect and display bodily processes, enabling an individual to then modify those processes. The basic requirements of a biofeedback system are a sensor which is capable of detecting a particular physiological reaction. In response to this, a processor creates an electrical impulse which is then displayed to the user.

The technique can be used to reduce autonomic effects, gain control over normally involuntary actions or re-educate voluntary movement after injury. A number of modalities can be used for biofeedback including skin responses, cardiovascular measurements, electroencephalography, and electromyography.

Electromyography (EMG) feedback is particularly valuable in the rehabilitation of muscle function. The electrical signal produced by motor unit firing is displayed visually or aurally. The subject then aims to reduce or increase motor unit recruitment to alter the feedback signal. This type of feedback may be used as motivation in rehabilitation strength training, or for postural re-education. The technique can also be used to re-educate muscle action sequences, for example in the treatment of shoulder instability (Beall, Diefenbach and Allen, 1987).

Skin reactions, such as galvanic skin response (GSR) and skin temperature, have been used extensively in relaxation training. The skin resistance is measured and amplified to give a feedback signal in GSR. As arousal or stress level is elevated, insensible sweating will increase, lowering the skin resistance and altering the signal. With temperature feedback, a thermistor is used to detect skin temperature changes occurring as a result of vasodilatation or vasoconstriction. With practice, the sympathetic activity controlling these changes can, to a certain extent, be controlled by the athlete.

Electroencephalogram (EEG) signals are useful when trying to initiate a relaxation response. When awake and alert, the brain emits electrical impulses in the beta frequencies (above 14 Hz), but when asleep, the frequencies reduce to the theta level (4–7 Hz) and still further to the delta level (below 4 Hz) during anaesthesia. Between the fully alert and sleeping states, there is a level of daydreaming or 'relaxed wakefulness' at the alpha level (7–14 Hz). This is the level of relaxation, and subjects can be trained using EEG biofeedback to stimulate the brain to produce waves at this level and so encourage relaxation. In addition, the mind is more susceptible to self-suggestion at the alpha level, and EEG feedback can be used prior to visualization techniques.

Motivation

Motivation is the desire that leads an individual to engage in, or sustain, a particular activity. Magill (1989) defined motivation as 'the causes of the initiation, maintenance and intensity of behaviour'. Factors which motivate often fulfil a need in an athlete, and needs will change and fluctuate with time. In order to motivate athletes to perform a particular task, and maintain the motivation, we must recognize the athlete's needs and act on them.

Both personal and social factors can act as motivators. Personal factors include such things as goals, physical sensations, and the way in which an athlete views him or herself. Social factors embrace considerations such as peer pressure, affiliation and rewards. The social and personal factors will merge to alter the meaning a situation has to an athlete, and it is this which will determine behaviours such as effort, persistence and performance (Lewthwaite, 1990).

Motivating factors may consist of both intrinsic and extrinsic rewards. An intrinsic reward relies on a person's own feelings, it is something internal. Athletes who train out of sheer enjoyment, or because they feel more competent when they do so, are intrinsically motivated. Extrinsic motivation relies on a reward which is outside the person. Winning a medal or cup is an extrinsic reward.

One of the problems with extrinsic motivation, is that an athlete can feel manipulated by the reward system, and have a sense that continual striving takes away their personal control (Rejeski and Kenney, 1988). To be effective, motivation must consist of a combination of both intrinsic and extrinsic rewards, which are carefully planned.

Three personal motivational factors, involving both intrinsic and extrinsic rewards, are important within the context of exercise and injury, and will be considered further. These are goal setting, belief in one's personal capability, and perceptual-affective experience (Lewthwaite, 1990).

Goal setting

Goals may be classified according to both type and timescale. Two types of goal are generally used within the context of sport. The first, task-involved, rely on the need to improve a skill or performance of an activity. The second, ego-involved, focus on the necessity to prove oneself and be judged as competent or at least avoid being judged incompetent. Various social and situational factors will influence goals, such as age, cultural background, peers, coaches, and performance evaluation.

The timescale during which a goal is to be achieved is also important, and goals may be either long term or short term. Long-term goals are the things an athlete wants to achieve as the end result of all his training. These may be dreams or aspirations, such as a young athlete wanting to compete in the Olympic games, or end results such as the injured athlete wanting to compete next season. Short-term goals are those which the athlete wants 'right now' and will affect his or her immediate performance.

A number of features are important to the goal setting process. First, a goal should be difficult enough to stretch an athlete, but at the same time be achievable. To do this, a goal must take into account the capabilities of an athlete, and will require knowledge of past experience and personality characteristics. Secondly, goals should be specific, rather than general. For example, a goal to perform ten repetitions with a specific weight is better than simply telling an athlete to 'do his best'. Feedback or knowledge of results (KR) is necessary to tell the athlete how he or she is performing with respect to the goal. Thirdly, a goal which is decided with the participation and agreement of the athlete is more effective. Often, when an ath-

lete is instrumental in the goal setting process, goals will be set to a higher standard. Some guidelines for goal setting are outlined in Table 3.5.

A number of authors have demonstrated the benefits of goal setting to performance. Locke and Bryan (1966) showed specific goals to be better than a general goal to 'do your best' on a lighting pattern task. The specific goal group not only performed better, but had a faster rate of performance improvement. Harari (1969) assessed performance on a 750-yard running task, and found goals which were specific to an athlete's own performance (individual goal) and which were difficult, to be most effective. Nelson (1978) showed goal setting to be effective on an elbow flexion strength test. Of four groups tested, the one which was given an age norm (meaningful goal) performed the best.

Belief in capability

The belief that one is capable of performing to a certain standard is an important intrinsic factor determining an athlete's motivation. Bandura (1982) described two types of self-confidence or 'self-efficacy' in this context. First, efficacy expectation. This is the belief that an individual can achieve something because of their innate abilities. For example, someone may believe that

Table 3.5 Guidelines for goal setting

A goal should be		
1	*Specific*	Specify a set number of repetitions or weight to be lifted, for example, rather than saying 'do your best'
2	*Meaningful*	Tell the athlete what the average score is and give them a reason for obtaining the goal
3	*Difficult*	A goal must stretch an athlete. If it is too easily obtained there is no reason for performance to improve
4	*Obtainable*	Failure to achieve a short-term goal over a number of trials will demotivate
5	*Measurable*	The athlete must know if he or she is achieving the goal and will require knowledge of results (KR)
6	*Individual*	Personality factors and previous performance should be taken into account to 'tune' the goal to the athlete
7	*Agreed*	Participation in the goal-making process is more effective

they have the 'will-power' to modify their eating habits and so lose weight, or the 'natural talent' to win a race. Secondly, Bandura referred to 'outcome expectations', or the belief that when one acts in a certain way, a particular result will follow. In the example of weight loss, the person displaying this characteristic would believe that changing eating habits will result in weight loss, whether they want them to or not.

Within the context of sports injury rehabilitation, it is not enough for an athlete undergoing rehabilitation to believe that a certain flexibility exercise will restore full range of movement (an outcome expectation). The athlete must also be encouraged to believe that he or she has the capacity to endure discomfort, and to persist with the exercise programme (efficacy expectation).

Perceptual-affective experience

The perception of effort, and the emotion attached to that effort can act as a motivation. People naturally tend to persist with activities which are enjoyable and are resistant to uncomfortable or painful actions, but the subjective definition of what is enjoyable varies greatly between individuals.

The standard subjective measure of exercise intensity is the rating of perceived exertion (RPE) or Borg scale (Borg, 1982; Table 3.6). This runs from 6 to 20 and is roughly based on the difference between resting and maximal heart rates (60–200 b.p.m.). Various central (cardiopulmonary) and peripheral (biochemical) physiological cues enable the athlete to rate his or her own exertion, but a number of psychosocial factors are also involved. Subjects tend to score lower on the RPE scale when exercising with others (Hardy, Hall and Prestholdt, 1986). Subjects appear to be influenced in the direction of another's response, perhaps to present themselves favourably. Studies with male subjects and female investigators have shown that the males tended to rate

Table 3.6 Rating of perceived exertion (RPE)

Original rating	Description
6	
7	Very, very light
8	
9	Very light
10	
11	Fairly light
12	
13	Somewhat hard
14	
15	Hard
16	
17	Very hard
18	
19	Very, very hard
20	

After Borg (1982).

themselves lower at intense workloads than when tested by a male experimenter (Boutcher, Fleisher-Curtian and Giles, 1988), suggesting that they were concerned to 'appear fit'. Female subjects, when tested by male experimenters, did not show the same variation in rating.

Although two subjects may rate a particular work intensity similarly, their emotional response to this workload may be entirely different. Someone who has not exercised before is likely to find intense exercise unpleasant (negative), whereas the athlete may find this same workload challenging (positive). Using an 11-point 'feeling scale' Hardy and Rejeski (1989) showed RPE to be directly related to past level of physical activity, and to the belief that exercise is an integral part of a healthy lifestyle. Furthermore, it has been shown (Lewthwaite, 1990) that feelings of aversion to intense exercise in children are negatively correlated to attraction to and involvement in sport.

Clearly the social context and the emotion attached to an exercise can act as a motivator. It is more likely that an athlete will work hard in an enjoyable group atmosphere than an isolated training session which he or she attends begrudgingly.

Psychological effects of exercise

Exercise and self-concept

Athletes and coaches usually associate exercise with the improvement of a number of physiological variables. In addition to these however, several psychological characteristics have also been shown to change as a result of participation in a regular exercise programme. Enhancement of self-confidence, self-esteem, and body image have been shown (Vincent, 1976; Sonstroem, 1984) and reductions in anxiety, depression, stress and tension have been demonstrated (Cooper, 1982). Of these variables, self-esteem, defined as 'the degree to which individuals feel positive about themselves' or a 'personal judgement of worthiness' would seem to be the one with the greatest potential for benefit from exercise (Sonstroem and Morgan, 1988).

Enhanced well-being

Athletes often claim that exercise makes them 'feel good', and the 'runners high' is a widely reported phenomenon. Reductions in stress and anxiety have been reported lasting for between 2 to 5 hours after the cessation of training (Morgan, 1985), and decreased depression has been demonstrated as a result of 6–20-week exercise programmes (Greist et al., 1979). In addition, altered states of consciousness have been described following distance running (Mandell, 1979). Weight training programmes have been shown to enhance self-concept in both male (Dishman and Gettman, 1981; Tucker, 1982) and female (Brown and Harrison, 1986) athletes. Three theories exist to explain these phenomena, the distraction hypothesis, and the production of monamines and endorphins.

The distraction hypothesis proposes that participation in vigorous exercise distracts the athlete from stress. Comparison between exercise, meditation and distraction show similar reductions in state anxiety (Bahrke and Morgan, 1978), but the effect resulting from exercise appears to last longer (Morgan, 1985).

Depression is also affected by exercise. Reductions in the monoamine chemicals noradrenaline and serotonin (5–HT) are associated with depressed states in humans, and these same chemicals have been shown to increase in rats subjected to chronic exercise (Brown et al., 1979). Increases in the release of endorphins and enkephalins, or slowing of the dissociation rates of these chemicals has also been proposed (Pert and Bowie, 1979). By measuring plasma levels of these chemicals or using opiate antagonists to neutralize them, researchers have demonstrated some association between exercise and endorphins. Carr et al. (1981) reported significant rises in beta-lipotrophin and beta-endorphin levels in female subjects exercising at intensities up to 100 W. Farrell et al. (1983) showed increases in plasma leucine-enkephalin-like activity from mean values of 22.2 pmol/ml to 26.1 pmol/ml following a ten-mile road race. Anxiety, measured on a profile of moods states (POMS) test was also shown to reduce.

It seems likely that these various physiological and psychological changes act synergistically in some way to produce the altered mood states associated with chronic exercise (Morgan, 1985).

Exercise addiction

The experience of exercise for an athlete, and the way in which this fits into the rest of his life, is one factor which determines whether or not an exercise becomes addictive (Crossman, Jamiesen and Henderson, 1987). Addiction is both physiological and psychological in nature and reflects that person's need for exercise. This need can be positive or negative. Positive addiction exists when an athlete receives some psychological or physical benefit from an activity, and is able to control the activity. The negatively addicted athlete is controlled by the activity and will experience severe negative affects (withdrawal) with a missed exercise bout. They often engage in an activity at the expense of their health, or other factors, such as relationships and career prospects. The negatively addicted athlete may be failing to gain approval from significant others and may shelter feelings of inadequacy or unattractiveness. This type of athlete often exercises alone or in isolation from the group. They experience feelings of enhanced self-concept and even euphoria during and immediately after exercising. Importantly, this individual is more likely to ignore pain or injury and work through this to complete a workout. In the same vane, they tend to be anxious if a workout is missed and almost appear to suffer 'withdrawal symptoms' (Table 3.7).

Learning skilled movement

Skill has been said to be behaviour which is purposeful and well organized. It is economical in terms of effort and acquired by practice and experience (Kent, 1994). In this section we will look at the types of skills available, and how to develop them effectively. In order to improve motor (movement) skills for both sports performance and rehabilitation, it is also necessary to have some knowledge of the psychological processes that an athlete goes through when deciding 'what to do' and 'what not to do' in any action.

Information processing

To fully appreciate the way in which an athlete uses information, we can imagine him as a computer, taking information in (input) performing a calculation or function with the information (processing), and then giving us data or action as a result (output). The processing that has occurred, involves three overlapping stages (Fig. 3.3). During the first stage, that of stimulus identification, information from a number of sources (such as auditory, visual, tactile and kinaesthetic) are analysed. Various components are put together such as size, shape and colour to identify an object as a ball, for

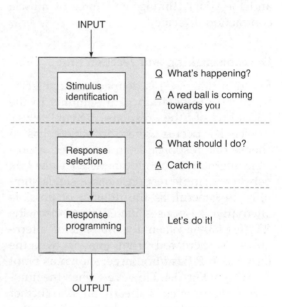

Figure 3.3 Stages of information processing.

Table 3.7   Characteristics of exercise addiction

The athlete may:
1   Perform several bouts of exercise per week for up to an hour at a time
2   Experience a high degree of positive effect after exercising
3   Exercise alone or isolate themselves when in a group
4   Be highly satisfied and less self-critical when exercising than at any other time
5   Experience a state of euphoria when exercising
6   Be more depressed/anxious/angry after missing a workout
7   Tend to ignore physical discomfort/injury in order to complete exercise regime

Adapted from Glasser (1976) and Anshel (1991).

example. Patterns of movement such as speed and direction are also detected. The knowledge gained (a representation of the stimulus) is passed on to the second stage, response selection.

The task now is to select an appropriate movement from those available to the athlete, so this stage may be seen as a link between the sensory and motor systems. Once a decision has been made concerning the movement, the third stage has begun. Response programming now has the task to organize the motor system to carry out the desired action. To do this, the brain and body must be readied for action. A motor programme must be retrieved and organized, and the order, timing, and force of muscle contraction directed.

Decision-making and reaction time

Reaction time (RT) is defined as the interval from the presentation of a stimulus to the initiation of the response (Kent, 1994). Choice RT occurs when an athlete has to choose one response from a number of possible alternatives, while simple RT is the link between a single response and a single stimulus. In general, as the number of possible alternative responses increases, so does the RT (Fig. 3.4). When the number of alternatives is increased from one or two, the increase in RT is very large, shown as point A (58%) in Fig. 3.4. However, when the number of alternatives is already high, to further increase them leads to only a small increase in RT shown as point B (3%) in Fig. 3.4. Clearly, to keep the number of choices to a minimum will ensure a faster reaction time.

An important factor in determining reaction time, is how well a stimulus and response seem to fit together naturally to an athlete (stimulus–response compatibility). For example, when driving a car, it seems natural to steer to the right to make the car move to the right. Moving the hands in the opposite direction (when reversing) initially seems 'awkward' or 'unnatural'. The more

compatible a stimulus and response, the less the choice RT. If a movement feels natural, it seem that we can perform it faster. We still get the relationship between the number of alternatives and RT described in Fig. 3.4, but the slope of the line is flatter.

Where a stimulus and response are not compatible, enough practice will still reduce the RT. For example, when we first learn to drive, steering when reversing is very hard. We have to turn the wheel to the right to make the car go to the left. With practice, however, the movement becomes easier, and professional drivers can perform this action easily. The type of practice is important however, the same stimulus must be used to evoke the same response (known as consistent mapping).

Anticipation is one method used to reduce RT. An experienced athlete can often predict what action will occur (spatial anticipation) and when it will occur (temporal anticipation). Predicting which shot an opponent will use to return a tennis ball with is an example of spatial anticipation, while predicting when a player is going to strike the ball when taking a football shot is an example of temporal anticipation. Anticipation allows an athlete to organize a movement sequence in advance so that when the relevant stimulus is received, the response is

Figure 3.4 The relationship between choice reaction time and the number of alternative movement responses (see text). After Schmidt (1991).

initiated with a shorter RT. The disadvantage with anticipation occurs when an athlete gets it wrong. If an athlete has predicted a movement incorrectly, they will have begun the wrong series of events for the response (an incorrect motor programme will have been 'switched on'). By the time the athlete realizes the mistake, they must inhibit or backtrack the action before they initiate the correct response.

Limitations of information processing

Stimuli received by the athlete can be processed either in a series (one after another), or in parallel (at the same time). Processing for stimulus identification occurs in parallel. We can see a ball approaching and hear the sound of the kick at the same time. Response selection may occur either in parallel (at the same time) or in series (one after the other). Actions which require large amounts of mental activity are normally processed in a series. This tends to be slow, attention demanding and voluntary, and is termed controlled processing (Table 3.8). On the other hand, familiar actions, those which have been practised over and over are the result of automatic processing. This is fast, not attention demanding, involuntary and occurs in parallel.

Response programming occurs in series, only one response being generated at a time. The combination of parallel processing in the early stages of information processing and serial processing in the later stages, creates a bottleneck (Fig. 3.5). If one response

Figure 3.5 The information processing bottleneck. Stimuli A and B are received together. A is processed first, the delay between the two being the psychological refractory period (PRP).

has already begun, and another stimulus is received, the second stimulus cannot evoke a response until the first is completed. The delay in responding to the second stimulus is called the psychological refractory period (PRP). Where the interval between two stimuli is short, the PRP will be longer because the response programming stage has only just begun. Where the interstimulus interval is longer, the response is already well on its way, so the PRP is shorter. If the interstimulus interval is very short, the athlete will deal with both stimuli as if they were one (a process called 'grouping'). The resultant response however will be different again.

Because the response selection processes occur in series, the continuous 'stream' of information received by the athlete results in 'chunks' of responses being produced at a rate of approximately three per second (Schmidt, 1991). The chunks are strung together to produce a smooth action (Fig. 3.6).

Types of skill

Skills may be classified into one of a number of categories (Table 3.9). Initially, skills may be either open or closed. During the performance of an open skill, the environment will vary and be unpredictable. An example is tackling in football. The player does not know which of several alternative move-

Table 3.8 Information processing in the response selection stage

Controlled processing	Automatic processing
Slow	Fast
Attention demanding	Not attention demanding
Serial	Parallel
Voluntary	Involuntary

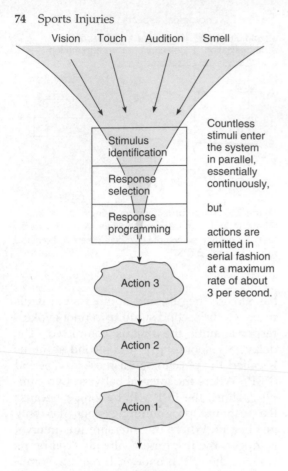

Vision   Touch   Audition   Smell

Stimulus identification

Response selection

Response programming

Action 3

Action 2

Action 1

Countless stimuli enter the system in parallel, essentially continuously,

but

actions are emitted in serial fashion at a maximum rate of about 3 per second.

Figure 3.6   Information is received in a continuous stream, but responses are produced in a series of 'chunks'. From Schmidt (1991).

ments his opponent will make. With a closed skill the opposite is true, the environment is stable and predictable, an example being swimming. Here, the same action is repeated over and over again and the environment in which it is performed remains the same. The difference between these two types of skill comes in the need to respond to variations in the environment, using perception and decision-making. In a closed skill, many of the motor decisions may be made in advance, and there is no need to make rapid modifications during the performance of an action.

The second classification deals not with environmental stimuli, but with the ongoing nature of the skill. A discrete skill is one (normally brief) which has a defined beginning and end, such as catching a ball. Continuous skills are played out over a period of time, such as swimming or running. Between these two extremes, are serial skills. These involve a group of discrete skills joined together, to make a new action. The various component skills involved are strung together in a specific sequence. An example is a gymnastic routine. Initially each discrete skill is separate, but with practice the linked skills proceed automatically.

The final classification concerns motor and cognitive skills. In short, cognitive skills must answer the question 'what to do' whereas motor skills answer 'how to do it'. With a cognitive skill the decisions about which movement to take are important, but not the complexity of the movement itself. An example would be a chess move, where the

Table 3.9   Skill types and examples

Open		Closed	
Unpredictable environment		Predictable environment	
Soccer tackle		Swimming	
Discrete	*Serial*		*Continuous*
Distinct beginning and end	Discrete actions linked together		No distinct beginning or end
Catching a ball	Gymnastic routine		Swimming or running
Cognitive		*Motor*	
'What should I do?'		'How should I do it?'	
Chess move		High jump	

physical action itself is quite simple, but the choice of which action to use is complex. At the other end of the continuum, motor skills focus on the quality of a movement action itself. The decision about which action to take has already been made. A good example is the high jump, where the athlete knows exactly which action to take, but the action itself is complex and the performance of this action will be the deciding factor for success.

The stages of skill learning

Motor (movement) skills involve an organized sequence of activities. There are three characteristic stages to motor skill learning (Fitts and Posner, 1967; Schmidt, 1991).

Stage I (cognitive)

This is the stage of understanding, where the athlete attempts to form an idea of the whole skill. The process is cognitive rather than motor in nature, and hence the title of this learning stage. The athlete is learning what to do (and importantly, what not to do), and how to do it. Environmental cues which later will go unnoticed are important to this early stage of learning. They provide an important frame of reference for building the new skill. For example, when learning a new dance step a person will often focus their attention on their foot position, which they later take for granted. An important aim of this stage is to utilize information from past learning. By grouping together already familiar movement sequences, an action which approximates the new skill is created. This stage is intensely demanding in terms of attention, and so simultaneous processing is not generally possible.

In this stage movements will be poorly coordinated. The athlete must concentrate intensely and will therefore tire easily. The therapist can assist by providing clear instructions and feedback. The athlete will need constant coaching and correction of the skill to prevent them practising mistakes.

Stage II (motor)

This is the stage of effective movement, when the athlete will try to make the motor programme more exact and match it to the demands of the new skill. The individual movements will gradually become more consistent and the athlete is now able to recognize their own mistakes. Self-practice (unsupervised) can now be allowed. Importantly, if unsupervised practice is allowed in stage I, when the athlete is unable to recognize mistakes, they will simply practise these mistakes and learn an incorrect motor sequence.

The dependence on visual and verbal cues (stage I) now gradually gives way to the reliance on proprioceptive information. Movements become more consistent ('grooved' or 'stable') and the athlete is able to work on the finer details of an action. As the action becomes more efficient, energy expenditure is reduced. A more refined motor programme is built to accomplish the action, and the athlete learns effective ways to deal with response-produced feedback. Environmental cues are used for timing and as anticipation develops, movements become smoother and less rushed.

The individual movement sequences used in stage I are now linked together to give a longer skill sequence. The actions must still be slow and precise with progression made only when the movement sequence is correct.

In stage I the environment was structured to simplify it and reduce the number of variables presented to the athlete. In this way, the athlete was able to focus all their attention inwards on the movement itself. For closed skills (predictable environment) this continues by practising the same movement in a process called fixation. With open skills (changing environment), however, variety now becomes a key factor. Some of the basic skill factors have been learnt and so they no longer require attention. To further develop this, the environment is changed to encourage the athlete to predict/anticipate how these changes will affect their performance (diversification). The aim is to select an appropriate response to the changing environmental cues (stimulus response compatibility). This reduces reaction/response time and is essential to move into stage III.

Stage III (automatic)

In this stage the action 'runs by itself' or becomes 'grooved'. Now, the action is fast and independent of attention demands. The motor sequences in this final stage are highly evolved, and a single programme can control the action for a relatively long period. The decreased demand on attention means that the subject is free to perform higher order cognitive activities, for example, game strategy in football or style considerations in dance. Little self-talk about actual body movements occurs, and in fact performance will almost always suffer if this type of self-talk is attempted (Schmidt, 1991). However, self-talk about higher order activities continues.

The disadvantage of autonomous action is that the skill is difficult to modify once it has started. Muscle reaction speed may be developed (e.g. balance board work for the ankle), with multiple repetitions being performed in a changing environment. For example, the athlete may be asked to maintain trunk stability (automatic) while catching a ball thrown to him at random (environment).

Because the autonomous stage does not require substantial cognitive investment, focusing on an automatic skill can reverse the learning process. The use of controlled processing in an automatic skill can result in 'choking', where an experienced athlete fails under pressure (Masters, 1992).

In addition, as the motor skill is highly evolved in the autonomous stage, further improvement will be minimal. However, some continual improvement will occur as physical and mental effort to produce the skill reduces. Attributes such as style and form may improve rather than actual physical performance.

Practice

Where a number of skills are to be learned, such as a variety of strokes in tennis for example, the choice is to teach them individually or as a whole, and to vary aspects of each skill or to hold them constant (Table 3.10).

Where an individual skill is taught and practised before moving onto another, 'blocked' practice is taking place. This enables the athlete to concentrate on a single task before moving on. Repeated practice is used without interruption enabling the athlete to correct mistakes and refine the skill. Alternatively, 'random' practice may be used (Magill and Hall, 1990). Now, all the tasks are practised in the same session, and the order in which they are practised is varied, so that on the whole the athlete never works on the same task in two consecutive bouts. In terms of learning, random practice is far more effective than blocked practice (Shea and Morgan, 1979; Goode and Magill, 1986). Performance of the single task actually improves more during a blocked practice session, but in competition the results of random practice are far better.

There are several reasons why random practice gives better overall performance than blocked practice. First, when a second task is learned, aspects of the first are forgotten and must be re-learned with each successive practice bout. In terms of learning this has advantages because with blocked prac-

Table 3.10 Practising skills

Blocked
Individual skills are practised in isolation
Random
Individual skills are mixed during practice
Constant
The dimensions of a skill are held constant
Variable
The dimensions of a skill vary

tice the solution to a skill problem is simply remembered and repeated (without the need for cognition) for each bout. With random practice, the solution must be generated each time, requiring a more problem-orientated process. Furthermore, learning is enhanced because the athlete is more actively involved in the changing tasks used in random practice, rather than the simple repetition of blocked practice. In addition, continually changing tasks makes them more distinct from each other, so reducing the tendency to confuse one task with another (Schmidt, 1991).

Another method which has proved successful is variable practice. Here, the same class of skill is practised (contrasting to random practice where different skill classes are used), but dimensions of the skill are varied. For example, different throwing distances in javelin, or different speeds of passing in soccer. With constant practice, the dimensions of a skill remain the same and the skill is repeated in exactly the same fashion.

Practical implications of skill learning

So how do we apply the theories to sport and rehabilitation? We can focus attention on the three stages of learning, and see how the various learning methods fit into these stages (Table 3.11).

In the verbal cognitive stage (stage I) simple actions are chosen. These should involve moving a limited number of joints, and should demand relatively low levels of coordination. The important factor at this stage is for the athlete to be able to perform the skill in some fashion, even if it is not perfect. Using motivation to give the athlete a reason to learn is important.

Initially, demonstration is used to familiarize the athlete with the movement required. It is far easier for an athlete to see a movement and repeat it (of a fashion) than to rely on a series of verbal instructions—allow the athlete to 'see it' rather than 'hear it', by demonstrating the action (or having a model demonstrate it) and saying 'do this'. Once the action is attempted, corrections can be made. If the athlete is unable to even approximate to the action, it should be split into a number of simpler components.

Any instructions which need to be given should be simple and short. The athletes' past experiences may be used to describe the skill, so that they see the similarity to the new skill. For example, when teaching the abdominal hollowing action, described on page 152, the instruction 'imagine you are coughing', or 'imagine someone is hitting you in the stomach' describes the action which is required.

At this stage of learning, blocked practice (single action) and constant practice (one dimension of this action) are more effective than random and variable practice—the message at this stage is to 'keep it simple'.

Feedback is vital at this early stage. It is used after each trial to correct mistakes and

Table 3.11 Practical implications of skill learning

Verbal/cognitive	Motor	Autonomous
Select a few simple skills	Refine the skill	Practice is the key
Demonstration important	Use random, variable practice	Develop the ability to predict a response from a given stimulus
Motivation to give 'reason to learn'	Too much feedback creates dependence	Use mental practice to control emotional states and build confidence
Feedback about performance quality		
Use blocked, constant practice		

avoid the athlete practising these again and again. Feedback about knowledge of performance (KP) rather than knowledge of results (KR) is given. This means that the way the action is carried out (quality of movement) is corrected rather than the outcome. In other words, it would be more important to give feedback about the action of shooting in football practice rather than whether the shot scored a goal. The feedback should be prescriptive (that is it contains advice about what to do to correct the fault), simple and positive.

During the motor stage, the athlete can produce an approximation of the required skill, and the aim now is to refine this and focus on long-term retention of the skill. When the movement pattern is well developed, we need to develop the athlete's ability to perform the action in differing situations. To do this we move from constant to variable practice. The athlete should gain experience of the skill in a variety of dimensions such as speed, distance and direction (and combinations of these) of throwing, for example. We can now use random practice to facilitate long-term retention of the task. The aim is to enable the athlete to shift between skills effectively. Extrinsic feedback (given verbally by the instructor) is used to help improve performance. One feature of the action is assessed in turn, and again the feedback is prescriptive. However, it is easy to give too much feedback and the athlete may become dependent on this. Feedback should only be given when the action is considerably better or worse than expected (known as 'bandwidth' feedback), and only after a set of trials. It is important to remember that in the motor stage the athlete can now recognize his or her own mistakes.

Finally, in the autonomous stage a high level of performance is being aimed at with few attention demands, freeing the performer to focus on other aspects of a game, for example. The essential element in developing automaticity is practice, either of the whole task or stereotyped segments of it. A second key feature of automaticity is being able to accurately predict which stimulus will lead to which response, and working with an experienced coach can greatly assist this. Automatic control is more likely to occur with actions where consistency is high. Mental practice (running through an action in the imagination) is important for automatic skill training. It allows an athlete to rehearse the sequence of the components of an action, and to learn to gain control of emotional states and reduce uncertainty about performance and negative self-talk.

References

Andersen, M.B. and Williams, J.M. (1988) A model of stress and athletic injury: prediction and prevention. *Journal of Sport and Exercise Psychology*, **10**, 294–306

Anderson, M.B. and Williams, J.M. (1993) Psychological risk factors: injury prediction and preventive measures. In *The Psychology of Sport Injury* (ed. J. Heil), Human Kinetics, Champaign, Illinois

Anshel, M.H. (1991) A psycho-behavioral analysis of addicted versus non-addicted male and female exercisers. *Journal of Sport Behaviour*, **14**(2), 145–154

Bahrke, M.S. and Morgan, W.P. (1978) Anxiety reduction following exercise and meditation. *Cognitive Therapy Research*, **2**, 323–333

Bandura, A. (1982) Self efficacy mechanisms in human agency. *American Psychologist*, **37**, 122–147

Beall, M.S., Diefenbach, G. and Allen, A. (1987) Electromyographic biofeedback in the treatment of voluntary posterior instability of the shoulder. *American Journal of Sports Medicine*, **15**, 175–178

Beecher, H.K. (1959) *Measurement of Subjective Responses*, Oxford University Press, Oxford

Borg, G.A.V. (1982) Psychological bases of physical exertion. *Medicine and Science in Sport and Exercise*, **14**(5), 377–381

Boutcher, S.H., Fleisher-Curtian, L.A. and Giles, S.D. (1988) The effects of self-presentation on perceived exertion. *Journal of Sport and Exercise Psychology*, **10**, 270–280

Bramwell, S., Masuda, M., Wagner, N. and Holmes, T. (1975). Psychosocial factors in athletic injuries. *Journal of Human Stress*, **1**, 6–20

Brown, B.S., Payne, T., Kim, C., Moore, G., Krebs, P. and Martin, W. (1979) Chronic response of rat brain nor-epinephrine and serotonin levels to endurance training. *Journal of Applied Physiology*, **46**, 19–23

Brown, R.D. and Harrison, J.M. (1986) The effects of a strength training program on the strength and self-concept of two female age groups. *Research Quarterly for Exercise and Sport*, **57**(4), 315–320

Carr, D.B., Bullen, B.A., Skrinar, G.S., Arnold, M.A., Rosenblatt, M., Beitins, I.Z., Martin, J.B. and McArthur, J.W. (1981) Physical conditioning facilitates the exercise-induced secretion of beta-endorphins and beta-lipotrophin in women. *New England Journal of Medicine*, **305**, 560–562

Charman, R.A. (1989) Pain theory and physiotherapy. *Physiotherapy*, **75**(5), 247–254

Clark, L.V. (1960) Effect of mental practice on the development of certain motor skills. *Research Quarterly*, **31**, 560–569

Coddington, R. and Troxell, T. (1980) The effects of emotional factors on football injury rates – a pilot study. *Journal of Human Stress*, **6**, 3–5

Cooper, K.H. (1982) *The Aerobics Programme for Total Well-being*, Bantam Publishers, New York

Cornwall, M.W., Melinda, P.B. and Barry, S. (1991) Effect of mental practice on isometric muscular strength. *Journal of Orthopaedic and Sports Physical Therapy*, **13**, 5

Crossman, J., Jamieson, J. and Henderson, L. (1987) Responses of competitive athletes to lay-offs in training: exercise addiction or psychological relief? *Journal of Sport Behaviour*, **10**(1), 28–38

Dishman, R.K. and Gettman, L.R. (1981) Psychological vigour and self-perceptions of increased strength. *Medicine and Science in Sports and Exercise*, **13**, 73–74

Eysenck, H.J (1957) *The Dynamics of Anxiety and Hysteria*, Routledge and Kegan Paul, London

Eysenck, H.J. (1967) *The Biological Basis of Personality*, C.C. Thomas, Springfield, Illinois

Fansler, C.L., Poff, C.L. and Shepard, K.F. (1985) Effects of mental practice on balance in elderly women. *Physical Therapy*, **65**, 1332–1338

Farrell, P.A., Gates, W.K., Morgan, W.P. and Pert, C.B. (1983) Plasma leucine enkephalin-like radioreceptor activity and tension-anxiety before and after competitive running. In *Biochemistry of Exercise* (eds H.G. Knuttgen, J.A. Vogel and J. Poortmans), Human Kinetics, Champaign, Illinois

Fitts, P.M., and Posner, M.I. (1967) *Human Performance*, Greenwood Press, Westport, Connecticut

Glasser, W. (1976) *Positive Addiction*, Harper and Row, New York

Goode, S. and Magill, R.A. (1986) The contextual interference effects in learning three badminton serves. *Research Quarterly for Exercise and Sport*, **57**, 308–314

Gordon, S., Milios, D. and Grove, J.R. (1991) Psychological aspects of the recovery process from sport injury: the perspective of sport physiotherapists. *Australian Journal of Science and Medicine in Sport*, **23**(2), 53–60

Greist, J.H., Klein, M.H., Eischens, R.R., Faris, J., Gurman, A.S. and Morgan, W.P. (1979) Running as treatment for depression. *Comprehensive Psychiatry*, **20**, 41–53

Griffiths, D. (1980) *Psychology and Medicine*, Macmillan, London

Harari, H. (1969) Levels of aspirations and athletic performance. *Perceptual and Motor Skills*, **28**, 519–524

Hardy, C.J. and Rejeski, W.J. (1989) Not what, but how one feels: the measurement of affect during exercise. *Journal of Sport and Exercise Psychology*, **11**, 304–317

Hardy, C.J., Hall, E.G. and Prestholdt, P.H. (1986) The mediational role of social influence in the perception of exertion. *Journal of Sport Psychology*, **8**, 88–104

Hertling, D. and Kessler, R.M. (1980) *Management of Common Musculoskeletal Disorders*, J.B. Lippincott, Philadelphia

Hertling, D. and Kessler, R.M. (1990) *Management of Common Musculoskeletal Disorders*, J.B. Lippincott, Philadelphia

Jackson, D.W., Jarrett, H., Bailey, D., Kausek, J., Swanson, J. and Powell, J.W. (1978) Injury prediction in the young athlete: a preliminary report. *American Journal of Sports Medicine*, **6**, 6–14

Jacobsen, E. (1929) *Progressive Relaxation*, University of Chicago Press, Chicago

Kennedy, S., Kiecolt-Glaser, J.K. and Glaser, R. (1988) Immunologic consequences of acute and chronic stressors: mediating role of interpersonal relationships. *British Journal of Medical Psychology*, **61**, 77–85

Kent, M. (1994) *The Oxford Dictionary of Sports Science and Medicine*, Oxford University Press, Oxford

Kerr, G. and Fowler, B. (1988) The relationship between psychological factors and sports injuries. *Sports Medicine*, **6**, 127–134

Kerr, G. and Minden, H. (1988) Psychological factors related to the occurrence of athletic injuries. *Journal of Sports Psychology*, **10**, 167–173

Lewthwaite, R. (1990) Motivational considerations in physical activity involvement. *Physical Therapy*, **70**(12), 808–819

Locke, E.A. and Bryan, J.F. (1966) Cognitive aspects of psychomotor performance. The effects of performance goals on levels of performance. *Journal of Applied Psychology*, **50**, 286–291

Lynn, R. and Eysenck, H.J. (1961) Tolerance for pain, extroversion, and neuroticism. *Perceptual and Motor Skills*, **12**, 161–162

Magill, R. A. (1989) *Motor Learning. Concepts and Applications*, WCB Publishers, Iowa

Magill, R.A. and Hall, K.G. (1990) A review of the contextual interference effect in motor skill acquisition. *Human Movement Science*, **9**, 241–289

Mandell, A.J. (1979) The second wind. *Psychiatric Annals*, **9**, 57–69

Masters, R.S.W. (1992) Knowledge, knerves and knowhow: the role of explicit versus implicit knowledge in the breakdown of a complex motor skill under pressure. *British Journal of Psychology*, **83**, 343–358

Morgan, W.P. (1985) Affective beneficence of vigorous physical activity. *Medicine and Science in Sports and Exercise*, **17**(1), 94–100

Nelson, J.K. (1978) Motivating effects of the use of norms and goals with endurance testing. *Research Quarterly*, **49**, 317–321

Pert, C.B. and Bowie, D.L. (1979) Behavioral manipulation of rats causes alterations in opiate receptor occupancy. In *Endorphins in Mental Health* (eds E. Usdin, W.E. Bunney and N.S. Kline), Oxford University Press, Oxford

Reilly, T. (1975) *An Ergonomic Evaluation of Occupational Stress in Professional Football*, Unpublished Doctoral Thesis, Liverpool Polytechnic

Rejeski, W.J. and Kenney, E.A. (1988) *Fitness Motivation. Preventing Participant Dropout*, Life Enhancement Publications, Champaign, Illinois

Sanderson, F.H. (1977) The psychology of the injury-prone athlete. *British Journal of Sports Medicine*, **11**, 56–57

Sanderson, F.H. (1981) The psychology of the injury-prone athlete. In *Sports Fitness and Sports Injuries* (ed. T. Reilly), Faber and Faber, London

Schmidt, R.A. (1991) *Motor Learning and Performance*, Human Kinetics, Champaign, Illinois

Schneider, W. and Fisk, A. (1983) Attension theory and mechanisms for skilled performance. In *Memory and Control of Action* (ed. S. Magill), North Lolland, New York

Shea, J.B. and Morgan, R.L. (1979) Contextual interference effects on the acquisition, retention, and transfer of a motor skill. *Journal of Experimental Psychology*, **5**, 179–187

Sonstroem, R.J. (1984) Exercise and self esteem. *Exercise and Sports Science Reviews*, **12**, 123–156

Sonstroem, R.J. and Morgan, W.P. (1988) Exercise and self-esteem: rational and model. *Medicine and Science in Sports and Exercise*, **21**(3), 329–337

Tucker, L.A. (1982) Effect of a weight training program on the self concept of college males. *Perceptual and Motor Skills*, **54**, 1055–1061

Vandell, R.A., Davis, R.A. and Clugston, H.A. (1943) The function of mental practice in the acquisition of motor skills. *Journal of General Psychology*, **29**, 243–250

Vincent, M.F. (1976) Comparison of self-concepts of college women, athletes and physical education majors. *Research Quarterly*, **47**, 218–225

Violon, A. and Gilurgea, D. (1984) Familial models for chronic pain. *Pain*, **18**, 199–203

Wiess, D.M. and Weiss, M.R. (1987) Psychological rehabilitation and physical injury: implications for the sports medicine team. *The Sport Psychologist*, **1**, 318–330

Williams, J.I. (1989) Illness behaviour to wellness behaviour. *Physiotherapy*, **75**(1), 2–7

Williams, J.M., Tonymon, P. and Anderson, M.B. (1991) Effects of stress, stressors, and coping resources on anxiety and peripheral narrowing. *Journal of Applied Sport Psychology*, **3**, 126–141

Yukelson, D. and Murphy, S. (1993) Psychological considerations in injury prevention. In *Sports Injuries* (ed. P.A.F.H. Renstrom), Blackwell Scientific, Oxford

4

Sports massage

Massage is one of the original core skills of physiotherapy (Copestake, 1917). Unfortunately, massage fell from popularity because of the belief that it was 'unscientific' and 'unproven' despite the clinical experience of thousands of practitioners over many decades. Thankfully, massage is making a re-emergence in the more fashionable guise of 'sports massage' (Ylinen and Cash, 1988; King, 1993), both within physiotherapy and through the development of massage therapists. Various massage procedures are used within sports physiotherapy, and most influence the tissues by stretching or compression, resulting in both reflex and mechanical effects. The classical massage procedures are outlined in Table 4.1.

Massage techniques

Effleurage

Two types of effleurage are used (Fig. 4.1), the first is a superficial stroking movement designed to produce a sensory reaction, either of relaxation (slow stroking) or stimulation (fast stroking). The second is a deep action aimed at assisting lymphatic and venous drainage. The tissue manipulation starts distally and proceeds proximally in the direction of the heart, for example, 'knee to groin' or 'elbow to axilla'. The prox-

imal portion of the limb is treated first to clear lymphatic and venous congestion. This will allow the tissue fluids mobilized by the distal massage to move against less restriction.

The therapist uses his or her hands either together, or separately with one supporting the other to create more force. Skin contact is maintained throughout the action, and as they move, the hands change shape to contour the limb. The whole of the hand, and not just the leading edge should apply the pressure, to avoid sticking or jerking.

The force for the movement should come from overall body motion and not simply arm strength. The therapist adopts a stance with one foot in front of the other (walk standing) and transfers his or her weight from the rear to the front foot. The arms and hands transmit, rather than create, the force. At the beginning of the action the elbows will be bent, and at the end, full reach is achieved by straightening the arms. At this end point a slight overpressure is applied and the movement pauses before being repeated.

Some therapists prefer to maintain skin contact with a light stroking action as the hand is returned to the starting position. The advantage of this technique is that the movement is continuous, but the disadvantage is that sometimes the light pressure can be uncomfortable to a ticklish athlete.

Table 4.1   Massage procedures

Effleurage
Unidirectional stroking movement travelling proximally

Petrissage
Soft tissue compression including kneading, picking up, wringing, rolling and shaking

Frictions
Small, deep, circular or transverse movements at specific anatomical sites

Tapotement
Percussive actions including clapping, hacking, beating, tapping, shaking and vibration

Figure 4.1   Effleurage. (a) Both hands cover the surface of the limb. (b) Reinforced hand for deeper pressure. (c) Thumb web used to contour limb. (d) Superficial stroking—the flat hands or fingertips are pulled towards the therapist.

A light effleurage movement may be used to begin massage, to spread oil and acclimatise the athlete to massage and help them to relax. In addition, the lightness of the touch helps the practitioner to feel altered areas of tissue tension which may then be focused on later. As effleurage proceeds, the depth of the movement can increase developing the superficial stroking action into deep longitudinal pressure.

Petrissage

Various petrissage movements are used (Fig. 4.2). In each case the hands maintain contact with the skin and do not glide over the skin surface except when progressing from one area to another. Kneading is a circular motion carried out by compressing the tissues against underlying structures. This may be performed with the flat of the hand, the heel of the hand, or the pads of the fingers and thumbs. The choice of contact area is dependent on the size of the

body part being treated and the depth of the manipulation being carried out. Pressure is applied on the upward part of the circle, and released on the downward portion. At this point the hand is moved, lightly brushing over the skin surface to maintain contact.

Picking up is performed by compressing, then lifting and squeezing the tissues. The therapists' thumb and thenar eminence work against the medial two or three fingers to compress rather than pinch. The web between the thumb and first finger stays in contact with the skin so that the whole lateral portion of the hand surrounds the athlete's tissues. The action is more nor-

Figure 4.2 Petrissage. (a) Picking up. (b) Kneading. (c) Wringing. (d) Skin rolling.

mally performed alternately, enabling the therapists hands to recover between tissue compressions.

In a wringing movement, both hands pick the tissues up (see above), and then work against each other pulling and pushing the tissues before they are released. The hands progress by gently 'walking' them up and down the body of the muscle. With large muscles, the finger tips face each other and the elbows are apart to create power, through the transmission of body sway. The whole of the hand grips the tissues in this case. For smaller muscles, the grip is confined to the thumb and fingers alone. Now, the fingers face forwards and the elbows are held in, the movement coming from the elbows and wrists only.

With rolling, the skin is lifted away from the underlying tissues, and rolled between the thumbs and fingers of both hands. The technique is usually used on large body areas which have flat expanses of skin, for example the back, abdomen and thigh. The flat of the hands are placed on the skin at a distance to the therapist. The hands are pulled towards the therapist to gather the skin up. As the skin bunches up, the thumbs press forwards

and adduct to present their combined inner surfaces as a flat surface against the skin roll. Along the length of the spine, continuous skin rolling may be used. Again, the fingers feed the skin towards the approaching thumbs, but this time the fingers 'walk' along the skin surface to allow a continuous movement. The heels of the hands must be kept down on the skin surface to avoid the thumb tips 'digging in' as the hands move forwards.

Muscle shaking is used within sports physiotherapy to reduce muscle tone and relax a muscle. This is useful following strenuous activity for example, or where muscle spasm is present due to pain. In addition, hypertonity, due to postural changes, may be usefully reduced using shaking prior to proprioceptive neuromuscular facilitation (PNF) stretching procedures. The terms shaking and vibration are often used to describe very similar techniques. From the point of view of this book, shaking affects the whole of a structure (rib cage, limb or muscle) while vibration affects only part of the structure, having a more local effect (Fig. 4.3).

For shaking, the flat of the hand is used with slight pressure lightly gripping the mus-

(a)   (b)

Figure 4.3 Vibration and shaking. (a) Vibration—applied locally. (b) Muscle shaking—flat of hand moves whole muscle belly.

cle belly. As muscle resistance to palpation reduces, deeper pressure is used. Using shaking on a dependent muscle, for example the calf or hamstrings in crook lying, has the advantage that gravity pulls the muscle away from the bone thus broadening the muscle. The practitioner has to exert less pressure therefore, to achieve a similar effect. Vibration differs from muscle shaking in that it is used locally with only the fingertips (singly or reinforced) transmitting the force. The effect is deeper and more focused than shaking with the force directed into, rather than along, the muscle. It is stimulatory in

nature and may be used over trigger points for example.

Frictions

With frictions, only the therapist's fingers or thumbs are used to give an accurate, deep, soft tissue manipulation (Fig. 4.4). The fingers should be held locked but not hyperextended. With small areas, the first and second fingers are used overlapping as one unit. Larger areas may require the use of all of the finger tips of one hand reinforced by

Figure 4.4 Frictional massage. (a) Deep transverse friction—single finger. (b) Reinforced finger. (c) Transverse friction of muscle belly. (d) Circular friction to break up oedema.

the other hand. The friction may either be circular or transverse.

Circular frictions are normally used to break up thickened oedema, particularly around a joint. Three or four circular actions are used, gradually increasing in depth depending on patient tolerance. Pressure is released and the hand moved to another position before the friction is resumed.

Transverse frictions are a specific manipulation technique pioneered by Cyriax (1941). The transverse friction is performed with the skin of the patient and the therapist's finger acting as a single unit. The action demands great anatomical accuracy and must be of sufficient depth and sweep to affect the desired tissues. Tendons are generally frictioned in a stretched position, while muscles are treated in relaxed inner range. The aim is to produce local hyperaemia, massage analgesia and a reduction in adherent scar tissue to allow broadening of a muscle belly or transverse movement of a tendon. Transverse frictions to the Achilles tendon are shown on page 299, of the shoulder tendons on page 419, and of the elbow on page 445.

Tapotement

The percussive movements may be used to stimulate, or for evacuation of a hollow cavity. Percussion for evacuation, such as that used in chest physiotherapy, is not within the context of this book.

For stimulating tapotement the hands are relaxed, and follow each other in a succession of alternating movements. With clapping, the wrists are flail and the cupped hand strikes the body creating a hollow (rather than slapping) sound. Hacking involves striking the skin with either the ulnar border of the hand (severe) or the back of the tips of the fingers by using a pronation/supination movement of the forearm (mild). Beating is performed with the ulnar border of the semi-closed fist and tapping with the finger tips. The percussion

techniques are used over bulky muscle areas but must avoid bony areas (spine of the scapula, patella) as these will be painful if struck (Fig. 4.5).

| Practical application of techniques |

The lower limb

Posterior thigh

Massage to the posterior aspect of the leg begins with the athlete lying prone with the knee slightly flexed to take the stretch off the popliteal structures. The shin is supported by a rolled towel. A towel is placed over both legs, and folded back to reveal the leg to be massaged. The towel covers the leg again to maintain body heat once leg massage has finished, and the other leg is uncovered and massaged in turn. Where swelling is the main concern, the massage procedures begin in the upper leg to clear the lymphatic vessels here before fluid is pushed into them by lower leg massage. Effleurage begins the movement. A skin inspection is carried out. Cuts are either protected by waterproof taping, or the practitioner must wear protective gloves. Where a skin lesion is large, massage should not proceed directly over the area. A small amount of gel or cream is placed on the practitioner's hand and warmed, through friction, before application.

Where increased muscle tone is detected, muscle shaking is used to aid relaxation. The palm may be placed across the fibres of the muscle with the shaking movement perpendicular to the leg (transverse shaking). Alternatively, with a smaller limb, the hand may grip the muscle belly with the fingers parallel to the muscle fibres (longitudinal shaking). The palm contact for the shaking procedure causes the whole muscle to vibrate, and the effect is general. Where a more local effect is required, the finger tips rather than the palm are used in a 'claw hand' contact for local vibration. The action is now direc-

Figure 4.5 Tapotement. (a) Clapping. (b) Hacking. (c) Beating.

ted downwards into the depth of the muscle rather than along its length.

The effleurage stroke begins over the popliteal fossa and proceeds up the centre of the thigh to the buttock crease. The second stroke is medial, and the third stroke is lateral, both ending at the buttock crease.

Petrissage strokes begin with palmar kneading, one hand reinforcing the other, and is carried out over the bulky middle

area of the hamstrings. Picking up is used over the length of the muscle with wringing and rolling used over the muscle bellies. In each case, the tissue manipulation begins just above the popliteal fossa and proceeds centrally, medially and laterally, the number of 'muscle strips' depending on the size of the athlete's leg.

Local massage to the adductors may be given with the athlete supine and the hip flexed, abducted and externally rotated. The knee then rests on a folded pillow or the therapist's pelvic rim with the far hand stabilizing the knee. Alternatively, half crook side lying may be chosen (Fig. 4.6). The near hand begins the massage with effleurage and shaking, moving from the medial epicondyle of the knee to the groin. Palmar kneading and picking up are used followed by deep effleurage along the length of the adductor fibres using the thumb pad. Transverse frictions, if required, may be given by altering the hand so that the dominant hand lies perpendicular to the thigh. Flicking, using the ulnar borders of the hands in a rapid alternating action, is the most appropriate percussion technique. Hacking can be painful due to the fusiform nature of the muscle, while clapping tends to be better carried out with the athlete in side lying (see below). The massage finishes with effleurage and the athlete's position lends itself well to the use of passive stretching techniques including contract–relax (see p. 120) for the short adductors. An alternative starting position, which allows the application of more pressure, is half crook side lying with the affected leg extended on the couch. The unaffected leg lies forwards

with the hip and knee flexed and the knee supported on a pillow to prevent pelvic and spinal rotation.

Calf and Achilles

The calf area is treated after the posterior thigh in cases of general massage where swelling is the major concern. The shin is supported on a folded towel, or the leg being treated may be hooked over the other leg. Effleurage and muscle shaking are used to begin the treatment. Superficial strokes are applied longitudinally from achilles to knee with the hands working side by side or one hand resting over the other depending on limb size. The stroking movement is localized by using the thumb pads placed side by side, with the movement directed along the muscle fibres (Fig. 4.7). Kneading is given to the muscle bellies only, with picking up and muscle rolling being especially useful in cases of consolidated oedema. Circular frictions are applied along each side of the achilles tendon. This may be applied with one finger supporting the other or using a light pinch grip massaging both sides of the Achilles at once.

Figure 4.6 Treating the adductors. (a) Thigh rests on therapist's pelvis. (b) Bent upper leg rests on rolled towel.

Figure 4.7   Calf treatment. (a) Localized stroking using thumb pads. (b) Effleurage using thumb web. (c) Massage of the peronei.

An alternative starting position is with the knee held flexed by the therapist's hand while the other hand supplies the effleurage stroke, with the web of the hand. The calf is then massaged in two or three sections depending on size. Where more pressure must be exerted, crook lying is the position of choice. The therapist sits on the couch and supports the athlete's foot against her thigh. Effleurage is given with one cupped hand over the other. The therapist can lean back to exert more pressure. Local stroking is then applied with the finger tips rather than the thumbs. In the crook lying position, the edge of tibialis posterior and the peronei may be massaged using either the finger tips or the thumb with the rest of the fingers stabilizing the hand.

Anterior thigh

Massage to the anterior thigh proceeds in a similar order to that of the posterior thigh. Less direct pressure is used due to the reduced muscle bulk, and percussion movements are rarely used. Finger kneading may be used effectively around the patella especially over the suprapatellar pouch in the case of local pooling of oedema within this area. Kneading is probably the most useful procedure over the quadriceps because of the ease with which the muscle bellies are picked up.

Shin

Massage is only applied to the peronei over the lateral aspect of the shin due to the lack of muscle over the medial tibia. The size of the lateral compartment dictates that the whole hand cannot be used. Effleurage is applied with the thumbs held side by side or with the fingers, with the thumb stabilizing the hand. Alternatively, the hypothenar eminence may be used in larger subjects.

The back

Lower back

The subject is in the prone lying position with a rolled towel beneath the shins to flex the knees and take the stretch off the sciatic nerve. If the lordosis is very deep, some subjects find it more comfortable to have a folded towel placed beneath the abdomen. Massage to the back may be given in any direction, and the practitioner does not need to work 'distal to proximal' as with the limbs. The massage begins with effleurage from the posterior iliac crest to the scapula (Fig. 4.8). The fingers follow the line of the erector spinae muscle fibres and cover the back in two or three sections, depending on the athlete's size. Lateral effleurage (lateralizing) then follows, from the spine around the trunk to the abdomen. Kneading with the palms and heels of the hands begins at the inferior angles of the scapulae and works down towards the sacrum with alternating pressure movements of the hands. The line follows the line of the erector spinae. Both kneading and picking up may be used over the quadratus lumborum. Transverse kneading may be used across the erector spinae with the finger tips pulling towards the therapist and the sides of the thumbs pushing away. Local finger stroking is used with

the thumbs pressing together and finger kneading is performed with the pads of the fingers along the length of the erector spinae, across the posterior rim of the pelvis, and along the posterior aspect of the lower ribs. Skin rolling is used from the ilium to the scapula and transversely around the circumference of the lower trunk.

Fascial stretching may be used to good effect in the lower spine. The forearms are crossed and the hands are placed flat over the back. The practitioner leans forwards and down exerting pressure and pressing the hands apart to impart and stretch on the lumbar fascia. The hand must not slide over the skin surface as this will cause painful friction, the skin and hand move as one unit.

The lower back massage finishes with effleurage and light finger stroking movements to aid relaxation.

Upper back

When applying upper back massage the therapist stands at the couch side and later changes position to the head of the couch facing caudally (Fig. 4.9). Effleurage begins over the trapezius in a diamond shape, from the inferior angle of the scapula to the occiput, out to the acromion and down to the inferior angle once more. Kneading with the heel of the hand is used from the occiput to lower scapula. Petrissage is especially useful over the middle fibres of trapezius with ringing and rolling both appropriate techniques. Kneading, using the pads of the fingers, is useful along the length of the cervical extensors and to the rhomboids and levator scapulae. If the shoulder is internally rotated (hand behind the back), the medial border of the scapula can be lifted from the ribcage and the side of the therapist's hand can be used to massage beneath the undersurface of the scapula (serratus anterior and subscapularis muscles). Hacking, clapping and flicking actions are used over the middle trapezius fibres only, the superficial bony

Figure 4.8 Lower back massage. (a) Effleurage following the line of the erector spinae. (b) Lateral effleurage. (c) Deep lateralizing. (d) Fascial stretch. (e) Kneading. (f) Transverse kneading. (g) Skin rolling.

Figure 4.9 Upper back massage. (a,b) For upper back massage the therapist stands at the couch side and later changes to the head end. (c) Kneading the middle fibres of trapezius. (d) With the shoulder internally rotated the medial border of the scapula is lifted. (e) Massage to the upper trapezius. (f) Sub-occipital techniques.

surfaces making these techniques inappropriate over the scapula and upper spines.

The therapist then transfers to the head of the couch. Kneading and pressure techniques to the middle fibres of trapezius are more effective from this position. In addition, finger kneading and friction may be carried out to the occiput. Where massage is required to the upper cervical and sub-occipital regions only, the athlete may be positioned supine, lying with the head supported on a folded towel. The therapist sits at the head end of the couch and using finger kneading and friction to the sub-occipital tissues. From this position, passive stretching techniques for the upper trapezius and levator scapulae may then be carried out.

The upper limb

Shoulder and upper arm

Arm and shoulder massage may be carried out in either sitting or supine positions (Fig. 4.10). When sitting, the athlete's arm is supported on a small table, and while lying the arm is supported on a pillow or folded towel. Alternatively, the arm may be usefully supported across the therapist's leg (covered by a folded towel) for certain upper arm and shoulder procedures. The treatment begins with effleurage, the therapist holding the athlete's hand for limb stability. The therapist anchors the athlete's near hand. The palm of the therapist's far hand rests over the extensor aspect of the athlete's hand to begin the effleurage stroke. The movement begins distally, with the therapist's far hand moving from the athlete's fifth finger along the ulnar aspect of the forearm, across the under edge of the upper arm to end at the axilla. For the second stroke, the athlete's forearm is moved into mid-pronation. The action begins at the back of the athlete's hand and covers the radial side of the forearm and side of the upper arm, to again end at the axilla. For the flexor aspect of the arm, the therapist changes hands so that the near hand carries out the massage stroke. The movement begins at the thumb, and glides along the radial side of the forearm and anterior aspect of the upper arm to the axilla. The next stroke begins over the athlete's palm, and proceeds over the flexor aspect of the forearm and inner edge of the upper arm to the axilla. The last effleurage stroke begins on the flexor aspect of the fifth finger and moves across the inner edge of the forearm and upper arm to the inner axilla.

Muscle shaking is performed using the same single-handed grip as effleurage. The deltoid and triceps are shaken using the outer hand, while the biceps is shaken using the inner hand. In each case the other hand holds the athlete's hand to stabilize the arm.

Kneading begins with the hands placed on the anterior and posterior aspects of the deltoid. The hands press together compressing the shoulder and work alternately in circular motions. The alternate movement continues down the length of the upper arm with the hands gripping biceps and triceps, and moving around the arm slightly to cover the flexor and extensor aspects of the forearm. Each hand moves along the skin only as the compression pressure is released. Thumb kneading may be used for the forearm, with the thumbs lying side by side. The pressure is transmitted with the length of the distal phalanx rather than the tip ('along' rather than 'in').

Picking up and muscle rolling may be performed single-handed or with both hands alternately. The single-handed action maintains the grip on the athlete's hand (or elbow in the case of shoulder treatment) for stability. The therapist's outer hand is used for procedures on the posterior deltoid, triceps, and forearm extensors, the inner hand for the anterior deltoid, biceps, and forearm flexors. Double-handed actions are used for the middle fibres of the deltoid following on from kneading for the upper fibres of trapezius (see above). The thumb and finger grip

Figure 4.10 Massage of the shoulder and upper arm. (a) Arm supported on table in sitting. (b) Supine lying. (c) Using the therapist's leg for support. (d) Effleurage using the thumb web. (e) Wringing the triceps. (f) Hacking the flexor aspect of the forearm.

must avoid placing pressure over the acromion.

Wringing is used over the bellies of the biceps and triceps. In the case of the biceps, the therapist stands in front of the athlete with the hands over the anterior position of the arm and the fingers placed medially. For the triceps, the hands cup the posterior portion of the arm, again with the fingers medially placed. The wringing action is carried out using the cupped hands in opposition. The forearm flexors are wrung using the thumb pads in opposition to the pads of the index and ring fingers.

Percussion techniques are performed first on the flexor aspect of the whole arm with the forearm supinated, and then on the extensor aspect with the forearm pronated. For the extensor aspect the therapist stands level with the athlete's waist and faces their head. With the subject's forearm pronated, the action works from the posterior axilla and posterior deltoid across the triceps and then to the forearm extensors. For the flexor aspect, the therapist changes position to stand above the athlete's arm facing their feet. The athlete's forearm is supinated and the action begins at the medial axilla, and works down the front of the deltoid, over the biceps and across the forearm flexors. The therapist must make sure that he or she avoids contact with bony prominences and superficial tendons at the shoulder and elbow.

Foot massage

Foot massage (Fig. 4.11) may be used following an injury where swelling and scar tissue are present. In addition, foot massage is particularly beneficial as an aid to relaxation. Reflexology is a specialized form of foot massage not covered in this book.

Foot massage is often combined with passive joint movement (physiological and accessory), because the joints of the foot often become stiff through the use of constricting footwear. The reader is referred to Maitland (1991) and Kaltenborn (1989) for details of the techniques.

Effleurage is given by starting with the hands cupping the foot, with the fingers resting medially. Initially, both hands move from the toes to the ankle. As the action becomes firmer, one hand remains stationary to support the foot while the other carries out the massage stroke. General kneading is carried out with one hand holding the toes and the other imparting pressure through the hypothenar eminence. More specific finger kneading and circular frictions are used for the interossei. Firm digital pressure is used over the sole of the foot with the thumb pads or single knuckle. Light percussion techniques (finger tapping) are used only over the medial longitudinal arch with the foot supported in slight plantarflexion. A stretching action is used for the metatarsals. The hands surround the foot with the thumbs on the plantar surface and the finger tips coming together on the dorsal surface. The action is to press the thumbs into the plantar surface of the metatarsal heads and pull the neighbouring metatarsal bones down with the fingers. Slow passive movements are then used to fully stretch the tissues. Each toe is tractioned in turn, and flexion, extension, abduction and adduction are used for each of the metatarsal phalangeal (MTP) joints. Circular frictions and finger kneading are used around the malleoli, and to each side of the Achilles tendon.

Effects of massage

Effects of massage are achieved through mechanical, physiological, and psychological processes, and the interrelation between these three. Compression and squeezing will improve venous and lymphatic drainage, visible when superficial vessels are massaged (Hollis, 1987). Interstitial pressure is increased and fluid absorbtion aided. Fresh blood will enter the area. The superficial skin response to vigorous massage is an axon

Figure 4.11 Foot massage. (a) Finger kneading. (b) Plantar kneading using the knuckles. (c) Deep digital pressure of the sole.

reflex. Redness results (flare) through dilatation of skin arterioles and slight swelling (wheal) occurs through increased permeability of the capillary wall, allowing tissue fluid to escape into the surrounding area. The deep response to vigorous massage, however, can be a reduction in blood flow, if muscle tone is increased and blood flow through the muscle reduces as a consequence.

Deep stroking and kneading of the calf for a 10-minute period has been shown to increase blood volume for 40 minutes (Bell, 1964), and blood pressure has been shown to

reduce following back massage (Barr and Taslitz, 1970). Intradermal dye injections have been used to show lymph flow improvements with massage (McMaster, 1937), and massage has been shown to be significantly better at improving lymph flow when compared to electrical stimulation and passive movements (Ladd, Kottke and Blanchard, 1952).

A decrease in the viscosity of both blood and plasma has been shown following a 20-minute whole body massage (Ernst et al., 1987). Studies of muscle tone using the Hoffman (H) reflex, have shown a decrease in H reflex amplitude during, but not following, massage (Morelli, Seabourn and Sullivan, 1990; Sullivan et al., 1991).

Short-term pain relief, particularly through friction massage, is thought to be brought about by the closure of the pain gate and stimulation of endogenous opinoids (Cyriax, 1980). Although in contrast, gentler techniques do not appear to give this response. No significant change has been shown in beta endorphin or beta lipotrophin levels on pain-free subjects using effleurage and petrissage of the back over a 30-minute period (Day, Mason and Chesrown, 1987).

Tissues are mobilized as they are moved over each other, and adhesions stretched with more forceful actions. Massage has been shown to aid recuperation from muscle fatigue (Balke, Anthony and Wyatt, 1989), and is commonly used both before and after exercise with this in view. Sports massage has been shown to be effective at reducing delayed onset muscle soreness (DOMS) when it is applied within two hours of eccentric exercise (Smith et al., 1994). Creatine kinase (CK) levels were reduced, and a slight increase in both neutrophil emigration and cortisol levels were noted. Stimulatory massage, however, may have the reverse effect. CK and lactate dehydrogenase (LDH) have been shown to increase significantly following vigorous whole body massage, possibly illustrating mechanical trauma to the muscles with resultant increased cell membrane activity (Arkko, Pakarinen and Kari-Koskinen, 1983). Tissue damage of this type has been used to argue the case for rigorous training for therapists applying massage to athletes (Callaghan, 1993).

Stimulatory mechanical massage has been shown to be ineffective at increasing blood flow and aiding recovery (Carafelli et al., 1990). This type of massage can cause muscle contraction through the initiation of a tonic vibration reflex, and will therefore reduce blood perfusion through the muscle.

Pre-competition sports massage has been shown to produce mainly psychological benefits. No significant change in stride frequency has been shown in groups of male sprinters with and without massage (Harmer, 1991). All subjects in this study reported a 'positive response' to massage and the authors claimed that the athletes were able to cope better with physical exertion. No improvement has been shown in exercise performance, with heart rate, cardiac output, and arteriovenous oxygen responses all failing to show significant differences between massage and non-massage groups (Boone, Cooper and Thompson, 1991).

References

Arkko, P.J., Pakarinen, A.J. and Kari-Koskinen, O. (1983) Effects of whole body massage on serum protein and hormone concentrations, enzyme activities and haematological parameters. *International Journal of Sports Medicine*, **4**, 265–267

Balke, B., Anthony, J. and Wyatt, F. (1989) The effects of massage treatment on exercise fatigue. *Clinical Sports Medicine*, **1**, 189–196

Barr, J.S. and Taslitz, N. (1970) Influence of back massage on autonomic functions. *Physical Therapy*, **50**, 1679–1691

Bell, A.J. (1964) Massage and the physiotherapist. *Physiotherapy*, **50**, 406–408

Boone, T., Cooper, R. and Thompson, W.R. (1991) A physiologic evaluation of the sports massage. *Athletic Training. Journal of the National Athletic Training Association of America*, **26**, 51–54

Callaghan, M.J. (1993) The role of massage in the management of the athlete: a review. *British Journal of Sports Medicine*, **27**(1), 28–33

Carafelli, E., Sim, J., Carolan, B. and Libesman, J. (1990) Vibratory massage and short term recovery from muscular fatigue. *International Journal of Sports Medicine*, **11**, 474–478

Copestake, B.M.G. (1917) *The Theory and Practice of Massage and Medical Gymnastics*. H. K. Lewis, London.

Cyriax, J (1941) *Massage, Manipulation and Local Anaesthesia*, Hamilton, London

Cyriax, J. (1980) *Textbook of Orthopaedic Medicine*, 10th edn, Baillière Tindall, London.

Day, J.A., Mason, R.R. and Chesrown, S.E. (1987) Effect of massage on serum level of B-endorphin and B-lipotrophin in healthy adults. *Physical Therapy*, **67**, 926–930

Ernst, E., Matrai, A., Magyarosy, I., Liebermeister, R.G.A., Eck, M. and Breu, M.C. (1987) Massages cause changes in blood fluidity. *Physiotherapy*, **73**, 43–45

Harmer, P.A. (1991) The effect of pre-performance massage on stride frequency in sprinters. *Athletic Training. Journal of the National Athletic Training Association of America*, **26**, 55–59

Hollis, M. (1987) *Massage for Therapists*, Blackwell Scientific Publications, Oxford

Kaltenborn, F.M. (1989) *Manual Mobilization of the Extremity Joints*, Olaf Norlis Bokhandel, Norway

King, R.K. (1993) *Performance Massage*, Human Kinetics, Champaign, Illinois

Ladd, M.P., Kottke, F.J. and Blanchard, R.S. (1952) Studies of the effect of massage on the flow of lymph from the foreleg of the dog. *Archives of Physical Medicine and Rehabilitation*, **33**(8), 971–973

Maitland, G.D. (1991) *Peripheral Manipulation*, 3rd edn, Butterworth-Heinemann, Oxford

McMaster, P.D. (1937) Changes in the cutaneous lymphatics of human beings and in the lymph flow under normal and pathological conditions. *Journal of Experimental Medicine*, **65**, 347

Morelli, M., Seabourn, D.E. and Sullivan, J. (1990) Changes in H-reflex amplitude during massage of triceps surae in healthy subjects. *Journal of Orthopaedics and Sports Physical Therapy*, **12**, 55–59

Smith, L.L., Keating, M.N., Holbert, D., Spratt, D.J., McCammon, M.R., Smith, S.S. and Israel, R.G. (1994) The effects of athletic massage on delayed onset muscle soreness, creatine kinase, and neutrophil count: a preliminary report. *Journal of Orthopaedics and Sports Physical Therapy*, **19**, 93–99

Sullivan, S.J., Williams, L.R.T., Seabourne, D.E. and Morelli, M. (1991) Effects of massage on alpha motoneuron excitability. *Physical Therapy*, **71**, 555–560

Ylinen, J. and Cash, M. (1988) *Sports Massage*, Stanley Paul, London

5

Taping in sport

Strapping or taping is used extensively in the prevention and treatment of sports injuries, and this chapter looks at the more common taping methods. The aim is to set out some fundamental principles of both tape application and the mechanisms by which taping achieves its effect. Where appropriate, specific strapping techniques are described in Section II of this book.

Taping materials

Various forms of tape are available, either elastic or inelastic. In general, elastic tape is used with injured contractile tissue to provide a graded resistance or compression. Inelastic tape is more often used with non-contractile tissue injuries to take the place of a ligament in reinforcing a joint. Zinc-oxide tape is the most common inelastic type. It is air permeable, allowing the skin to breath and some moisture to escape through the tape. The tape is backed with a strong adhesive which may be a hypoallergenic formation. The tape strength is largely dependent on the number of individual threads per inch, a value known as the thread count (Lutz et al., 1993). The higher quality tapes generally have a higher thread count and are therefore stronger and less affected by body heat and moisture. The edge of zinc-oxide taping may be serrated to make tearing off strips of tape during application easier.

The elastic tapes may be either adhesive backed or adherent. Adhesive elastic tapes will normally stretch both longitudinally and transversely. Typically, this type of tape will recoil to 125% of its original length when initially stretched lengthways (Austin, Gwynn-Brett and Marshall, 1994). However, multiple stretching will cause the tape to fatigue. Rather than tensile strength, elastic tape has good compression qualities and will pull on the skin if applied pre-stretched.

Adherent or cohesive tapes are normally impregnated with latex, enabling them to stick to themselves rather than to the athlete's skin. This feature makes the cohesive tapes reusable to a certain extent, giving cost savings. Most tapes are water repellent to some degree, but the latex coated cohesive tapes may also be water resistant enabling an athlete to bathe with them on and so maintain fitness by exercising in water.

Beneath the tape, padding materials are used to protect the skin or bony prominences and to fill in superficial anatomical cavities. The padding may be either foam or fibre based. Polyester urethane foam underwrap is used to prevent tape adhering to the skin and to provide a more even compression. Fibre padding such as orthopaedic felt, or its synthetic equivalent, is used where thicker packing is required. These have the advantage that they may be cut and shaped. A variety of taping supplies are listed in Table 5.1.

Splinting or bracing materials vary from thermoplastic materials used to support unstable joints to anatomical braces used to immobilize a joint, especially after surgery. In addition, a variety of elasticated stockinets and purpose-designed braces are available for most major joints. Elasticated braces may be shaped to accommodate the contours of the joint. For example, knee sleeves may be open to reduce compression over the patellar area, while ankle braces are shaped to contour the foot and lower shin. These braces offer compression to prevent pooling of oedema and heighten confidence in a body part through proprioceptive enhancement. Braces may be made of neoprene where the

Table 5.1 Taping supplies

Taping and padding materials
Zinc-oxide tape (various sizes)
Elastic tape (various sizes)
Cohesive tape (various)
Waterproof tape
Felt and foam padding (various thicknesses)
Underwrap
Tubular elasticated bandage (various sizes)
Blister protectors
Cotton gauze squares (sterile and non-sterile)
Sterile plasters (various sizes)
Paraffin gauze

Skin care preparations
Adhesive spray
Adhesive remover
Antiseptic solution and ointment
Moisturizing skin cream
Skin toughener spray
Petroleum jelly

Instruments/apparatus
Razor and soap
Tape cutters, bandage scissors, sharp/blunt
  scissors
Cotton wool, cotton-tipped applicators
Surgical gloves

From Norris (1994), with permission.

additional advantage of heat retention is useful. Metal or plastic stays are often built into braces to make them more robust.

Application

Skin preparation

The limb is generally positioned with the injured structure, or part to be protected, in a shortened position. For example, the lateral ligament of the ankle is strapped with the joint held everted and dorsiflexed. Where a general limitation of all movements is required at a joint, the functional mid-range position is chosen.

The contact between the skin and strapping should be as firm as possible to prevent excessive movement which may lead to skin abrasion. Anything that reduces this skin contact will result in a loss of adhesiveness. Substances which are secreted or excreted from the skin, such as the hydrolipid film, dead epidermal cells, and sweat, will stick to the tape rather than allowing direct skin contact. Clean and dry skin is therefore a requirement for good adhesion.

Some athletes will have hypersensitivity to components within the strapping and may show severe allergic reactions. Chemical skin reactions are more likely with strong zinc-oxide adhesive than with hypoallergenic preparations based on polyacrylate. Where this type of adhesive still causes irritation, cohesive strapping is chosen. Mechanical irritation can result if the drag of the strapping exceeds the elastic properties of the skin, or if the strapping starts to slip and 'burn' the skin.

Before tape is applied, the body area and skin condition is inspected. Sensation and circulation of the skin should be assessed before and after tape application. Minor scratches and abrasions can be protected by petroleum jelly or paraffin gauze, while larger areas should be covered by a sterile dressing. It must be remembered, however, that in cases of a large wound, first aid is required and not simply taping.

The skin is lightly shaved or the hair flattened down and an underwrap applied. Skin preparation products such as tincture of benzoin or adhesive spray can be useful where strapping fixation is poor. The use of underwrap does allow the strapping to be applied onto non-shaved skin, but the cutaneous stimulation is likely to be less than with direct skin application. This may make underwrap better where mechanical rather than functional strapping is used. Superficial skin damage occurs more commonly over areas of soft skin, such as within the popliteal and cubital fossae. In addition, taping over unprotected bony prominences can lead to pressure points if the tape is applied too tightly. This is common over the base of the fifth metatarsal with forefoot taping for example.

Tape application

Tape may be either cut or torn prior to application. To cut tape, it should be loosely folded over the lower blade of the scissors with the non-adhesive face inwards (Fig. 5.1a). If the adhesive face is directed outwards, the tape will stick to the scissors and jam between the blades. When tearing tape, speed rather than strength is the deciding factor. The tape should be stretched over the tips of the thumbs with the non-adhesive face inwards. The thumbs should be held together, and one hand twisted against the other with the aim of rapidly breaking the tape edge (Fig. 5.1b). The faster the action, the less strength required.

In many circumstances, the strapping is applied along the line of the tissue fibres, so knowledge of the underlying anatomy is obviously important. The aim is to reduce the movement which stresses the injured tissues, but allow a near normal range of motion in other directions.

Tape may either be applied in a number of individual strips or as a continuous roll. Application in strips has the advantage of accuracy both in terms of the underlying anatomy and the tension applied to the individual strips. It can, however, be slow. Continuous application, while being considerably quicker, uses more tape and can make tension difficult to control.

Where strapping is applied in layers, the overlap between successive pieces is normally half the width of the tape. This ensures that the tape layers do not part with movement of the body (Adams, 1985). Gapping of the tape can trap skin between the tape layers causing skin damage. The tape should be applied smoothly and moulded to the anatomical contours of the body part. Creases should be avoided as these will create pressure spots. Tape is secured to the skin via anchoring strips (Fig. 5.2a). These are either elastic or inelastic strips applied

(a)

(b)

Figure 5.1   Tape may be either cut or torn prior to application.

Figure 5.2 (a) Anchor; (b) reins; (c) stirrup and (d) fixing strips. From Norris (1994).

directly to the skin without traction. Care must be taken not to compress the skin as the anchor tape is surrounding the limb and can easily impair the circulation. From the anchors, reins or stirrups may be attached, under traction. A rein travels between two anchor strips (Fig. 5.2b), while a stirrup is a U-shaped loop which passes beneath a body part, for example under the heel and up either side of the shin (Fig. 5.2c). The reins or stirrups are applied along the length of anatomical structures or to pull a joint into a particular position. They relieve stress from ligaments or perform the actions which a muscle would perform were it to contract. Care must be taken to avoid tape slippage which can lead to a friction burn of the skin. The reins are therefore attached to the anchor strips or skin by secure fixing strips. These run at 90° to the reins and attach in a semi-circular fashion, not surrounding the limb (Fig. 5.2d). Once the main skeleton of the taping has been formed, the components are supported by casting strips to hold the reins in place and perform a firm cover for the tape. An additional protective layer may be provided by a piece of elasticated stockinet placed over the whole taping. A glossary of terms used when taping is shown in Table 5.2.

Table 5.2 Glossary of taping terms

Anchor	The first tape strips applied to the skin, for the attachment of additional tape
Butterfly	Tape strips applied from a single fixed point and fanning out
Buttress	Material used to support or limit movement
Casting strips	Tape placed over reins to hold them firm
Continuous taping	A single length of tape wound around a structure repeatedly
Fixing strip	Tape used to make reins secure
Lock	Inelastic tape which secures an anatomical structure
Padding	Foam or fibre-based material used to protect bony prominences or fill superficial cavities
Rein	A strip of tape travelling between two anchor points
Skin toughener	Skin preparation products such as tincture of benzoin or spray adhesive
Stirrup	A U-shaped loop of tape
Strip taping	Applying a number of individual strips of tape
Underwrap	Thin polyester urethane foam placed beneath tape to protect the skin

From Norris (1994), with permission.

The aim of functional taping is not to immobilize the limb completely. Instead, movement which stresses the injured tissues is reduced, while a near normal range of motion is allowed in other directions. This allows the athlete to continue with modified and reduced intensity training while protecting those tissues damaged during the original injury. In addition, the tape may be used to re-educate movement giving the athlete feedback (see below). To achieve this, the limb is positioned with the injured structure to be protected in a shortened position. For example, the lateral ligament of the ankle is strapped with the joint held everted and dorsiflexed. Where a general limitation of all movements is required at a joint, the functional mid-range position is chosen.

Aftercare and tape removal

The athlete must be observed for two or three minutes after taping application to ensure against circulatory complications. The finger or toe nail of the treated limb should be firmly pressed and released to ensure that colour returns readily, demonstrating that an adequate blood flow is reaching the nail bed. However, even with correctly applied strapping complications may occur later, so the athlete must be warned to remove the strapping immediately in the presence of skin discoloration in the fingers or toes, increasing swelling, increasing pain, or numbness/tingling. Both passive and active joint movements are performed to ensure that the tape limits the range of motion correctly, and that it stays on.

The strapping is removed by lifting the end and pressing the skin down to form a tunnel. A tape cutter or bandage scissors are then used (lubricate the tip of the cutter) to cut the tape. The tape should be pulled back on itself and the skin pressed down at the same time to avoid too much skin traction. Residual adhesive should be cleaned from the skin. Frequent tape removal and re-application will increase skin irritation, as will tape slippage which can lead to a skin burn. Each time the tape is taken off, some of the protective corneum is stripped, so the skin must be protected with a moisturising cream over the treated area.

Taping mechanisms

Taping appears to achieve its effects by both mechanical and functional mechanisms. Mechanically, the range of motion at the joint is reduced by taping and the force required to displace the joint is increased. Radiographic studies of static talar tilt and anterior displacement, for example, have shown significant movement reductions with ankle taping (Larsen, 1984; Vaes et al., 1985). Electrogoniometry has also been used to demonstrate reduced inversion/eversion and plantar flexion during active exercise with the ankle taped (Laughman et al., 1980; Fumich et al., 1981). The limitation to movement is quickly reduced as the tape degrades with body heat and moisture. Forty percent of the supportive strength of ankle tape is lost after just ten minutes of vigorous exercise (Rarick et al., 1962). In addition, the typical tensile strength of zinc-oxide tape is considerably less than the tensile strength of the anterior talofibular ligament for example (Andreasson and Edberg, 1983; Attarian, McCrackin and Devito, 1983), meaning that multiple layer application is required to secure the joint effectively. Although the mechanical stabilizing effect of tape is reduced following exercise, taping has been shown to reduce the incidence of ankle injuries (Garrick and Requa, 1973; Ekstrand, Gillquist and Liljedahl, 1983). Clearly, another mechanism must be working to aid joint stability.

The additional mechanism may be an enhancement in functional stabilization of a joint through skin stimulation. Two mechanisms seem to act here, first, direct reflex stimulation, and secondly a learning process.

Activation of a cutaneous reflex response is a familiar occurrence, and is demonstrated in both the abdominal reflex and the flexor withdrawal response. Cutaneous stimulation causes muscle contraction within the region of the stimulant. It is possible that the stimulation of adhesive tape, and particularly the drag caused by the tape on the skin with movement, will initiate this response, as cutaneous receptors can stimulate proprioceptive reflexes (Darton, Lippold and Shahani, 1985). Peroneal reaction time has been shown to shorten with taping application (Karlsson and Andreasson, 1992) and the peroneus brevis has been shown to function for a longer period at the end of the swing phase of gait (Glick, Gordon and Nishimoto, 1976). In addition, during single leg standing, peroneal muscle activity has been shown to be significantly greater in taped than in non-taped ankles (Loos and Boelens, 1984).

Ankle proprioception has been shown to be enhanced by taping (Robbins, Waked and Rappel, 1995). Using a series of angled blocks, subjects were asked to estimate perceived slope direction and amplitude. Absolute foot position error was 4.11° for subjects wearing athletic footwear, 3.13° for those wearing taping and athletic footwear and 1.96° for barefoot athletes. When compared to the barefoot condition, untaped subjects wearing athletic footwear were 107.5% worse and taped subjects were 58.1% worse. This study demonstrated not just the ability of taping to enhance proprioception, but the detrimental effect of athletic footwear on proprioception (see p. 334).

The other way cutaneous stimulation seems to work is by reminding the athlete not to perform an unwanted action. Skin drag is uncomfortable, and can be used to great effect to correct faulty technique through feedback. In this situation, the athlete learns to adjust muscle control to prevent the skin drag (McLean, 1989). A good example is the avoidance of repeated flexion of the lumbar spine. Strips of pre-stretched elastic adhesive tape placed either side of the spine will drag on the skin as the athlete flexes, reminding him or her to avoid this action.

This cutaneous stimulation of underlying protective mechanisms may be used in other regions. For example, it is unlikely that a mechanical strapping could immobilize the hamstrings sufficiently to prevent tearing while still allowing unhindered function. However, elastic adhesive tape applied pre-stretched along the length of the muscle may remind the athlete not to overstretch and could therefore be useful in the subacute phase of injury to this body part.

Uses

Strapping in sport is normally used either to prevent injury or to promote the safe use of an injured body part, and may be used at any stage of healing. Its use in the acute phase of an injury must be treated with caution. Although its protective function is useful, accumulation of swelling and the need for regular inspection of the body part usually make the use of compression bandages or inflatable splints more appropriate. The aim of taping in the sub-acute phase of injury is to support the injured structure, by reducing the range of motion of actions which place stress on the damaged tissues. The use of functional taping should allow near normal movements in ranges other than those which stress the injury.

The great majority of publications describe strapping to the ankle, with particular reference to the lateral ligament, perhaps because this is one of the most commonly injured areas in sport. Reduction in the rate of ankle injuries following strapping application has been shown by a number of authors. Studying a population of 2562 college basketball players, Garrick and Requa (1973) showed an injury rate for non-strapped ankles of 32.8 sprains per 1000 players. This reduced dramatically to 14.7/1000 when a basketweave strapping with heel-lock was used. When the effect of strapping was studied on players who had previous ankle sprains, the injury rate reduced from 27.7/1000 to 16.4/1000. Ekstrand, Gillquist and Liljedahl (1983) taped half the previously injured, or unstable ankles, of Swedish football players. After a six-month period, those taped had no lateral ligament injuries to the ankle, but those without taping had suffered nine ligament injuries.

Some therapists believe that restricting movement at one joint by the use of taping may throw stress on other joints in the limb, although the evidence for this is inconclusive. Ankle taping has been shown to cause the heel to lift sooner in the stance phase of barefoot walking. In non-taped athletes, heel lift has been shown to occur at 71.5% of the stance phase, but at 67.1% in those athletes who wore ankle taping (Carmines et al., 1988). This alteration of the biomechanics may adversely affect the metatarsophalangeal joints (particularly the first) increasing forefoot stress. This could make turf toe a contraindication to ankle taping. Neither Glick, Gordon and Nishimoto (1976) nor Garrick and Requa (1973) found any increase in knee injuries as a result of ankle taping in their subjects.

Taping examples

Three procedures will be used as illustrative example here. The first is the use of reins to support the plantarfascia, secondly, the use of proprioceptive taping to reduce lumbar flexion in low back pain, and thirdly, the use of padding and anatomical taping in the treatment of a lateral ligament sprain to the ankle.

Use of check reins

The plantarfascia is taped with the foot in its neutral position as plantarflexion places the structure on stretch (see p. 332). The skin is sprayed with skin preparation to improve

tape adhesion. Anchor strips of 5-cm zinc-oxide tape are placed across the plantar aspect of the forefoot covering the first and fifth metatarsal heads. The strip runs to the dorsal surface of the first and fifth metatarsals but does not encircle the foot. A second anchor is placed around the calcaneum and a third below the heel pad to cover the whole of the heal. Three strips of zinc-oxide tape are then used as reins from the heel, fanning out towards the forefoot. When the patient weight bears, the taping should prevent the foot from flattening completely, and take the stretch off the plantarfascia.

Fixing strips may be used, and placed at 90° to the reins. Each strip starts and finishes at the edge of the dorsum of the foot.

Proprioceptive taping for postural re-education

In cases of lumbar pain, where a large component of the condition is due to stress accumulation through repeated bending, proprioceptive taping is used to remind the patient not to flex the lumbar spine, but to move at the hips instead (see p. 166). The patient lies prone, and two strips of adhesive fleece net taping are placed over the erector spinae at each side of the spine, with the skin relaxed, from the crest of the ilium to the lower thoracic region. On top this two 5-cm strips of zinc-oxide tape are placed to stretch the skin. The tape is adhered to the lower thoracic region and then gently pulled caudally to traction the skin. Only slight skin bunching should be noticed. Once the tape has set, it will restrict lumbar flexion by pulling on the skin, and encourage the patient to perform the 'hip hinge' action when bending. (Fig. 5.10).

Anatomical taping with padding

Padding and anatomical taping are used to support the ankle after tearing of the anterior talo-fibular ligament. Underwrap is wound

Table 5.3 Taping procedures used in later chapters

Taping used	Figure and page number
Turf toe	Fig. 14.3 p. 319
Plantar fascia	Fig. 14.6 p. 322
Heel pad	Fig. 14.7 p. 323
Correction of patellar position	Fig. 11.9 p. 248
Patellar fat pad	Fig. 11.38 p. 285
Acromioclavicular	Fig. 19.9 p. 411
Proprioceptive shoulder taping	Fig. 19.21 p. 428

around the foot and ankle from the metatarsal heads to a point 20 cm above the malleoli. Plantarflexion and inversion are the movements which must be limited to reduce stress on the healing ligament. To achieve this a felt or foam rubber wedge is placed beneath the calcaneum with the larger side placed laterally to evert the rearfoot. A felt horse shoe is placed beneath and to the sides of the lateral malleolus to avoid oedematous pooling and to create an automassage effect when walking. Two strips of 5-cm zinc-oxide tape are used as heel locks. These are adhered medially and pulled laterally to force the ankle joint into eversion.

A figure of eight is then used to lock the ankle and 5-cm elastic tape is used (continuous) to add compression. The tape begins over the tubercle of the fifth metatarsal and is pulled over the dorsum of the foot and around the forefoot forcing the foot into eversion. As the tape emerges laterally, once more it is pulled tightly over the medial malleolus to pull the foot into dorsiflexion. The tape winds behind the calcaneum and then across the dorsum of the foot overlapping the first

Figure 5.3 Calf and Achilles. Place elastic anchors around the mid-foot and calf, and a felt heel raise below the heel. Tape with the athlete prone and the foot plantarflexed. Three reins run between the foot and calf to maintain the plantarflexed position.

Figure 5.4 Elbow. Begin with the arm slightly flexed. Place elastic anchors around the forearm and upper arm. Reins cross the elbow to maintain flexion. Apply several layers as required.

Figure 5.5 Wrist. Begin with the wrist slightly flexed. Place anchors around the hand and mid-forearm. Reins link the two anchors, on the palmar surface of the forearm. The taping may be reinforced by fixing strips around the wrist.

Figure 5.6 Thumb. Hold the thumb slightly flexed and adducted to protect against an over extension injury. Using 2 cm zinc-oxide tape, loop around the wrist (loosely) and then continue a figure-of-eight around the thumb and back onto the wrist. Ensure that the wrist loop is not overtight.

Figure 5.7 (a) Ankle (strip taping). Place elastic reins around the forefoot and mid-calf. Place the first stirrup from the calf rein, and beneath the heel. Place a second stirrup from the forefoot rein around the calcaneum. Alternate stirrups building up a 'basket weave' taping. (b) Ankle (continuous taping). Evert and dorsiflex the foot (for an inversion injury). Begin the taping on the outer edge of the foot. Take it across the dorsum of the foot, and beneath the sole pulling the foot into eversion. Loop around the lower shin forming a figure of eight. Leave the heel free to enable the athlete to wear a shoe.

Medial aspect of knee

Lowback

Figure 5.8   Medial aspect of knee. Begin with the knee slightly flexed. Place elastic anchors around the upper calf and lower thigh. Join these with several layers of overlapping zinc-oxide taping, crossing on the joint line.

Figure 5.10   Lowback. Begin with the spine in lordosis. Place overlapping strips of zinc-oxide taping either side of the spine, to provide skin feedback to flexion.

Thigh

(a)

(b)

Figure 5.9   Thigh. (a) Place elastic tape around the thigh to compress the area. (b) Reinforce with zinc-oxide reins lengthways, to provide resistance to overstretch.

piece of taping by one-half. Tension is placed on the tape to pull the foot into dorsiflexion once more and the tape passes over the achilles to finish on the dorsum of the foot. Here, the edge of the tape is held down by a small piece of 5-cm zinc-oxide tape. Gaps or 'windows' between the tape should be avoided to guard against blister formation.

Table 5.3 lists the taping proceedures used in the clinical chapters of this book, while Figs 5.3–5.10 illustrate some common taping techniques used in sport.

References

Adams, I. (1985) *Strapping in Sport*, Johnson and Johnson wound care, Ballière Tindall, London

Andreasson, G. and Edberg, B. (1983) Rheological properties of medical tape used to prevent athletic injuries. *Textile Research Journal*, **53**, 225–230

Attarian, D.E., McCrackin, H.J. and Devito, D.P. (1985) Biomechanical characteristics of human ankle ligaments. *Foot and Ankle*, **6**, 54–58

Austin, K.A., Gwynn-Brett, K.A. and Marshall, S.C. (1994) *Illustrated Guide to Taping Techniques*, Mosby Year Book/Wolfe Medical, London

Carmines, D.V., Nunley, J.A., McElhaney, J.H. (1988) Effects of ankle taping on the motion and loading pattern of the foot for walking subjects. *Journal of Orthopaedic Research*, **6**, 223–229

Darton, K., Lippold, O.C.J. and Shahani, M. (1985) Long latency spinal reflexes in humans. *Journal of Neurophysiology*, **53**, 1604–1608

Ekstrand, J., Gillquist, J. and Liljedahl, S. (1983) Prevention of soccer injuries. *American Journal of Sports Medicine*, **11**, 116–120

Fumich, R.M., Ellison, A.E., Geurin, G.J. and Grace, P.D. (1981) The measured effect of taping on combined foot and ankle motion before and after exercise. *American Journal of Sports Medicine*, **9**, 165–170

Garrick, J.G. and Requa, R.K. (1973) Role of external support in the prevention of ankle sprains. *Medicine and Science in Sports and Exercise*, **5**, 200–203

Glick, J.M., Gordon, R.B. and Nishimoto, D. (1976) The prevention and treatment of ankle injuries. *American Journal of Sports Medicine*, **4**, 13–14

Karlsson, J. and Andreasson, G.O. (1992) The effect of external ankle support in chronic lateral ankle joint instability. An electromyographic study. *American Journal of Sports Medicine*, **20**(3), 257–261

Larsen, E. (1984) Taping the ankle for chronic instability. *Acta Orthopaedica Scandinavica*, **55**, 551–553

Laughman, R.K., Carr, T.A., Chao, E.Y., Youdas, J.W. and Sim, F. (1980) Three dimensional kinematics of the taped ankle before and after exercise. *American Journal of Sports Medicine*, **8**, 425–431

Loos, T. and Boelens, P. (1984) The effect of ankle tape on lower limb muscle activity. *International Journal of Sports Medicine*, **5**, (Suppl.) 45–46

Lutz, G.E., Barnes, R.P., Wickiewicz, T.L. and Renstrom, P.A.F.H. (1993) Prophylactic athletic taping. In *Sports Injuries* (Volume IV of the encyclopaedia of sports medicine) (ed. P.A.F.H. Renstrom), Blackwell Scientific, Oxford

McLean, D.A. (1989) Use of adhesive strapping in sport. *British Journal of Sports Medicine*, **23**(3), 147–149

Norris, C.M. (1994) Taping: components, application and mechanisms. *Sports Exercise and Injury*, **1**, 14–17

Rarick, G.L., Bigley, G., Karst, R. and Malina, R.M. (1962) The measurable support of the ankle joint by conventional methods of taping. *Journal of Bone and Joint Surgery*, **44A**, 1183–1190

Robbins, S., Waked, E. and Rappel, R. (1995) Ankle taping improves proprioception before and after exercise in young men. *British Journal of Sports Medicine*, **29**(4), 242–247

Vaes, P., De Boeck, H., Handelberg, F. and Opdecam, P. (1985) Comparative radiologic study of the influence of ankle joint bandages on ankle stability. *American Journal of Sports Medicine*, **13**(1), 46–50

6

Physical training and injury

Principles of training

In any form of training the body is exposed to a workload or physical stress at an intensity, duration and frequency sufficient to cause physical change. To achieve a training effect, the body must be overloaded, that is, exposed to a physical stress which is greater than that encountered in everyday living. The response to this training stress is catabolism, the breakdown of metabolic fuels or tissues. Following the catabolic response, an excessive tissue adaptation occurs, anabolism, causing the tissues affected to increase (Astrand and Rodahl, 1986).

As fitness improves, the intensity of the load which is required to produce a training effect will increase. Adaptation to the load occurs, and so further improvement will only occur if the training intensity is increased. Physical activity in itself is therefore not synonymous with physical training (Astrand and Rodahl, 1986). A training effect will only occur if an activity is sufficiently demanding.

In addition to a minimum intensity, the training load must be continued for a certain duration. High intensity training which is too brief may not allow time for the physical adaptations required by the body. The frequency of training, that is, how often it is carried out, is also important. Training is a stimulus which causes an anabolic adapta-

tion. This adaptation will take time, and so adequate recovery must be allowed between training sessions for the body tissues to modify themselves. The type of training will dictate the type of tissue adaptation which occurs, a principle known as specificity (McCafferty and Horvath, 1977) (see below).

Training effects are not permanent. The motor system adapts to the level (overload) and type (specificity) of stress that is imposed on it. If the stress is removed, and training ceases, the motor system will again adapt to the new, now lower, level of stress and detraining will occur. This transient nature of training adaptation is known as the reversibility principle (Thorstensson, 1977; Enoka, 1994).

When training for aerobic (cardiopulmonary) fitness or stamina, exercise intensity may be assessed by measuring heart rate or maximal oxygen uptake (VO_2 max). The American College of Sports Medicine (1978) recommended the quantity and quality of exercise required to develop and maintain aerobic fitness and body composition. A training frequency of three to five days per week is required, at an intensity of 60% to 90% of the maximum heart rate reserve, or 50%–85% VO_2 max. This should be carried out for a duration of 15–60 minutes, and be continuous or rhythmical in nature. These recommendations were later updated

(ACSM, 1990) to include the provision of resistance training. One set of 8–12 repetitions was recommended with 8–10 exercises for the major muscles groups, for two days per week.

Fitness

Physical fitness has been defined as a set of attributes that relate to the ability of people to perform physical activity (McArdle et al., 1991) or the ability of a person to function efficiently and effectively to enjoy leisure, to be healthy, to resist hypokinetic disease, and to cope with emergency situations (Kent, 1994).

Fitness can be thought of as a continuum from optimal fitness at one side through average fitness to complete lack of fitness and death (Fig. 6.1). The exact components of fitness required to make an individual optimally efficient and effective will be determined largely by the physical activity to be performed.

Fitness may be subdivided into two types. Task (performance)-related fitness is that required for sport and within occupational activities. Health-related fitness includes components which are associated with some aspect of health. Physical training will improve fitness, but may not always enhance

health. Extreme development of any one of the fitness components, in isolation, will upset the delicate balance between the components and may actually be detrimental to health. For example, excessive development of flexibility will lead to hyperflexibility and, when strength lags behind, instability. Excessive development of strength may reduce range of motion leaving an athlete 'muscle bound'. Favouring some muscles to the detriment of others will often lead to a change in the equilibrium point (resting position) of a joint.

Fitness components

The fitness components may be conveniently defined as 'S' factors (Table 6.1). The term stamina is used to encompass both cardiopulmonary and local muscle endurance. Cardiopulmonary endurance is associated with a reduced risk of coronary heart disease (Ashton and Davies, 1986), and local muscle endurance is a factor in any sustained activity, especially joint stability. Suppleness (flexibility) and strength (see below) are concerned with the health of the musculoskeletal system, to maintain both range of movement and joint integrity. Speed (rate of movement) and power (rate of doing work) are both needed in later stage rehabilitation as part of proprioceptive training (see p. 171). Skill training is important, not just for sports specific actions, but for the skill of individual movement such as scapulo-humeral rhythm or gait re-education for example. The principles of skill training and their

| Death | Average fitness | Optimal fitness |

Figure 6.1 The fitness continuum.

Table 6.1 'S' factors of fitness

Factor	Concept
Stamina	Cardiopulmonary and local muscle endurance
Suppleness	Passive and active flexibility
Strength	Isometric, isotonic (concentric and eccentric) isokinetic strength
Speed	Speed (rate of movement) and power (rate of doing work)
Skill	Motor skill
Specificity	Overload must match tissue adaptation required
Spirit	Psychological aspects of injury, including illness behaviour

relevance to rehabilitation are discussed on page 71.

Specificity refers to the SAID principle, that is 'specific adaptation to imposed demands'. The change taking place in the body of an athlete (adaptation) as a result of training (the imposed demand) will be determined by the type of training which is used, and will be specific to it.

Specificity applies to strength and power development, but also to the energy systems used while exercising. A particular cardio-pulmonary training programme will cause specific training adaptations. Aerobic fitness developed on a cycle ergometer, for example, will differ slightly from that obtained while running.

It is important, therefore, that training matches, as accurately as possible, the action which the athlete will use in a sport, in terms of joint range, muscle work, energy system, and skill.

Spirit covers the psychological implications of both performance and injury recovery as is covered in Chapter 3.

Warm-up

Many athletes conscientiously warm-up in the belief that they will protect themselves against injury, and enhance their sporting performance. Whilst neither of these beliefs have been conclusively proven, there is mounting evidence in the literature to suggest that both may contain elements of truth. This section does not attempt to be a full review of the subject, but will draw on some of the many studies concerning warm-up to illustrate important points.

Warm-up types

Warm-up may be either passive, involving an external heat source, or active, involving body heat. An active warm-up, in turn, may be general, using the whole body, or specific, working only those body parts to be used in competition.

Many external heat sources are suitable for a passive warm-up. Common types used by athletes include hot baths or showers, and saunas. Clinically, physiotherapists use a number of modalities including hot packs, whirlpool baths, and electrotherapy (short-wave diathermy in particular). Benefits are claimed to result from the increase in tissue temperature, and physical performance has been improved using this type of warm-up.

Carlile (1956) showed improvements in swimming times after hot showers (8 minutes at 40°C). Davies and Young (1983) warmed the triceps surae muscle group with hot water baths, and showed increases in peak power output with cycling and jumping tasks. Sargeant (1987) also used water baths, and showed increases in peak force and power of 11% after heating, and reductions of up to 21% after cooling.

With a passive warm-up, no significant active body movement is used, and little energy is expended. Subsequent physical work will not therefore be impaired due to depletion of energy stores (Shellock and Prentice, 1985). This type of warm-up can be useful clinically, when active movement is either not desirable or not possible.

General warm-ups are the type most commonly used in sport. The overall body temperature is raised by active exercise, increasing the temperature of the deep muscles and body core. Richards (1968) compared different durations of stool stepping as an active warm-up, before a vertical jump task. Short, one- and two-minute warm-ups improved performance by 23%, while a four-minute period had no effect. A six-minute warm-up reduced performance by 27%, presumably through fatigue.

Specific warm-up involves movements which are to be used in actual competition, but at a reduced intensity. Rehearsal of body movement takes place, and the specific tissues directly involved in the activity are heated. This type of warm-up would seem especially appropriate for events requiring highly skilled and coordinated actions, and some research is available to support this view. DeVries (1959) compared passive (hot showers and massage), active (calisthenics) and specific (swimming) warm-up prior to a swimming task and showed significant improvement in performance only after the specific warm-up.

Effects of warm-up

The effects of warm-up seem to be physiological, psychological and biomechanical. Physiological effects are largely due to increases in tissue temperature, while psychological effects are mainly due to practice. Biomechanical effects are achieved by alterations in the tissue response to mechanical strain.

Cardiovascular changes

The change from a relaxed resting state to a higher training level should be gradual, to avoid suddenly stressing the cardiovascular system. Equally, to stop training quickly, and reduce cardiac output too rapidly can compromise venous return.

A warm-up of sufficient intensity will cause an alteration in regional blood flow. When resting, only 15–20% of the total blood flow goes to the skeletal muscles, but after about 10 minutes of general exercise this figure is increased to 70–75% (Renstrom and Kannus, 1992). During a warm-up, blood flow is increased to active muscles, and reduced to visceral tissues, earlier than would occur without a warm-up. Increased blood flow causes the delivery of nutrients and removal of metabolic wastes to be enhanced (Karvonen, 1978).

Barnard et al. (1973) examined the effects of sudden strenuous exercise on men with no symptoms of cardiac problems. Each subject ran vigorously on a treadmill for 10–15 seconds without a warm-up. In 70% of these subjects, abnormal changes were seen on an ECG trace, indicative of subendocardial ischaemia. These changes were reduced, or even abolished, when a warm-up was performed before activity. Similarly, the effect of sudden onset exercise on blood pressure was improved. Average systolic blood pressures of 168 mmHg were seen without warm-up and these reduced to 140 mmHg when warm-up preceded exercise.

One of the reasons for these changes is that the adaptation of the coronary blood flow to strenuous exercise is not instantaneous. The cardiac output is unable to increase quickly enough to meet the demands of sudden high intensity work (Astrand and Rodahl, 1986), and a warm-up gives the cardiovascular system time to respond.

Tissue temperature

The ability to perform physical work is improved by elevated temperature (Bergh and Ekblom, 1979a). Warm-up prior to maximal exercise will enable the adaptations necessary for these changes, to occur sooner.

Oxygen dissociation from haemoglobin is more rapid and complete, and oxygen release from myoglobin is greater at higher temperatures (Astrand and Rodahl, 1986). The critical level of various metabolic processes is lowered, causing an acceleration in metabolic rate and a more efficient usage of substrates. Muscle contraction is more rapid and forceful (Bergh, 1980). The sensitivity of nerve receptors and speed of transmission of nervous impulses are both increased as temperature rises (Astrand and Rodahl, 1986). This more rapid transmission of kinaesthetic signals is particularly important when complex highly skilled movements are used. These temperature-dependent changes are summarized in Table 6.2.

The increased tissue temperature created by a warm-up will alter the force–velocity curve of a muscle (see p. 17). The effect is to shift the curve to the right by 12% for each 1°C increase in temperature (Enoka, 1994). The change in contraction velocity (maximal

Table 6.2   Tissue changes with increased temperature

1   Increased speed of contraction and relaxation of muscle
2   Increased force of muscle contraction
3   Greater mechanical efficiency due to lowered viscous resistance within the muscles
4   Haemoglobin releases oxygen more easily at higher temperature, therefore oxygen utilization by muscle is improved
5   Similar effects with myoglobin
6   Nerve and muscle metabolism is improved. If a specific warm-up is used, motor unit recruitment for maximum activities is facilitated
7   Dilatation of local vascular bed leads to increased blood flow through active tissues
8   Lower critical level of metabolic reactions

velocity of shortening) results in an increase in peak power output of the muscle (Fig. 6.2).

Large temperature changes have been shown to affect maximal isometric force. Cooling the hand muscles to 15°C reduced maximum isometric force by 30%

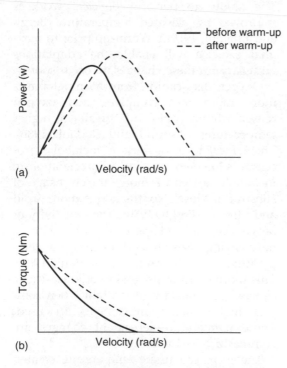

(a)   Velocity (rad/s)

(b)   Velocity (rad/s)

Figure 6.2   Effect of tissue temperature increase due to warm-up. (a) Peak power is increased demonstrated by increased height obtained on vertical jump test. (b) Maximum velocity of shortening increased and torque–velocity curve shifts to the right. Adapted from Enoka (1994).

(Ranatunga, Sharpe and Turnbull, 1987) while warming the quadriceps changed maximal isometric torque from 262 Nm at 30.4°C to 312 Nm at 38.5°C, an increase of 2.4%/°C (Bergh and Ekblom, 1979b).

Mobilization hypothesis

In the initial period of intense exercise, high amounts of energy are required immediately. The anaerobic reserves are quickly used up, and the aerobic system has not yet become fully functional. The difference between the energy needed, and that which can be supplied, is known as the oxygen deficit, and represents stored energy, and the build up of metabolic wastes (Fig. 6.3). When exercise stops, the body continues to provide energy aerobically to replenish the energy stores and metabolize waste products which have accumulated. This, in turn, creates the oxygen debt.

Gutin and Stewart (1971) argued that a function of warm-up was to mobilize the body's cardiovascular system to reach a steady state. As warm-up was stopped, a brief rest period before competition allowed the oxygen debt to be repaid, without letting the cardiovascular system return to normal levels. When competition commenced, the oxygen deficit would be smaller, and some anaerobic energy would be available to the athlete at the end of exercise.

Gutin et al. (1976) asked subjects to pedal a cycle ergometer at an intensity sufficient to

Figure 6.3 The effect of warm-up on oxygen deficit.

produce a heart rate of 140 b.p.m., a rate which they claimed equated with a 50-60% VO_2 max. The subjects' performance in a subsequent exercise task was significantly better than a control group who did not undertake a warm-up; a result possibly due to the mechanism described above.

A rest period is essential after the warm-up, to allow the oxygen debt to be repaid. But, following rest, the body must be kept warm to maintain the warm-up effects until the athlete competes. As an illustration, Andzel and Gutin (1976) used bench stepping both as a warm-up and exercise task. A 30 or 60 second rest after the warm-up resulted in improved performance, but when no rest period followed the warm-up, performance remained unchanged.

How long should a warm-up last, and what intensity of exercise should be used? A number of papers have addressed these questions. Andzel (1982) compared warm-up periods at an intensity sufficient to produce a heart rate of 120 and 140 b.p.m., followed by a 30-second rest period.

Performance was significantly better with the 140 b.p.m. group. Richards (1968) argued that while some warm-ups would enhance performance, others could interfere with performance if fatigue set in. By varying the length of stool stepping, she concluded that a 1 or 2-minute warm-up was superior to a 4 or 6-minute period in her study, Bonner (1974) saw similar effects by altering warm-up periods with a static cycle task. Where performance was reduced in these examples, the workload was obviously too high. Sargeant and Dolan (1987) compared warm-up periods with changing intensity assessed by percentage of VO_2 max, and concluded that a 39% VO_2 max intensity was superior to a warm-up at 56% VO_2 max.

Unfortunately there are no hard and fast rules to guide the athlete in terms of warm-up duration and intensity, but, generally, once the heart rate has reached about 140 b.p.m., this should be sustained for 2–3 minutes. This workload should be sufficient to induce light sweating, and is appropriate for the cardiopulmonary part of the warm-up. Obviously, the time taken to achieve this heart rate will depend on exercise intensity and fitness level, so the total warm-up period will be considerably longer.

Biomechanical effects

Safran et al. (1988) showed that a greater force and length of stretch was required to tear isometrically preconditioned muscles (Fig. 6.4). They claimed that the rise in temperature occurring during the warm-up period could alter the viscosity of the connective tissue within the muscle, and that isometric contractions caused a stretch at the musculotendinous junction. LaBan (1962) showed a 1.5% increase in the length of a stretched tendon following a temperature increase to 42.5°C. Warren, Lehmann and Koblanski (1971) demonstrated increases of 5.8% in length and 58% in force to failure for tendons heated to 45°C.

Figure 6.4 The effect of warm-up on tissue failure. After Safran et al. (1988).

Shellock and Prentice (1985) argued that muscle elasticity is dependent on blood saturation. They claimed that cold muscles with lower blood saturation levels were therefore more susceptible to injury. Fluids exhibit higher viscosity with lower temperatures, and so joint inertia will be greater when the synovial fluid of a joint is colder.

Changes have also been noted in structural stiffness of muscle following warm-up and exercise. Immediately following activity, muscle stiffness is increased, but can be significantly reduced by stretching. The increase in stiffness is thought to result from thixotrophy (Enoka, 1994), the property exhibited by materials whereby they become more fluid when disturbed (shaken). Within muscle, stable bonds are formed between actin and myosin filaments. The bonds are increased following activity, but disengaged by stretching. This has important implications for both warm-up and cool down. Warm-up will help minimize general muscle stiffness, while cool down will reduce the actin and myocin bonding which remains following exercise (see also DOMS p. 138).

Psychological effects

Psychological aspects of warm-up fall broadly into two categories. First, there are psychological effects of a physical warm-up which will be dealt with below. Secondly, aspects of sports psychology, such as visua-lization and imagery, which are dealt with in the section on sports psychology related to injury.

Two psychological factors are important in the context of warm-up, these are rehearsal and arousal. Rehearsal will only take place when an athlete performs a specific warm-up, with actions relevant to the sport to be performed in competition. During the warm-up, the athlete is re-familiarizing him or herself with the skilled movements required by a sport. Confidence is improved, and the athlete may be more relaxed following this practice.

When an athlete is performing a skilled task, if he or she rests and then resumes the same task, his or her performance may suffer. This phenomenon is called warm-up decrement (WUD), and is well documented (Adams, 1961; Nacson and Schmidt, 1971; Schmidt, 1982).

A number of explanations have been suggested to account for WUD. At a basic level it is seen as simply forgetting an aspect of the motor skill. Nacson and Schmidt (1971) suggested that WUD results from a loss of 'activity set'. They claimed that a number of variables such as arousal level and attention had to be adjusted (tuned) to a specific task. With practice, the adjustments reach an optimal level, which is reduced with rest. They showed that WUD could be reduced if, during the rest period, a completely different movement was practised. This second movement could not contribute to the memory of the first task, but did require a similar activity set to the original skill.

So far, we have dealt with skills which were practised during the warm-up period to improve subsequent sporting performance. When the practice of one task improves performance on another, positive transfer is occurring. However, if during a warm-up skills are practised which are different to those needed for competition, they may interfere with the learning process and *negative transfer* can occur. Here, performance suffers because a slightly different skill, with a different activity set, is remembered. An example would be practising tennis strokes with a racquet of different weight and size to that of the one used in competition.

The second psychological effect of warm-up is that of arousal. The relationship between level of arousal and performance, is demonstrated by the inverted-U hypothesis (Fig. 6.5). In a plot of arousal level against performance, initially increased arousal correlates initially with improved performance. But, as arousal continues to increase, an optimal level is reached. Above this point, further arousal is detrimental to performance.

The point of optimum arousal is related to the psychological profile of the athlete, and the complexity of the task to be performed. Activities which require fine muscular control (such as archery) or involve important decision-making (such as wicket keeping) generally require lower arousal levels. Where actions involve gross muscular actions without fine control and without complex decision-making (power lifting for example) a higher level of arousal is generally required.

The function of warm-up, therefore, must be to psychologically prepare the athlete, and place him at the level of arousal appropriate to the task to be undertaken. A highly motivated (aroused) athlete may need to be relaxed prior to a complex activity. Conversely, a poorly motivated athlete, due to compete in a strength event, may need his arousal level increased, by 'psyching' him up.

Warm-up technique

The intensity and duration of the warm-up period will depend on the type of activity to be undertaken and the athlete's fitness. A fitter athlete competing at a high level will take longer to warm-up as his thermoregulatory system will be more efficient.

During cold weather it will take longer for the body's core temperature to increase, and so the warm-up should be longer or more vigorous. Hogberg and Ljunggren (1947) showed a 15-minute warm-up to be more effective than a shorter five-minute period, but found the effects were not increased when the warm-up period was stretched to half an hour. DeVries (1980) suggested a warm-up of sufficient intensity and duration to raise the body's core temperature by 1–2°C. This, he argued, was enough to induce mild sweating. Warm-up effects may persist for 45–80 minutes, the time variation being dependent on the rate of heat loss.

General warm-up exercises include jogging, light aerobics, and callisthenics. Each must be hard enough to cause mild sweating, but not so intense as to exhaust the athlete. These should be followed by specific warm-up movements mimicking the actions to be carried out in competition. Examples for squash would be gentle flowing arm actions holding a racquet, gradually building up to full forearm and backhand movements.

At the beginning of the warm-up, joints are only moved in the mid-range. As warm-up continues, a greater range of movement is sought until the limb moves freely through full range. The exercises are progressive and should always feel comfortable and without strain.

Flexibility training (see below) should not be practised at the beginning of a warm-up

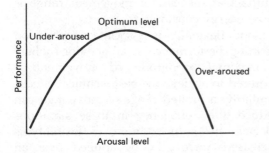

Figure 6.5 Relationship between arousal and performance.

(Sapega et al., 1981). The benefits of elevated tissue temperature on flexibility make it more productive to perform stretching exercises after a warm-up period. However, flexibility exercises should be used within the first part of a training session, especially in sports requiring a large range of motion. This is particularly important, for example, in gymnastics, dance, the martial arts, and certain track and field athletic events. In these cases, a warm-up is performed first, followed by flexibility exercises. The latter are progressed in range of motion until the range used is equal to that expected in competition.

Warm-down

On cessation of exercise it is important to reverse the processes which occurred during the warm-up. The heart is no longer helped by the rhythmic contraction and relaxation of the leg muscles. Consequently, to stop intense exercise immediately will increase the demand on the cardiovascular system causing the heart rate to rise. Metabolic waste products formed during exercise, such as lactic acid, will no longer be carried away from the working area with so much vigour. Instead they will remain in the area causing pain. This is thought to be one possible cause of delayed onset muscle fatigue (Byrnes and Clarkson, 1985). Flushing the area with fresh blood by performing a gentle warm down can reduce this effect.

Flexibility training

Flexibility has been defined as the range of movement possible at a specific joint or series of articulations (Cureton, 1941) or the amount or 'amplitude' of joint movement and the general absence of stiffness (Reilly, 1981).

Two types of flexibility are generally recognized, static and dynamic. Static (or extent) flexibility refers to the amount of movement obtained by passively moving a limb to a maximum degree. Dynamic flexibility is concerned with the amount of active movement possible as a result of muscle contraction. The concern here is not so much the degree of movement present, as the ease with which it is obtained. This type of flexibility is probably more important in speed events (Hardy and Jones, 1986).

Dynamic flexibility must not be confused with agility, which can be defined as the ability to rapidly change the direction of either the whole body or individual body parts without loss of balance (Borms, 1984).

Effects of flexibility training

Flexibility training is generally thought to achieve effects in two broad areas, that of performance enhancement and injury prevention, and these two will be addressed.

Improved performance

To achieve maximal performance, a limb must be able to move through a non-restricted range of motion (Shellock and Prentice, 1985). In sprinting, for example, lack of adequate dynamic flexibility could result in a reduced stride length with possible reductions in sprinting speed. In addition, greater resistance to movement through increased joint inertia and muscle stiffness at the end of movement range is more energy consuming.

Good flexibility is associated with good sporting performance in all activities where a maximal amplitude of movement is required to achieve the best technical effects. Similarly, a limited range of movement can reduce work efficiency in these situations (Borms, 1984). In addition, if flexibility is increased, force may be applied over an increased distance (Reilly, 1981), thus facilitating acceleration of an implement.

Injury prevention

Cureton (1941) was one of the first to suggest that flexibility training may condition muscles, ligaments, and fascia to greater tensile strength and elasticity, leading to injury prevention. Holt, Travis and Okita (1970) proposed that increased flexibility of the hip extensors and low back muscles could result in fewer injuries with activities of daily living, while DeVries (1962) argued that the maintenance of adequate joint mobility helps to prevent or relieve soft tissue pain.

Ekstrand and Gillquist (1982), and Ekstrand et al. (1983) asserted that muscle tightness may predispose athletes to certain injuries, and suggested that the type of training programmes undertaken could affect the number of injuries suffered. Netball players, who had not warmed up have been shown to have an increased risk of injury (Hopper, 1986), while warming up and stretching have been shown to be important factors in the prevention of hamstring injuries in Australian football (Seward and Patrick, 1992).

Tightness occurs in muscle groups in set patterns, with the biarticular muscles (mobilizers, see p. 144) showing a greater tendency to shorten. For example, of the hip extensors it is the hamstrings (biarticular) rather than the gluteals (uniarticular) which commonly show tightness and injury through tearing. Tightness of the muscle may pull a joint out of alignment altering the equilibrium point of the joint and predisposing to joint injury. Further details of this type of change or 'muscle imbalance' is given on pages 144–159.

Muscle reflexes

Kisner and Colby (1990) argued that the term flexibility may be interchanged with elasticity, and refers to the ability of a muscle to relax and yield to stretch. This definition fails to take account of the importance of joint structures in flexibility, but does indicate the importance of muscle function when applying stretching exercises.

Three muscle reflexes are important when using flexibility training, the stretch reflex, autogenic inhibition, and reciprocal inhibition (Table 6.3).

When a muscle is stretched, elongation is detected by the muscle spindle afferent nerve fibres. These receptors send impulses to the dorsal roots of the spinal cord, and a reflex is caused which contracts the extrafusal fibres of the same muscle, in opposition to the original stretching force. The reflex is therefore facilitatory. The stretch imposed may be either sudden (as in a knee jerk reflex), where the muscle responds to a change in velocity, or prolonged (as with postural sway), where the muscle measures the change in length.

In addition to the muscle spindle, the Golgi tendon organ (GTO) in the muscle tendon will also register stretch. Both these receptors are affected by changes in muscle

Table 6.3   Muscle reflexes and stretching

Stretch reflex Responds to: —change in velocity (phasic) (e.g. knee jerk reflex) —change in length (postural) (e.g. body sway)	Facilitatory ($\uparrow$ tone)
Autogenic inhibition (the reverse stretch reflex) —Golgi tendon organ (GTO) measures tension	Inhibitory ($\downarrow$ tone)
Reciprocal innervation —Agonist contracts, antagonist relaxes to allow movement	Inhibitory ($\downarrow$ tone)

length, but the GTO is also receptive to changes in muscle tension (Bray et al., 1986).

When a muscle is stretched, there is a corresponding stretch of the muscle spindle. But, if the stretch lasts for longer than 6 seconds, the GTO registers not only the change of length of the muscle, but also the alteration in tension in the muscle tendon. The GTO will then cause a reflex relaxation of the muscle, a process known as autogenic inhibition or the reverse stretch reflex. This has a protective function, causing the muscle to relax and allowing it to stretch before it is damaged. It is therefore inhibitory.

Stretching which involves short jerking movements will tighten the muscle through the stretch reflex, while movements lasting for longer than 6 seconds will allow the muscle to relax again through stimulation of the GTO, which will override the stretch reflex. When a muscle is tensed, a reflex relaxation of the antagonist will occur, a process known as reciprocal inhibition. If, for example, the biceps muscle contracts to flex the elbow, its antagonist, the triceps, must relax to allow the movement to occur.

Techniques of flexibility

Five methods of stretching are generally recognized, static, ballistic, active and two proprioceptive neuromuscular facilitation (PNF) techniques (Table 6.4).

During static stretching, a muscle is stretched to the point of discomfort and held there for an extended period. Ballistic stretching involves taking the limb to its end of movement range, and adding repetitive bouncing movements, usually for a period of about 30 seconds (Hardy and Jones, 1986). This method is no longer as popular as it was, because of the suggestion that injury may result from abrupt stretching of soft tissues (Etnyre and Lee, 1987). Although not recommended for regular training, ballistic stretching does have a place in the final stages of rehabilitation (see below). Active stretching involves pulling a limb into full inner range so that the antagonist muscle is stretched passively while the agonist is strengthened. This type of stretch is important when correcting muscle imbalance (see p. 155). The inner range contraction is used to shorten a lengthened (lax) muscle while the shortened muscle is stretched using a functionally relevant movement.

PNF techniques have been adopted by the sporting world from neurological physiotherapy treatments. These techniques use alternating contractions and relaxations of muscles and capitalize on the various muscle reflexes to achieve a greater level of relaxation during the stretch.

Two PNF techniques are used, contract-relax (CR) and contract-relax-agonist-contract (CRAC). The CR technique involves lengthening a muscle until a comfortable stretch is felt. From this position, the muscle is isometrically contracted, and held for a set period. The muscle is relaxed, and then taken to a new lengthened position until the full stretch is again felt by the subject. The rationale behind the CR method is that the contracted muscle will relax as a result of

Table 6.4 Summary of stretching techniques

1	Ballistic—rapid jerking actions at end of range to force the tissues to stretch
2	Static stretching (SS)—slowly and passively stretching the muscle to full range, and maintaining this stretched position with continual tension
3	Active stretch—contract the agonist muscle to full inner range to impart a stretch on the antagonist
4	Contract-relax (CR)—isometrically contracting the stretched muscle, and then relaxing and passively stretching the muscle still further. This action is usually performed by a partner
5	Contract-relax-agonist-contract (CRAC)—the same as CR except that during the final stages of the stretching phase, the muscle opposite the one being stretched is contracted

autogenic inhibition, as the GTO fires to inhibit tension. Some authors argue that a maximal isometric contraction is needed to initiate relaxation through the GTO mechanism (Janda, 1992). Others recommend the use of minimal isometric contractions (Lewit, 1991) which seem more appropriate in situations where pain is present.

With the CRAC method, the muscle is stretched as above, but in the final stages of the stretch, the opposing muscle groups are isometrically contracted as the stretch is applied, to make use of reciprocal inhibition of the agonist, and reduce its tension. Of these techniques, PNF stretches have been shown to be more effective (Holt, Travis and Okita, 1970; Cornelius and Hinson, 1980; Holt and Smith, 1983; Etnyre and Abraham, 1986), with CRAC methods generally being better than CR.

These various procedures may be illustrated with a common hamstring stretch. A ballistic stretch could involve keeping the leg straight and vigorously reaching for the toes with a bouncing action, for example repeated toe touching in standing or long sitting. The rapid action may tighten the muscle, but stretches other soft tissues including the non-contractile muscle elements, muscle tendons, and ligaments surrounding the hip, knee and spine. In addition, repeated spinal flexion, in this particular exercise, may increase intradiscal pressure within the lumbar discs placing the athlete in danger of discal migration (McKenzie, 1981) or discal herniation.

A static stretch performed in this position would involve reaching towards the toes, holding the movement, and allowing the muscle to relax and 'give'. Various authors have given guidelines for the optimal holding period, and Borms et al. (1987) suggest a ten-second duration as optimal for improving coxa-femoral flexibility.

An active stretch could be performed by standing, holding on to a wallbar for support, and lifting the straight leg upwards using the force of the hip flexors.

The CR technique for the hamstrings could be performed with an athlete lying on his or her back. The athlete's leg is lifted by a training partner, keeping the knee straight. After holding the stretch for ten seconds, the athlete contracts his hamstrings by pulling the straight leg down towards the floor against his partner's resistance. The tension is kept on for 10–20 seconds, a sufficient time to allow the GTO to override the stretch reflex. The tension is then released, and the stretch reapplied by the training partner.

This stretch is taken further by applying the CRAC procedure. This time, as the stretch is applied, the athlete tries to increase the stretch himself by pulling the straight leg up towards his head, tensing his hip flexors. In so doing, the hamstrings are relaxed still further through reciprocal inhibition, and the stretch becomes more effective. A variety of general flexibility exercises are illustrated in Fig. 6.6. Permission is given for this page to be photocopied and handed out to athletes. The exercises to be used may be ticked in the boxes provided. More details on stretching exercise are given in Norris (1994).

Factors affecting flexibility

The amount of movement present at a joint during a stretch (amplitude) is affected by internal (body) and external (environmental) factors. Internal factors include the bony contours of the joint. These will differ between individuals, and in certain pathologies such a arthritis, movement will decrease as bone formation changes. These factors cannot readily be affected by flexibility training, but must be taken into consideration when prescribing stretching programmes, especially with the elderly and during rehabilitation.

Other internal factors include volume of surrounding tissue, an obese individual frequently being less flexible than a lean one. Muscle tissue, tendons, and joint capsules

Figure 6.6 Stretching exercises. Tick (✓) exercises to be used.

are other internal factors which may result in movement limitation. Johns and Wright (1982) indicated that 47% of mid-range stiffness is due to the joint capsule, 41% due to muscle fascial sheaths, 10% due to the tendon, and 2% due to the skin. Other factors include cartilage, and viscosity of joint fluid (Holland, 1968).

Sapega et al. (1981) argued that the relative contributions of various soft tissues to passive resistance vary between joints. However, they pointed out that when a muscle is relaxed, it is the connective tissue framework of the muscle and not the myofibrillar elements themselves which provide passive resistance. Consequently they concluded that connective tissue is the major structure limiting joint motion (especially where adhesions are present) and should therefore be the target for stretching procedures.

Temperature is one external factor which affects flexibility (Harris, 1969), and we have seen that increases in tissue temperature can result in reductions in synovial fluid viscosity and increased soft tissue extensibility (LaBan, 1962).

At a temperature of approximately 40°C a thermal transition of collagen occurs, allowing a greater plastic deformation when stretched (Rigby, 1964). Elastic (recoverable) deformation of connective tissue is favoured by high-force short duration stretching with tissue at normal body temperature or slightly cooled, while plastic deformation (permanent lengthening) is greater with lower-force, longer-duration stretching at elevated temperatures. If the tissue is then allowed to cool in this stretched position, results are noticeably better (Sapega et al., 1981).

Individual variations in body structure can have apparent affects on flexibility. Individuals with long slender limbs are likely to be more flexible than shorter individuals with thicker musculature. However, good flexibility in one joint does not guarantee similar attributes in other joints, because flexibility has been shown to be joint specific (Harris, 1969).

In general, flexibility decreases with age (Harris, 1969), although between individuals this trend is very much dependent on activity levels and other lifestyle factors (Borms, 1984). A general belief is that girls are more flexible than boys, but it is not clear whether this is due to body structure or social and environmental influences (Goldberg, Saranitia and Witman, 1980).

Therapeutic stretching

When stretching is used as a manual therapy to mobilize a joint after injury or surgery, the various techniques will be combined. If muscle spasm is the limiting factor, ice may be used to limit the pain and and this may be combined with PNF stretching (cryostretch procedures). However, to stretch connective tissue effectively, higher than normal temperatures are required, so heat is the modality of choice, where muscle spasm does not limit movement.

The ability of the heat source to reach the tissue to be stretched must be considered, and this will largely depend on the tissue depth and vascularity. In the forearm, temperature elevations of 7°F have been produced by 20 minutes of hot water immersion (Barcroft and Ebholm, 1943), and ultrasound produced a mean temperature elevation of 9°F in muscle near the femoral shaft in the human thigh (Lehmann, DeLateur and Silverman, 1966). Intra-articular knee temperatures have been effectively raised in both canine and human subjects by hot water immersion, shortwave, and microwave diathermy (Sapega et al., 1981).

After heating, pulley systems and weights may be used to apply a passive stretch to an immobile joint where adhesions limit movement.

Sapega et al. (1981) recommended a stretching period of 20–60 minutes for the knee joint, with several 30-second breaks, during which full range movements are carried out. In addition, they used biofeedback from an audible electromyographic device over the quadriceps to encourage maintenance of muscle relaxation. Following passive stretching, the joint was cooled for 15 minutes with crushed ice while maintaining the stretching force.

Strength training

Strength is the ability to overcome a resistance, it is the maximum tension which a muscle can produce (McArdle, Katch and Katch, 1986). Strength is usually measured as the torque exerted in a single maximal isometric contraction of unrestricted duration (Enoka, 1994). However, clinically it is important to define the type of strength by prefacing the term with the category of muscle contraction which was used. We should therefore talk of isometric or isotonic strength, rather than simply strength alone.

Adaptation to resistance training

Muscular contraction involves a combination of physiological and neurological processes, and consequently adaptations to resistance training are both myogenic (structural) and neurogenic (seen on EMG only) in nature.

Myogenic changes

One of the most noticeable myogenic adaptations to resistance exercise is increased muscle size or hypertrophy. Increased cross-sectional area has been found to result from an increase in size of individual muscle fibres. Luithi et al. (1986) found an increase of 8.4% in cross-sectional area of the vastus lateralis following a 6-week period of resistance exercise.

The increase in size occurs in both type I (slow twitch) and type II (fast twitch) fibres. Selective hypertrophy can occur, causing just the type I or just the type II fibres to increase in size, the ratio between the two

fibre types remaining the same (see also p. 145). In normal adults the ratio is about 1:1 or 2:1, but in competitive bodybuilders ratios as high as 6:1 have been found, compared to 0:1 in sprinters (Astrand and Rodahl, 1986). In addition, heavy resistance training has been shown to increase the proportion of type IIA (fast oxidative glycolytic) fibres (Bandy, Lovelace-Chandler and McKitrick-Bandy, 1990). Of greater dispute is the possibility of muscle fibre splitting (hyperplasia) in humans. A greater number of muscle fibres is seen in competitive bodybuilders, but this is thought to be a congenital feature of the more successful athletes (Bandy, Lovelace-Chandler and McKitrick-Bandy, 1990). Most authors agree that the increase in cross-sectional area following resistance training is the result of hypertrophy rather than hyperplasia.

In addition to the increase in fibre size, which occurs with hypertrophy, connective tissue proliferation is also seen (McArdle, Katch and Katch, 1986). Thickening of the muscle's connective tissue support, and that of the musculo-tendinous junction may reduce the risk of soft tissue trauma.

Endurance training has long been known to increase the number of mitochondria and the capillary density (number per square millimetre of tissue). However, resistance training is thought to lead to hypertrophy without a significant increase in the number of capillaries (Astrand and Rodahl, 1986). As the number of capillaries stays the same, but the size of the muscle tissue increases, the capillary density is reduced. Each capillary must now supply a greater fibre area with oxygen and nutrients, a factor which may account for the relatively poor aerobic capacity of athletes who train solely for strength.

Alterations in muscle energy stores have been reported following resistance training programmes. Increased intramuscular stores of adenosine triphosphate (ATP) and creatine phosphate (CP) have been reported

(MacDougall et al., 1977). Similarly, increases in two of the enzymes of anaerobic glycolysis (phosphofructokinase and lactate dehydrogenase) have been reported (Costill et al., 1979). Increases in phosphogen stores and the enzymes of anaerobic glycolysis could be expected to prolong the maintenance of a maximal muscle contraction (Bandy, Lovelace-Chandler and McKitrick-Bandy, 1990).

Neurogenic changes

Significant strength gains may be made at the beginning of a strength training programme without noticeable changes in muscle size. The increase in strength is thought to be the result of more efficient activation of the motor units (Astrand and Rodahl, 1986). As Sale (1988) stated 'strength has been said to be determined not only by the quantity and quality of the involved muscle mass, but also by the extent to which the muscle mass has been activated'.

Increased EMG activity occurs during maximal muscle contraction following a resistance training programme, indicating an increased recruitment of motor units and a greater firing rate (Bandy, Lovelace-Chandler and McKitrick-Bandy, 1990). For a muscle to produce its greatest force, all of the motor units it contains must be recruited. Normally, high threshold motor units are only recruited in periods of extreme need, with the smaller motor units being recruited first. The small slow oxidative (SO) fibres are recruited at low force levels, while the fast glycolytic (FG) fibre may not be recruited until 90% of maximum force production is reached. Between these two extremes lower threshold FG and fast oxidative glycolytic (FOG) fibres are recruited (Fig. 6.7a).

In addition to enhanced recruitment, an increase in firing rate (frequency) of motor units is also seen. A single nerve impulse will cause an isolated twitch response, while a number of impulses are required to produce a sustained contraction (Fig. 6.7b). The greater the excitation of a motoneurone the greater the firing rate of the motor unit in impulses per second (Hz). Motor units fire at rates of between 10–60 Hz, with large increases in force seen for small increases in frequency at the lower end of the spectrum. At the higher end (Fig. 6.7c), increasing the frequency of motor unit excitation has little effect on force production.

With strength training, a subject may gain the ability to recruit the large motor units more easily and so increase the muscle force production. In addition, the firing rate of the motor units utilized in a contraction may be enhanced with training.

Motor unit synchronization (groups of motor units being activated together) has been shown to be greater in strength athletes than control subjects, and is likely to increase as a result of a resistance training programme. This change is more likely to increase the rate of force development rather than peak force itself (Sale, 1988).

Evidence for neural adaptation following strength training comes from EMG studies which show increased activation of prime movers, as a result of improved skill and coordination. For example, during plyometric exercise (see p. 128) the high stretch load can result in a period of inhibition at the start of the eccentric phase while the trained individual shows facilitation possibly as an adaptation of reflex response (Sale, 1992).

Activation of the prime mover may be limited by insufficient motivation, or inhibition. During new strength tasks, excessive co-contraction may occur to stabilize and protect the moving joints. Simultaneous contraction of the antagonist will reduce the force output of the agonist through reciprocal inhibition. Training could reduce the co-contraction and allow greater activation of the agonist muscle group resulting in a greater force output (Sale, 1988).

Such inhibition may explain the phenomenon of *bilateral deficit* (Sale, 1992). In a weight-training exercise, which requires the

Figure 6.7 Neural adaptation to strength training. (a) The size of motor unit recruitment. The small slow twitch oxidative (SO) motor units are recruited at low force levels. The largest high threshold fast twitch glycolytic (FG) are not recruited until 90% maximal force is obtained. Between these two extremes are the lower threshold FG units and the fast twitch oxidative glycolytic (FOG). For each line, the low point shows the recruitment threshold, and the high point shows the maximum firing rate obtained with maximum contraction force. (b) Effect of firing rate on muscle force. A single impulse from the axon to the muscle creates a twitch contraction giving a low force output. A high frequency train of impulses (high firing rate) creates a longer tetanic contraction, giving a force which is 10 times greater. (c) Force – frequency curve. At low frequencies small increases in frequency give very large increases in force. At high frequencies the reverse is true, and doubling the frequency from 50 Hz to 100 Hz gives virtually no corresponding increase in force. From Sale (1992).

simultaneous use of both limbs (for example, the squat, leg press, or arm pressing movements), the total force which a subject can produce is often considerably less than the sum of the force of the individual limbs acting alone. In contrast to this inhibitory interlimb effect, *cross-education* represents an overflow of chronic changes from the work-ing muscle to the non-working muscle. This is commonly seen in rehabilitation where an injured muscle may be enhanced by working its uninjured counterpart. Both bilateral deficit and cross-education represent neural adaptation as there are often no significant morphological changes.

Increases in load may occur in resistance training without substantial elevations in strength. Rutherford (1988) cited an example of subjects training on a leg extension exercise. Improvements of 200% in load lifted were accompanied by strength increases of only 11%. He argued that increased coordination of muscles used as 'fixators' in the leg extension movement could account for the improved weight training ability.

Whatever the exact mechanisms involved, it seems clear that neural adaptation is largely responsible for the initial strength gains following a resistance training programme. Gains made later on are more likely to result from muscle hypertrophy. In addition, neural adaptation is likely to be one of the factors leading to specificity of strength training.

Specificity of strength training

Maximum force production from a muscle is then a result of a blend of myogenic and neurogenic adaptations which are specific to a particular movement pattern. Improvements in contractile properties, such as maximum force, velocity of shortening and rate of tension development, can vary with the type of contraction used in training (McArdle, Katch and Katch, 1986). Training a muscle to perform in a particular movement is not simply a question of overloading it against a resistance. For example, strengthening the leg muscles with a squatting exercise will not increase the performance on a leg extension movement to the same degree as training the same muscles on a leg extension bench. To strengthen a muscle for a specific movement, an exercise must mimic the movement as closely as possible. Similarly, strength gains resulting from isometric training will be specific to the joint angle at which the training was carried out.

Training a muscle at a specific velocity will result in strength gains at speeds close to, or less than, the training velocity (Rutherford, 1988), a phenomenon known as velocity specificity. One explanation of this principle is

that before training, subjects are unable to produce maximal contractions at all velocities, and through practice they learn to fully activate their prime movers only at the velocities used during training.

Another possibility is preferential hypertrophy of one fibre type. There is little evidence for transformation of one fibre type to another, except following electrical stimulation. Preferential hypertrophy of type II fibres does occur, but at both fast and slow velocities, so the neural explanation seems more likely.

Muscle work

Muscle contractions may be categorized into two types, static (isometric) where the limb segments do not move, and dynamic (isotonic) where movement does occur. The term isotonic (same tension) is confusing however, because as the limb segments move, leverage forces change and the muscle tension varies continually.

Dynamic contractions may be subdivided into either concentric (muscle shortening) or eccentric (muscle lengthening). Isokinetic contractions are dynamic (and may be concentric or eccentric), but the speed of contraction is held constant, by continually varying the resistance. Isokinetic systems do not permit acceleration, the speed being held constant. Isoacceleration (Westing, Seger and Thorstensson, 1991) involves a subject working against a preset acceleration (concentric) or deceleration (eccentric).

The term 'isotonic' has come to be used to describe a concentric or eccentric contraction performed using free weights or a machine which offers a fixed resistance, and this convention is adhered to in this book for clarity.

During concentric contractions, alterations in leverage of the limb throughout the movement mean that the resistance imposed can be no greater than the weakest part of the muscle force curve. If the resistance exceeds the weakest point, the movement is not completed, and the subject reaches a 'sticking point'. The force generated with concentric exercise cannot therefore be maximal throughout the range.

Eccentric training

During an eccentric contraction the muscle is lengthening under active tension. Eccentric contractions are frequently used to resist gravity, the muscles being used as a 'brake'. Tensions developed during eccentric contractions are greater than those of concentric or isometric contractions, leading some authors to argue that the training effect is superior (Darden, 1975).

Greater strength increases have been demonstrated using eccentric training in comparison with concentric activity. Subjects working eccentrically for six repetitions at 120% of the concentric 1RM have been shown to produce equivalent strength gains to those performing 10 repetitions at 80% of 1RM (Johnson et al., 1976). However, the amount of muscle soreness (DOMS) encountered with pure eccentric work makes it more appropriate to start a training period with concentric contractions and progress to eccentric contractions in the final stages. In addition, training specificity and safety considerations make eccentric training in isolation less desirable.

Greater force is produced when concentric contractions are immediately preceded by eccentric contractions, due in part to the recovery of elastic energy from the series and parallel elastic components of the muscle. In running, for example, as the speed increases, the amount of force produced by muscle contraction itself will proportionally reduce (force–velocity trade-off). To compensate, the part played by elastic recoil of the muscle increases (Cavagna, 1977; Stanton and Purdam, 1989) giving the athlete 'spring in his step'.

Plyometrics

Rapid eccentric contraction used immediately before an explosive concentric action forms the basis of plyometric training. This type of training was first used in Eastern block countries in the development of speed (Verhoshanski and Chornonson, 1967). The movements involve a pre-stretch of a muscle, followed by a rapid contraction causing the athlete to move in the opposite direction. Effects are achieved in both the contractile and inert structures of the muscle.

The rapid stretch of the muscle stimulates a stretch reflex, which in turn generates greater tension within the lengthening muscle fibres. In addition to increased tension, the release of stored energy within the elastic components of the muscle makes the concentric contraction greater than it would be in isolation.

Increased tension will in turn stimulate golgi tendon organ (GTO) activity, inhibiting excitation of the contracting muscle. Desensitization of the GTO has been suggested as a possible mechanism by which plyometrics allows greater force production (Bosco and Komi, 1979).

The use of muscle contraction involving acceleration in the concentric phase and deceleration in the eccentric phase more closely matches the normal function seen in sport, and therefore has advantages in terms of training specificity. However, the rapid movements involved are not suitable in early stage training as they can be relatively uncontrolled. Machinery is becoming available which offers a combination of the safety inherent in an isokinetic system and the functional advantages of positive and negative acceleration (Seger et al., 1988; Westing, Seger and Thorstensson, 1991). In addition, the use of 'inertial training' apparatus (Voight and Draovitch, 1991), in which the weight resistance travels horizontally, makes acceleration followed by deceleration more convenient.

Practical considerations of plyometric training

Plyometric exercise is only effective when the concentric contraction occurs immediately following the pre-stretch cycle. If there is a pause in activity, some of the benefits are lost as elastic energy is wasted, and the effect of the stretch reflex is altered (Voight and Draovitch, 1991). This type of training is intense, and should only be used after a thorough warm-up, and usually at the end of an exercise programme. To perform plyometrics the athlete needs a good strength base, and his proprioceptive activity should be tested using single leg standing and single leg half squats (eyes closed, position maintained for 30 seconds) before training commences. Any detriment in proprioception may cause the athlete to fall as fatigue sets in. Safety considerations including proper clothing and footwear, and a firm non-slip sports surface are essential.

Three types of exercises are normally used, in-place, short-response, and long-response. In-place activities include such things as standing jumps, drop jumps and hopping. Short-response actions are those such as the standing broad jump, standing triple jump, and box jumps. Long-response movements include bounding, hopping, and repeated hurdle jumps. Various plyometric exercises are shown in Fig. 6.8, and in the rehabilitation examples within the clinical chapters of this book.

Although plyometric activity is primarily used for lower limb training, is does have an important place for the upper limb and trunk. Overhead throwing actions using a medicine ball, and throwing and catching from a bent-knee sit up position are examples of this.

Resistance may be added to increase the overload on the working muscles as the plyometric activity is used. Vertical jumps may be performed using light dumb-bells, or a squat/leg press machine, and horizontal movements (lateral jumps, side hops) can be overloaded using an elastic cord.

Plyometrics has its use in late stage rehabilitation, and functional pre-competitive

Figure 6.8 Examples of plyometric exercises.

testing following injury. The adaptations produced by this type of activity within a previously injured muscle are likely to make it more capable of withstanding explosive effort as encountered in sprinting and jumping activities for example. This, in turn, may reduce the risk of re-injury. Using heavy resistance exercise in late stage rehabilitation of the injured athlete may allow the limb to regain lost strength, but without plyometric activity it is likely that the limb could still break down in the competitive situation, because the strength activity does not match the speed and power of the action to be used on the field of play.

Isometric training

The term isometric literally means the same or constant (iso) length (metric). Tension is developed, but no change occurs in the external length of the muscle, and there is no movement of the object or limb segment. The external resistance can therefore be equal to the maximum tension the muscle can generate.

Isometric contractions will increase strength, but only at the joint angle at which the training is carried out (Fleck and Schutt, 1985). For more general strength training, a variety of joint angles must be used. It takes approximately four seconds for the muscle to reach maximal tension, and this contraction should be maintained for 6 seconds (Astrand and Rodahl, 1986).

The use of purely isometric training would seem to be more appropriate at the start of a rehabilitation programme, where a patient's range of movement has to be limited. As soon as dynamic muscle work can be performed safely and effectively, this should form the mainstay of the strength training programme.

Isokinetics

The fundamental feature of an isokinetic contraction, is the lack of acceleration. Speed is held constant, the name isokinetic literally meaning, iso (constant) kinetic (speed). The resistance encountered from an isokinetic system will equal the force generated by the muscles of the exercising limb. Consequently, the tension developed by a muscle exercising isokinetically can be maximal at all joint angles throughout the range of movement, providing a resistance which is totally accommodating.

Strength gains will be velocity specific (see above), and gains made at slow speeds do not carry over to movements faster than the training velocity. The faster movements used in isokinetics can reduce training time. In addition, muscle soreness following this type of exercise is minimal. The effort a subject produces can be difficult to judge, unless an accurate feedback system is available. The feedback system is also essential to maintain extrinsic motivation to perform at maximal levels.

A number of authors have indicated that strength gains using an isokinetic resistance system are superior to those from an isotonic system. However, this type of comparison is difficult because of the number of variables involved, and the results are inconclusive.

Resistance training methods

Exercise progression

As with exercise in general, strength training requires a muscle to be 'overloaded' or worked at a resistance greater than that normally encountered (Hellbrandt and Houtz, 1956). This may be achieved in a number of ways, the most common of which in the context of sports injuries is weight training.

To increase the overload placed on a muscle, and progress the exercise, a number of methods may be employed, as listed below.

1 Resistance
2 Leverage
3 Isolation
4 Gravity
5 Sets/repetitions

6   Rest interval
7   Frequency of training
8   Speed of movement
9   Range of motion
10 Duration of exercise
11 Type of muscle work
12 Group action of muscles
13 Starting length of muscle
14 Momentum/inertia

Increasing the resistance, exercise duration, and frequency will make the exercise harder, as will reducing the rest interval. Altering the effect of gravity, by inclining or declining a bench will affect the point of maximal leverage. Changing the length of the lever arm will also alter the resistance, for example arm abduction performed in the standing position will be harder with a weight bag in the hand than with one fastened to the elbow.

The relationship between length–tension and force–velocity (see above) means that altering the starting length of a muscle or the speed of movement will change the overload. For example, when performing a sit-up exercise the hip flexors and abdominal flexors will work. By bending the hips, the work of the hip flexors will be reduced, increasing the overload of the abdominal flexors.

As the speed of movement increases, the force output from the muscle is reduced. In addition, more rapid actions have more momentum and are therefore harder to stop (a safety consideration) and are performed with ballistic muscle actions.

The type of muscle work (isometric or isotonic) and the function of the muscle (agonist/fixator, etc.) can be used to great effect, as can the range of movement. Initial rehabilitation exercises, where range of movement is limited, tend to be isometric in nature, progressing to isotonic and increasing the range of motion. The motor skill involved with group muscle action makes it vital that a muscle is not simply worked as a prime mover, but as a fixator and synergist as well.

The combination of repetitions (number of complete executions of an exercise) and sets (number of repetitions grouped together) in weight training is the subject of considerable debate. In general, low numbers of repetitions have been traditionally used to increase strength while higher numbers have been favoured for endurance.

Research evidence to support this practice is conflicting. Berger (1962) found that athletes who trained for four, six and eight repetitions showed significantly greater gains in strength than those training for two, ten or twelve repetitions. Clarke and Stull (1970) and Stull and Clarke (1970) showed that both types of training produced gains in both strength and endurance. However, if both types of training produce an equal gain in strength and endurance, clearly using low repetitions is more economical in terms of time.

A number of combinations of sets and repetitions have been developed, the most widely used probably being that of DeLorme and Watkins (1948).

Weight training programmes

DeLorme and Watkins

This method requires the user to first discover the maximum weight which can be lifted ten times—the 10 repetition maximum (10RM). The programme then consists of three sets of ten repetitions at percentages of this maximal value, as follows:

1   1st set, 10 repetitions at 50% of 10RM
2   2nd set, 10 repetitions at 75% of 10RM
3   3rd set, 10 repetitions at 100% of 10RM.

The DeLorme and Watkins programme enables the movement to be rehearsed before a maximal contraction is required, perhaps recognizing the importance of neurogenic factors in strength performance.

Pyramid system

In this routine, the number of repetitions performed with each set is reduced as the weight increases, the subject working on a 'light to heavy' system. This results in the athlete performing a few repetitions to fatigue when the muscle is thoroughly warm. An example is given below:

1 1st set, 12 repetitions at 50% maximum
2 2nd set, 8 repetitions at 65% maximum
3 3rd set, 6 repetitions at 75% maximum, or to fatigue.

Oxford technique

This is the reverse of the pyramid system, now the user adopts a 'heavy to light' system starting by performing 10 repetitions at their 10RM and reducing to 75% and 50% of this value.

1 1st set, 10 repetitions at 100% 10RM
2 2nd set, 10 repetitions at 75% 10RM
3 3rd set, 10 repetitions at 50% 10RM.

The Oxford technique (Zinovieff, 1951) works on the principle that as the muscle fatigues, the weight should be reduced to take account of the reduction in force output.

DAPRE technique

Knight (1979) recommended that the resistance to be lifted should be based on previous performance. The technique of daily adjusted progressive resistance exercise (DAPRE) determines when, and by how much, to increase the weight and allows for individual differences in the rate of strength development as shown below.

1 1st set, 10 repetitions 50% working weight
2 2nd set, 6 repetitions 75% working weight
3 3rd set, maximum number of repetitions with working weight
4 4th set, maximum number of repetitions with adjusted working weight

Four sets are performed as indicated in Table 6.5, the first two sets being ten and then six repetitions with one half and then three quarters of the 'working weight'. This is roughly a 6RM, and is determined from previous performance. In the third set, the weight is adjusted depending on the number of repetitions which could be performed. For example, if in the third set the athlete is able to lift the weight only five times, the weight used in the fourth set will be the same. If he or she were able to perform ten repetitions in the third set, the weight is increased by 2.5 to 5 kg. The number of repetitions performed during the fourth set with this adjusted weight determine the new working weight to be used in the next training session.

High intensity strength training

For a muscle to work maximally, during the final set an athlete should not stop training simply because a certain number of repetitions have been performed, but only when no more can be performed. In this way voli-

Table 6.5 Guidelines for adjusting weight in the DAPRE technique

Number of repetitions performed in third set	Adjusted working weight (fourth set)	Next session
-2	Deduct 2.5–5 kg	Deduct 2.5–5 kg
3–4	Deduct 0–2.5 kg	Same weight
5–6	Same weight	Add 2.5–5 kg
7–10	Add 2.5–5 kg	Add 2.5–7.5 kg
10–11	Add 5–7.5 kg	Add 5–10 kg

tional fatigue rather than number of repetitions determines the extent of the set.

If maximal work can be performed in a single set, multiple sets may not be necessary. Various authors (Hurley et al., 1984a and b; Messier and Dill, 1985; Braith et al., 1989) have shown that high intensity weight training using a single set of seven to ten repetitions performed to volitional fatigue can produce strength gains comparable to traditional multiset systems.

Braith et al. (1989) found that a single set of high intensity exercise was effective in developing isometric strength. A training programme consisting of one set of 7–10 repetitions, with maximal effort resulted in isometric strength gains greater than those achieved by other authors (O'Shea, 1963; Smith and Melton, 1981), with traditional multiset programmes.

Hurley et al. (1984a) showed strength increases of 33% for lower body and 50% for upper body, when using a single set of 8–12 repetitions performed to volitional fatigue. Silvester et al. (1982) found that one set of arm curls performed to volitional fatigue was as effective at increasing biceps strength as three sets at maximal weights.

Messier and Dill (1985) also showed a single set performed to volitional fatigue produced greater mean values of amount of weight lifted, than three sets at sub-maximal weight. The duration of training in this study was 20 minutes, compared to 50 minutes required for a multiple set programme.

High intensity strength training, although effective, may not be appropriate for early rehabilitation when pain will limit the intensity of training which an athlete is capable of.

Circuit training

Circuit training (Morgan and Adamson, 1962) consists of a series of exercises performed in a continuous sequence, with a minimum rest period in between. Initially, an individual carries out a performance test on each exercise to his or her maximum capacity. The score obtained determines the number of repetitions to be performed during training. In this manner individuals of differing fitness levels are able to train together, each performing the same exercises but at different levels of difficulty.

A variety of free exercises or apparatus may be used, incorporating different fitness components. Exercises for strength (push ups, chins) may be interspersed with flexibility (straight leg raise), stamina (jogging), speed (throwing a medicine ball) and skill (flamingo balance). Specificity of training may be enhanced by mimicking the actions involved in a particular sport. For example, a circuit may be set up on a football pitch involving short sprints, zig-zag running, dribbling skills and shooting skills, in addition to upper body and trunk work. The circuit may be progressed by altering the frequency (number of complete circuits), intensity (resistance, percentage of VO_2 max, range of motion) or duration (number of repetitions) of the various exercises. Either the number of repetitions may be dictated, in which case the aim is to complete the circuit as quickly as possible, or the time is specified with the aim of performing the greatest number of repetitions. An example of a typical circuit is given in Fig. 6.9.

One specific type of exercise may be used, as with circuit weight training (CWT) using only resistance training apparatus. Less emphasis is placed on heavy overload or a single muscle group, and instead a more general fitness programme is obtained. CWT involves alternating the body part worked (arms/legs/trunk) to prevent fatigue of one muscle group. Various types of work–rest ratio may be used. Typical combinations would be eight or more exercises, with a weight of 40–55% 1RM. As many repetitions as possible should be performed for 30 seconds, with a rest of 15 seconds (McArdle, Katch and Katch, 1986).

Hamstring stretch
(20)
(30)
(40) seconds hold.
Hold position for (seconds)

Sit-up with knees bent
(10)
(12)
(15) repetitions

Chins (5)
(7)
(9) repetitions

Lunge (10)
(12)
(15) repetitions

Alternate leg thrust (15)
(20)
(25) repetitions

Spinal extension   (8)
(10)
(12) repetitions

Zig-zag between cones
(5)
(8)
(10) repetitions

Flamingo balance
(20)
(30)
(40) seconds hold

Push up (10)
(15)
(20) repetitions

Figure 6.9 Circuit training. Example of a general circuit, with values for beginners (top), intermediates (middle) and advanced (bottom) athletes.

Increase in cardiopulmonary (CP) fitness has been shown with CWT, but it is dependent on rest period, exercise intensity, exercise type and total work. Allen, Byrd and Smith (1976) failed to show significant changes in VO_2 max using 30-second work and 60-second rest periods, the long rest period allowing too much recovery. A programme using a shorter rest period (15 seconds) showed an increase of 11% VO_2 max in women but no significant change in men (Wilmore, Parr and Girandola, 1978). Here, the rest period was short enough, but the exercise intensity for the men was not adequate. The women worked at 87.6% of their VO_2 max, but the men at only 78.2% of theirs. Longer training programmes have been shown to produce better results in terms of VO_2 max improvement (Pollock et al., 1969), and Gettman, Ayres and Pollock,

(1978) showed a 3.5% increase in VO_2 max after a 20-week CWT programme. Subjects performed at 50% of their maximum strength in a 30-minute programme, which progressed from 10 to 20 repetitions with a rest period which was reduced from 30 to 20 seconds.

Slow speed (60°/s) isokinetic CWT has been shown to be better than high speed (120°/s) training at increasing cardiopulmonary fitness (Gettman and Ayres, 1978). This reflects the importance of the total work performed during the circuit. Athletes using slow speed training worked for a longer period than those using the high speed programme.

Improvements in VO_2 max are not as great with CWT as with running. Average values after a 20-week programme being 3.5% for CWT compared with 35% for running (Gettman and Pollock, 1981). However, the real value of CWT is to maintain cardiopulmonary fitness when an athlete is unable to run or perform other cardiopulmonary fitness activities due to lower limb injury. In a study comparing CWT with running, Gettman, Ayres and Pollock (1979) examined subjects who worked for 8-week periods firstly at CWT, then on a running programme, and finally on either running or CWT. Improvement in VO_2 max obtained by running were preserved with CWT, and both groups maintained cardiopulmonary fitness to the same levels. Increases in lean body mass, reductions in bodyfat, and strength improvements have all been shown with CWT (Gettman and Pollock, 1981).

Kinetic chain exercise

Movement of the limbs occurs as a kinetic chain. Several joints arranged in sequence move together to produce a complex motor action. If the terminal joint in the kinetic chain can move freely, the chain is open. If this same joint is unable to move independently because if faces a significant resistance, the action constitutes a closed kinetic chain. Most functional activities involving the lower limb in sport are performed using a closed kinetic chain. Walking, running, jumping, and rising from a sitting position are all examples of closed kinetic chain activities. The only open kinetic chain activity of the lower limb normally used in sport is kicking.

We have seen the importance of exercise specificity in terms of muscle work and energy system, but the exercise must also be specific to the type of kinetic chain action used. To exercise the quadriceps on a leg extension bench (open chain) does not accurately reflect the demands placed on the lower limb with running and jumping (closed chain). As many of the adaptations produced during resistance training, particularly in the first four weeks of training, are neurogenic in nature the mismatch in movement patterns could detrimentally affect the athlete's performance (Palmitier, Scott and Chao, 1991).

A common open chain movement used in knee training is the seated leg extension exercise. The muscles primarily responsible for this action are the quadriceps. Contrast this to the closed chain movement of the squat. When the leg extends to raise the body from the squatting position the hamstrings extend the hip and assist in knee extension as the foot is stabilized. This co-contraction (co-activation) greatly reduces the anterior shear forces acting on the knee, and is of particular importance in the rehabilitation of anterior cruciate ligament (ACL) repairs (see p. 260).

Several additional differences exist between open (single joint or 'isolation') and closed chain (multijoint or 'general') exercises in resistance training. In an open chain action, movement occurs mainly distal to the joint axis, whereas with a closed chain action motion is both proximal and distal to the joint. An open chain action primarily emphasizes concentric work, but a closed chain movement brings a more balanced action of concentric, eccentric and isometric contractions into play.

Proprioceptive neuromuscular facilitation

This technique uses mass movement patterns to more closely simulate normal activity. Proprioceptive neuromuscular facilitation (PNF) techniques combine movements in diagonal patterns utilizing one of each of the following, flexion/extension, adduction/abduction and internal/external rotation. The various combinations for the upper and lower limbs are summarized in Fig. 6.10.

Each diagonal movement takes advantage of the anatomical position of the major muscles involved in the action, enabling them to completely shorten from a fully stretched starting position (Voss, Ionta and Myers, 1985). For example, flexion-adduction-external rotation of the leg is accomplished primarily by those muscles which are anteriorly and medially positioned. The component of the combined action which stretches the muscle most will determine the muscles action. Therefore, in the example above, a muscle may act primarily as a flexor, sec-ondly as an adductor and thirdly as an external rotator. For example, to achieve the greatest stretch on psoas, the leg is positioned in extension, abduction and internal rotation, and contracted to its shortest position by the opposing action (flexion-adduction-external rotation).

In addition to the position of the muscle, the timing of the muscle contraction is important. Normal timing aims at a smooth maximum contraction throughout the range, using accommodating manual resistance. Rotation begins the action, and the movement continues initially with the distal joints and then the proximal. Instead of normal timing, 'timing for emphasis' may be used. This technique employs the principle of irradiation or overflow to allow the athlete's stronger muscles to facilitate the weaker ones. This may be achieved by using manual resistance to prevent the strongest muscles in a group from moving the limb on their own. As the movement is performed, a greater resistance is offered to the stronger muscles in the hope that some stimulus will overflow to the weaker muscles encouraging them to contract more forcefully.

The third method is that of slow reversals. This uses the principle of successive induction, which demonstrates that immediately following a flexor withdrawal reflex the extensor thrust is stronger. Carrying this over to volitional movement, the motion required is immediately preceded by an action exactly opposite with the result that the final pattern is produced more strongly (Atkinson, 1986).

These techniques, although originally designed for use with patients suffering from neurological conditions, adapt well to the rehabilitation of sports injuries. For example, with lower limb re-strengthening a flexion-adduction-lateral rotation movement may be combined with knee extension. This movement is far more functional than a simple leg extension action using a multistation weight training machine. Where quadriceps weakness is the major problem, the

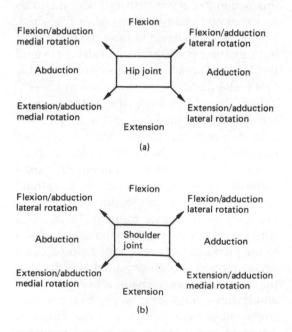

Figure 6.10   PNF patterns. (a) Hip joint. (b) Shoulder joint. After Hollis (1977).

'timing for emphasis' procedure may be used to focus on the knee extensors. Similarly, extension-abduction-medial rotation, combined with knee flexion may be used to precede the movement in a 'slow reversal' technique. Initially, manual resistance is used, but as rehabilitation progresses, a weight and pulley system may be used attaching a strap around the foot and ankle.

The use of muscle reflexes to facilitate stretching with PNF techniques such as contract-relax (CR) and contract-relax-agonist-contract (CRAC) is described on p. 120.

Implications for rehabilitation

The evidence on mixtures of sets, repetitions and types of muscle work indicates that no single combination yields optimal gains for everyone. In early rehabilitation, where range of motion is severely limited, isometric exercise is useful. Performing this type of exercise in inner range will contribute to joint stability, and it is important that this be obtained before resisted movement is begun.

Because isometric gains are joint angle specific, resistance training should progress rapidly to involve all types of muscle work. At the beginning of a weight-training programme we have seen that neurogenic changes predominate. Practising the skilled movement involved in the exercise is therefore important at this stage, so multiset regimes are likely to be more successful. As rehabilitation progresses, all the fitness components must be worked. Power and speed are important and should be combined with rapid eccentric contractions in plyometric routines. Cardiopulmonary fitness may be maintained using circuit weight training, where lower limb injury prevents activities such as running, cycling or swimming.

For pure strength gains, high intensity programmes are more suitable for well-motivated individuals. Those who are poorly motivated may not be able to perform maximally in one set and so would be better to stay on more traditional multiset programmes.

For a weight training exercise to be maximal throughout the range of motion, the resistance offered to the muscle must change. Some form of accommodating resistance provided by an asymmetric cam or electronic braking system may be useful. Alternatively, free weights using bodybuilding techniques such as 'forced repetitions' and 'cheating repetitions' can be used. Here, a training partner or body swing, respectively, is used to take the weight through the point of maximal leverage traditionally called the 'sticking point'.

Specificity of training makes it of paramount importance that exercise mimics as closely as possible the function which will be required of the athlete. At this stage sports specific skills should be practised in preference to pure strength work.

Muscle pain

Muscle pain occurs under normal circumstances with exercise, and does not necessarily indicate injury. Two types of pain are generally recognized. First, pain which occurs during exercise, but disappears when the activity stops (ischaemic pain). Secondly, with unaccustomed exercise, discomfort may not occur immediately afterwards, but pain comes on a number of days later (delayed onset muscle soreness).

Ischaemic muscle pain

Pain of this type begins in the working muscle and increases in intensity as exercise continues. It disappears when exercise stops and generally leaves no after-effects. The rise in intramuscular pressure during exercise can compress the blood vessels running through a muscle producing ischaemic pain.

The accumulation of metabolites is generally accepted to be the cause of the pain. Lactic acid is often cited as the culprit, but patients who are unable to produce lactic acid (McArdles syndrome) still suffer ischaemic pain. Histamine, acetylcholine, serotonin (5–HT), potassium and bradykinin are the most likely agents to cause the pain of ischaemia (Newham, 1991).

Delayed onset muscle soreness

Delayed onset muscle soreness (DOMS) is residual muscle pain which occurs 24–48 hours following unaccustomed bouts of intense exercise. Eccentric muscle work, and exercise with a long muscle length have been shown to increase the intensity of the delayed onset soreness (Talag, 1973; Newman et al., 1983; Clarkson and Byrnes, 1986; Jones, Newham and Torgan, 1989). A number of possibilities exist for the cause of this pain, and it is probable that a combination of factors occur, the contribution of each being related to activity type and individual differences.

Mechanical trauma can develop as a result of the high tensions developed during eccentric contractions (Newman et al., 1983). More trauma is likely with eccentric work than with other muscle actions, because the tensions created during eccentric contraction are usually greater. In a study of downhill running, increases in creatine kinase and myoglobin were seen, suggesting that structural damage was occurring within the muscle (Byrnes and Clarkson, 1985).

Disruption seems to be to the connective tissue elements, rather than the contractile tissue within the active muscles. McArdle, Katch and Katch (1986) cited an example where hydroxyproline, a product of connective tissue breakdown, was detected in the urine of subjects suffering from DOMS. They suggested that this is indicative of damage around the muscle or an imbalance of collagen metabolism. This disruption, and similar damage to tendons within the musculotendinous unit can give rise to pain (Abraham, 1979; McArdle, Katch and Katch, 1986). The connective tissue surrounding the muscle, when damaged, becomes more permeable allowing excess leakage of muscle enzymes and an increased uptake of injected radio-isotopes (Newham, 1991).

Unaccustomed exercise can also produce a build-up of metabolites within the working muscle. This in turn will give rise to osmotic changes in the cellular environment of the muscle resulting in fluid retention and subsequent pressure on sensory nerves. Similarly, ischaemia of the working muscle can occur leading to an accumulation of pain (p) substance, bringing on reflex muscle spasm (DeVries, 1961; Abraham, 1977).

Metabolite build-up or ischaemia is thought to be partially responsible for the pain of DOMS, but is unlikely to be the sole cause of the condition (Byrnes and Clarkson, 1985; McArdle, Katch and Katch, 1986).

A number of methods have been suggested to relieve DOMS. Stretching has been shown to reduce pain in the anterior tibial muscles (DeVries, 1961). Increasing the blood flow to the muscle during the warm down period is also helpful. This can be achieved by gentle exercise, hot showers, or massage. In each case, a possible mechanism of relief is that of flushing fresh blood through the muscle to remove metabolic wastes, and pumping the lymphatic vessels to remove local oedema and reduce interstitial pressure.

Muscle fatigue

Muscular fatigue has been defined by Edwards (1981) as 'a failure to maintain the required or expected force', during muscular contraction. Changes in muscle function associated with fatigue include loss of force or power output, slowing of relaxation, changes in contractile characteristics, and alterations in electrical properties (Gibson and Edwards, 1985).

Two basic mechanisms of fatigue have been described, central and peripheral.

Central fatigue refers to changes occurring proximal to the motor neurone, and involves neural and psychological changes such as motivation, and recruitment. Peripheral fatigue involves the motor unit itself, and occurs chiefly through exhaustion of the muscle energy supplies. The type and intensity of activity being performed will decide whether central and peripheral fatigue occur separately or in combination.

If a subject is told to push as hard as he or she can for as long as possible, without feedback, his or her force output will fall due to fatigue. If central fatigue occurs, more force can only be generated when the muscle is stimulated electrically.

Traditionally, fatigue types have been studied by comparing forces generated by maximum stimulated contraction (MStC), with those of maximal voluntary contractions (MVC). In unfatigued muscle, the MVC is the same as the MStC. With central fatigue, the force produced during MVC is less than that from an MStC, while in peripheral fatigue there is no difference between force of MVC and MStC (Bigland-Ritchie, 1981).

Peripheral fatigue can be further categorized into high and low frequency types. The natural firing frequencies of normal voluntary contractions are approximately 5–30 Hz. High frequency fatigue occurs when a muscle is stimulated at high frequencies between 50–100 Hz, while low frequency fatigue is the loss of force at low stimulation frequencies between 10 and 40 Hz.

References

Abraham, W.M. (1977) Factors in delayed onset muscle soreness. *Medicine and Science in Sports*, **9**(1), 11–20

Abraham, W.M. (1979) Exercise induced muscle soreness. *Physician and Sports Medicine*, **7**(10), 57–60

Adams, J.A. (1961) The second facet of forgetting. A review of warm-up decrement. *Psychological Bulletin*, **58**, 257–273

Allen, T.E., Byrd, R.J. and Smith, D.P. (1976) Hemodynamic consequences of circuit weight training. *Research Quarterly*, **47**, 299–306

American College of Sports Medicine (1978) The recommended quantity and quality of exercise for developing and maintaining fitness in healthy adults. *Medicine and Science in Sports and Exercise*, **10**, VII–X

American College of Sports Medicine (1990) The recommended quantity and quality of exercise for developing and maintaining cardiorespiratory and muscular fitness in healthy adults. *Medicine and Science in Sports and Exercise*, **22**, 265–274

Andzel W.D. (1982) One mile run performance as a function of prior exercise. *Journal of Sports Medicine*, **22**, 80–84

Andzel, W.D. and Gutin, B. (1976) Prior exercise and endurance performance: a test of the mobilisation hypothesis. *Research Quarterly*, **47**(3), 269–276

Ashton, D. and Davies, B. (1986) *Why Exercise?* Basil Blackwell, London

Astrand, P-O. and Rodahl, K. (1986) *Textbook of Work Physiology*, McGraw-Hill, Maidenhead

Atkinson, H.W. (1986) Principles of treatment. In *Cash's Textbook of Neurology for Physiotherapists*, 4th edn (ed. P.A. Downie), Faber and Faber, London. pp. 147–219

Bandy, W.D., Lovelace-Chandler, V. and McKitrick-Bandy, B. (1990) Adaptation of skeletal muscle to resistance training. *Journal of Orthopaedic and Sports Physical Therapy*, **12**(6), 248–255

Barcroft, H. and Ebholm, O.G. (1943) The effect of temperature on blood flow and deep temperature in the human forearm. *Journal of Physiology*, **102**, 5–20

Barnard, R.J., Gardner, G.W., Diaco, N.V., MacAlpin, R.N. and Kattus, A.A. (1973) Cardiovascular responses to sudden strenuous exercise: Heart rate, blood pressure, and ECG. *Journal of Applied Physiology*, **34**, 883

Berger, R.A. (1962) Effect of varied weight training programmes of strength. *Research Quarterly*, **33**, 168–181

Bergh, U. (1980) Human power at subnormal body temperatures. *Acta Physiologica Scandinavica*, **478**(Suppl.), 1–39

Bergh, U. and Ekblom B. (1979a) Physical performance and peak aerobic power at different body temperatures. *Journal of Applied Physiology*, **46**, 885–889

Bergh, U. and Ekblom, B. (1979b) Influence of muscle temperature on maximal muscle strength and power output in human skeletal muscles. *Acta Physiologica Scandinavica*, **107**, 33–37

Bigland-Ritchie, B. (1981) EMG and fatigue of human voluntary and stimulated contractions. In *Human Muscle Fatigue: Physiological Mechanisms* (eds R. Porter and J. Whelan), Ciba Foundation Symposium 82, Pitman Medical, London

Bonner, H.W. (1974) Preliminary exercise: a two-factor theory. *Research Quarterly*, **45**, 138–147

Borms, J. (1984) Importance of flexibility in overall physical fitness. *International Journal of Physical Education*, **11**, 2

Borms, J., Van Roy, P., Santens, J-P. and Haentjens, A. (1987) Optimal duration of static exercises for improvement of coxofemoral flexibility. *Journal of Sports Science*, **5**, 39–47

Bosco, C. and Komi, P.V. (1979) Potentiation of the mechanical behaviour of the human skeletal muscle through pre-stretching. *Acta Physiologica Scandinavica*, **106**, 467

Bray, J.J., Cragg, P.A., Macknight, A.D.C., Mills, R.G. and Taylor, D.W. (1986) *Lecture Notes on Human Physiology*, Blackwell Scientific, Oxford

Byrnes, W.C. and Clarkson, M.C. (1985) Delayed onset muscle soreness following repeated bouts of downhill running. *Journal of Applied Physiology*, **59**, 283

Carlile, F. (1956) Effect of preliminary passive warming on swimming performance. *Research Quarterly*, **27**(2), 143–151

Cavagna, G.A. (1977) Storage and utilisation of elastic energy in skeletal muscle. *Exercise and Sports Sciences Reviews*, **5**, 89–129

Clarke, D.H. and Stull, G.A. (1970) Endurance training as a determinant of strength and fatigability. *Research Quarterly*, **41**, 19–26

Clarkson, P.M. and Byrnes, K.M. (1986) Muscle soreness and serum creatine kinase activity following isometric, eccentric, and concentric exercise. *International Journal of Sports Medicine*, **7**, 152–155

Cornelius, W.L. and Hinson, M.M. (1980) The relationship between isometric contraction of hip extensors and subsequent flexibility in males. *Journal of Sports Medicine and Physical Fitness*, **20**, 75–80

Costill, D.L., Fink, W.J., Getchell, L.H., Ivy, J.L. and Witzmann, F.A. (1979) Lipid metabolism in muscle of endurance trained males and females. *Journal of Applied Physiology: Respiratory, Environmental and Exercise Physiology*, **47**, 787

Cureton, T.K. (1941) Flexibility as an aspect of physical fitness. *Research Quarterly*, **12**(Suppl.), 381–390

Darden, E. (1975) Positive and negative work. *Scholastic Coach*, **45**, 6–12 and 85–86

Davies, C.T.M. and Young, K. (1983) Effect of temperature on contractile properties and muscle power of triceps surae in humans. *Journal of Applied Physiology*, **55**, 191–195

DeLorme, T. and Watkins, A. (1948) Techniques of progressive resistance exercise. *Archives of Physical Medicine and Rehabilitation*, **29**, 263–273

DeVries, H.A. (1959) Effects of various warm-up procedures on 100 yard times of competitive swimmers. *Research Quarterly*, **30**, 11–20

DeVries, H.A. (1961) Prevention of muscular distress after exercise. *Research Quarterly*, **32**, 177

DeVries, H.A. (1962) Evaluation of static stretching procedures for improvement of flexibility. *Research Quarterly*, **33**, 222–229

DeVries. H.A. (1980) *Physiology of Exercise for Physical Education and Athletics*, William C. Brown, Dubuque

Edwards, R.H.T. (1981) Human muscle function and fatigue. In *Human Muscle Fatigue: Physiological Mechanisms* (eds R. Porter and J. Whelan), Ciba Foundation Symposium 82, Pitman Medical, London

Ekstrand, J. and Gillquist, J. (1982) The frequency of muscle tightness and injuries in soccer players. *American Journal of Sports Medicine*, **10** (March–April), 75–78

Ekstrand, J., Gillquist, J., Moller, M. et al. (1983) Incidence of soccer injuries and their relation to training and team success. *American Journal of Sports Medicine*, **11**, (March–April) 63–67

Enoka, R.M. (1994) *Neuromechanical Basis of Kinesiology*, 2nd edn, Human Kinetics, Champaign, Illinois

Etnyre, B.R. and Abraham, L.D. (1986) H-reflex changes during static stretching and two variations of proprioceptive neuromuscular facilitation techniques. *Electroencephalography and Clinical Neurophysiology*, **63**, 174–179

Etnyre, B.R. and Lee E.J. (1987) Comments on proprioceptive neuromuscular facilitation stretching. *Research Quarterly for Exercise and Sport*, **58**(2), 184–188

Fleck, S.J. and Schutt, R.C. (1985) Types of strength training. *Clinics in Sports Medicine*, **4**(1), 159–169

Gettman, L.R. and Ayres, J.J. (1978) Aerobic changes through 10 weeks of slow and fast speed isokinetic training (abstract). *Medicine and Science in Sports and Exercise*, **10**, 47

Gettman, L.R. and Pollock, M.L. (1981) Circuit weight training: A critical review of its physiological benefits. *The Physician and Sports Medicine*, **9**(1), 44–60

Gettman, L.R., Ayres, J.J. and Pollock, M.L. (1978) The effect of circuit weight training on strength, cardiorespiratory function, and body composition of adult men. *Medicine and Science in Sports and Exercise*, **10**, 171–176

Gettman, L.R., Ayres, J.J. and Pollock, M.L. (1979) Physiological effects on adult men of circuit strength training and jogging. *Archives of Physical Medicine and Rehabilitation*, **60**, 115–120

Gibson, H. and Edwards, R.H.T. (1985) Muscular exercise and fatigue. *Sports Medicine*, **2**, 120–132

Goldberg, B., Saranitia, A. and Witman, P. (1980) Preparticipation sports assessment – an objective evaluation. *Pediatrics*, **66**, 736–745

Gutin, B. and Stewart, K. (1971) Prior exercise and endurance. Physiology meeting. Springfield, Mass. Cited in Gutin et al. (1976)

Gutin, B., Stewart, K., Lewis, S. and Kruper, J. (1976) Oxygen consumption in the first stages of strenuous work as a function of prior exercise. *Journal of Sports Medicine*, **9**, 60–65

Hardy, L. and Jones, D. (1986) Dynamic flexibility and proprioceptive neuromuscular facilitation. *Research Quarterly for Exercise and Sport*, **57**, 150–153

Harris, M.L. (1969) Flexibility: a review of the literature. *Physical Therapy*, **49**(6), 591–601

Hellebrandt and Houtz (1956) Mechanics of muscle training in man: experimental demonstration of the overload principle. *Physical Therapy Review*, **36**, 371–383

Hogberg, P. and Ljunggren, O. (1947) Uppvarmningens inverkan på lopprestationerna. *Svensk Idrott*, **40**

Holland, G.L. (1968) The physiology of flexibility: a review of the literature. In *Kinesiology Review*, pp. 49–62

Hollis, M. (1977) *Practical Exercise Therapy*, Blackwell Scientific, Oxford

Holt, L.E. and Smith, R. (1983) The effect of selected stretching programs on active and passive flexibility. Del Mar, CA: Research Center for Sport

Holt, L.E., Travis, T.T. and Okita, T. (1970) Comparative study of three stretching techinuqes. *Perceptual and Motor Skills*, **31**, 611–616

Hopper, D. (1986) A survey of netball injuries and conditions related to these injuries. *Australian Journal of Physiotherapy*, **32**(4), 231–239

Hurley, B.F., Hagberg, J.M., Allen, W.K., Seals, D.R., Young, J.C., Cuddihee, R.T. and Holloszy, J.O. (1984a) Effect of training on blood lactate levels during submaximal exercise. *Journal of Applied Physiology: Respiratory Environment, and Exercise Physiology*, **56**, 1260

Hurley, B.F., Seals, D.R., Ehsani, A.A., Cartier, L.J., Dalsky, G.P., Hagberg, J.M. and Holloszy, J.O. (1984b) Effects of high-intensity strength training on cardiovascular function. *Medicine and Science in Sports and Exercise*, **16**(5), 483–488

Janda, V. (1992) *Muscle and Back Pain – Assessment and Treatment of Impaired Movement Patterns and Motor Recruitment*, Associated Course to the 5th International Symposium of the Physical Medicine Research Foundation, Oxford

Johnson, B.L, Adamezyk, J.W, Tenmore, K.O and Stromme, S.B. (1976) A comparison of concentric and eccentric muscle training. *Medicine and Science in Sports and Exercise*, **8**, 35–38

Jones, D.A., Newham, D.J. and Torgan, C. (1989) Mechanical influences on long standing human muscle fatigue and delayed onset muscle pain. *Journal of Physiology*, **224**, 173–186

Karvonen, J. (1978) Warming up and its physiological effects. Acta Universitatis Ouluensis. Series D, No. 31. *Pharmacologica et Physiologica*, No. 6

Kent, M. (1994) *The Oxford Dictionary of Sports Science and Medicine*, Oxford University Press, Oxford

Kisner, C. and Colby, L.A. (1990) *Therapeutic Exercise. Foundations and Techniques*, Davis, Philadelphia

Knight, K.L. (1979) Knee rehabilitation by the daily adjustable progressive resistance exercise technique. *American Journal of Sports Medicine*, **7**, 336

LaBan, M.M. (1962) Collagen tissue: implications of its response to stress in vitro. *Archives of Physical Medicine and Rehabilitation*, **43**, 461–466

Lewit K. (1991) *Manipulative Therapy in Rehabilitation of the Locomotor System*, 2nd edn, Butterworth-Heinemann, Oxford

Luithi, J.M., Howald, H., Claasen, H., Rosler, K., Vock, P. and Hoppeler, H. (1986) Structural changes in skeletal muscle tissue with heavy resistance exercise. *International Journal of Sports Medicine*, **7**, 1399–1403

MacDougall, J.D., Ward, G.R., Sale, D.G. and Sutton, J.R. (1977) Biochemical adaptation of human skeletal muscle in heavy resistance training and immobilization. *Journal of Applied Physiology*, **43**, 700–703

McArdle, W.D., Katch, F.I. and Katch, V.L. (1986) *Exercise Physiology. Energy, Nutrition, and Human Performance*, Lea and Febiger, Philadelphia

McCafferty, W.B. and Horvath, S.M. (1977) Specificity of exercise and specificity of training: a subcellular review. *Research Quarterly*, **48**, 358–371

McKenzie, R.A. (1981) *The Lumbar Spine. Mechanical Diagnosis and Therapy*, Spinal Publications, Lower Hutt, New Zealand

Messier, S.P. and Dill, M.E. (1985) Alteration in strength and maximal oxygen uptake consequent to Nautilus circuit weight training. *Research Quarterly*, **56**(4), 345–351

Morgan, R.E. and Adamson, G.T. (1962) *Circuit Training*, G. Bell and Sons, London

Nacson, J. and Schmidt, R.A. (1971) The activity-set hypothesis for warmup decrement. *Journal of Motor Behavior*, **3**, 1–15

Newham, D.J. (1991) Skeletal muscle pain and exercise. *Physiotherapy*, **77**, (1) 66–70

Newman, D.J., Mills, K.R., Quigley, B.M. and Edwards, R.H.T. (1983) Pain and fatigue after concentric and eccentric muscle contractions. *Clinical Science*, **64**, 55–62

Norris, C.M. (1994) *Flexibility. Principles and Practice*. A&C Black, London

O'Shea, P. (1963) Effects of selected weight training programs on the development of strength and muscle hypertrophy. *Research Quarterly*, **37**, 95–102

Palmitier, R.A., An, K., Scott, S.G. and Chao, E.Y.S. (1991) Kinetic chain exercise in knee rehabilitation. *Sports Medicine*, **11**(6), 402–413

Pollock, M.L., Cureton, T.K. and Greniger, L. (1969) Effects of frequency of training on working capacity, cardiovascular function and body composition of adult men. *Medicine and Science in Sports*, **1**, 70–74

Ranatunga, K.W., Sharpe, B. and Turnbull, B. (1987) Contractions of a human skeletal muscle at different temperatures. *Journal of Physiology*, **390**, 383–395

Reilly, T. (1981) The concept, measurement and development of flexibility. In *Sports Fitness and Sports Injuries* (ed. T. Reilly), Faber and Faber, London

Renstrom, P. and Kannus, P. (1992) Prevention of injuries in endurance athletes. In *Endurance in Sport* (eds R.J. Shephard and P.O. Astrand), IOC Medical Commission Publication, Blackwell Scientific, Oxford, pp. 325–350

Richards, D.K. (1968) A two factor theory of the warmup in jumping performance. *Research Quarterly*, **39**, 668–673

Rigby, B. (1964) The effect of mechanical extension under the thermal stability of collagen. *Biochimica et Biophysica Acta*, **79**, 634–636

Rutherford, O.M. (1988) Muscular coordination and strength training. Implications for injury rehabilitation. *Sports Medicine*, **5**, 196–202

Safran, M.R., Garrett, W.E., Seaber, A.V., Glisson, R.R. and Ribbecsk, B.M. (1988) The role of warmup in muscular injury prevention. *American Journal of Sports Medicine*, **16**(2) 123–129

Sale, D.G. (1988) Neural adaptation to resistance training. *Medicine and Science in Sports and Exercise*, **20**(5), 135–145

Sale, D.G. (1992) Neural adaptation to strength training. In *Strength and Power in Sport* (ed. P.V. Komi), IOC Medical Publication, Blackwell Scientific, Oxford

Sapega, A.A., Quedenfel, T.C., Moyer, R.A. and Butler R.A. (1981) Biophysical factors in range of motion exercise. *The Physician and Sports Medicine*, **9**(12), 57–65

Sargeant, A.J. (1987) Effect of muscle temperature on leg extension force and short term power output in humans. *European Journal of Applied Physiology*, **56**, 693–698

Sargeant, A.J. and Dolan, P. (1987) Effect of prior exercise on maximal short term power output in humans. *Journal of Applied Physiology*, **63**, 1475–1480

Schmidt, R.A. (1982) *Motor Control and Learning*, Human Kinetics, Champaign, Illinois

Seger, J.Y., Westing, S.H., Hanson, M., Karlson, E. and Ekblom, B. (1988) A new dynamometer measuring concentric and eccentric muscle strength in accelerated, decelerated, or isokinetic movements. *European Journal of Applied Physiology*, **57**, 526–530

Seward, H.G. and Patrick, J. (1992) A three year survey of Victorian football league injuries. *Australian Journal of Medicine and Science in Sport*, **24**(2), 51–54

Shellcok, F.G. and Prentice, W.E. (1985) Warming up and stretching for improved physical performance and prevention of sports related injuries. *Sports Medicine*, **2**, 267–278

Silvester, L.J., Stiggins, C., McGown, C. and Bryce, G. (1982) The effect of variable resistance and free-weight training programs on strength. *National Strength and Conditioning Association Journal*, **3**, 30-33

Smith, M.J. and Melton, P. (1981) Isokinetic versus isotonic variable resistance training. *Amercian Journal of Sports Medicine*, **9**(4), 275–279

Stanton, P. and Purdam, C. (1989) Hamstring injuries in sprinting – the role of eccentric exercise. *Journal of Orthopaedic and Sports Physical Therapy*, **10** (9)

Stull, G.A. and Clarke, D.H. (1970) High resistance low repetition training as a determiner of strength and fatigability. *Research Quarterly*, **41**, 189–193

Talag, T.S. (1973) Residual muscular soreness as influenced by concentric, eccentric, and static contractions. *Research Quarterly*, **44**(4), 458–469

Thorstensson, A. (1977) Observations on strength training and detraining. *Acta Physiologica Scandinavica*, **100**, 491–493

Verhoshanski, Y. and Chornonson, G. (1967) Jump exercises in sprint training. *Track and Field Quarterly*, **9**, 1909

Voight, M.L. and Draovitch, P. (1991) Plyometrics. In *Eccentric Muscle Training in Sports and Orthopaedics* (ed. M. Albert), Churchill Livingstone, London

Voss, D.E., Ionta, M.K. and Myers, B.J. (1985) *Proprioceptive Neuromuscular Facilitation: Patterns and Techniques*, Harper and Row, Philadelphia

Warren, C.G., Lehmann, J.F. and Koblanski, J.N. (1971) Elongation of rat tail tendon: effect of load and temperature. *Archives of Physical Medicine and Rehabilitation*, **51**, 465–474

Westing, S.H., Seger, J.Y. and Thorstensson, A. (1991) Isoacceleration: a new concept of resistive exercise. *Medicine and Science in Sports and Exercise*, **23**(5), 631–635

Wilmore, J.H., Parr, R.B. and Girandola, R.N. (1978) Physiological alterations consequent to circuit weight training. *Medicine and Science in Sports and Exercise*, **10**, 79–84

Zinovieff, A.N. (1951) Heavy resistance exercise, the Oxford technique. *British Journal of Physical Medicine*, **14**, 129

7

Exercise therapy

Structure vs function

Often, a student physiotherapist, new to soft tissue injury management, will focus their attention purely on structure. Equipped with a vast knowledge of anatomy they try to find which single structure has been injured. If it is a muscle tear, for example, they may note the muscle's origin and insertion and treat the muscle in isolation. When it comes to exercise, they consider the muscle's action and give this action as an exercise of some type. For example, if the hamstring muscles are torn, exercises are often given which simply involve flexing the knee against resistance and performing a toe-touching movement to stretch the muscle.

As experience is gained, the clinical physiotherapist realizes the error of this reductionist approach. If the body is reduced to a number of simple components, rehabilitation of a sporting injury is largely ineffective. The muscle may strengthen or increase in flexibility, for example, but the ability of the patient to perform the adaptations of daily living (ADL), and the athlete to participate in sport, often remains poor. The athlete with a hamstring tear treated in this way will very often find pain relieved mainly through the passage of time, but when they return to sport the injury simply recurs.

On the other hand, rather than reducing the body to simple structural components, if movement quality is the starting point for rehabilitation, the athlete's ability is rapidly enhanced. Instead of considering the textbook anatomy of an area, if the therapist asks the simple question 'how does this injury affect the athlete?' the answer will often guide the rehabilitation programme perfectly.

The functional decrement which the patient is suffering becomes the central focus, rather than the structural damage, and as a consequence, rehabilitation is considerably more successful. The athlete with the hamstring injury described above may well lack strength and flexibility, and in the early stages of rehabilitation, simple single plane motions may suffice. But if the therapist considers the function of the hamstrings in the closed kinetic chain position, the action of the muscle in ballistic movements, and the stresses imposed on a two-joint muscle, a whole series of exercises become available.

Through this approach the therapist can break away from standard lists of exercises which fail to take account of the needs of the individual. Instead of the athlete grinding away in boredom at endless repetitions of a movement, exercise therapy can become vibrant and challenging. The end result is a more rewarding period of rehabilitation for both athlete and therapist.

The aim of this chapter is therefore to develop the theme of 'functional exercise therapy', and we will begin by looking at muscle imbalance.

Muscle imbalance

Basic concepts

Changes in muscle length or strength occur throughout the body in set patterns rather than purely at random. The relationship between the tone and length of muscles around a joint is known as muscle imbalance and has been described by a number of authors (Janda and Schmid, 1980; Sahrmann, 1987; Richardson, 1992; Kendall et al., 1993; Comerford, 1995; Norris, 1995a). Muscles may be broadly classified into two types, those whose actions are mainly to stabilize a joint and approximate the joint surfaces, and those responsible more for movement, which more effectively develop angular rotation. The main differences between the two types of muscles is shown in Table 7.1.

The stability muscles tend to be more deeply placed while the mobilizers are superficial. In addition, mobilizers are often biarticular muscles. For example, in the leg the rectus femoris is classified as a mobilizer, while the quadriceps are stabilizers. Stabilizer function is more slow twitch (type I) or tonic in nature, while that of the mobilizers tends towards fast twitch (type II) phasic action. This physiology suits the functional requirements of the muscles enabling mobilizers to contract and build maximal tension rapidly, but to fatigue quickly. The stabilizers build tension slowly and perform well at lower tensions over longer periods, being more fatigue resistant.

Stabilizer muscles are better activated in closed kinetic chain actions, where movement occurs proximally on a distally stabilized segment. Mobilizer function is more effective in an open chain situation, where free movement occurs without distal fixation. The structure and functional characteristics of the two muscle categories makes the stabilizers better equipped for postural holding and anti-gravity function. The mobilizers are better set up for rapid ballistic movements.

Two of the fundamental changes seen in the muscle imbalance process include tightening of the mobilizer (two-joint) muscles and loss of endurance within the inner range for the stabilizer (single-joint) muscles. These two changes are used as tests for the degree of muscle imbalance. The combination of length and tension changes alter muscle pull around a joint and so pull the joint out of alignment. Changes in body segment alignment and the ability to perform movements, which dissociate one body segment from another, form the bases of the third type of test used when assessing muscle imbalance (Fig. 7.1).

The mixture of tightness and weakness seen in the muscle imbalance process alters body segment alignment and changes the equilibrium point of a joint. In addition, imbalance leads to lack of accurate segmen-

Table 7.1   Muscle types (basic classification)

Stability	Movement
Deep	Superficial
Slow twitch	Fast twitch
One joint	Two joint
Weaken and lengthen	Tighten and shorten
Inhibited	Preferential recruitment

Figure 7.1   Assessing muscle imbalance.

tal control. The combination of stiffness (hypoflexibility) in one body segment and laxity (hyperflexibility) in an adjacent body segment leads to the establishment of relative flexibility (White and Sahrmann, 1994). In a chain of movement the body seems to take the path of least resistance, with the more flexible segment moving first and furthest. If we take as an illustration two pieces of rubber tubing (Fig. 7.2) of unequal strengths. When the movement begins at C and A is fixed, the more flexible area B–C moves more. This will still be the case if C is held still and A moves.

Taking this example into the body, Fig. 7.3 shows a toe-touching exercise. The two areas of interest with relation to relative stiffness are the hamstrings and lumbar spine tissues. As we flex forwards, movement should occur through a combination of anterior pelvic tilt and lumbar spine flexion (see p. 165). Subjects often have tight hamstrings and looser lumbar spine tissues due to excessive bending during everyday activities. During this flexion action, greater movement and, therefore, greater tissue strain will always occur at the lumbar spine. Relative stiffness, in this case, makes the toe-touching exercise ineffective as a hamstring stretch unless the trunk muscles are tightened to stabilize the lumbar spine.

Muscle adaptation

Muscle adaptation to reduced usage has been extensively studied using immobilized limbs (Appell, 1990). The greatest tissue

Figure 7.3 Relative stiffness in the body. (a) Tighter hamstrings, more lax spinal tissues. (b) Forward flexion should combine pelvis tilt and spinal flexion equally. (c) Tight hamstrings limit pelvic tilt, throwing stress on the more lax spinal tissues.

changes occur within the first days of disuse. Strength loss has been shown to be as much as 6% per day for the first eight days with little further loss after this period (Muller, 1970). Greater reduction in size and loss of numbers is seen in type I fibres, with a parallel increase in type II fibres, demonstrating selective atrophy of type I fibres (Templeton et al., 1984). However, not all muscles show an equal amount of type I fibre atrophy. Atrophy is largely related to change in use relative to normal function, with the initial percentage of type I fibres that a muscle contains being a good indicator of likely atrophy pattern. Those muscles with a predominantly anti-gravity function, which cross one joint and have a large proportion of type I fibres, show greatest selective atrophy (e.g. soleus and vastus medialis). Those predominantly slow anti-gravity muscles which cross multiple joints are next in order of atrophy (e.g.

Figure 7.2 Relative stiffness. When the cord is stretched, the tighter segment (A–B) moves less than the looser segment (B–C).

erector spinae), while last are phasic, predominantly fast type II muscles which can be immobilized with less loss of strength (e.g. biceps) (Lieber, 1992).

These three categories of muscles have led to stabilizers being subdivided into primary and secondary types (Jull, 1994) as shown in Fig. 7.4. Examples of the three types include multifidus, transversus abdominus and vastus medialis oblique as primary stabilizers. The gluteals and oblique abdominals are classified as secondary stabilizers, while rectus femoris and the hamstrings are mobilizers, only acting as stabilizers in conditions of extreme need.

The primary stabilizers have very deep attachments, lying close to the axis of rotation of the joint. In this position they are unable to contribute any significant torque, but will approximate the joint. In addition, many of these smaller muscles have important proprioceptive functions (Bastide et al., 1989). The secondary stabilizers are the main torque producers, being large monoarticular muscles attaching via extensive aponeuroses. Their multipennate fibre arrangement makes them powerful and able to absorb large amounts of force through eccentric action. The mobilizers are fusiform in shape, with

a less powerful fibre arrangement, but one which is designed for producing large ranges of motion. In addition, the mobilizers are biarticular muscles, which have their own unique biomechanical characteristics (see p. 17).

Selective changes in muscle may also occur as a result of training (Richardson and Bullock, 1986). In the knee, rapid flexion–extension actions have been shown to selectively increase activity in the rectus femoris and hamstrings (biarticular) but not in the vasti (monoarticular). In this study, comparing speeds of 75°/s and 195°/s, mean muscle activity for the rectus femoris increased from 23.0 uV to 69.9 uV. In contrast, muscle activity for the vastus medialis increased from 35.5 uV to only 42.3 uV (Fig. 7.5). The pattern of muscle activity was also noticeably different in this study after training. At the fastest speeds the rectus femoris and hamstrings displayed phasic (on and off) activity while the vastus medialis showed a tonic (continuous) pattern (Fig. 7.6).

Even in the more functional closed kinetic chain position similar changes have been found (Ng and Richardson, 1990). A four-week training period of rapid plantar flexion in standing gave significant increases in

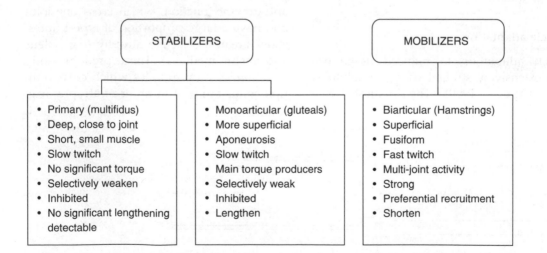

Figure 7.4 Muscle types (extended classification). After Jull (1994).

Figure 7.5 Changes in muscle activity with increases in speed. From Richardson and Bullock (1986).

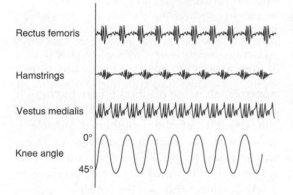

Figure 7.6 Pattern of muscle activity during rapid alternating knee flexion–extension. Biarticular muscles are phasic, monoarticular muscles are tonic. Redrawn from Richardson and Bullock (1986).

jump height (gastrocnemius, biarticular) but also significant loses of static function of the soleus (monoarticular).

Changes in muscle length

Chronic muscle lengthening

Stabilizer muscles tend to 'weaken' (sag) whereas mobilizers tend to 'shorten' (tighten). Taking these responses further, primary stabilizers will react quickly to pain and swelling, by inhibition. Swelling has been shown to cause a reflex inhibition of

muscles in the knee (de Andrade et al., 1965; Stokes and Young, 1984). In addition, marked asymmetry of the multifidus has been shown using real-time ultrasound imaging (Hides et al., 1994). The cross-sectional area (CSA) of the multifidus was substantially reduced at the level of lumbar lesion. The authors suggested that the mechanism for the CSA reduction was inhibition through perceived pain via a long loop reflex.

In addition to changes in muscle bulk, alteration in fibre type has been shown in the multifidus with low back pain (LBP) patients (Biedermann et al., 1991). A reduced ratio of slow twitch to fast twitch muscle fibres was shown, possibly as an adaptive response by the muscle to changes in functional demand placed upon it. Furthermore, injury may have caused a shift in the recruitment patterns of the motor units of the paraspinal muscles, with the fast twitch motor units being recruited before the slow twitch units.

The transversus abdominus shows a similar response in the chronic LBP patient. Normally, this muscle acts as a primary stabilizer of the lumbar spine (Jull, 1994). It is active in both flexion and extension of the lumbar spine (Cresswell et al., 1992) and during action of the upper limb and lower limb in multiple directions (Hodges, Richardson and Jull, 1996). In addition, contraction of transversus abdominus precedes that of the other abdominal and lumbar extensor muscles (Cresswell, Oddsson and Thorstensson, 1994; Hodges and Richardson, 1996a). Following LBP, transversus abdominus function changes considerably (Hodges and Richardson, 1995; Hodges, Richardson and Jull, 1996). Timing of onset of transversus contraction is delayed by a mean of 129 ms, while the action of the other abdominals is largely unchanged.

The secondary stabilizer muscles show a tendency to lengthen and weaken. As postural muscles they almost seem to give way to the pull of gravity and 'sag'. This reaction has been termed stretch weakness (Kendall et al., 1993). The muscle has remained in an elongated position, beyond its normal resting position, but within its normal range. This is differentiated from overstretch where the muscle is simply elongated or stretched beyond its normal range.

The length–tension relationship of a muscle (see p. 18) dictates that a stretched muscle, where the actin and myosin filaments are pulled apart, can exert less force than a muscle at normal resting length. Where the stretch is maintained, however, this short-term response (reduced force output) changes to a long-term adaptation. The muscle tries to move its actin and myosin filaments closer together, and to do this, it must add more sarcomeres to the ends of the muscle (Fig. 7.7). This adaptation, known as an increase in serial sarcomere number (SSN), changes the nature of the length tension curve.

Long-term elongation of this type causes a muscle to lengthen by the addition of up to 20% more sarcomeres (Gossman et al., 1982). The length–tension curve of an adaptively lengthened muscle moves to the right (Fig. 7.8). The peak tension that such a muscle can produce in the laboratory situation is up to 35% greater than that of a normal length muscle (Williams and Goldspink, 1978). However, this peak tension occurs at

Figure 7.8 Effects of immobilizing a muscle in shortened and lengthened positions. The normal length–tension curve (control) moves to the right for a lengthened muscle, giving it a peak tension some 35% greater than the control (point A). When tested in an inner range position however (point B), the muscle tests weaker than normal. After Gossman et al. (1982).

approximately the position where the muscle has been immobilized (point A, Fig. 7.8). If the strength of the lengthened muscle is tested with the joint in mid-range or inner-range (point B, Fig. 7.8), as is common clinical practice, the muscle cannot produce its peak tension, and so the muscle appears 'weak'. For this reason, manual muscle tests have been described as being more accurate indicators of positional (rather than total) strength (Sahrmann, 1987).

In the laboratory situation the lengthened muscle will return to its optimal length within approximately one week if once more placed in a shortened position (Goldspink, 1992). Clinically, restoration of optimal length may be achieved by either immobilizing the muscle in its physiological rest position (Kendall et al., 1993), and/or exercising it in its shortened (inner-range) position (Sahrmann, 1990). Enhancement of strength is not the priority in this situation, indeed the load on the muscle may need to be reduced to ensure correct alignment of the various body segments and correct performance of the relevant movement pattern.

SSN may be responsible partly for changes in muscle strength without parallel changes

Figure 7.7 Muscle length adaptation. (a) Normal muscle length. (b) Stretched muscle—filaments move apart and muscle loses tension. (c) Adaptation by increase in serial sarcomere number (SSN), normal filament alignment restored, muscle length permanently increased.

in hypertrophy (Koh, 1995). SSN exhibits marked plasticity and may be influenced by a number of factors. For example, immobilization of rabbit plantarflexors in a lengthened position showed an 8% increase in SSN in only 4 days, while applying electrical stimulation to increase muscle force showed an even greater increase (Williams et al., 1986). Stretching a muscle appears to have a greater effect on SSN than does immobilization in a shortened position. Following immobilization in a shortened position for 2 weeks, the mouse soleus has been shown to decrease SSN by almost 20% (Williams, 1990). However, stretching for just 1 hour per day in this study, not only eliminated the SSN reduction, but actually produced nearly a 10% increase in SSN. An eccentric stimulus appears to cause a greater adaptation of SSN than a concentric stimulus. Morgan and Lynn (1994) subjected rats to uphill or downhill running, and showed SSN in the vastus intermedius to be 12% greater in the eccentric trained rats after 1 week. It has been suggested that if SSN adaptation occurs in humans, strength training may produce such a change if it were performed at a joint angle different from that at which the maximal force is produced during normal activity (Koh, 1995).

Rather than being weak, the lengthened muscle lacks the ability to maintain a full contraction within inner range. This shows up clinically as a difference between the active and passive inner ranges. If the joint is passively placed in full anatomical inner range, the subject is unable to hold the position. Sometimes the position cannot be held at all, but more usually the contraction cannot be sustained, indicating a lack in slow twitch endurance capacity.

Clinically, reduction of muscle length is seen as the enhanced ability to hold an inner-range contraction. This may or may not represent a reduction in SSN, but is a required functional improvement in postural control. Muscle shortening has been shown in the dorsiflexors of horseriders. Clearly,

this position is not held permanently as with splinting, but rather shows a training response. Following pregnancy, SSN increases in the rectus abdominus in combination with diastasis. Again, the length of the muscle gradually reduces in the months following birth. Inner-range training, then, is likely to shorten a lengthened muscle (Goldspink, 1996).

Inner-range holding ability

The ability of a stabilizer muscle to maintain an isometric contraction at low load over a period of time is vital to its anti-gravity function (Richardson, 1992). This may be assessed by using the classic muscle test position (see Appendix) and asking the subject to maintain a contraction in full inner range (Richardson and Sims, 1991). The important factor in the assessment is the length of time a static hold can be maintained without jerky (phasic) movements occurring. In each case the limb is placed passively into full inner range. When released, if the limb drops, the passive range of motion differs from the active range, which is an important indicator of poor stabilizer function. Full stabilizing function is achieved when a subject can maintain the inner-range position for 10 repetitions each of 10 seconds duration (Jull, 1994). Often the first two or three repetitions are performed normally, and it is only with further repetition that the deficit becomes apparent.

Tests for the major stabilizing muscles of the trunk, pelvic and shoulder girdle areas, including transversus abdominus, gluteus medius, gluteus maximus, the deep neck flexors and the lower trapezius are described below.

Lower limb

The iliopsoas is assessed in the sitting position. The patient flexes the hip while maintaining a 90° knee flexion so that the foot is lifted clear of the ground (Fig. 7.9a).

The gluteus maximus in assessed in prone lying with the knee flexed to 90°. The hip is lifted to inner-range extension and held (Fig. 7.9b).

The gluteus medius is tested in side lying with the knee flexed. The action is combined with hip abduction, with slight lateral rotation to emphasize the posterior fibres of the muscle (Fig. 7.9c).

Cervical spine

For the cervical spine the essential stabilizers are the deep neck flexors. These are retrained in the supine position using pressure biofeedback with the cuff placed behind the head or upper cervical spine (Jull, 1994). The aim is to achieve sub-occipital rather than lower cervical flexion. The action is a minimal flexion or 'nodding' action of the head alone, avoiding forceful actions or lifting the head from the couch (see p. 393).

Upper trunk

A blanket assessment of scapular stability may be usefully made in prone falling (Fig. 7.10). Slowly lowering (eccentric push-up) will often reveal inappropriate movement of the scapula in the first phase of the action. The scapulae should remain apart, and firmly fixed to the thoracic wall throughout the movement. Scapular movement outward and upward indicates lack of stability (Janda, 1994). If the scapulae fall together, the rhomboids and levator scapulae are dominant (Kendall et al., 1993). True winging, apparent through lifting of the medial edge of the scapula, represents serratus anterior inactivity.

Scapular stability is enhanced by restoring the functional capacity of the lower trapezius and serratus anterior, which as stability muscles often show reduced activity and length-

Figure 7.9 Inner range holding of the lower limb. (a) Iliopsoas, (b) gluteus maximum, (c) gluteus medius (posterior fibres).

Figure 7.10 Eccentric push-up as a global assessment of scapulo-thoracic stability. (a) Athlete slowly lowers from a push-up position—note position of scapula. (b) Scapulae should remain apart and fixed to the rib cage as body is lowered. (c) Scapulae fall together if rhomboids and levator scapulae are dominant. (d) True winging. The medial edge of the scapulae lift.

ening. Surface electromyography (sEMG) may be used with the active electrode placed over the lower trapezius. The patient is placed in prone lying and his or her scapula is passively positioned into its neutral position by the therapist. This often requires retraction and depression to neutralize the protraction/elevation often found (Fig. 7.11). The patient is encouraged to hold this position through his own muscle activity, gaining feedback from the sEMG readout. Enough muscle activity should be used to keep the anterior aspect of the shoulder off the treatment couch, but not to retract the scapulae. Once this position can be maintained actively, the holding time is built up until the patient can perform 10 repetitions, holding each for 10 seconds.

The scapular force couples may be maximally challenged using a side-lying braced position (Wilk and Arrigo, 1993). The patient begins in side lying with the arm flexed/abducted to 90° and internally rotated. The hand is now flat on the couch with the fingers pointing towards the patient. Scapular fixation is maintained against the rhythmic stabilization provided by the therapist in all planes.

Figure 7.11 Enhancing scapulo-thoracic stability. (a) Scapular repositioning. (b) Rhythmic stabilization. (c) Trunk rocking. (d) Arm movement progressions.

The next stage is to introduce a limited range of movements of the humerus onto the now stable base of the scapular thoracic joint. Initially, the patient assumes elbow support prone lying to work the shoulder in closed kinetic chain format. He or she moves his or her body over the arm forward and backwards and side to side to create closed chain flexion/extension and abduction/adduction. At all times the scapula must remain in contact with the thorax. The patient is now moved to the edge of the couch so the affected arm hangs over the couch side. Maintaining scapula thoracic stability, inner-range movements in all three planes are used in an attempt to automatize stability (see p. 77).

The starting position is now changed to sitting or standing and inner-range movements are used with sEMG monitoring of the lower trapezius. Home exercises may be used by asking the patient to place the thumb of his or her opposite hand beneath his inferior scapular angle. He or she then gently keeps the inferior ankle pressed against the thumb (retraction and depression) while performing inner-range movements.

These initial actions, where stabilization ability is being re-educated, must keep the arm below 30° abduction to prevent scapular movement. Later, greater glenohumeral range may be used as the patient can control scapulo-thoracic movement.

The scapulo-thoracic muscles may be selectively strengthened using the individual exercises shown in Fig. 7.12.

Lower trunk

Inner-range holding of the trunk begins with the abdominal hollowing action. The patient begins in the prone kneeling starting position. As the transversus has horizontally aligned fibres, this action allows the abdominal muscles to sag, giving stretch facilitation. The patient focuses their attention on their umbilicus and is instructed to pull the umbi-licus 'in and up' while breathing normally (Fig. 7.13a). This action has been shown to dissociate activity in the internal obliques and transversus from that of rectus abdominus (Richardson et al., 1992). This makes the exercise useful for re-educating the stabilizing function of the abdominals where rectus abdominus has become the dominant muscle of the group.

To facilitate learning multisensory cueing is used (Miller and Medeiros, 1987) to increase the sensory input to the patient. Auditory cues can be provided by the therapist speaking to the subject and giving feedback about performance. Visual cues are given by encouraging the subject to look at the muscles as they function, and by using a mirror. Kinaesthetic cueing is accomplished by encouraging the subject to 'feel' the particular action, for example, asking them to 'feel the stomach being pulled in'. Tactile cues are provided by the therapist touching the subject's abdomen as muscle contraction begins.

Several errors can occur when a patient practises abdominal hollowing. Essentially, the rib cage, shoulders and pelvis should remain still throughout the action. The contour of the abdomen will flatten if a deep breath is taken and held, but the therapist should see the chest expansion involved (Fig. 7.13b). Where this occurs, the patient is instructed to exhale and hold this chest position as the exercise is performed. Placing a belt around the lower chest is useful to give feedback about chest movement (Richardson and Hodges, 1996).

Another substitution action is to use the external oblique to brace the abdomen. However, these muscles will pull on the lower ribs and depress them at the same time, slightly flexing the thoracic spine. A horizontal skin crease is often visible across the upper abdomen (Fig. 7.13c). Where this occurs, the patient is encouraged to perform pelvic floor contraction at the same time as abdominal hollowing. Simultaneous contraction of the gluteus maximus must be avoided with this action, as this will teach an inap-

Muscle	Suggested exercises
Serratus anterior	Scapular plane abduction, push-up, end-range shoulder flexion in prones, serratus anterior punch
Upper trapezius	Shoulder shrugs, scapular plane abductions
Middle trapezius	Rowing, shoulder elevation and hyper extension in standing, shoulder abduction and flexion in prones, scapular retraction with horizontal abduction of the externally rotated shoulder in prone
Lower trapezius	Scapular plane abduction and rowing, shoulder depression and retraction in sitting, elevation of the externally rotated arm which is positioned diagonally between flexion and abduction
Levator scapulae	Shoulder elevation, abduction, flexion, rowing
Rhomboids	Rowings, shoulder retraction, elevation and abduction, scapular retraction with horizontal abduction of the interanlly rotated shoulder in prone
Latissimus dorsi	Press-ups, lateral pull
Pectoralis major	Press-ups
Pectoralis minor	Press-ups

Figure 7.12 Exercises to selectively strengthen the scapulo-thoracic muscles. After Kamker et al. (1993).

Figure 7.13 Abdominal hollowing. (a) Normal. The subject pulls the umbilicus in and up, drawing in the lower abdomen. (b) Incorrect. The subject takes a deep breath in, raising the ribs to stretch the abdominal muscles to produce flattening. (c) Incorrect. The subject using the external oblique to brace the abdomen. The lower ribs are depressed and the slight flexion caused a horizontal skin crease across the upper abdomen.

propriate motor pattern for trunk stability during dynamic sports activity.

Restoration of the abdominal hollowing mechanism can also be enhanced by the use of pressure biofeedback (Chattanooga Group Limited, Bicester, England). The biofeedback unit consists of a rubber bladder and pressure gauge similar to a sphygmomanometer.

In prone lying, the pressure biofeedback unit is placed beneath the abdomen with the lower edge of the bladder level with the anterior superior iliac spines, and the centre of the bladder over the umbilicus (Fig. 7.14a). The unit is inflated to 70 mmHg, and abdominal hollowing is performed. The aim is to reduce the pressure reading on the biofeedback unit by 6–10 mmHg, and to be able to maintain this contraction to repetition (10 repetitions of 10 second hold) to ensure that endurance of the target muscles is adequate (Richardson and Hodges, 1996).

As a further test a crook lying position is used. The bladder of the unit is placed beneath the subject's lumbar spine and inflated to show a constant figure of 40 mmHg. The subject is instructed to contract the abdominal muscles without performing a posterior pelvic tilt (Fig. 7.14b). If the lordosis is unchanged, a constant pressure is shown on the pressure unit. Increasing pressure shows flattening of the lordosis (lumbar flexion), while reducing pressure shows increased lordosis (lumbar extension). Excessive motion in either direction represents loss of lumbar stability. Alteration of starting position and the addition of simultaneous limb movement encourages body awareness and movement control.

The ability of the deep abdominals to maintain spinal stability may be accurately assessed using the heel slide manoeuvre (Fig. 7.14c). The subject starts in crook lying with the spine in a neutral position and the pressure biofeedback unit positioned beneath the lower spine. One leg is then gradually straightened, sliding the heel along the ground to take the weight of the leg. During this action, the hip flexors are working eccentrically and pulling on the pelvis and lumbar spine. If the strong pull of these muscles is sufficient to displace the pelvis, the pelvic tilt is noticeable by palpation

(a)

(b)

(c)

Figure 7.14 Use of pressure biofeedback. (a) Prone lying abdominal hollowing assessment. (b) Assessing change in the depth of the lordosis during abdominal hollowing. (c) The heel slide to test lumbar stability.

of the anterior superior iliac spine (ASIS) and by an alteration of the pressure biofeedback unit. The action must be completed without using the substitution actions described above.

Measurement and enhancement of multifidus function is begun in prone lying. The fibres of multifidus (Fig. 7.15a) are palpated medial to the longissimus at L4 and L5 levels. The spinous processes are identified and the fingers then slide laterally into the hollow between the spinous process and the longissimus bulk. The difference in muscle consistency is assessed, and then the patient's ability to isometrically contract the multifidus in a 'setting' action is determined. The patient is encouraged to use multifidus setting in a sitting position with a neutral lumbar spine. Palpation is with the therapist's thumb and knuckle of the first finger placed on either side of the lumbar spinous process at any one level. The instruction to the patient is to 'feel the muscle swelling' without actively flexing the lumbar spine (Fig. 7.15b). The patient's own thumbs may be used to give feedback for home practice. sEMG can also be used as the multifidus is superficial at this level. Enhancement of multifidus function as part of manual therapy (using rhythmic stabilization in side lying) is described on p. 365.

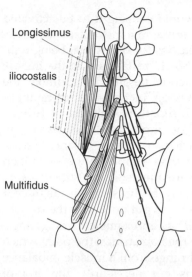

Figure 7.15   (a) The fascicles of multifidus in the lumbar spine.

Figure 7.15   (b) Multifidus facilitation in sitting.

Muscle shortening

Mobilizer muscles have long fusiform shapes and, as such, show a tendency to tighten. Tightness in the hamstrings, for example (mobilizers, biarticular), is often seen while tightness in the gluteals (stabilizers, monoarticular) is rare. As well as reducing range of motion, the tightened muscle is more likely to develop painful trigger points (Travell and Simons, 1983) These are small hypersensitive regions within a muscle which stimulate afferent nerve fibres causing pain. The sensation created is a deep tenderness with an overlying increase in tone creating a palp-

ably tender band of muscle. When palpated deeply, the trigger point creates a local muscle spasm giving the 'jump sign' (Janda, 1993). The irritability threshold of a tight muscle is lowered causing it to be activated earlier than normal in a movement sequence. One of the reasons for this is that being tight there is less 'slack' to take up in the muscle before contraction begins. In addition, the muscles shows an increased afferent input via the stretch receptors (Sahrmann, 1990).

Tightness of mobilizer muscles is an important factor in muscle balance assessment. Rather than simply range of motion however, we are interested in a subject's ability to maintain body segment alignment while the stretch is put on. Using the straight leg raise (SLR) as an example of range measurement for the hamstrings, the point which indicates full range from a muscle imbalance perspective is not necessarily the end of available motion for the leg, but the point at which hamstring tension is sufficiently high to cause the pelvis to tilt (see below).

The lower limb

The tests used to assess muscle length may also be used to stretch a muscle if it is found to be tight. The three key movements to assess restriction of pelvic motion are the modified Thomas test, the SLR, and the Ober test. If any of the movements reproduce the patient's pain it is relevant, and if the range is significantly less than the optimal value given, the muscle will require specific stretching.

With the Thomas test (Fig. 7.16), the patient begins in crook lying at the end of the couch. The knees are brought to the chest and the back flattened to a point where the sacrum just begins to lift away from the couch surface but no further. One leg is held close to the chest to maintain the pelvic position and the other leg is straightened over the couch end. An optimal alignment exists when the femur lies horizontally, and aligned to the sagittal plane (no abduction). The tibia should lie vertically (90° knee flexion) and be aligned with the sagittal plane (no hip rotation) as shown in Fig. 7.16. If the femur rests above the horizontal

and the knee is flexed less than 90°, tightness may be present in either the iliopsoas or rectus femoris. If the rectus is tight, straightening the knee will take the stretch off the muscle and the leg will drop down. If the knee is straightened and the leg stays in place, it indicates tightness in the iliopsoas.

The modified Ober test begins in side lying (Fig. 7.17). The test assesses the length of the tensor fascia lata providing the pelvis remains in a neutral position. In side lying, the lower leg is bent to improve stability and

Thomas test

(a)

(b)

(c)

Figure 7.16 Thomas test. (a) Normal. (b) Tight rectus femoris—hip flexed, but femur drops down as leg is straightened. (c) Tibia should be vertical—deviation from this position indicates femoral rotation.

Figure 7.17   Ober test. (a) With pelvis neutral, upper leg should stay in extension and adduct past the horizontal. (b) A false reading is obtained if the pelvis is allowed to tip and the lumbar spine to laterally flex.

the therapist stabilizes the pelvis to avoid lateral pelvic dipping. The couch should be low enough to allow pressure to be placed through the iliac crest in the direction of the lower shoulder. Maintaining the neutral pelvic position, the hip is abducted and extended to 15°. It is then adducted while maintaining extension. An optimal length for an athlete would be seen when the upper leg is able to lower to couch level (Fig. 7.17). Where hip extension is limited, the test can still be carried out, but the hip tightness must be assessed further to determine if it is muscular, capsular, or osteological in nature.

The hamstrings are assessed by two actions, the straight leg raise (SLR) and the tripod test (Fig. 7.18). For the SLR, the anterior rim of the pelvis is palpated to note the point at which the pelvis begins to posteriorly tilt due to hamstring tightness. This is the point at which a stable base is no longer being provided for the hamstrings to stretch against and is perhaps more relevant than full passive range pressing against a fully posteriorly tilted pelvis. The tripod test again assesses the interplay between hamstring flexibility and lumbar stability. In the sitting position (feet off the floor) one leg is straightened, two measures are noted, first, the point at which posterior pelvic tilting

occurs, and finally the total range of combined motion at both hip and knee. For optimal performance, the lumbar spine should remain neutral and allow the knee to straighten to within 10° of full extension while the femur remains horizontal.

Figure 7.18   Assessing the effect hamstring tightness on pelvic tilt. (a) Straight leg raise—the beginning of posterior pelvic tilt marks the loss of alignment. (b) Tripod test—as the leg is straightened the pelvis posteriorly tilts.

Where muscle tightness is found, the test exercises may be used as starting positions for stretching. Before stretching tight muscles, we must ensure that excessive strain will not be placed on adjacent body parts through relative stiffness. This often requires some stability work before beginning the stretch. Passive static stretching is used initially, followed by contract–relax (see p. 120). Finally the opposing muscles are shortened to full inner range to stretch the antagonist actively. From the Thomas test position the hip is flexed slightly and the knee extended against the resistance of limb weight alone. The position is held for 20–30 seconds and the leg is then lowered to a new stretched position. The opposing knee must remain tightly gripped to the chest to ensure the posterior pelvic tilt is maintained throughout the exercise. An alternative exercise to stretch the hip flexors while re-educating spinal stability is the half lunge (Fig. 7.19a). The half-kneeling position is taken up, with one hand placed on a chair to aid balance, the other pressing into the lumbar spine on the side of the dependent leg. The abdominal hollowing procedure is performed and is held throughout the exercise to maintain a neutral position of the lumbar spine. To impart the stretch, the body lunges forwards, forcing the dependent hip into extension while avoiding increasing the lordosis.

In the Ober test position the ilio-tibial band (ITB) is stretched. However, this exercise is only effective if the subject is able to stabilize the pelvis against frontal movement by

Figure 7.19   Hip flexibility exercises. (a) Half lung. (b) Hip hitching in standing. (c) Hip hitching is maintained (pull pelvis up against hand) as upper leg is lowered into adduction. (d) Active knee extension (holding thigh). (e) Active knee extension (press thigh against hand). (f) Active knee extension in sitting—the tripod test.

maintaining a contraction of the quadratus lumborum and ipsilateral obliques. To re-educate this action, the subject is first taught a hip-hitching action in standing (Fig. 7.19b) to be repeated in lying. Finally, hip-hitching is performed and the subject maintains the contraction of the trunk side flexors on the side of the upper leg, as this leg is lowered into adduction and slight extension (Fig. 7.19c).

The hamstrings are initially stretched in the SLR test position. Exercise one (Fig. 7.19d) is the active knee extension (AKE) manoeuvre, where the upper leg is held in 90° hip flexion and the leg is straightened. An alternative is to straighten the leg in 160° hip flexion and then actively pull the straight leg up to 90° hip flexion without allowing the knee to bend (Fig. 7.19e). This combines inner-range shortening of the hip flexors with lengthening of the hip extensors. Finally, the tripod test position combines lumbar stability with mobilizer lengthening in a functional starting position (Fig. 7.19f). The subject begins sitting on the edge of a couch with the feet off the floor. An upright sitting posture is taken with the lumbar spine in its neutral position. This position is maintained throughout the exercise by performing abdominal hollowing. The leg is now straightened to stretch the hamstrings against the stable base of the unmoving pelvis.

The upper limb

Neck side flexion combined with other movements is a key movement for the trapezius, sternomastoid and anterior scalenes (Fig. 7.20). Side flexion away from the tight muscle, combined with neck flexion, stretches the trapezius. The levator scapulae is stretched by the same movement, but this time adding rotation away from the muscle being stretched. At the same time the shoulder is depressed. Elevation of the shoulder represents loss of scapulo-thoracic stability and is a sign that end range has been

reached. The sternomastoid is stretched by combining side flexion away, and rotation towards, the muscle being tested. The anterior scalene is stretched initially by manual pressure on the first rib combined with side flexion away from the muscle. Further stretch is placed on the muscle by rotating towards the muscle and extending the lower cervical spine by performing a full chin-tuck action. The rhomboids are stretched by actively stabilizing the scapula and flexing the arms to 90° and protracting. The arms are then crossed to the elbows.

In supine lying, the pectoralis major and minor and latissimus dorsi may be tested (Fig. 7.21). When lying supine, the posterior border of the acromion should rest no more than 2–3 finger breadths above the surface of the couch. A greater gap, combined with resistance to posterior shoulder girdle glide and painful direct palpation, represents tightness in the pectoralis minor. The pectoralis major is assessed by arm abduction. The sternal portion of the muscle is assessed with the arm at 120° abduction. When released, it should rest level with the couch. The clavicular portion is evaluated by lowering the arm over the couch side into extension/abduction, 80–90° extension is the norm. Latissimus dorsi is stretched by taking the arm overhead into flexion/abduction to couch level. In addition, latissimus dorsi may be stretched in standing. The back is flattened against the wall and the shoulder flexed, adducted and externally rotated (Koala stretch).

Posture

The combination of altered muscle length and function will be noticeable as a change in body alignment to both static (posture) and dynamic (segmental control) assessment.

Standing posture is assessed in comparison to a standard reference line (Kendall et al., 1993). The subject is positioned with a plumb-line passing just in front of their lat-

(a)

(b)

(c)

Figure 7.20 Neck side flexion tests. (a) Trapezius and levator scapulae (see text), (b) sternomastoid, (c) anterior scalene.

Figure 7.21   Supine lying tests. (a) Pectoralis minor, (b) pectoralis major (sternal portion), (c) pectoralis major (clavicular portion), (d) latissimus dorsi.

eral malleolus. In an ideal posture this line should pass just anterior to the mid-line of the knee, and then through the greater trochanter, bodies of the lumbar vertebrae, shoulder joint, bodies of the cervical vertebrae, and the lobe of the ear (Fig. 7.22).

When viewed from the front, with the feet three inches apart, the line should bisect the body into two equal halves. The anterior superior iliac spines (ASIS) should be approximately in the same horizontal plane, and the pubis and ASIS should be in the same vertical plane (Kendall et al., 1993). This alignment defines the neutral lumbo-pelvic alignment as one of 5° to the horizontal.

Anatomical landmarks are compared for horizontal level on the right and left sides of the body, and include the knee creases, buttock creases, pelvic rim, inferior angle of the scapulae, acromion processes, ears, and the external occipital protruberences. In addition, the alignment of the spinous processes and rib angles are observed, with minor scoliosis becoming more evident when assessed in Adam's position. The distance between the arms and the trunk (keyhole), skin creases, and unequal muscle bulk are indicators of asymmetry requiring closer examination. Foot and ankle alignment are also assessed.

Anterior superior iliac
spine and pubic bone
in vertical alignment

Figure 7.22 The standard reference line for posture.
After Kendall et al. (1993).

When compared to this standard line, four posture types are commonly seen (Fig. 7.23). In the lordotic posture anterior pelvic tilt is excessive. The abdominal muscles and gluteals are typically lengthened and of poor tone. The hip flexors may shorten, and pelvic tilt is limited by tightness in the overactive and tight hamstrings. In an extreme lordotic posture, seen in chronic obesity, the lumbar spine rests in extension with the lumbar facet joints impacted and the elastic recoil of the hamstrings allowing the pelvis to hang. This posture equates with the pelvic crossed syndrome described by Janda and Schmid (1980). The lordotic posture is commonly seen in young gymnasts and dancers. In addition, it is the posture most noticeable after childbirth.

In the sway back posture the pelvis remains level, but the hip joint is pushed forward of the posture line. The hip is effec-tively extended, lengthening the hip flexors, and the body 'hangs' on the hip ligaments. The lordosis is now longer and more shallow than in the lordotic posture, and may extend up to the mid-thoracic spine. In addition, there is typically a noticeable crease where the direction of movement changes at a single spinal level, rather than through several, as is the case with the lordotic posture. A patient with this posture will often be able to point to the exact point of pain which normally occurs after prolonged standing. The sway back posture may be combined with dominance of one leg in standing ('hanging on the hip'), especially in the adolescent. Now, weakness in the gluteus medius allows the pelvis to tip laterally, a situation partially compensated by increased tone in the tensor fascia lata. Shortening is seen in the ilio-tibial band (ITB) with a prominent groove apparent on the lateral aspect of the thigh.

With the flat back posture, the main problem is lack of mobility in the lumbar spine and a flattening of the lordosis. This posture reflects the extension dysfunction described by McKenzie (1981). The pelvis is posteriorly tilted in comparison to the reference line, and the lumbar tissues are often thickened and immobile.

In the kyphotic posture the shoulder joint moves anteriorly to the posture line and the thoracic kyphosis is increased. In an optimal upper body alignment (Table 7.2) the scapulae should be approximately three finger breadths from the spine and the medial borders of the scapulae should be vertical. Optimal positioning of the shoulder is assessed by comparing the head of the humerus in relation to the acromion process. In optimal positioning, no more than one-third of the humeral head should be anterior to the point of the acromion. The humerus should be held with the cubital fossa at 45° to the sagittal plane in relaxed standing. A greater angle than this indicates excessive medial rotation, indicative of tightness in the medial rotators (especially the pectoralis major) and lengthening of the lateral rotators.

(a) Lordotic

Body segment alignment

Pelvis is anteriorly tilted with lordosis increased.
Knees are hyperextended

Elongated and weak

Anterior abdominals.
Hamstrings may lengthen initially or shorten to compensate where posture has been present for some time

Short and strong

Low back and hip flexors

(b) Kypholordotic

Body segment alignment

Head held towards the cervical spine hyperextended.
Scapulae may be abducted.
Increased lumbar lordosis, and increased thoracic kyphosis.
Pelvic anteriorly placed
body segment

Elongated and weak

Neck flexors, upper erector spinae.
External oblique.
If scapulae are abducted, middle and lower trapezius

Short and strong

Neck extensors and hip flexors.
If scapulae are abducted, serratus anterior, pectoralis major and/or minor, upper trapezius

(c) Sway Back

Body segment alignment

Long kyphosis with pelvis the most anterior body segment, hip joint moves forwards of posture line.
Low lumbar area flattens.
Pelvis neutral. Hip and knee joints hyperextended. Where subject stands predominately on one leg pelvis will be down to non favoured side.
Favoured leg appears longer in standing only

Elongated and weak

One hip joint flexors. External oblique.
Upper extensors. Neck flexors.
Where on leg is favoured, gluteus medius (especially posterior fibres) on favoured side

Short and strong

Low back musculature short but not strong. Where one leg is favoured, tensor fascia lata is strong and iliotibial band is tight on favoured side

(d) Flat Back

Body segment alignment

Loss or lordosis with pelvis in posterior tilt

Elongated and weak

One joint hip flexors

Short and strong

Hamstrings,
Abdominals may be strong, with back muscles slightly elongated

Figure 7.23 Posture types and muscle imbalance. When a subject is viewed from the side and compared to a standard posture line, four main posture types may be found. These are associated with shortened and lengthened muscles as shown. After Kendall et al. (1993).

Table 7.2 Alignment of the shoulder girdle

From behind	From the side
Medial border of scapula vertical	Line from ear canal to centre of shoulder joint
Medial border of scapula no more than three finger breadths from the spinous processes	No more than one third of head of humerus anterior to acromion
Spine of scapula T3/T4 level, inferior angle at T7	Humerus held with cubital fossa 45° to sagittal plane
Scapula flat against chest wall	

Deviation from this ideal is often described as a 'round shouldered' posture, a blanket term which covers a number of scenarios. Tightness in the anterior structures will pull the shoulder forwards, away from the posture line. The weight of the arm moves further from the centre of gravity of the upper body, dramatically increasing the leverage forces transmitted to the thorax. Eventually, the thoracic kyphosis will increase as a result. Tightness in the pectoralis minor pulls on the coracoid process tilting the scapula forwards superiorly (Fig. 7.24a). Tightness in the pectoralis major causes a combination of excessive medial rotation at the glenohumeral joint with anterior displacement of the humeral head (Fig. 7.24b). Excessive abduction of the scapula (Fig. 7.24c) and downward rotation (Fig. 7.24d) may result from lengthening of the lower trapezius and serratus anterior. Excessive elevation (Fig. 7.24e) and upward rotation (Fig. 7.24f) may result from tightness in the upper fibres of trapezius.

Segmental control

The ability to dissociate the movement of one body segment from that of a neighbouring segment is dependent on stabilization ability and adequate mobilizer length. The central features of segmental control require the pelvis to tilt independently of the lumbar spine in both frontal and sagittal planes, the shoulder girdle and thoracic spine to move in relation to each other, and the upper and lower portions of the cervical spine to move in a controlled fashion.

Lumbo-pelvic rhythm

The combination of movements of the hip on the pelvis, and the lumbar spine on the pelvis increases the range of motion of this body area. In forward flexion in standing, for example, when the legs are straight, movement of the pelvis on the hip is limited to about 90° hip flexion. Any further movement, allowing the subject to touch the ground, must occur at the lumbar spine. In this example the body is acting as an open kinetic chain and the pelvis and lumbar spine are rotating in the same direction. Anterior tilt of the pelvis is accompanied by lumbar flexion (Fig. 7.25a). In the upright posture, the foot and shoulders are static and so spinal movement acts in a closed kinetic chain. In this situation, movement of the pelvis and lumbar spine (lumbo-pelvic rhythm) occur in opposite directions (Fig. 7.25b). Now, an anteriorly tilted pelvis is compensated by lumbar extension to maintain the head and shoulders in an upright orientation. The relationship between various pelvic

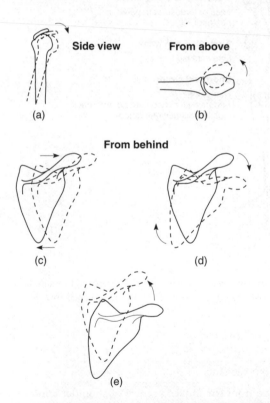

Figure 7.24 Postural changes around the shoulder. (a) Superior tilt of the scapula. (b) Medial rotation and anterior displacement of the gleno-humeral joint. (c) Abduction. (d) Downward rotation. (e) Elevation and upward rotation.

Figure 7.25 Lumbo-pelvic rhythm. (a) Lumbo-pelvic rhythm in open chain formation occurs in the same direction. Anterior pelvic tilt accompanies lumbar flexion. (b) Lumbo-pelvic rhythm in closed kinetic chain formation occurs in opposite directions. Anterior pelvic tilt is compensated by lumbar extension. From Norris (1996).

movements and the corresponding hip joint action is shown in Table 7.3.

For lumbo-pelvic rhythm to function correctly, hip flexion should be greater than lumbar flexion, and occur first during functional activities. In subjects where there is a history of back pain, however, the reverse situation often occurs leading to stress through repeated flexion of the lumbar spine.

In the lower trunk, the ability to dissociate lumbar movement from pelvic movement is important, and is often lost in the chronic low back pain patient. Three exercises are

used to assess lumbo-pelvic rhythm. In the first (Fig. 7.26) the subject stands side on to a wallbar for support. Hip flexion is then performed to beyond 90°. The movement should ideally occur in three phases. Initially, there should be no pelvic movement, with phase I consisting of hip flexion alone. During phase II the pelvis should begin to posteriorly tilt but the lumbar spine movement should not be excessive. In phase III no further hip or pelvic movement is available and the final position is obtained by lumbar flexion alone. Where control of lumbo-pelvic rhythm is poor, lumbar flexion often occurs early in phase I, with thoracic movement noticeable as the subject dips the chest downwards towards the knee. Once detected, this same movement is used to re-educate pelvic control, with the subject actively stabilizing the

Figure 7.26 Lumbo-pelvic rhythm: standing. (a) Hip flexes, no pelvic or lumbar movement. (b) Posterior rotation of pelvis begins as hip approaches 90°. Lordosis flattens. (c) Maximum hip and pelvic motion. Lumbar flexion completes movement. (d) Incorrect: pelvic rotation and lumbar flexion occurs immediately.

Table 7.3 **Relationship of pelvis, hip joint, and lumbar spine during right lower-extremity weight-bearing and upright posture**

Pelvic motion	Accompanying hip joint motion	Compensatory lumbar motion
Anterior pelvic tilt	Hip flexion	Lumbar extension
Posterior pelvic tilt	Hip extension	Lumbar flexion
Lateral pelvic tilt (pelvic drop)	Right hip adduction	Right lateral flexion
Lateral pelvic tilt (hip hitch)	Right hip abduction	Left lateral flexion
Forward rotation	Right hip MR	Rotation to the left
Backward rotation	Right hip LR	Rotation to the right

MR—medial rotation, LR—lateral rotation. From Norkin and Levangie (1992).

pelvis and initially performing hip flexion to only 10–20°.

Lumbo-pelvic rhythm is further assessed in prone kneeling (Fig. 7.27). From this position the subject sits back onto the ankles. Again, the action should occur in three phases. In phase I no lumbar or pelvic movement should occur. In phase II hip, pelvis and lumbar spine should all move, and in phase III lumbar flexion and some thoracic flexion finishes the action. Faulty lumbo-pelvic rhythm often shows up as lumbar flexion occurring immediately.

The hip hinge movement is the final action (Fig. 7.28). This measures the subject's ability to isolate pelvic motion from that of the lumbar spine. Initially, forward flexion is assessed, and the relative contribution of anterior pelvic tilt to this movement is important. With normal lumbo-pelvic rhythm, anterior pelvic tilt reduces the amount of lumbar flexion required to reach downwards to waist height. Where pelvic tilt is limited, greater lumbar flexion is required, and throughout the day the number of lumbar flexion movements is greatly increased leading to accumulated stress on the body tissues in this area. The subject is re-trained to maintain the neutral lumbar position and flex the hip on the fixed foot. To release tension from the hamstrings, the knees should be slightly unlocked as the movement begins.

Pelvic motion in the frontal plane

Pelvic motion control in the frontal plane represents the Trendelenburg sign (see Fig.

Figure 7.28 Hip hinge movement. (a) Correct: knees unlock, pelvis rotates anteriorly. Neutral lumbar position maintained. (b) Incorrect: pelvis fixed, flexion occurs to spine only.

9.7, p. 216). When the body weight is supported on one leg, the hip abductors (mainly gluteus medius) of the supporting leg work to prevent the pelvis dipping. Their action, combined with that of quadratus lumborum of the contralateral leg, can dip the pelvis upwards on the free leg side, effectively adducting the hip on the supporting side. Where these muscles are unable to hold an inner-range contraction, the pelvis is seen to dip downwards towards the lifted leg, effectively adducting the weight-bearing limb.

In the non-weight-bearing situation, inactivity of the gluteus medius shows as a false hip abduction movement. Normally, when the upper leg is lifted from side lying, the pelvis remains level and the hip moves on this stable base (Fig. 7.29). When the hip abductors are weak, the subject is unable to abduct the leg correctly. Instead, the pelvis is laterally tilted through the action of the trunk side flexors. Although the leg lifts, the rela-

| (a) Phase I | (b) Phase II | (c) Phase III | (d) Incorrect method |

Figure 7.27 Lumbo-pelvic rhythm: kneeling. (a) Phase I. Hip flexion alone. (b) Phase II. Posterior pelvic tilt and hip flexion combined. (c) Phase III. Lumbar flexion completes movement. (d) Incorrect: lumbar flexion and posterior pelvic tilt occur immediately.

Figure 7.29 Pelvic alignment during hip abduction. (a) Correct: pelvis remains stable as hip abducts. (b) Incorrect: pelvis tilts laterally on spine giving false appearances of hip abduction.

tionship between the femur and pelvis remains unchanged, with close inspection showing the movement isolated to the lower spine.

Scapulo-humeral rhythm

Motion of the shoulder girdle, as a whole, changes the position of the glenoid fossa, placing it in the most favourable location for the maximum range of humeral movement. When the glenoid cavity moves, it does so in an arc, the diameter of which is the length of the clavicle (Palastanga et al., 1989). The medial border of the scapula moves in a similar, but smaller arc and as a consequence the positions of the shoulder girdle structures change in relation to each other.

As the scapula moves medially and laterally towards and away from the vertebral column, the curvature of the rib cage forces the scapula to change from a frontal to a more sagittal position. This, in turn, alters the direction in which the glenoid cavity faces. With elevation, the scapula is accom-

panied by some rotation, the glenoid cavity gradually pointing further upwards as the scapula gets higher.

With both shoulder abduction and flexion, the clavicle axially rotates. As the scapula twists, the coracoclavicular ligament 'winds up' and tightens, causing the clavicle itself to rotate. For this reason a diminished range of movement at either the acromioclavicular (AC) or sternoclavicular (SC) joints, which reduces clavicular rotation, will also impair scapular and therefore gleno-humeral motion.

Movement of the arm into abduction may be divided into three overlapping stages (Table 7.4). In stage I, no movement of the scapula should occur. As the arm abducts, lateral rotation may be detected by palpation of the bicipital groove (intertubercular sulcus). If the humerus is maintained in a neutral position, abduction in the frontal plane is limited to about 90°. Laterally rotating the humerus increases this range to 120° (Lucas, 1973). When the arm is elevated in the sagittal plane, abduction is accompanied by medial rotation due to tightness in the coraco-humeral ligament (Gagey et al., 1987). No rotation is required for elevation in the scapular plane (30–45° anterior to the frontal plane). In this position, the joint capsule does not undergo torsion, and the deltoid and supraspinatus are optimally aligned.

At the beginning of abduction in the frontal plane, slight approximation of the humerus should occur (maximum 3 mm) to overcome the weight of the arm as the fibres of the joint capsule are taken off stretch, and no longer support the arm through elastic recoil. No noticeable elevation of the shoulder should occur, unless the upper fibres of trapezius dominate the movement. The instantaneous axis of rotation in stage I is near the root of scapular spine, and moves superiorly and laterally as abduction progresses.

By the beginning of stage II, from 30° of abduction, the scapula should be upwardly rotating to maintain clearance between the

Table 7.4 Movement of the arm into abduction

Stage one
Gleno-humeral movement alone for first 30°, inferior angle of scapula should not move

Maximum of 3 mm upward displacement of the humeral head (through the pull of deltoid), rotator cuff limits further shift

Lateral rotation of the humerus (detected as movement of the bicipital groove) occurs by the end of stage one

Stage two
Scapular elevation and upward rotation points glenoid cavity towards the ceiling

Humeral head glides inferiorly by 90° revealing a sulcus

Stage three
Scapula slides around rib cage and thoracic spine flattens

Inferior angle of scapula should not protrude further than 1 cm from chest wall

acromion and the approaching greater tuberosity of the humerus. Scapular rotation in the beginning of stage I occurs as a result of elevation of the clavicle on the SC joint. Between 80–140° the instantaneous axis of rotation (IAR) migrates towards the AC joint along the upper central scapular area. Movement at this stage is then due to elevation of the clavicle on the SC joint and rotation of the scapula on the clavicle at the AC joint. Movement of the scapula and humerus occur in a ratio of about 1:2.

Scapular rotation occurs as a result of force-couples between the various muscles attached to the scapula (Fig. 7.30). Upward (lateral) rotation, accompanying shoulder joint abduction or flexion, is brought about by contraction of the upper and lower fibres of trapezius and the lower digitation of serratus anterior. Serratus anterior is probably the most important of the group, pulling powerfully on the inferior border of the scapula as trapezius lifts the lateral end of the clavicle and acromion process. If serratus anterior and the lower fibres of trapezius are ineffective, the upper trapezius will dominate the movement. In this case, these fibres show increased tone and can be tight. As the abduction moves into stage II, the moment

arm of lower trapezius is lengthened and this portion of the muscle becomes increasingly active in the movement.

Downward (medial) rotation frequently occurs as a result of eccentric action of the above muscles. However, in activities such as hanging and chinning a beam, active scapular rotation is accomplished by levator scapulae and the rhomboids pulling upwards on the medial side of the scapula together with pectoralis minor pulling the coracoid process down. In cases where these muscles are tight or overactive, upward rotation of the scapula will be limited during abduction.

As scapular rotation progresses, lateral rotation of the humerus should be apparent as the cubital fossa and thumb orientate towards the ceiling. Ineffective scapular upward rotators, especially lengthening of the lower fibres of trapezius, will prevent correct orientation of the glenoid and increase the risk of impingement. Tightness in the medial rotators, especially the pectoralis major and subscapularis, combined with lengthening and weakness of the lateral rotators may lead to delayed lateral rotation at the gleno-humeral joint resulting in impingement of the greater tuberosity against the inferior acromion.

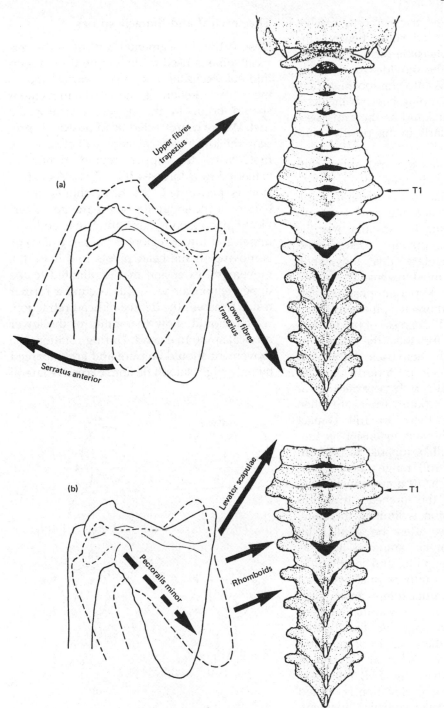

Figure 7.30 Muscle-force couples which create scapular rotation. (a) Lateral rotation. (b) Medial rotation. From Palastanga, Field and Soames (1989), with permission.

During stage II, as the humerus reaches 90° abduction, its head slides beneath the acromion, and a noticeable dip is formed in the skin. Failure of the shoulder musculature to pull the humerus into this position may result in the head slipping beneath the acromion with a sudden thud as the arm raises above 90° and similarly in this position during descent.

During stage III, as the arm approaches 120° abduction, no further movement is available from the gleno-humeral joint. Further range to reach the arm overhead is achieved by sliding the scapula over the thorax into further upward rotation and abduction. To facilitate this movement, the thoracic spine must reverse its kyphosis and flatten. A kyphotic posture, and inflexibility in the thoracic spine will therefore limit the final degrees of abduction. As a simple test for this, the patient is asked to stand with their back flat against a wall with the pelvis posteriorly tilted to avoid any possibility of hyperextension at the lumbar spine. Both arms are then abducted, keeping them in full contact with the wall. If thoracic extension is limited, the patient will be unable to perform pure abduction to full range. Instead, the arm moves through flexion–abduction to bring it in front of the forehead. In conditions where abduction is limited, therefore, greater range may often be gained by mobilizing the thoracic spine as well as working on the gleno-humeral joint.

As the arm moves into its final overhead position and the scapula rotates maximally, the inferior angle of the scapula juts out through the outer edge of the thorax. However, no more than 1–2 cm of the inferior angle should be visible at this point. During this final phase the IAR moves to the AC joint. Clavicular elevation is limited by tension in the costoclavicular ligament. As the coracoid process moves away from the clavicle, tension in this ligament causes dorsal rotation of the clavicle about its long axis.

The cervical and thoracic spines

Observation of segmental control of the cervical spine is used to determine the division into sub-occipital and lower cervical movement. As flexion is initiated, movement should occur in the upper cervical spine first. Where a protracted head posture is present, the lower cervical spine will often move first, with the upper region remaining extended in a lordosis (Fig. 7.31). As extension is performed, the head should move back over the shoulders before the upper cervical spine extends, indicating that both the upper and lower region of the cervical spine is moving. If the head pivots to initiate the movement, extension may be limited to the upper region alone. If this occurs, a further test is to assess the degree of head retraction, which should show the ability of the lower cervical spine to extend. During rotation, the movement should be pure and accompanied by only slight lateral flexion. Excessive lateral

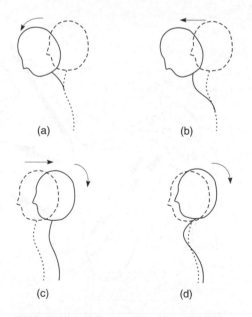

Figure 7.31 Movement of the cervical spine. (a) Upper cervical flexion—axial rotation. (b) Lower cervical flexion, upper extension with translation of joints. (c) Extension occurs in upper and lower cervical region. (d) Extension in upper cervical region only.

flexion indicates a possible tightness in the levator scapulae and/or the scalenes. If these muscles are tight, and are limiting rotation, shrugging the shoulders (and so relaxing the muscles) will increase the available range of rotation.

The thoracic spine is assessed with the subject sitting over the couch end. The subject should be able to reverse (flatten) the thoracic kyphosis as extension is attempted. Rotation movements should be symmetrical. Emphasis is placed on the upper thoracic region when thoracic rotation is combined with cervical rotation. The mid-thoracic region is tested with the arms folded, while the lower thoracic region is emphasized by placing the patient's arms overhead and pulling through the thoracolumbar fascia.

Restoration of muscle balance

Three elements combine to restore muscle balance: correction of segmental control, increasing core stability, and lengthening tight muscles. The order in which these are used will depend on the patient's symptoms.

Tight muscles may inhibit their antagonists (Jull and Janda, 1987) and often develop painful trigger points. This is especially the case in the upper limb. Furthermore, through relative flexibility (see p. 145) a tight muscle will throw stress onto a hyperflexible body segment causing tissue stress and pain. Elimination of tightness and re-development of stability, coupled with correction of segmental movement, is therefore a key aim of treatment.

Where pain is a prominent factor, the elimination of this pain may be the primary aim of treatment. Pain which occurs through muscle spasm, or through trigger points in tight muscle, may be relieved by treatment aimed at reducing muscle tone. This can be achieved by modalities or manual therapy, and will often involve the use of stretching.

Where pain is the result of persistence over stress on a hypermobile segment, the initial treatment should be aimed at segmental control and stability. Stability may have to be applied passively at first (through taping or splinting) until sufficient control of the muscular stabilizing system has been gained.

Finally, where the tissues themselves are normal, but poor alignment has become habitual (particularly in adolescent athletes), coordination and alignment training may be all that is required. This will necessitate close inspection and regular feedback, and the use of a video in these cases is of great value.

Proprioceptive training

Background to proprioceptive training

Proprioception has been defined as a specialized variation of touch encompassing the sensations of both joint movement and joint position (Lephart and Fu, 1995). During acute injury, proprioception may play a protective role by reflex muscular splinting. The reflex, initiated by displacement of mechanoreceptors and muscles spindles, occurs far more rapidly than that brought about by pain (nociception) (Barrack and Skinner, 1990). Joint effusion contributes to a reduction in mechanoreceptor discharge resulting in inhibition of muscular contraction. This is especially seen in the vastus medialis (VMO) of the knee for example, where just 60 ml of intra-articular effusion may result in 30–50% inhibition of quadriceps contraction (Kennedy et al., 1982). Proprioceptive deficits have also been shown to parallel joint degeneration (Barrett, Cobb and Bentley, 1991), but it is unclear whether this occurs as a result of degeneration, or is in fact part of its aetiology (Lephart and Fu, 1995).

From a clinical standpoint, proprioception may be seen to consist of three interrelating components (Beard et al., 1994) (Fig. 7.32), representing activity at spinal, brain-stem, and higher centre levels (Tyldesley and Grieve, 1989).

Each component is assessed by a variety of different tests (Lephart and Fu, 1995). First,

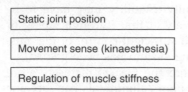

Figure 7.32 Components of proprioception.

static joint position sense is used to maintain posture and balance at brain-stem level. Input for these actions is from joint proprioception, the vestibular centres in the ears, and from the eyes. Balance and postural exercise with the eyes open and/or closed may be used to enhance static joint position sense. This component is commonly measured by tests which address reproduction of passive positioning (RPP) and reproduction of active positioning (RAP). The subject is required to return the joint to its start position after either an active or passive movement.

Secondly, kinaesthetic awareness or 'movement awareness' is a result of higher centre activity. This component encompasses the detection of both joint displacement and velocity change. It is commonly assessed by measuring the threshold to detection of passive motion (TTDPM), the subject simply stating when he or she feels movement has begun. Once movement has been detected through kinaesthetic awareness, motor programmes may be performed automatically in many cases (see p. 76). Consciously performed joint positioning activities, especially at end range, will enhance the development of automatic control and cognitive awareness (Lephart and Fu, 1995).

Finally, closed loop efferent activity is required for reflex (spinal) activity and regulation of muscle stiffness, leading to dynamic joint stability. This type of activity underlies all movements by supplying reflex splinting when a joint is stressed. Damage to joint receptors has been shown to affect co-contraction of muscles and reduce joint sta-

bility. This, in turn, can lead to an increase in the likelihood of injury (Tyldesley and Grieve, 1989).

Proprioception is enhanced at this level through the initiation of reflex joint stabilization, using activities which involve sudden alterations in joint position. Reflex stabilization is therefore assessed through measurement of the onset of muscle contraction in relation to joint displacement (see p. 00). The aim is to see if the muscles are able to limit joint displacement and effectively stabilize the joint.

Using TTDPM and RPP, Barrack and Skinner (1984) found decreased kinaesthesia with increasing age. In general, our highly mechanized western society may fail to impose the variety of movements which an individual requires for optimal musculoskeletal health. This reduced movement 'vocabulary' decreases the proprioceptive stimulation needed for skilled motor action (Jull and Janda, 1987). After injury, proprioceptive input is further reduced due to prolonged inactivity and damage to proprioceptive nerve endings within the injured tissues. A number of authors have stressed the importance of proprioceptive training in rehabilitation following injury to the knee (Barrack and Skinner, 1983; Beard et al., 1994), ankle (Freeman et al., 1965; Lentell et al., 1990; Konradsen and Ravn, 1990) and shoulder (Smith and Brunolli, 1990; Lephart et al., 1994). The functional importance of proprioceptive training has also been emphasized during rehabilitation of the spine (Lewit, 1991; Irion, 1992; Norris, 1995a), although its use in spinal rehabilitation is less common than for other areas of the body.

Proprioception may be enhanced with training. Barrack and Skinner (1983) found enhanced kinaesthesia in trained dancers, and Lephart and Fu (1995) demonstrated the same in intercollegiate gymnasts. Both of these types of athletes practice free exercise using body weight as resistance and use complex multi-joint activities. This type of training would seem appropriate for proprioceptive rehabilitation.

Training techniques

Proprioceptive training involves highly skilled actions, often performed at speed, with the aim of gaining automatization of movements for reflex stabilization. Proprioceptive training combines the principles of skill learning with the three aspects of proprioception described above. The stages of skill training are described on pp. 75–78. Essentially, exercises are progressed in terms of speed and complexity aiming at quality of movement execution rather than simple overload. Multiple sensory inputs are used to improve the sense of both static position and movement. Once this has been achieved, dynamic stability exercises may be used.

Proprioceptive training involves complex coordination and may be split into three closely interrelating components (Table 7.5). Training begins by splitting complex movements into a number of simple component sequences, with the choice of exercise being determined by the functional requirements of the patient. Splitting the movement in this way enables the athlete to focus their attention selectively on a single action, making learning far easier. In this first stage, actions must be slow and precise with the emphasis on control of the correct body position. The rate of movement is progressed, while maintaining accuracy, and the simple movement components are linked together to form the total activity sequence (Tropp, Alaranta and Renstrom, 1993). The athlete must stop when they become fatigued, failure to do so will often lead to practice of incorrect exercise technique and negative transfer effects (p. 116). Movement of other body parts draws the athlete's attention away from the conscious control of the core action, and assists in the development of automatic actions. To gain true automaticity of a movement sequence thousands of repetitions are needed. Rather than practising isolated exercises to repetition, functional activities should be built into an athlete's activities of daily living (ADL).

Using proprioceptive training of the ankle as an example, single leg standing may begin followed by single leg standing with 1/4 squat activities, and finally the same base activity with throwing and catching. This

Table 7.5 Proprioceptive training

Increase awareness of correct pattern
Split complex movement sequence into simple components
Increase awareness by passive movement using multisensory input

Gain voluntary control of movement pattern
Use multisensory stimulation during demonstration and performance of exercise
Start with slow precise movements
Stop exercising when patient becomes fatigued
Continually correct movement pattern passively
Progress exercise only when movement pattern is correct
Patient must perform independently before proceeding to more advanced actions
Link simple tasks to form more complex actions

Gain automatic control of movement
Progress speed while maintaining accuracy of movement
Perform multiple repetitions of movement sequence
Perform actions with other body parts while maintaining accurate stability in the affected body part

From Norris (1995b).

could be built into an athlete's daily activities (ADL) by performing simple home exercises such as cleaning the teeth while standing on one leg!

Once an action can be performed correctly on a stable surface, the subject may be positioned on a moving base of support. The subject must now use not just joint position and movement sense, but anticipation of body displacement requiring reflex stabilization. Initially, the labile surface should involve uniaxial movements, for example a rocker board. Placing the pivot of this type of board in the frontal plane will work the flexion and extension reaction, while placing the pivot in the sagittal plane will work abduction and adduction. If the pivot is then placed diagonally, movements will be bi-axial in nature. Progression is made to the wobble board where the pivot point is dome-shaped to allow tri-axial motion. Other apparatus useful for balance work and muscle reaction includes the large diameter (65 cm) gymnastic ball, the mini-trampette, the 'Fitter' ski-training device (Fitter International Inc., Calgary, Alberta, Canada) and the 'slide trainer' (Forsa Fitness Equipment, London, England). In each case, as the patient is pushed off balance, the aim is to maintain stabilization and enhance both movement detection and closed-loop reflex muscular stabilization. These actions must be built into an athlete's normal training programme rather than isolated from it.

Examples of proprioceptive training for the ankle, knee, shoulder and spine are given on pp. 311, 266, 435, and 366 respectively.

Kinetic chain exercise

Movement of the limbs occurs as a kinetic chain. Several joints arranged in sequence move together to produce a complex motor action. If the terminal joint in the kinetic chain can move freely, the chain is open. If this same joint is unable to move indepen-dently, because it faces a significant resistance, the action constitutes a closed kinetic chain. Most functional activities in sport involving the lower limb are performed using a closed kinetic chain. Walking, running, jumping and rising from a sitting position are all examples of closed kinetic chain activities. The only open kinetic chain activity of the lower limb normally used in sport is kicking.

We have seen the importance of exercise specificity in terms of muscle work and energy system, but the exercise must also be specific to the type of kinetic chain action used. To exercise the quadriceps on a leg extension bench (open chain) does not accurately reflect the demands placed on the lower limb with running and jumping (closed chain). As many of the adaptations produced during resistance training, particularly in the first four weeks of training, are neurogenic in nature the mismatch in movement patterns could detrimentally affect the athlete's performance (Palmitier et al., 1991).

A common open chain movement used in knee training is the seated leg extension exercise. The muscles primarily responsible for this action are the quadriceps. Contrast this to the closed chain movement of the squat. When the leg extends to raise the body from the squatting position the hamstrings extend the hip and assist in knee extension as the foot is stabilized. This co-contraction (co-activation) greatly reduces the anterior shear forces acting on the knee, and is of particular importance in the rehabilitation of ACL repairs.

Several additional differences exist between open (single joint or 'isolation') and closed chain (multi-joint or 'general') exercises in resistance training. In an open chain action, movement occurs mainly distal to the joint axis, whereas with a closed chain action motion is both proximal and distal to the joint. An open chain action primarily emphasizes concentric work, but a closed chain movement brings a more balanced action of concentric, eccentric and isometric contractions into play. Closed kinetic chain exercises for the shoulder are described on p. 436.

Mid-section training in sports

Training the abdominal region is fraught with danger. Athletes often adhere to traditional exercises and training methods with almost religious fervour. Many of these exercises, however, lack sound scientific foundation. To be able to develop more appropriate exercises for the trunk, we must first have to understand what traditional exercises achieve. To this end we will begin by briefly analysing two traditional types of exercise, the 'sit-up' and 'leg-raise'.

Function of the abdominal muscles

The rectus abdominus and lateral fibres of external oblique may be considered as the prime movers of trunk flexion, while the internal oblique and transversus abdominus are the major stabilizers (Miller and Medeiros, 1987). The rectus and external oblique are superficial muscles which often dominate trunk actions, while the transversus and internal oblique are more deeply placed and patients often show an inability to contract them voluntarily.

The rectus abdominus will flex the trunk by approximating the pelvis and rib cage. EMG investigation has shown the supra-umbilical portion to be emphasized by trunk flexion, while activity in the infra-umbilical portion is greater in positions where a posterior pelvic tilt is held (Lipetz and Gutin, 1970; Guimaraes et al., 1991). Internal oblique and transversus are activated by abdominal hollowing actions (Richardson et al., 1992), and the transversus acts at the initiation of movement to stabilize the trunk in overhead and lower limb actions (Hodges and Richardson, 1996a).

In sport, the abdominal muscles essentially function to stabilize the trunk and provide a firm base of support for the arms and legs to work against. If stability is poor (in relation to total power of the athlete), limb actions will cause displacement of the pelvis and trunk. This can be compared to a car tyre skidding on ice, where some of the energy required for forward motion is lost. In the same way, if trunk stability is poor, limb power will suffer and additional stress is placed on the spinal tissues if they move to full end range. If we take an overhead pressing movement as an example (Fig. 7.33), if the pelvis tilts forward and the spine hollows (full extension), trunk stability comes from facet joint approximation and elastic recoil of non-contractile tissues (passive stability)

(a)   (b)

Figure 7.33   Trunk stability in overhead pressing actions. (a) Abdominals pulled in tight, pelvis level. Trunk actively stable, reducing stress on lumbar tissues. (b) Abdominals lax, pelvis tilted. Trunk passively stable, increasing stress on lumbar tissues.

rather than from muscle action (active stability) (see p. 363). Therefore, the fundamental key to safe and effective abdominal training in sport is to train for trunk stability before training for trunk muscle performance.

Analysis of conventional exercises

Two exercises underlie most abdominal training, the sit-up and leg-raise. These movements must be briefly analysed to determine their usefulness.

The sit-up

The sit-up is essentially an action where an athlete comes from a supine lying to a long sitting position by performing hip flexion, usually with trunk flexion. There are several modifications of this action which will be dealt with below.

In a classic sit-up, as soon as the head lifts, activity is seen in the rectus abdominus (Walters and Partridge, 1957), and as a consequence the rib cage is depressed anteriorly. This initial period of flexion emphasizes the supra-umbilical portion of the rectus, the infra-umbilical portion and the internal oblique contracting later (Kendall and McCreary, 1983). As the internal oblique contracts, it pulls on the lower ribs, causing the ribs to flare out and so increase the infra-sternal angle.

One of the problems that poorly toned individuals face is bow stringing of the abdominals, which is often seen at the initiation of the sit-up action. For the superficial abdominals (rectus abdominus and external oblique) to pull flat, the deep abdominals (transversus abdominus and internal oblique) must be strong enough to perform an abdominal hollowing action and act as stabilizers. Where the deep abdominals are weak and the superficial abdominals are lengthened), the abdominal wall will be seen to dome and the athlete may lift the trunk with the lumbar spine extended or flat rather than flexed (Fig. 7.34).

Figure 7.34 Trunk alignment during a sit-up exercise. (a) Deep abdominals pull abdominal wall flat. (b) Deep abdominals allow abdominal wall to 'dome', lengthened superficial abdominals allow anterior pelvic tilt, and hollow back.

Fixation of the pelvis is provided by the hip flexors, especially iliacus through its attachment to the pelvic rim. The strong pull of the hip flexors is partially counteracted by the pull of the lateral fibres of external oblique and the infra-umbilical portion of the rectus abdominus, which tend to tilt the pelvis posteriorly. Action of the external oblique, if powerful enough, will compress the ribs and reduce the infra-sternal angle once more (Kendall and McCreary, 1983).

In a poorly conditioned subject, the initial movement in a sit-up may be a momentary posterior tilting of the pelvis by action of the hip extensors. This will pre-stretch the hip flexors, giving them a mechanical advantage before hip flexion occurs. During this phase the abdominal muscles work eccentrically (Ricci, Marchetti and Figura, 1981).

Effects of foot fixation
If the sit-up action is attempted from the supine lying position without allowing trunk flexion, there is a tendency for the legs to lift up from the supporting surface.

This occurs because the legs constitute roughly one third of the body weight and the trunk two thirds.

As the abdominal muscles flex the spine, the centre of gravity of the upper body is moved caudally. Movement of the centre of gravity in this fashion reduces the lever arm of the trunk enabling the subject to sit up without the legs lifting (Fig. 7.35).

In cases where the abdominal muscles are weak, maximum spinal flexion will not occur and so the lever arm of the trunk remains long. Now, the greater weight and lever arm of the trunk causes it to remain on the floor and the legs are seen to lift.

If the feet are fixed, the hip flexors can now pull powerfully without causing the legs to lift. In addition, the act of foot fixation itself may facilitate the iliopsoas (Janda and Schmid, 1980). Foot fixation requires the subject to pull against the fixation point by active dorsiflexion. This process stimulates the gait pattern at heel contact increasing activity in the tibialis anterior, quadriceps and iliopsoas, a pattern known as flexor synergy (Atkinson, 1986).

Modifications of the sit-up

THE BENT KNEE SIT-UP AND TRUNK CURL

The bent knee sit-up is performed from the crook-lying starting position, with the knees flexed to 90° and hips flexed to 45°. The action is one of trunk flexion followed by,

or performed with, hip flexion. The trunk curl is performed from the same starting position, but no hip flexion occurs, the lumbar spine remaining in contact with the supporting surface. The bench-curl is performed from a starting position of 90° hip flexion, the shin being supported on a bench or chair.

Bending the knees and hips to alter the starting position of the sit-up will affect both the passive and active actions of the hip flexors, and the biomechanics of the lumbar spine. In supine lying, the iliopsoas is on stretch, and aligned with the horizontal (Fig. 7.36). In this position, vertebral compression is at its greatest as the muscle contracts, and trunk lifting is at a mechanical disadvantage. The ratio of lifting to compression is therefore approximately 1:10 (Watson, 1983). As the knees are flexed, the iliopsoas is pulled more vertically and so the ratio of trunk lifting to vertebral compression is reduced to 2:5 in crook lying and 1:1 in bench lying.

With 45° hip flexion, tension development in the iliopsoas has been shown to be 70–80% of its maximum, while with the hips and knees flexed to 90° this figure reduces to between 40 and 50% (Johnson and Reid, 1991).

Pull of iliopsoas

Trunk lifting

Vertebral compression
2:5

1:10

3.3:3.3

Figure 7.36 Mechanical advantage of iliopsoas during the sit-up. As the hip is flexed, the moment arm of the iliopsoas is lengthened. The muscle can therefore complete the sit-up action by using less force, and so vertebral compression is reduced. From Norris (1994a).

Figure 7.35 Changing leverage of the trunk. As the trunk flexes, the centre of gravity of the upper body moves closer to the hip, reducing the leverage effect. From Norris (1994a).

However, passive tension developed by the iliopsoas due to elastic recoil must also be considered. If the hips are flexed, the iliopsoas will not be fully stretched, and will not be able to passively limit the posterior tilt of the pelvis. Instead, to fix the pelvis and provide a stable base for the abdominals to pull on, the hip flexors will contract earlier in the sit-up action. This contraction, although occurring earlier, will be of reduced intensity (Walters and Partridge, 1957) due to the length–tension relationship of the muscle.

With the legs straight in the traditional sit-up position, the iliopsoas is stretched, and can passively limit posterior tilting of the pelvis. However, in this stretched position, the iliopsoas is capable of exerting greater force during hip flexion. If the abdominal muscles are too weak to maintain the position of the pelvis, the stronger hip flexors will hyperextend the lumbar spine and cause the pelvis to tilt forwards, lengthening the abdominals, and hyperextending the lumbar spine. This type of action is, therefore, unsuitable for postural re-education if the aim is to shorten posturally lengthened abdominal muscles.

Straight-leg raising

The bilateral straight leg raise has been shown to create only slight activity in the upper rectus, although the lower rectus contributes a greater proportion of the total abdominal work than with the sit-up (Lipetz and Gutin, 1970). The rectus works isometrically to fix the pelvis against the strong pull of iliopsoas (Silvermetz, 1990). The force of contraction of the iliopsoas is at its maximum when the lever arm of the leg is greatest, near the horizontal, and reduces as the leg is lifted towards the vertical.

In subjects with weaker abdominals, the pelvis will tilt and the lumbar spine will hyperextend. This forced hyperextension will dramatically increase stress on the facet joints particularly in the lumbar spine. The movement is likely to be limited by impaction of the inferior articular processes on the laminae of the vertebrae below, or in some cases by contact between the spinous processes (Twomey and Taylor, 1987). Where this action occurs rapidly, damage may result to the facet joint structures. Once contact has occurred between the facet and lamina, further loading will cause axial rotation of the superior vertebra (Yang and King, 1984). The superior vertebra pivots, causing the inferior articular process to move backwards overstretching the joint capsule.

Modification of straight-leg raising

As none of the abdominal muscles actually cross the hip, they are not prime movers of the straight-leg raising movement. However, the action is an important one as it emphasizes the pelvic stabilizing function of the infra-umbilical portion of the rectus abdominus, and lateral external oblique.

A number of exercises serve as modifications of the bilateral straight-leg raise to reduce the stress on the lumbar spine. The first action is the heel slide (Fig. 7.37a). From a crook-lying starting position an abdominal hollowing action is performed to stabilize the spine (p. 152). From this position, one leg is straightened while keeping the heel on the ground and sliding the leg into extension.

The second movement is leg lowering (Fig. 7.37b). For this exercise the subject lies supine with the hips flexed to 90° but the knees extended. From this position, the legs are lowered by eccentric action of the hip flexors to a point where the pelvis begins to tilt. Immediately this occurs, the legs are brought up again to 90° hip flexion. The advantage of this exercise over the standard straight-leg raise is one of changing leverage. With the standard leg-raising action, the subject starts from a point of maximum leverage on the leg, forcing the hip flexors and abdominals to work maximally straight

Figure 7.37 Modifications of the straight leg raise. (a) The heel slide. (b) Leg lowering. (c) Pelvic raise. (d) Leg raise from wallbar hanging position.

away. With leg lowering, the starting position is one of minimum leverage as the legs are held vertically. As the legs are lowered away from the vertical, leverage increases but the subject is able to control the decent of the legs and avoid the position of maximal leverage which would cause the spine to hyperextend. In cases where subjects find the leg lowering difficult to control, the knees should be bent, to reduce leverage on the leg, or the subject can perform the exercise close to a wall, so the legs cannot be lowered fully.

The third modification of the straight-leg raise is the bench-lying pelvic raise (Fig. 7.37c). Here, the subject starts the action in bench lying and maintains 90° hip and knee flexion throughout the movement. The arms are held by the sides to give counterforce and aid general stability. The action is to flex the lumbar spine, keeping the legs relatively inactive, and lift the buttocks from the ground. Although the lumbar spine is flexed,

as with the trunk curl, the movement occurs from 'below upwards' with the L5–S1 joint moving first followed by flexion of each successively higher lumbar segment. The reverse movement (above downwards) is seen with trunk-curling actions (McKenzie, 1981).

Finally, performing the actions from a wallbar hanging position (Fig. 7.37d) places the trunk vertically, reducing the leverage forces on the lumbar spine considerably, and providing traction. Initially, the athlete is required to hold a neutral pelvic position, preventing anterior tilt of the pelvis, and being encouraged to 'press the small of the back into the wallbars'. The action is then progressed to one of hip and knee flexion, bringing the bent knees up to a point where 90° hip flexion is achieved, but still keeping the lumbar spine in contact with the wallbars. The final progression is to stop knee and hip movement, and flex the lumbar spine to lift the back away from the support of the wallbars. This action, although working the abdominals hard, will also strengthen and possibly shorten the hip flexors.

Functional Load Abdominal Training

Functional Load Abdominal Training (FLAT) is an exercise regime based on active spinal stabilization techniques used for trunk rehabilitation (Norris, 1995a, 1995b). In stage I of the FLAT programme, contraction of the internal oblique and transversus abdominus is re-educated using the abdominal hollowing exercise in a variety of starting positions (see p. 365).

If the subject has lengthened abdominals, these are shortened by performing an inner range holding movement. This action is a modification of the trunk curl to combine three actions (Norris, 1994a, 1994b). The subject posteriorly tilts the pelvis, performs abdominal hollowing, and depresses the rib cage while exhaling (Fig. 7.38). Maximum trunk flexion is attempted, providing this is not contraindicated by lumbar pathology. If abdominal lengthening has occurred, the subject will show a greater passive range of motion than active range of motion to lumbar flexion. To correct this, an eccentric action is used. The subject uses his or her finger tips on the outside of the knees to pull themselves into full passive lumbar flexion. They set the abdominal muscles and

attempt to hold this position as they let their hand grip relax. Initially, they will only be able to decelerate the lowering action using an eccentric contraction of the target muscles. As muscle adaptation occurs, the movement will become more controlled and slower. Eventually an isometric hold will become possible and finally a concentric action. Once this is achieved, full range exercise is begun, using slow movements building up to a total repetition time of 10–30 seconds.

The second exercise uses leg and pelvic motion on a fixed trunk to increase the emphasis on the lower abdominals (Lipetz and Gutin, 1970; Guimaraes et al., 1991). The subject begins the action in crook lying and draws the knees right up onto the chest (Fig. 7.39). The action is then a posterior pelvic tilt combined with abdominal hollowing to flex the lower lumbar spine and raise the sacrum off the supporting surface. Again the repetition time is gradually increased to 10–30 seconds. Because both of these exercises flex the lumbar spine, a passive extension action, such as extension in lying and anterior pelvic tilting, should be performed at the end of the exercise bout to compensate for flexion stresses.

The FLAT programme progresses through a series of exercises designed to minimize stress on the passive spinal tissues while maximizing overload on the target muscles (Fig. 7.40). The reader is referred to Norris (1997) for further details.

TRUNK CURL SEQUENCE

1. Pevic tilt
2. Hollowing
3. Fingers to heels

Figure 7.38   Trunk curl sequence.

PELVIC RAISE

Figure 7.39   Pelvic raise.

(a)

(b)

(c)

(d)

(e)

Figure 7.40 Abdominal training exercises. (a) Abdominal hollowing. (b) Heel slide. (c) Pelvic raise. (d) Bench curl (crunch). (e) Curl with twist. From Norris (1997).

References

Appell, H.J. (1990) Muscular atrophy following immobilisation: a review. *Sports Medicine*, **10**, 42

Atkinson H.W. (1986) Principles of treatment. In *Cash's Textbook of Neurology for Physiotherapists*, 4th edn (ed. P.A. Downie), Faber and Faber, London

Barrack, R.L. and Skinner, H.B. (1990) The sensory function of knee ligaments. In *Knee Ligaments: Structure, Function, and Injury* (ed. D. Daniel). Raven Press

Barrack, R.L., Skinner H.B. and Buckley, S.L. (1989) Proprioception in the anterior cruciate deficient knee. *American Journal of Sports Medicine*, **17**, 1–6

Barrett, D.S., Cobb, A.G. and Bentley, G. (1991) Joint proprioception in normal, osteoarthritic, and replaced knees. *Journal of Bone and Joint Surgery*, **73B**, 53–56

Bastide, G., Zadeh, J. and Lefebvre, D. (1989) Are the 'little muscles' what we think they are? *Surgical and Radiological Anatomy*, **11**, 255–256

Beard, D.J., Kyberd, P.J., O'Connor, J.J., Fergusson, C.M. and Dodd, C.A.F. (1994) Reflex hamstring contraction latency in anterior cruciate ligament deficiency. *Journal of Orthopaedic Research*, **12**(2), 219–228

Biedermann, H.J., Shanks, G.L., Forrest, W.J. and Inglis, J. (1991) Power spectrum analyses of electromyographic activity. *Spine*, **16**(10), 1179–1184

Comerford, M. (1995) *Muscle Imbalance*, Course notes. Nottingham School of Physiotherapy.

Cresswell, A.G., Grundstrom, H. and Thorstensson, A. (1992) Observations on intra-abdominal pressure and patterns of abdominal intra-muscular activity in man. *Acta Physiologica Scandinavica*, **144**(4), 409–418

Cresswell, A.G., Oddsson, L. and Thorstensson, A. (1994) The influence of sudden perturbations on trunk muscle activity and intra abdominal pressure while standing. *Experimental Brain Research*, **98**, 336–341

de Andrade, J.R., Grant, C. and Dixon, A. (1965) Joint distention and reflex muscle inhibition in the knee. *Journal of Bone and Joint Surgery*, **47**(A), 313–322

Freeman, M.A.R., Dean, M.R.E. and Hanham, I.W.F. (1965) The etiology and prevention of functional instability of the foot. *Journal of Bone and Joint Surgery 1965b*, **47B**, 678–685

Goldspink, G. (1996) Personal communication.

Goldspink, G. (1992) Cellular and molecular aspects of adaptation in skeletal muscle. In *Strength and Power in Sport* (ed. P.V. Komi), Blackwell, Oxford

Gossman, M.R., Sahrmann, S.A. and Rose, S.J. (1982) Review of length associated changes in muscle. *Physical Therapy*, **62**(12), 1799–1808

Guimaraes, A.C.S., Vaz, M.A., De Campos, M.I.A. and Marantes, R. (1991) The contribution of the rectus abdominus and rectus femoris in twelve selected abdominal exercises. *Journal of Sports Medicine and Physical Fitness*, **31**(2), 222–230

Hides, J.A., Stokes, M.J., Saide, M., Jull, G.A. and Cooper, D.H. (1994) Evidence of lumbar multifidus muscle wasting ipsilateral to symptoms in patients with acute/subacute low back pain. *Spine*, **19**(2), 165–172

Hodges, P.W. and Richardson, C.A. (1995) Neuromotor dysfunction of the trunk musculature in low back pain patients. In *Proceedings of the World Confederation of Physical Therapists Congress*, Washington

Hodges, P.W. and Richardson, C.A. (1996a) Contraction of transversus abdominus invariably precedes movement of the upper and lower limb. In *Proceedings of the 6th International Conference of the International Federation of Orthopaedic Manipulative Therapists (IFOMT)*, Lillehammer, Norway

Hodges, P.W. and Richardson, C.A. (1996b) Inefficient muscular stabilisation of the lumbar spine associated with low back pain: A motor control evaluation of transversus abdominus. *Spine*, **21/22**, 2640–2650

Hodges, P., Richardson, C. and Jull, G. (1996) Evaluation of the relationship between laboratory and clinical tests of transversus abdominus function. *Physiotherapy Research International*, **1**, (1) 30–40

Irion, J.M. (1992) Use of the gym ball in rehabilitation of spinal dysfunction. *Orthopaedic Physical Therapy Clinics of North America*, Oxford, pp. 375–398

Janda, V. (1993) Muscle strength in relation to muscle length, pain and muscle imbalance. In *Muscle Strength. International Perspectives in Physical Therapy* (ed. K. Harms-Ringdahl), **8**, Churchill Livingstone, Edinburgh

Janda, V. (1994) Muscles and motor control in cervicogenic disorders: Assessment and management. In *Physical Therapy of the Cervical and Thoracic Spine*

(ed. R. Grant), 2nd edn, Churchill Livingstone, Edinburgh

Janda, V. and Schmid, H.J.A. (1980) Muscles as a pathogenic factor in backpain. *Proceedings of the International Federation of Orthopaedic Manipulative Therapists*, 4th conference, New Zealand, pp. 17–18

Johnson, C. and Reid, J.G. (1991) Lumbar compressive and shear forces during various trunk curl-up exercises. *Clinical Biomechanics*, **6**, 97–104

Jull, G.A. (1994) Headaches of cervical origin. In *Physical Therapy of the Cervical and Thoracic Spine* (ed. R. Grant), Churchill Livingstone, New York

Jull, G.A. and Janda, V. (1987) Muscles and motor control in low back pain: Assessment and management. In *Physical Therapy of the Low Back* (ed. L.T. Twomey), Churchill Livingstone, New York

Kamkar, A., Irrgang, J.L., and Whitney, S.L. (1993) Nonoperative management of secondary shoulder impingement syndrome. *Journal of Orthopedic and Sports Physical Therapy*, **17**(5), 212–224

Kendall, F.P. and McCreary, E.K. (1983) *Muscle Testing and Function*, 3rd edn, Baltimore, Williams and Wilkins

Kendall, F.P., McCreary, E.K. and Provance, P.G. (1993) *Muscles. Testing and Function*, 4th edn, Baltimore, Williams and Wilkins

Kennedy, J.C., Alexander, I.J. and Hayes, K.C. (1982) Nerve supply of the human knee and its functional importance. *American Journal of Sports Medicine*, **10**, 329

Koh, T.J. (1995) Do adaptations in serial sarcomere number occur with strength training? *Human Movement Science*, **14**, 61–77

Konradsen, L. and Ravn, J.B. (1990) Ankle instability caused by prolonged peroneal reaction time. *Acta Orthopedica Scandinavica*, **61**(5), 388–390

Lentell, G.L., Katzman, L.L. and Walters, M.R. (1990) The relationship between muscle function and ankle stability. *Journal of Orthopaedic and Sports Physical Therapy*, **11**, 605–611

Lephart, S.M. and Fu, F.H. (1995) The role of proprioception in the treatment of sports injuries. *Sports Exercise and Injury*, **1**(2), 96–102

Lephart, S.M., Warner, J.P., Borsa, P.A. and Fu, F.H. (1994) Proprioception of the shoulder in normal, unstable, and surgical individuals. *Journal of Shoulder and Elbow Surgery*, **3**(4), 371–381

Lewit, K. (1991) *Manipulative Therapy in Rehabilitation of the Locomotor System*, 2nd edn, Butterworth-Heinemann, Oxford

Lieber, R.L. (1992) *Skeletal Muscle Structure and Function*. Williams and Wilkins, Baltimore

Lipetz, S. and Gutin, B. (1970) An electromyographic study of four abdominal exercises. *Medicine and Science in Sports and Exercise*, **2**, 35–38

Lucas, D.B. (1973) Biomechanics of the shoulder joint. *Archives of Surgery*, **107**, 425–432

McKenzie, R.A. (1981) *The Lumbar Spine. Mechanical Diagnosis and Therapy*, Spinal Publications, Lower Hutt, New Zealand

Miller, M.I. and Medeiros, J.M. (1987) Recruitment of internal oblique and transversus abdominus muscles during the eccentric phase of the curl-up exercise. *Physical Therapy*, **67**, 1213–1217

Morgan, D.L. and Lynn, R. (1994) Decline running produces more sarcomeres in rat vastus intermedius muscle fibers than does incline running. *Journal of Applied Physiology*, **77**, 1439–1444

Muller, E.A. (1970) Influence of training and of inactivity on muscle strength. *Archives of Physical Medicine and Rehabilitation*, **51**, 449–462

Ng, G. and Richardson, C.A. (1990) The effects of training triceps surae using progressive speed loading. *Physiotherapy Practice*, **6**, 77–84

Norkin, C.C. and Levangie, P.K. (1992) *Joint Structure and Function*, 2nd edn, F.A. Davis, Philadelphia

Norris, C.M. (1994a) Abdominal training. Dangers and exercise modifications. *Physiotherapy in Sport*, **14**(5), 10–14

Norris, C.M. (1994b) A flat stomach – the right way. *Exercise Magazine*, November 1994

Norris, C.M. (1995a) Spinal stabilisation. *Physiotherapy*, **81**(2), 1–4

Norris, C.M. (1995b) Spinal stabilisation, 5. An exercise programme to enhance lumbar stabilisation. *Physiotherapy*, **81**(3), 31–39

Norris, C.M. (1997) *Abdominal Training*, A&C Black, London

Palastanga, N., Field, D. and Soames, R. (1989) *Anatomy and Human Movement*, Butterworth-Heinemann, Oxford

Palmitier, R.A., An, K., Scott, S.G. and Chao, E.Y.S. (1991) Kinetic chain exercise in knee rehabilitation. *Sports Medicine*, **11**(6), 402–413

Ricci, B., Marchetti, M. and Figura, F. (1981) Biomechanics of sit-up exercises. *Medicine and Science in Sports and Exercise*, **13**, 54–59

Richardson, C.A. (1992) Muscle imbalance: Principles of treatment and assessment. *Proceedings of the New Zealand Society of Physiotherapists Challenges Conference*, Christchurch, New Zealand

Richardson, C.A. and Bullock, M.I. (1986) Changes in muscle activity during fast, alternating flexion–extension movements of the knee. *Scandinavian Journal of Rehabilitation Medicine*, **18**, 51–58

Richardson, C.A. and Hodges, P. (1996) *New advances in exercise to rehabilitate spinal stabilisation*, Course notes, Edinburgh

Richardson, C.A. and Sims, K. (1991) An inner range holding contraction: An objective measure of stabilizing function of an antigravity muscle. *Proceedings of the World Confederation for Physical Therapy 11th International Congress*, London

Richardson, C., Jull, G., Toppenburg, R. and Comerford, M. (1992) Techniques for active lumbar stabilisation for spinal protection: A pilot study. *Australian Journal of Physiotherapy*, **38**(2), 105–112

Sahrmann, S.A. (1987) Posture and muscle imbalance: Faulty lumbar-pelvic alignment and associated musculoskeletal pain syndromes. *Postgraduate Advances in Physical Therapy*, Forum Medicum, Berryville, Virginia

Sahrmann, S.A. (1990) Diagnosis and treatment of movement-related pain syndromes associated with muscle and movement imbalances. Course notes. Washington university

Silvermetz, M.A. (1990) Pathokinesiology of supine double leg lifts as an abdominal strengthener and suggested alternative exercises. *Athletic Training*, **25**, 17–22

Smith, R.L. and Brunolli, J. (1990) Shoulder kinaesthesia after anterior glenohumeral joint dislocation. *Physical Therapy*, **69**, 106–112

Stokes, M. and Young, A. (1984) The contribution of reflex inhibition to arthrogenous muscle weakness. *Clinical Science*, **67**, 7–14

Templeton, G.H., Padalino, M., Manton, J., Glasberg, M. and Silver, C.J. (1984) Influence of suspension hypokinesia on rat soleus muscle. *Journal of Applied Physiology*, **56**, 278–286

Travell, J.G. and Simons, D.G. (1983) *Myofascial Pain and Dysfunction*, Williams and Wilkins, Baltimore

Tropp H., Alaranta H. and Renstrom, P.A.F.H. (1993) Proprioception and coordination training in injury prevention. In *Sports Injuries. Basic Principles of Prevention and Care* (ed. P.A.F.H. Renstrom), IOC Medical Commission, Blackwell Scientific, London

Twomey, L.T. and Taylor, J.R. (1987) Lumbar posture, movement and mechanics. In *Physical Therapy of the Low Back* (eds L.T. Twomey and J.R. Taylor), Churchill Livingstone, Edinburgh

Tyldesley, B. and Grieve, J.I. (1989) *Muscles, Nerves and Movement: Kinesiology in Daily Living*, Blackwell Scientific, Oxford

Walters, C. and Partridge, M. (1957) Electromyographic study of the differential abdominal muscles during exercise. *American Journal of Physical Medicine*, **36**, 259–268

Watson, J (1983) *An Introduction to Mechanics of Human Movement*, MTP Press, Lancaster

White, S.G. and Sahrmann, S.A. (1994) A movement system balance approach to management of musculoskeletal pain. In *Physical Therapy of the Cervical and Thoracic Spine* (ed. R. Grant), Churchill Livingstone, New York

Wilk, K.E. and Arrigo, C. (1993) Current concepts in the rehabilitation of the athletic shoulder. *Journal of Orthopedic and Sports Physical Therapy*, **18**(1), 365–378

Williams, P.E. (1990) Use of intermittent stretch in the prevention of serial sarcomere loss in immobilised muscle. *Annals of the Rheumatic Diseases*, **49**, 316–317

Williams, P.E. and Goldspink, G. (1978) Changes in sarcomere length and physiological properties in immobilized muscle. *Journal of Anatomy*, **127**, 459–468

Williams, P., Watt, P., Bicik, V. and Goldspink, G. (1986) Effect of stretch combined with electrical stimulation on the type of sarcomeres produced at the ends of muscle fibers. *Experimental Neurology*, **93**, 500–509

Yang K.H. and King, A.I. (1984) Mechanism of facet load transmission as a hypothesis for low-back pain. *Spine*, **9**, 557–565

8

First contact management

Injury prevention

Injury prevention should perhaps be the most important topic within the field of sports medicine. The term 'prevention' is normally used in the context of sports injuries to refer to any measure which can stop an injury occurring. But the processes of prevention also play an important role in arresting the exacerbation of a current injury, and ensuring that the same injury does not recur.

The causes of sports injuries are many and varied. Williams and Sperryn (1976) implicated failure in technique, faulty sports equipment, poor physical fitness, inadequate warm-up and psychological factors. Taimela, Kujala and Osterman (1990) divided injury risk factors into intrinsic and extrinsic groups as shown in Table 8.1.

Some factors will clearly affect athletes differently, and certain elements are more important in one sport than another. However, in general the more risk factors an athlete shows, the more likely he or she is to be injured. Consequently, the aim of the coach or practitioner should be to reduce these risk factors to a minimum.

Warm-up

The subject of warm-up is dealt with in depth in Chapter 6. A general warm-up, intense enough to induce mild sweating without causing fatigue, is important for injury prevention. The general activity should be followed by a specific warm-up designed to produce a suitable arousal level in the athlete, and to rehearse any complex skills which will be used later in competition.

Joints, muscles, and other soft tissues should be extended through their full physiological range before competition. However, it is important that flexibility training in itself be separate to, and follow after a warm-up.

It is also important that vigourous exercise does not end abruptly, but slows gradually during a cool down period. This period allows the cardiopulmonary system to return to resting levels without placing undue stress on the body. In addition, delayed onset muscle soreness (DOMS) may be reduced by flushing fresh blood into the muscles previously worked during exercise, and removing waste products. To achieve an increase in muscle perfusion, the activity must involve rhythmic muscle pumping actions of low intensity. The use of post-event massage in this context is described on p. 97.

Fitness

All the components of fitness are required for injury prevention (see p. 111), and importantly, a balance should exist between each. For example, increased flexibility without a

Table 8.1 Injury risk factors

Extrinsic
Organization and management
Type of sport
Training errors
Environment
Equipment

Intrinsic
Age
Gender
Somatotype
Local anatomy and biomechanics
Fitness
Physical symmetry
Joint integrity
Motor control (skill)
Psychological/psychosocial factors

Adapted from Taimela et al. (1990).

similar increase in strength may leave a joint hypermobile or unstable and increase the risk of injury. Similarly, strength and muscle bulk increases without adequate flexibility and skill can leave an athlete 'muscle bound' and lacking agility.

Symmetry of muscle development and range of motion is also important. Athletes who exercise unilaterally, for example throwers, must take care that they redress the imbalance caused by their sport with a suitable strength training programme. Unequal muscle development across a single joint or series of joints may alter specific body segment alignment and general posture. Similarly, unequal training within an antagonistic pair of muscles will cause imbalance.

It is also important that training accurately reflects the physical demands of a sport, and exercise be specific to the physiological adaptations that the sport requires (SAID principle, see p. 112). Sports requiring speed and power, for example, will suffer if only strength is included in training. The 'strong' athlete who has trained exclusively with heavy weight training is open to injury when rapid explosive actions are used in

sport. This is because the skills involved in the two actions are very different.

Psychological factors

Athletes of a certain psychological type may be more predisposed to injury and the sports coach must recognize this. Equally, during particularly stressful periods, or when life pressures outside the sporting context are great, athletes who do not normally get injured may start to have problems. These concepts are dealt with in Chapter 3, but all coaches and practitioners working with sports teams must get to know their athletes. Realizing that a player is having problems with his or her spouse, or has recently had a family bereavement is vital to 'total player management'.

Equipment and environment

All athletes are under pressure to buy particular sportswear. Professional athletes may receive sponsorship, and amateur athletes (particularly children) will respond to changing fashions. It is important to emphasize to the athlete that sports equipment should be comfortable and functional. If a particular shoe or item of clothing does not fit correctly, another should be tried, the fit being more important than the type.

The field of play should also be the focus of attention, particularly in amateur sport. Before training, both the environment and equipment should be inspected by the coach. If, for example, a child falls on a broken bottle that no one realized was there, part of the responsibility lies with the coach for not checking the area beforehand.

Another aspect of 'environment' that warrants attention is the other players. Variability of young athletes grouped by chronological age rather than biological (physiological) age may be tremendous. This is especially true at the onset of puberty, where a relatively narrow age range of two years in a grouping of 9–11 year olds will give a large size variation. It was these variations (at the time within the child labour market) which gave rise to the use of physiological age groupings based on pubic hair development (Crampton, 1908).

Table 8.2 shows the difference between age, size and a selection of performance variables in small and large youth ice hockey players in the same league. It is clearly a risk to have a 37 kg athlete able to produce an impact force of just over 1000 N competing against a 74 kg athlete capable of producing an (almost double) impact force of 1700 N.

Self-assessment of maturity can be made using secondary sex characteristics including external genitalia and pubic hair in males, and breasts, pubic hair, and menarche in females (Malina and Beunen, 1996). There is obviously a potential problem of under- and over-estimation (by the athlete or others) to remain with peers or to gain a competitive advantage, but the threat of random testing by medical staff should control this.

Rules

In professional sport, rule changes have had a dramatic effect, particularly with head injuries. However, the local youth club under-12 team must also have a firm policy of sports regulation. Where children are involved, it is important to lay down firm rules concerning safety and equipment. The coach who tries to

Table 8.2 Age, size and performance variables of youth ice-hockey players

	Small	Large
Variable	Mean	Mean
Age (years)	13.4	14.0
Weight (kg)	37.1	74.3
Stature (cm)	147.4	178.9
Grip strength (kg)	27.7	56.5
Maximal speed (m/s)	7.6	8.3
Impact force (N)	1010.0	1722.0
Speed at impact (m/s)	3.2	3.7

Adapted from Roy et al. (1989).

be popular by allowing a 'free for all' is really being irresponsible and is likely to be the cause of injury.

Screening

The subject of physical screening of youngsters in sport is one which attracts much discussion. A variety of anatomical abnormalities may develop largely unnoticed to the layperson. However, these can often be readily identified by the sports medicine practitioner with a series of annual screening tests. Posture (p. 15), flexibility (p. 122) and strength (p. 131) can all be measured using fairly simple field tests. These can be incorporated into a training session and educational period for youngsters, at the beginning of a season.

First aid

First aid treatment marks the beginning of the rehabilitation process. Correct management at this stage can reduce the severity of an injury and so shorten the time an athlete is away from sport. More importantly, effective first aid can save lives. In this section, a number of first aid methods relevant to the injured sportsperson are described. All therapists involved with sports injuries management are recommended to obtain certification in cardiopulmonary resuscitation (CPR) and basic first aid.

The unconscious athlete

Unconsciousness is the result of an interruption of normal brain activity. The most common cause in sport is concussion. The first decision to be made with an unconscious athlete is whether he or she is still breathing. If not, resuscitation must be started *immediately*.

If the athlete is breathing, the severity of loss of consciousness should be assessed. Response of the eyes, body movements and speech all give clues to the level of consciousness. Table 8.3 shows a number of responses which may be tested. In addition, pulse and respiratory rate and depth should be noted, as any sudden change is important.

Concussion

Concussion occurs when the brain is rapidly 'shaken', and the condition can be present even though the patient is still conscious. Often, the period of unconsciousness is so brief that it may go unnoticed, and there is only transient memory loss. This is frequently the case with contact injuries where an athlete collides with another and hits his or her head.

After such an incident, an athlete should only be allowed to continue if he did not lose consciousness. Tests such as the ability to stand up without assistance, stand alone with eyes closed, and run to a mark and change direction rapidly are all useful (Walkden, 1981). Even then, the athlete should be regularly checked.

Caution must always be exercised with concussion injuries. Unfortunately, the practitioner or coach who has to decide whether to allow an athlete to continue playing has no way of knowing if secondary brain damage is going to develop. At the time of injury, bleeding may have occurred which could accumulate and give rise to a subdural haematoma.

Table 8.3 Response testing in the unconscious athlete

Do the eyes open:
spontaneously
to speech
to pain
Does the athlete move:
to verbal command
to painful stimulus
Is the athlete's speech:
normal
confused
inappropriate
incomprehensible

If the athlete remains unconscious, he or she should be placed in the recovery position until an ambulance is available to take him or her to hospital. If there is bleeding or discharge from an ear, the athlete should be turned so that the affected ear is dependent. Nothing should be given by mouth, and the athlete should not be left unattended. Testing for responses should continue regularly (every 10 minutes or less) and any changes in the athlete's condition should be recorded.

The cumulative effects of concussion are important, in sports such as boxing, steeplechase, and football (Corsellis, 1974; Sortland, Tysvaer and Storli, 1989; McLatchie, 1993). EEG disturbances due to neuronal damage through repeated trauma are seen, especially where a series of EEGs are performed. In addition, neuropsychological performance is impaired, often in the presence of a normal CT scan (McLatchie, Brooks and Galbraith, 1987).

Epilepsy

If an epileptic athlete loses consciousness, he or she may fit. Rigidity may last for a few seconds and cyanosis of the mouth and lips can occur. The athlete should be protected by clearing a space around him or her. Any tight clothing around the neck should be loosened, and something soft placed under his or her head.

No attempt should be made to move the athlete, or restrain the athlete, and nothing should be given by mouth until he or she has fully recovered. No object should be placed in the mouth of a fitting athlete as they may choke. In addition, it has been known for an epileptic to break a tooth in this way and inhale it.

Diabetic coma

In diabetes mellitus both hyperglycaemia and hypoglycaemia may give rise to unconsciousness. Hyperglycaemia usually develops gradually and so is rarely a first aid problem.

With intense unaccustomed exercise, the blood sugar level may fall, and hypoglycaemia can then result. An athlete may initially feel faint, dizzy or light-headed, and may be confused or disorientated. The skin becomes pale, the pulse rapid, and sweating occurs. Breathing often becomes shallow, and muscle tremor may be apparent. The level of consciousness drops rapidly.

If the athlete is conscious a rapidly metabolized sugar (glucose tablet or sugary drink) will help, together with some slowly absorbed carbohydrate (bread) to prevent recurrent blood glucose fall. If the athlete is unconscious, nothing should be given and hospital treatment should be sought. If the coma is due to hypoglycaemia, the response to sugar is usually rapid and the danger of secondary symptoms is averted. If hyperglycaemic coma is present, slightly more sugar will not harm the patient (Sperryn, 1985).

Resuscitation

With an unconscious subject who is not breathing, or in whom no heart beat can be detected, it is vital that these processes be restored or sustained until hospital treatment is available. In all cases, help must be summoned as soon as possible. A basic mnemonic usefully describes the course of action: ABC — airway, breathing, circulation.

Airway

If breathing is noisy, or not present, the airway may be blocked. This can occur if the tongue has fallen back and is covering the airway, or if the airway is narrowed due to the position of the head. Absence of the gagging reflex may allow saliva or vomit to accumulate at the back of the throat and block the airway. The subject's chin should be pulled forwards and the head tilted back (Fig. 8.1a). This will open the airway. If breathing is still noisy, the head should be turned to one side keeping the head well back, providing cervical injury is not suspected.

Foreign matter may be cleared from the mouth by sweeping two fingers around the inside the mouth (Fig. 8.1b). The practitioner should look, listen and feel for signs of respiratory movements (Fig. 8.1c). If these are not present, artificial ventilation is required.

Breathing

When the airway is cleared, the subject should be laid supine, and mouth to mouth, or mouth to nose ventilation given. In small children the nose and mouth may be used together. The subject's mouth is opened wide and his or her nose pinched close, at the same time keeping the subject's head well back (Fig. 8.2a). The practitioner breathes out directly into the subject's mouth, making sure a good seal is maintained between his or her own lips and the subject's mouth. The chest should be observed to assess lung inflation (Fig. 8.2b). If this does not occur, the airway may still be blocked, in which case the head should be re-adjusted and the artificial ventilation resumed. If no chest movement occurs this time, the subject should be treated with an abdominal thrust as though choking (see below).

After two lung inflations, the carotid pulse (lying between the larynx and the anterior edge of the sternomastoid) should be tested (Fig. 8.2c). This will only be present if the systolic blood pressure is at least 60 mmHg. If a pulse is present, but breathing has not commenced, artificial ventilation should be continued at a rate of 10 inflations per minute. If the pulse is not detected, external chest compression is required.

Circulation

For external chest compression, the subject should be supine on a firm surface. The practitioner kneels to one side, and places the

Figure 8.1   Opening the airway. (a) Pull the athlete's chin forwards and tilt the head back. (b) Clear away foreign matter by turning the head to the side and sweeping two fingers around inside the mouth. (c) Look, listen and feel for signs of respiratory movements.

heel of one hand, reinforced by the other, over the subject's lower sternum (Fig. 8.3a). Keeping the elbows locked, a downwards pressure is exerted onto the patient's sternum by the practitioner leaning downwards and pushing through straight arms (Fig. 8.3b). The force used should be sufficient to depress the sternum by 4–5 cm. The pressure is released and the procedure repeated 15 times. Following this, attention is again focused on the mouth and two breaths of artificial ventilation are given. This sequence of 15 repetitions of external chest compression and two breaths of artificial ventilation continues until hospitalization is available, or the subject recovers. The carotid pulse is checked after one minute and then after

each third minute. When the pulse returns, chest compression is stopped. If breathing returns and is sustained, the subject is placed into the recovery position.

If an assistant is available, resuscitation may be carried out with one person performing chest compression and the other artificial respiration. The rate is then five compressions to one inflation (Fig. 8.3c).

A number of resuscitation aids are available. Some consist of a plastic sheet, mouthpiece and valve which covers the face of the subject and holds the mouth open. Plastic airways themselves are helpful to hold the tongue away from the back of the throat, and airways with a valve to stop the passage of saliva to the practitioner are also available.

Figure 8.2 Breathing. (a) Open the athlete's mouth, pinch his or her nose closed and tilt the head back. (b) Breathe directly into the athlete's mouth and observe his or her chest movements. (c) Test the carotid pulse.

All airways have the potential to damage the soft palate and should only be used after appropriate training.

Recovery position

When an unconscious athlete is breathing and shows a regular pulse, he or she should be placed into the recovery position (*First Aid Manual*, 1995). In this position, the chin is lifted forwards to keep the airway clear and open, the head is lower than the body so fluids will drain from the mouth avoiding the possibility of them being inhaled. The athlete's hand supports the head and protects it from the ground, and the arm and leg are bent, increasing stability and prevent-

ing the body rolling forwards. The side-lying position avoids the chest compression of the prone position, making breathing easier.

The athlete is rolled into the recovery position in five stages (Fig. 8.4), making sure that the open airway remains a priority throughout the movement. In stage I, the practitioner kneels to the side of the athlete at waist level. The athlete's airway is opened (gum shield removed) by pulling the chin forwards and tilting the head back. If there is time, objects such as the athlete's spectacles, keys in the pocket, and any cord in or around the neck (stopwatch, whistle, etc.) should be removed. The nearest arm is bent to 90° at the elbow and shoulder, and supinated to bring the palm forward facing at the side of the head

Figure 8.3 Circulation. (a) One hand, reinforced by the other, is placed over the athlete's sternum. (b) Keeping the elbows locked, a downwards pressure is exerted to depress the sternum by 4–5 cm. (c) With an assistant, one person performs chest compression, and the other artificial respiration.

('oath' position). For stage II, the athlete's other arm is brought across the chest and his or her hands held together against his near cheek throughout the remaining stages to support and protect the head. In stage III the athlete's far leg is grasped over the lower hamstrings to flex it and pull the bent knee towards the practitioner. The foot remains on the floor to take the weight of the limb and avoid lifting stress on the practitioner. In stage IV the athlete's knee is pulled towards the practitioner to roll the athlete onto his side. The practitioner's knees prevent the athlete from rolling too far. Finally, in stage V the athlete's chin is pulled forwards to

clear the tongue from the throat and assist drainage. Final adjustments are made to the athlete's hand beneath his cheek to maintain correct head alignment, and to the athlete's upper leg (flexed at 90° to both hip and knee) for maximum stability.

If the limbs cannot be bent, the side-lying position may be maintained by placing a rolled blanket or similar item below the athlete along one side of his or her body.

Skin wounds

Skin wounds are common injuries in sport, especially when athletes train on hard sur-

Figure 8.4   Moving an athlete into the recovery position. Stage I: open airway, remove any obstructing objects, straighten legs and kneel at the athlete's waist, bend near arm into oath position. Stage II: bring far arm across chest to side of face, and maintain this position throughout. Stage III: grasp far leg, bend knee and pull it towards you. Stage IV: roll the athlete towards you, blocking him or her with your knees. Stage V: adjust the head position to ensure a clear airway, adjust upper leg position to ensure whole body stability.

faces. When treating skin wounds, the practitioner must protect him or herself against contact with blood or tissue fluids. If the practitioner has grazes, sores, or open wounds on the hands or forearms, these must be covered with a waterproof adhesive dressing. Disposable gloves should always be used when treating skin wounds of any type. Where gloves are not available, ask the athlete to dress his or her own wound under the practitioner's supervision. If the athlete is unconscious and gloves are not available, the practitioner should improvise and place his or her hands in plastic bags.

As described in Chapter 2, wounds may be either open or closed, depending on whether the epidermis has been completely penetrated. With closed wounds, such as abrasions and gravel burns, the aim is to prevent infection and remove any foreign material. The injured area is cleaned with 0.5% chlorhexidine or a mixture of chlorhexidine and cetrimide, and grit or other material removed with sterile forceps. If an athlete is known to be allergic to chlorhexidine, sterile water should be used instead. Exposed areas may be left without a dressing, as air will assist healing. If an abrasion cannot be left exposed, it should be dressed with a single layer of paraffin gauze and a dry dressing (or a dry dressing alone for small wounds). The area should be checked every 48 hours to ensure there is no infection and that healing is progressing. When a practitioner decides that a player must continue until the end of the match, a wound may be sprayed with antiseptic dry spray, and the area bandaged with a cohesive (non-adhesive) tape which is impermeable to blood.

Open wounds, such as lacerations and puncture wounds, are more serious. The amount of bleeding which occurs is dependent on the site of the injury and the depth of the wound, arterial damage will obviously give profuse bleeding. The first priority is to stop bleeding with direct pressure over the wound and elevation of the injured limb. Pressure should be given with a sterile (or at least clean) dressing, or the patient's hand, and maintained for at least 10 minutes to allow blood clotting.

Some minor lacerations may be cleaned and closed with sterile adhesive strips or dumb-bell sutures. These have the advantage that no local anaesthetic is needed for their application, and they avoid the risk of stitch marks and suture tearing of the skin.

More extensive wounds may require suturing. When deeper tissues have been damaged, suturing in layers may be required. The deep layers being sutured with catgut and the skin closed with silk. Because of the risk of infection, all but the most minor open skin wounds should be managed in a hospital casualty department. In cases where bleeding is profuse, the patient may need to be treated for shock by lying him or her flat and elevating the lower limbs, until he or she can be removed to hospital.

All skin wounds run the risk of tetanus infection, so an injured athlete who sustains a major injury may require a full course of tetanus prophylaxis. This consists of three injections of 0.5 ml tetanus toxoid. The first is given at the time of injury, the second 6 weeks later and the third 6 months after the first. If an athlete is not sure of the time interval since his last tetanus injection (or if a course has been given within the last 12 months), a booster dose of 0.5 ml toxoid may be given after injury as a precaution.

Soft tissue injury

The initial aim with a soft tissue injury is to protect the area from further harm and slow the inflammatory process. A simple mnemonic for first contact treatment is RICE: rest, ice, compression, elevation.

Rest

The immediate first aid concern (assuming a life-threatening situation does not exist) is to protect the injured body part from further injury. This may simply mean rest, or splinting/strapping in the case of an injured joint to limit movement. Inflatable splints are invaluable here for fast immobilization to permit safe removal to hospital. Details on strapping are given in Chapter 5.

During the acute phase of inflammation, the athlete should rest. However, rather than complete rest, 'functional rest' is to be preferred. Here, any activity which stresses the injured tissue is avoided, but other activities are allowed. In the sub-acute phase, the injured tissues themselves should be allowed to move gently, to produce a strong mobile scar, and to allow collagen fibres to align in the direction of stress (Sterns, 1940; Burri, Helbing and Spier, 1973; Cyriax, 1982). Total rest of an injured body part may lead to increased adhesions. In addition, a haphazard arrangement of collagen fibres within the newly formed scar will result in a reduction of tensile strength.

More vigorous general exercise is to be encouraged, with the injured body part still protected. This will help maintain general cardiopulmonary fitness and the condition of the non-injured tissues.

Ice

Ice, or cold application, is used to slow the metabolic rate of the injured tissue and reduce hypoxic tissue damage (Knight, 1989). Furthermore, the production of cold-induced analgesia is desirable. An ice pack should be kept on for 15–20 minutes and reapplied every two hours for the first two days following injury.

If no ice is available, cold water is of use, but the tissue temperature changes are not as great as with ice, and so hypoxic damage is not prevented as efficiently. The use of ice is covered later in this chapter.

Compression

Compression is used in combination with cold to reduce swelling. Compression should be sufficient to limit the formation of oedema but not to compromise the blood flow to the area. The circulation distal to the compression should be checked by observing skin coloration. In addition, a finger-nail or toe-nail should be squeezed on the injured limb which has been compressed. The subungual skin will go white with compression and the normal pink coloration should return a few seconds after pressure is released, illustrating that adequate circulation is reaching the nailbed.

Elevation

Gravity will pull swelling into a dependent limb, so elevation should be used to aid lymphatic drainage. The limb need only be elevated above the level of the heart. Athletes with lower limb injuries, particularly to the ankle, should be encouraged to keep the leg elevated on a stool when sitting throughout the day. In addition, gentle isometric or short range isotonic exercise is useful to stimulate the muscle pump and aid venous return and lymphatic drainage.

A combination of the above treatment techniques will produce the best results. Cold compresses can easily be applied with lint soaked in iced water and wrapped around the limb. A polythene bag covers the wet lint and an elastic tubular bandage covers both. The compress is reapplied every 2 or 3 minutes as its temperature rises. The limb is elevated and isometric exercise performed at a rate of one contraction every three to five seconds. Various cryogel impregnated bandages are commercially available which perform a similar job. Flaked ice in a towelling bag may be applied flat with an elastic bandage over the top. Again, elevation and muscle pump exercise is required.

Fractures

Fractures should only receive treatment after breathing has been restored and bleeding stopped. If a fracture is present, squeezing the area or gentle limb movements will usually cause pain. If the accident was not seen, and the athlete has not moved, a screening examination is required. The 'squeeze technique' is used. This procedure, where a body area is compressed to assess pain and bony contour, starts at the head, and then moves to the neck, shoulders and arms and so on until the whole body has been assessed. The experienced practitioner can carry out such an examination in 30–60 seconds.

If a fracture is found, the injured bone should be immobilized by splinting. A number of options exist. Several emergency splints are on the market, and sports clubs should be encouraged to have these available. The various types include inflatable splints, cardboard splints, backslabs and slings. If none of these are available, improvization is the order of the day. Broom handles, hockey sticks and ski poles are all useful splints, and with lower limb fractures using the other leg is also effective. In each case the limb should be gently straightened (if pain is not intense) and immobilized.

Injuries to the shoulder/clavicle or forearm fractures are best immobilized across the chest in a sling. Where the elbow cannot be bent, the straight arm is fixed at the side of the chest, by straps around the pelvis, waist and chest.

The question of whether an injury is a fracture or not often arises in sport. Observation will show any obvious deformity, and palpation by squeezing will usually elicit intense pain, considerably more than with a soft tissue injury. In addition, bleeding is normally more profuse. However, the only way to be totally sure is to view a radiograph of the affected limb.

Dislocations and subluxations

The most common joints dislocated in sport are the fingers and shoulder. No attempt should be made to reduce a shoulder dislocation because of the danger of damage to the axillary nerve (but see p. 428). Finger dislocations may be reduced easily, and this can lead to a underestimation of their potential severity. If light traction applied along the length of the bone causes the joint to relocate, this action is justified. Reduction later will need to be carried out under anaesthetic, as muscle spasm will have set in. There are two potential dangers of injury management on the field using the age old 'pull it, tape it, and play on' attitude. First, a fracture may have occurred near the joint line which will only reveal itself on X-ray. For this reason, even if the joint is successfully reduced, an X-ray is desirable (Walkden, 1981). Secondly, the final injury result may be jeopardized by early aggressive management (Reid, 1992). Misplaced taping may subject the injury to rotatory or angulatory stress leading to mala-

lignment, and increased/accumulating swelling may lead to additional joint stiffness.

Genital injury

Injury to the genitalia is common in the male, and a suitable box should be worn to offer some degree of protection. Bruising to the scrotum may occur by direct contact with another player or apparatus. The pain from such an injury is often incapacitating. Application of a cold sponge or ice may give some relief. If blood occurs in the urine after this injury, the player should seek medical attention.

Torsion of the testicles may occur in cycling, particularly in teenagers, and priapism (persistent erection) has been reported due to vascular obstruction (Sperryn, 1985). In both cases, medical attention is required.

Injury to the female genitalia may similarly occur through direct trauma causing contusion and possible pubic fracture, especially after a fall onto gymnastic apparatus. In addition, water-skiing may cause vaginal injury through forced douching. Female water-skiers are well-advised to protect the pudendal region by wearing a wet suit and not a bathing costume. Immediate gynaecological assistance is required.

Choking

Choking occurs when the act of swallowing forces something over the entrance to the trachea rather than into the oesophagus. Two first aid procedures may be used. Initially, the athlete should be bent forwards and firmly slapped with the flat of the hand between the shoulder blades five times. If this fails to dislodge the item, an abdominal thrust (Heimlich manoeuvre) may be used. Here, sharp pressure is placed over the upper abdomen in an attempt to rapidly increase abdominal pressure and simulate a cough.

The victim may be lying supine in which case the thrust can be through the straight arms of the practitioner. In standing, the practitioner wraps his arms around the victim and forces the heels of his hands up and into the victim's abdomen. The manoeuvre must be sharp and hard, and may be repeated five times (Fig. 8.5).

Five back slaps may be used alternating with five abdominal thrusts until the obstruction is removed. If the athlete loses consciousness, relaxation of muscle spasm may release the obstruction, so check to see if spontaneous breathing has resumed.

Cramp, stitch and winding

A sudden blow to the solar plexus may affect the sympathetic nerve centre in this region, causing a transient contusion (Reid, 1992). A momentary paralysis of the diaphragm may occur with spasm of the abdominal muscles, causing the player to be 'winded' (Fowler, 1981). Respiration is impaired and nausea may ensue. The player will almost always fall to the ground if the blow was severe, and should be left in the side-lying position until recovered. Reassurance is all that is required and a cold sponge to the nape of the neck may sometimes help. The injury occurs when the athlete is off-guard and the abdominal muscles are relaxed, so there is a danger of intra-abdominal injury (rib or visceral). For this reason, a winded player should be carefully observed for the remaining practice period or game.

Figure 8.5   Abdominal thrust technique for choking (Heimlich manoeuvre). (a) Standing position, (b) lying position.

Cramps can be a particular problem to athletes because they are so unpredictable. The terms cramp or spasm are used to imply a painful, sustained, and involuntary muscle contraction. It is important to realize that cramps are symptoms of some underlying fault. They may be the result of nerve entrapment, or metabolic disorder, and so, if persistent, the athlete should seek medical attention.

A number of possible causes have been suggested (Benda, 1989). Fluid loss, low glucose, electrolyte imbalance, training faults and fatigue have all been implicated. Cramps affect many different categories of people. Well-conditioned athletes are at risk, as are sedentary individuals who often complain of cramps in bed at night. The unfit individual who suddenly embarks on a vigorous keep-fit routine is particularly at risk.

Fluid loss will occur with profuse sweating, and athletes are best advised to take small amounts of water throughout a training period. Large amounts taken when cramp has occurred are not generally as effective, and lead to a bloated feeling.

Electrolyte imbalance altering the excitability of motor units is another possible cause (Fowler, 1981), and both potassium and salt may be involved. Some athletes use electrolyte drinks, but those containing a lot of sugar should be avoided, as should salt tablets. Salt will draw fluid out of the circulatory system, and sugar will slow fluid absorption. If salt or potassium is to be taken, it should be incorporated into the diet as a preventive measure. Potassium-rich foods such as bananas and oranges, and salty foods are suitable.

Pain relief and reduction of muscle spasm may be achieved by the use of ice and stretching. Ice is used to produce cold analgesia, and then slow stretching is carried out. Contraction of the antagonist muscle will help relax the cramped muscle through reciprocal inhibition. Direct pressure over the pain trigger point of the muscle, and deep massage using kneading techniques can both be effective with some athletes.

Stitch is pain which occurs in the upper abdomen. It occurs more often after a heavy meal and is common in runners. It is generally made worse by expiration and relieved slightly be inspiration. A number of possibilities exist as to its cause. After a heavy meal, the mesentery must bear excessive weight, and the liver is full of blood. This may give rise to minor internal bleeding. A reduction in oxygen supply to the diaphragm, or alterations in blood flow to the spleen and liver have also been suggested (Peterson and Renstrom, 1986).

Diaphragmatic breathing should be encouraged, allowing the abdominal wall to protrude during inspiration. The athlete should lean away from the affected side, or reach overhead with the arm on the affected side, both to stretch the area out. Some athletes report relief by squeezing a hard object in their hand, but the relief mechanism for this technique is puzzling.

Spinal injury

Sport accounts for 10–15% of severe spinal injuries, and unfortunately a significant number of these are made worse by incorrect management. Descriptions exist of patients who became quadriplegic after being able to move their limbs at the time of accident, and of individuals presenting with unstable neck fractures two weeks after injury (Garrick and Webb, 1990). A lack of neurological signs does not rule out spinal injury, and the safest approach is to assume that any player who has sustained substantial head or neck trauma has an unstable fracture until this has been disproven radiologically. Even with more minor trauma, unless the athlete is alert and able to demonstrate full range pain-free neck motion without neurological signs, he or she may still have sustained bony injury. The advice is clear; when in doubt immobilize the neck and refer the athlete for further investigation.

Where severe trauma to the spine has occurred, the athlete should not be moved unless he is in a life-threatening situation. If movement is necessary the aim is to prevent further injury to the spine. The position in which the athlete is found should be maintained unless priorities of airway or circulation demand otherwise. Initial treatment follows the ABC protocol, and if movement is required the head and body should be fully supported and moved as one. The therapist maintains the head position by placing his hands over the patient's ears. Three assistants kneel at one side of the athlete and two at the other side. The patient may be rolled in one piece (log roll) onto his or her side into the recovery position.

When an athlete is wearing a helmet (motorcycle or football) it should only be removed where airway obstruction or fire occurs (Meyer and Daniel, 1985). An assistant stabilizes the head by placing his or her hands around the athlete's neck. The practitioner unfastens the chin strap and grips the helmet at either side of the rim, spreading this outwards. The helmet is slowly removed by applying traction from below as the assistant continues to stabilize the athlete's neck. When the helmet has been removed, traction is reapplied to the head and maintained until a backboard is in place.

Environment and injury

Thermal stress

The human functions best at temperatures between 36.5 and 40.0°C (Astrand and Rodahl, 1986), and the body will try to keep itself within this region, to maintain equilibrium in the body core. When the external temperature rises, sweating occurs to try to lower body temperature, and when the external temperature is lower than the ideal, shivering starts in an attempt to increase body temperature through metabolic activity.

Heat is exchanged between the body and external environment through convection, conduction and radiation, and through the evaporation of water from the skin surface and respiratory passages. Heat loss through radiation occurs without contact between the body and the object receiving the heat, providing the environment is cooler than the body. In situations where the temperature of the environment exceeds that of the body, radiant heat energy is absorbed from the surroundings, and heat loss must occur by evaporation. Conduction involves direct contact between objects, and is particularly important in water. The rate of heat loss by convection is largely dependent on the rate of movement of air (or water) over the body surface. Accidental immersion in cold water will result in rapid heat loss. This will be made worse by attempting to swim rather than waiting for help, as the moving water passing the body results in greater heat loss through convection. The cooling effect of temperature and wind speed combined is represented by the wind chill factor. When it is cold and windy, air touching the body surface becomes warmed by body heat, but is immediately taken away to be replaced by cold air once more. Table 8.4 shows the wind chill index at various temperatures and wind speeds. It can be seen that a temperature of 10°F is equivalent to −25°F when the wind is blowing at 20 mph. This speed can easily be achieved on a blustery winter's day by running at 8 mph into a 12 mph headwind. In addition, when more body surface is exposed heat total loss is greater. Thirty to forty percent of the loss of body heat occurs through the head, so wearing a hat in a cold windy environment is essential.

Evaporation provides the most effective means of heat loss from the body. For each litre of water which is lost by evaporation of sweat and moisture from the respiratory passages, 580 kcal is lost from the body (McArdle, Katch and Katch, 1986). The total amount of sweat lost will be determined largely by the amount of skin exposed, the air

Table 8.4   The wind chill index

Ambient temperature (°F**)														
40	35	30	25	20	15	10	5	0	−5	−10	−15	−20	−25	−30
Equivalent temperature (°F)														

Wind Speed (mph)

	40	35	30	25	20	15	10	5	0	−5	−10	−15	−20	−25	−30
Calm	40	35	30	25	20	15	10	5	0	−5	−10	−15	−20	−25	−30
5	37	33	27	21	16	12	6	1	−5	−11	−15	−20	−26	−31	−35
10	28	21	16	9	4	−2	−9	−15	−21	−27	−33	−38	−46	−52	−58
15	22	16	11	1	−5	−11	−18	−25	−36	−40	−45	−51	−58	−65	−70
20	18	12	3	−4	−10	−17	−25	−32	−39	−46	−53	−60	−67	−76	−81
25	16	7	0	−7	−15	−22	−29	−37	−44	−52	−59	−67	−74	−83	−89
30	13	5	−2	−11	−18	−26	−33	−41	−48	−56	−63	−70	−79	−87	−94
35	11	3	−4	−13	−20	−27	−35	−43	−49	−60	−67	−72	−82	−90	−98
*40	10	1	−6	−15	−21	−29	−37	−45	−53	−62	−69	−76	−85	−94	−101

Little danger | Danger | Great danger

* Convective heat loss at wind speeds above 40 mph have little additional effect on body cooling.
**°C = 0.556 (°F − 32)

From McArdle, Katch and Katch (1986), with permission.

temperature and humidity, and the speed of air currents surrounding the body. Water loss through sweating can be as much as two litres per hour. This must be compensated for by fluid intake, but during vigorous exercise only about 800 ml of fluid can be emptied by the stomach (McArdle, Katch and Katch, 1986), so the payback is never complete. In addition, various factors can affect the ability of the body to take fluids up. A 10% glucose solution, for example, will reduce the rate of fluid uptake by 40%, so the use of glucose drinks to replace fluid alone is not logical. When glucose loss rather than fluid loss is the concern, these drinks may be of use, but it should be noted that it can take as much as 30 minutes for the ingested glucose to reach the working muscle. The use of complex (polymerized) sugars may be of greater value in this respect.

Heat illness

Heat illness occurs in the form of cramp, exhaustion, and finally, heat stroke. Heat cramps occur after exercise in the particular muscles worked, probably due to electrolyte imbalance. Adding salt to meals in the periods before heat exposure is a useful precaution, but taking salt once cramp has occurred is not effective. Furthermore, ingestion of large amounts of salt is not well tolerated unless accompanied by large amounts of water which in turn results in a bloated feeling.

In those not acclimatized to hot weather, heat exhaustion can occur. This is thought to occur by ineffective adjustment of the circulation, combined with excessive fluid loss, which in turn results in lowered blood volume (McArdle, Katch and Katch, 1986).

Blood pooling results, usually in the periphery, leading to a reduction in cardiac output. Symptoms include a weak rapid pulse, low blood pressure, headache, dizziness and general malaise. The athlete will recover if exercise is stopped and he or she is moved to a cool environment. Fluids should be given.

Heat-stroke is a more serious condition, requiring medical attention. It is a failure of the thermoregulatory systems of the body, causing sweating to cease, and the skin to become dry and hot. The body temperature rises to dangerous levels, and death can result. Body core temperature must be lowered, and treatment includes ice application and whole body immersion in cold water.

Cold illness

In water, athletes with greater body fat percentages perform well as they have additional insulation, as witnessed by the endomorphic tendencies of most cross-Channel swimmers. However, most humans do not acclimatize well to cold, and the response is usually one of avoidance, by producing a warmer microclimate with clothing and local environmental changes. Heat loss can be reduced by shunting blood from the periphery (shell) to the central area (core) of the body. However, prolonged peripheral vasocontriction during cold causes circulatory deprivation to the exposed parts and can cause severe tissue damage through ischaemic cold injury. Early sensations include numbness, tingling and burning sensations in the fingers, toes, nose and ear lobes. Neuromuscular function deteriorates, so that motor performance is impaired, as witnessed by a loss of finger strength and dexterity.

Frost-bite may occur when ice crystals form in the peripheral tissues giving ulceration. First degree frost-bite affects the superficial layer of the skin, while second degree frost-bite involves the formation of skin blisters filled with exudate. Third degree frost-bite results when the deeper areas are frozen, including the subcutaneous tissues and muscle. Rapid freezing causes ice crystals to form within the cells, resulting in cellular damage and, ultimately, necrosis. Slow freezing occurs to the tissue fluids, but solutes are not involved in the freezing process. This increases the osmotic pressure of the extracellular fluid, and pulls liquid out from the cells causing exudate formation (Astrand and Rodahl, 1986).

If first and second degree damage has occurred, gentle re-warming is required, with any blisters being left untouched. The athlete should be sheltered, any restricting clothing should be loosened, and warm drinks given. Activity to increase metabolic heating is useful. Third degree frost-bite requires urgent hospitalization.

In addition to general cold injury, damage to the eyes may occur in events such as cross-country skiing and downhill skiing, with the combination of severe cold and wind. The blinking reflex may be impaired, reducing the nourishment to the cornea, and causing transitory damage (Kolstad and Opsahl, 1979).

Hypothermia occurs when the body core temperature drops below 35°C (Astrand and Rodahl, 1986), the temperature being measured rectally. Initial exposure to cold causes shivering, an autonomic response to generate heat through muscular activity. As the temperature drops further the athlete may become disorientated and may hallucinate. Further temperature reduction can cause loss of consciousness, with weak pulse and respiration. Reflexes are lost, pupil dilation occurs, and cardiac arrhythmias can occur.

Management in the field is by gradual body re-warming. Rapid re-heating can cause the core temperature to fall lower, due to the return of cold venous blood from the extremities to the core.

Clothing and temperature regulation

As the body temperature rises with exercise, sweating should be aided by wearing loose clothing which encourages air circulation around the body, and by clothing which allows the passage of moisture through it and away from the body (wicking). In addition, dark clothing radiates and absorbs heat well, whereas light clothing reflects heat.

In a cold climate, the athlete should wear fibrous materials and a number of layers of clothing to try to trap air as an insulation within the material of the garment. A hat should be warn to reduce heat loss from the head. As clothing becomes wet, it can lose as much as 90% of its insulating properties, because water conducts heat much more effectively than air. Cold weather clothing should ideally permit the passage of water vapour, but not air.

Sports clothing can be effectively combined in three layers. The inner layer consists usually of shorts and a vest made of a fibre which is water permeable but non-absorbent. The seams of the inner layer must be positioned so that no abrasion is caused between the clothing and the athlete's skin.

The intermediate layer offers greater heat insulation properties, and is usually fibrous (wool or cotton) or fleecy. Modern materials have removed the need for bulk to provide insulating properties, and the intermediate layer should not restrict movement. The outer or 'shell' layer is waterproof, but should preferably still allow the passage of moisture from the body. This layer should also be strong enough to resist ripping, and be conveniently removed. Zips or other fasteners around the ankles facilitate the removal of the shell garment without the need to remove sports shoes.

Pressure stress

Gas pressure

The pressure exerted on a diver when underwater can cause injury. Water is largely noncompressible, and so the weight of the mass of water on top of the diver combines with the atmospheric pressure at the surface. At surface level, the pressure is normally one atmosphere (760 mmHg), but as the diver descends the pressure increases by this value every 10 metres. Consequently, a diver at a depth of 20 metres is subjected to three atmospheres pressure (two from the water, one from the air). The body tissues are themselves largely non-compressible, but the air-filled cavities are at risk. These include particularly the lungs and respiratory passages, sinuses and middle ear.

Boyle's law dictates that the volume of a gas is inversely proportional to the pressure exerted on it. Thus, the volume of air in the lungs is halved as the pressure is doubled by descending underwater to a depth of two atmospheres. Underwater breathing systems supply air or a mixture of gases to the diver at high enough pressures to compensate for the effect of water depth.

However, the gas pressure itself can give problems as the diver ascends, and the gas expands. If the diver takes a deep breath and ascends without breathing out, the gas inspired will expand as the pressure upon it reduces. This can occur when a novice diver panics, takes a deep breath, and swims rapidly to the surface. Expansion can cause lung tissue to rupture, and air bubbles to be forced into the pulmonary venous system causing an air embolus. This will pass to the systemic circulation and eventually to the brain, causing symptoms of confusion and blurred vision if mild, and unconsciousness or death if severe.

If the lung tissue ruptures and air bursts through the pleural sac, a pneumothorax will occur. Between the chest cavity and lung, an air pocket is formed which will expand as the diver ascends. This gas expansion will cause lung collapse. Pressure damage to the eye and ear is covered in Chapter 18.

Gas concentration

Alteration in gas pressure will also change the partial pressures of each of the gases in a diver's compressed air tanks. Nitrogen, for example, increases in partial pressure by 600 mmHg for every 10 metres that the diver descends. The net flow of nitrogen through the alveolar membranes increases, and at a depth of 20 metres the body tissues will contain roughly three times as much nitrogen as they did on the surface (McArdle, Katch and Katch, 1986). This increase in quantity of nitrogen can give rise to nitrogen narcosis. Here, the diver first enters a state of euphoria similar to being drunk, later, numbing sensations are produced in the limbs, and the condition may prove fatal (Astrand and Rodahl 1986). For this reason the time and depth of a dive are generally limited to about one hour at depths of 30 metres.

Nitrogen diffuses and leaves the body tissues very slowly. If pressure is suddenly reduced by a diver ascending too rapidly, or decompression in an aircraft, nitrogen is released from the tissues as gas bubbles. These build up in the small blood vessels and restrict blood flow, giving muscle and joint pain and even paralysis — a condition known as 'the bends'. Avoidance is through slow ascent, or replacing nitrogen by helium and allowing the diver to breath a nitrogen–helium gas mixture. This mixture will also prevent nitrogen narcosis, and is the choice for deeper diving.

Altitude

At high altitudes the situation is reversed, with the air density reducing with height. At a height of 5500 m the air pressure is about half that at sea level, and this gives a corresponding reduction in partial pressure of oxygen (PO_2). The amount of oxygen carried by the blood reduces, and exercise performance is impaired.

The body's immediate response to the thinner air at altitude is an increase in respiratory drive giving hyperventilation, and an increase in blood flow, witnessed by an increased cardiac output (especially heart rate) by as much as 50% above resting sea-level values.

During the first few days of training at altitude, mountain sickness may occur. The symptoms are headache (most common), dizziness, nausea and vomiting (less common). Appetite can become suppressed, and a diet low in salt but high in carbohydrate is best tolerated. The cool dry air of mountainous regions can give mild dehydration resulting in soreness and drying of the mouth, lips and throat.

Acclimatization periods to high altitudes are largely dependent on the altitude itself. Improvements may be seen within a few days, but total acclimatization may take between 4–6 weeks. Two weeks is normally sufficient for altitudes up to 2300 m, with an additional week added for every 610 m increase (McArdle, Katch and Katch, 1986).

Cryotherapy

Cold or ice is probably the most convenient modality available for the treatment of sports injuries. Ice is a low-cost and effective treatment, but its ready availability can lead to misuse with the potential for injury.

Effects

Cryotherapy may be used both in the immediate treatment of sports injuries, and in later rehabilitation. During immediate treatment, the aim is to limit the body's response to injury, in particular hypoxic tissue damage, swelling, pain and muscle spasm. Later, during the rehabilitation phase, the aims change. Then, the goal is to restore function, and at that stage, the effects of other techniques such as exercise and manual therapy can be augmented by ice application.

Ice is often used in combination with rest, compression and elevation (RICE) as an effective initial treatment of sports injuries. Ice alone has been shown to be effective in the treatment of ankle injuries (Hocutt et al., 1983), but is usually more effective when used to treat soft tissue injuries in conjunction with compression (Santiensteban, 1990). As shown in Fig. 8.6, a combination of mild pressure and cooling (10 mmHg and 15–25°C) has been shown to produce significant reductions in artificially induced inflammation (Sloan, Giddings and Hain, 1988). The main effects of cryotherapy are outlined in Table 8.5.

During immediate treatment, the most important effect is often claimed to be a reduction in blood flow through the local capillary network. However, blood clotting will usually seal these damaged vessels within 3–5 minutes of injury (Knight, 1989), about the same time as it takes to get an athlete off the sports field and into the treatment room. Consequently, when an athlete is first seen, local bleeding may have stopped. For this reason decreased tissue metabolism is now thought to be a more important effect of cryotherapy during the immediate treatment of sports injuries (Knight, 1989; McLean, 1989). After injury, further tissue damage occurs through local hypoxia secondary to a disruption in blood flow. A reduction in metabolic rate and oxygen requirement is seen with ice treatment (Abramson et al., 1957), and this gives the body cells a better chance to survive for the period they are without oxygen, almost in a

Table 8.5 Physiological changes within cooled tissue

Decreased metabolism
Decreased circulation
Transient increase followed by decreased pain
Decreased muscle spasm
Decreased inflammation
Increased stiffness

From Knight (1989).

state of 'temporary hibernation' (Knight, 1989).

Circulatory changes occur during ice application, and are the subject of some debate. Blood flow has been shown to decrease during cold application and remain reduced for up to 45 minutes after treatment (Knight, Bryant and Halvorsen, 1981). Cold applications produce an easily observed reactive hyperaemia of the skin, but deeper vasodilatation may not occur during therapeutic cooling (Knight, 1989). Certainly the cyclical skin changes (the hunting response), originally described by Lewis (1930), have been shown to occur only in fingers which have been cooled to 20°C prior to ice water immersion (Knight et al., 1980).

The immediate response to ice application is a short-lived (5–60 s) dull pain, which is more intense with some individuals than others. Following this, pain reduction occurs through a reduction in nerve conductivity (Tepperman and Devlin, 1983), and stimulation of pain receptors (Halvorson, 1990). With immersion in iced water a second pain sensation is sometimes felt, followed by after-pain when the body part is removed from the ice bath (Fig. 8.7). The intensity of pain that an athlete feels is related to both the temperature imposed on the tissues, and the rate of temperature change or 'thermal gradient' (Wolf and Hardy, 1941; Croze and Duclaux, 1978). A slow application of ice immersion will normally abolish cold-induced pain (Knight, 1995).

Local cooling depresses muscle spindle activity (Mense, 1978; Halvorson, 1990) and so muscle spasm initiated through gamma

Figure 8.6 Combined pressure and cooling to reduce swelling. From Sloan, Giddings and Hain (1988) and Reid (1992).

Figure 8.7   Pain sensations following body part immersion in iced water. From Knight (1995).

nerve stimulation can be reduced. Inflammation is thought to be reduced by ice application (Schmidt et al., 1979), and joint viscosity has been shown to increase, and with it joint stiffness (Knight, 1989).

Cryotherapy techniques

Common cold applications include the use of flaked ice in towelling or plastic bags, cold compression, ice massage, cold sprays, ice baths, and cryogel or chemical packs.

The choice between the various methods is often dependent on cost and convenience. Ice soaks are better for uneven and small body parts, such as the hand and foot. With this technique some ice should be left floating on the surface of the water throughout the treatment to ensure that a low enough temperature is maintained.

Ice packs are better for larger tissue areas such as the knee, hip and shoulder. Flaked ice in a plastic bag will give a lower tissue temperature than ice in a towelling bag, with the towelling providing insulation. Although mild frost-bite is unusual (Knight, 1989) the body part should be regularly inspected. Wet towelling provides less insulation, but will still not give tissue temperatures as low as ice within a plastic bag. Knight (1989) claimed that two layers

of dry wrap placed below an ice pack resulted in ankle temperatures which were 16°C higher after a 30-minute application than when ice was applied directly to the skin. Wetting the wraps gave temperatures which were 5.7°C higher than direct application. These temperature differences may, however, be of use where a patient demonstrates ice sensitivity.

Cryogel bags usually give a lower temperature than flaked ice, depending on the freezer setting used. Placing this type of pack directly on the skin should be avoided, as mild frost-bite has been repeatedly observed (Knight, 1989). Chemical packs have the advantage of convenience, and are easily carried by athletes themselves. However, they rarely produce temperatures which are low enough, and the temperature reduction which does occur is usually too short-lived. Some packs also have the potential for chemical burns if punctured.

Similarly, temperature changes produced by cold sprays are slight and short-term. The place of cold sprays is really as a stimulant for use with spray stretch techniques. Here, the vapocoolant spray (usually fluromethane) is applied as a jet, either to overcome guarding muscle spasm or to treat irritable trigger points (Travell and Simons, 1983).

Ice or cold can be combined with compression to good effect. Several methods exist, including the use of elasticated bandage around a layer of ice, or a similar ice layer below a compression (IPC) boot. Machines which produce continuous cold air, or iced water and compression are also available.

Ice massage is particularly useful for pain relief of smaller tissue areas. Massage is carried out until cold anaesthesia ensues. Usual sensations are of cold, then burning, deep aching and finally numbness (Halvorson, 1990). Once numbness has occurred, no additional skin sensation follows with more prolonged treatment, but underlying tissue temperature will continue to fall.

During the immediate treatment of sports injuries ice should preferably be applied within 5–10 minutes of injury, but certainly as soon as possible, and kept on for 20–30 minutes. Re-application is made every 2 hours, it taking 2–4 hours for the ankle, knee, forearm and thigh to return to pre-application temperature (Knight, 1989). Ice may have no effect on joint swelling once intra-articular effusion has formed (McLean, 1989).

Cryostretch and cryokinetics are additional rehabilitation procedures involving the use of ice (Knight, 1995). Cryostretch is the combination of cold application to relieve pain (Kowal, 1983) and reduce muscle spasm, and stretching to increase mobility. Ice is applied until cold anaesthesia is present, and stretching is carried out for as long as numbness lasts. Cryokinetics is the combination of cold therapy with active exercise. Cold is used to reduce pain and allow active exercise to be performed earlier than would otherwise be possible. The benefits of the therapy are from the exercise itself rather than the ice application.

Dangers of ice application

The two main dangers with ice application are frost-bite and nerve palsy. Frost-bite occurs when local tissues freeze. Direct cellular damage occurs due to ice crystal formation and indirect damage occurs due to dehydration as water moves out of the cells to form extracellular crystals. In addition, vascular damage may also occur during the thawing process due to platelet aggregation and vessel occlusion. The intensity of the tissue response can also vary from minor erythema and swelling (frost-nip), blister formation (second degree or superficial frost-bite), damage to subcutaneous tissues (third degree or full thickness frost-bite) and tissue damage so severe that the body part is lost (fourth degree or deep frost-bite). Ebholm et al. (1957) reported mild frost-bite in subjects following ice water immersion of the forearm, and Proulx (1976) reported frost-bite in the first metatarsal following continuous ice pack application. Frost-bite is far more common when cold gel packs are used (Stevens and D'Angelo, 1978). These will often be cooled far below 0°C, and so should not be applied for longer than 30 minutes, and should not be used in conjunction with compression. Gel packs should be wrapped in a damp cloth to reduce the likelihood of injury (Knight, 1995).

Nerve palsy has been reported by several authors, at the fibular head, elbow and shoulder (Drez, Faust and Evans, 1981; Collins, Storey and Peterson, 1986; Green, Zachazewski and Jordan, 1989; Malone et al., 1992). Total motor and sensory loss can occur when tissue temperatures reduce to between 0–5°C. Nerve palsy is more common when compression is used with ice, and when chemical ice packs are used rather than crushed ice packs. Most incidences recover quickly providing no necrosis has occurred, with sensory function returning before motor function (Knight, 1995).

References

Abramson, D.L., Kahn, A., Tuck, S., Turman, G.A., Rejal, H. and Fleisher, C.J. (1957) Relationship between a range of tissue temperature and local oxygen consumption in the resting forearm. *Laboratory Clinical Medicine*, **59**, 789–793

Astrand, P-O. and Rodahl, K. (1986) *Textbook of Work Physiology*, 3rd edn, McGraw-Hill, Maidenhead

Benda, C. (1989) Outwitting muscle cramps – is it possible? *Physician and Sports Medicine*, **17**(9), 173–178

Burri, C., Helbing, G. and Spier, W. (1973) Rehabilitation of knee ligament injuries. In *The Knee*, Springer, New York

Collins, K., Storey, M. and Peterson, K. (1986) Peroneal nerve palsy after cryotherapy. *Physician and Sports Medicine*, **14**, 105–108

Corsellis, J.A.N. (1974) Brain damage in sport. *Lancet*, **i**, 401–402

Crampton, C.W. (1908) Physiological age — a fundamental principle. *American Physical Education Review*, **13**, 141–154

Croze, S. and Duclaux, R. (1978) Thermal pain in humans: influence of the rate of stimulation. *Brain Research*, **157**, 418–421

Cyriax, J. (1982) *Textbook of Orthopaedic Medicine*, Vol one, 8th edn, Baillière Tindall, London

Drez, D., Faust, D.C. and Evans, I.P. (1981) Cryotherapy and nerve palsy. *American Journal of Sports Medicine*, **9**, 256–257

Ebholm, O.G., Fox, R.H., Lewis, H.E. and MacPherson, H.E. (1957) Cold injury. *Journal of Physiology*, **139**, 14–15

First Aid Manual (1995) 6th edn, Dorling Kindersley, London

Fowler, J.A. (1981) First aid in sport. In *Sports Fitness and Sports Injuries* (ed. T. Reilly), Faber and Faber, London, pp. 253–258

Garrick, J.G. and Webb, D.R (1990) *Sports Injuries: Diagnosis and Management*, W.B. Saunders, Philadelphia

Green, G.A., Zachazewski, J.E. and Jordan, S.E. (1989) Peroneal nerve palsy induced by cryotherapy. *Physician and Sports Medicine*, **17**, 63–70

Halvorson, G.A. (1990) Therapeutic heat and cold for athletic injuries. *Physician and Sports Medicine*, **18**(5),

Hocutt, J.E., Jaffe, R., Rylander, C.R. and Bebbe, J.K. (1983) Cryotherapy in ankle sprains. *American Journal of Sports Medicine*, **10**, 316–319

Knight, K.L. (1989) Cryotherapy in sports injury management. In *International Perspectives in Physical Therapy*, 4 (ed. V. Grisogono), pp. 163–185

Knight, K.L. (1995) *Cryotherapy in Sport Injury Management*, Human Kinetics, Champaign, Illinois

Knight, K.L., Bryant, K.S. and Halvorsen, J. (1981) Circulatory changes in the forearm in 1, 5, 10 and 15°C water (Abs). *International Journal of Sports Medicine*, **4**, 281

Knight, K.L., Aquino, J., Johannes, S.M. and Urban, C.D. (1980) A reexamination of Lewis' cold induced vasodilation in the finger and the ankle. *Athletic Training*, **15**, 24–27

Kolstad, A. and Opsahl, R. (1979) Cold injury to the corneal epithelium, a case of blurred vision in cross-country skiers. *Acta Ophthalmology*, **48**, 789

Kowal, M.A. (1983) Review of the physiological effects of cryotherapy. *Journal of Orthopaedic and Sports Physical Therapy*, **5**, 66–73

Lewis, T.S. (1930) Observations upon the reactions of the vessels of the human skin to cold. *Heart*, **15**, 177–208

Malina, R.M. and Beunen, G. (1996) Matching of opponents in youth sports. In *The Child and Adolescent Athlete, Encyclopaedia of Sports Medicine (IV)* (ed. O. Bar-Or), Blackwell Scientific, Oxford

Malone, T., Englehardt, D.L., Kirkpatrick, J.S. and Bassett, F.H. (1992) Nerve injury in athletes caused by cryotherapy. *Journal of Athletic Training*, **27**, 235–237

McArdle, W.D., Katch, F.I. and Katch, V.L. (1986) *Exercise Physiology. Energy, Nutrition, and Human Performance*, Lea and Febiger, Philadelphia

McLatchie, G.R. (1993) Risks and injuries in combat sports. In *The Soft Tissues. Trauma and Sports Injuries* (eds G.R. McLatchie and C.M.E. Lennnox), Butterworth-Heinemann, Oxford

McLatchie, G.R., Brooks, N. and Galbraith, S. (1987) Clinical neurological examination, neuropsychology, electroencephalography and computed tomographic head scanning in active amateur boxers. *Journal of Neurology, Neurosurgery and Psychiatry*, **50**, 96–99

McLean, D.A. (1989) The use of cold and superficial heat in the treatment of soft tissue injuries. *British Journal of Sports Medicine*, **23**(1), 53–54

Mense, S. (1978) Effects of temperature on the discharges of muscle spindles and tendon organs. *Pflugers Archives*, **374**, 159–166

Meyer, R.D. and Daniel, W.W. (1985) The biomechanics of helmets and helmet removal. *Journal of Trauma*, **25**, 329–332

Peterson, L. and Renstrom, P. (1986) *Sports Injuries*, Martin Dunitz, London

Proulx, R.P. (1976) Southern California frostbite. *Journal of American College of Emergency Physicians*, **5**, 618

Reid, D.C. (1992) *Sports Injury Assessment and Rehabilitation*, Churchill Livingstone, London

Roy, M.A., Bernard, D., Roy, B. and Marcotte, G. (1989) Body checking in Pee Wee hockey. *Physician and Sports Medicine*, **17**(3), 119–126

Santiesteban, A.J. (1990) Physical agents and musculoskeletal pain. In *Orthopaedic and Sports Physical Therapy*, 2nd edn (ed. J.A. Gould), C.V. Mosby, St Louis

Schmidt, K.L., Ott, V.R., Rocher, G. and Schaller, H. (1979) Heat cold and inflammation (a review). *Zeitschrift fur Rheumatologie*, **38**, 391–404

Sloan, J.P., Giddings, P. and Hain, R. (1988) Effects of cold and compression on edema. *Physician and Sports Medicine*, **16**, 116

Sortland, U., Tysvaer, A.T. and Storli, O.V. (1989) Association football injuries to the brain – a neurological and encephalographic study of former football players. *Neuroradiology*, **31**, 44

Sperryn, P.N. (1985) *Sport and Medicine*, Butterworth-Heinemann, Oxford

Sterns, M.L. (1940) Studies on development of connective tissue in transparent chambers in rabbits ear. *American Journal of Anatomy*, **67**, 55

Stevens, D.M. and D'Angelo, J.V. (1978) Frostbite due to improper use of frozen gel packs. *New England Journal of Medicine*, **299**, 1415

Taimela, S., Kujala, U.M. and Osterman, K. (1990) Intrinsic risk factors and athletic injuries. *Sports Medicine*, **9**(4), 205–215

Tepperman, P.S. and Devlin, M. (1983) Therapeutic heat and cold. *Postgraduate Medicine*, **73**, 69

Travell, J. G. and Simons, D.G. (1983) *Myofascial Pain and Dysfunction: The Trigger Point Manual*, Williams and Wilkins, Baltimore

Walkden, L. (1981) Immediate post-injury considerations in games. In *Sports Fitness and Sports Injuries* (ed. T. Reilly), Faber and Faber, London, pp. 247–252

Williams, J.G.P. and Sperryn, P.N. (1976) *Sports Medicine*, Edward Arnold, London

Wolf, S. and Hardy, J.D. (1941) Studies on pain: observations on pain due to local cooling and factors involved in the 'Cold pressor' effect. *Journal of Clinical Investigation*, **20**, 521–533

9

Biomechanics of the lower limb during gait

Most sporting activities involve the movement of the human body over distance. An understanding of the biomechanical factors which affect gait is therefore fundamental to the prevention and management of sports injuries. Abnormal forces placed on the body through alterations in normal running or walking can cause injury. In addition, rehabilitation of lower limb injuries, if it is to be successful, must involve the restoration of correct gait. Failure to do so may impair performance and leave the athlete open to further problems.

Closed and open motion

Motion at a joint is often described anatomically as though it occurred in isolation, yet functionally, isolated joint movements rarely occur. The limbs or trunk may be considered as moveable chains, the links of which are the joints themselves. Movement of one of the joints causes an effect on the other links in the chain, and so other joints respond.

Open chain motion occurs when the proximal bone segment in a limb is fixed but the distal segment remains free. Closed chain motion is the reverse. Both the proximal and distal bone segments are fixed, and movement occurs between the two. When we evaluate a joint within a limb in open chain motion, the movement of the bony segment occurs distal to the joint being studied. Movement within a closed chain will occur both proximally and distally to the joint being studied.

Muscle function is also different in open and closed chain motion. Take, as an example, dorsiflexion of the foot. Open chain dorsiflexion, for example sitting in a chair and pulling the foot upwards, results from concentric action of the anterior tibial muscles. Closed chain dorsiflexion, such as occurs in walking as the body weight moves forward over the foot, involves eccentric action of the calf muscles.

Joint movements

Hip joint

The hip joint is the articulation between the head of the femur and the acetabulum. In standing, the femoral head is not completely covered by the acetabulum. This occurs in a position which mimics a quadruped stance, hip flexion to 90°, abduction to 5°, and lateral rotation to 10°. Hip flexion is free, being limited by soft tissue contact, but extension is usually limited to about 30°. Common values for abduction and adduction are 45° each, given a total range of rotation of 90°.

In single leg standing, forces of 1.8–3 times body weight have been recorded at the hip, while in the stance phase of walking, forces between 3.3 and 5.5 times body weight have been measured. With running, higher forces would be expected (Palastanga, Field and Soames, 1989). The hip passes through one flexion/extension movement during the running cycle. The limit of flexion occurs within the middle of the swing phase, and the limit of extension just before the end of the stance phase.

Knee joint

The knee joint articulation is between the condyles of the femur and tibia. The posterior surface of the patella and the patellar surface of the femur is usually considered in the knee complex. The neutral position of the knee is full extension. From this position, approximately 140° of flexion is possible in the average subject. In full extension, no transverse plane motion is possible, but as the knee flexes rotation can occur.

During the last 15° of extension, the femur medially rotates on a fixed tibia, or if the tibia is free it will laterally rotate to bring the bones into close pack formation and lock the knee (the screw home mechanism). Flexion progresses as a combination of rolling and gliding movements of the femoral condyles. At the beginning of flexion, rolling occurs alone, and as flexion increases the amount of gliding increases, until at the end of range, gliding is the only movement present.

The medial condyle only rolls for the first 10–15° of flexion while the lateral condyle continues until 20° flexion, and at the same time the two menisci deform. This range of motion is the amount required during normal gait, and means that the knee is more stable (no gliding movement) during this functional range. Beyond 20° flexion, the knee becomes looser as the part of the femoral condyles now involved in the articulation is smaller. As a result the knee ligaments relax, and a wider range of rotation is available.

During walking, forces between two and four times body weight are taken by the knee. Peak forces correspond to hamstring, quadriceps and gastrocnemius contraction, and occur at heel strike and during propulsion. In jumping, forces may approach 24 times body weight (Palastanga, Field and Soames, 1989). The knee flexes and extends twice during running. At initial contact the knee is extended, and it flexes during midstance to absorb shock. As toe-off is reached, the knee extends again to provide propulsion and flexes as part of the swing phase.

Ankle joint

The ankle or talocrural joint consists of the trochlea surface of the talus and the distal ends of the tibia and fibula. The talar trochlea is wider anteriorly, and so plantar flexion is more free than dorsiflexion, average values being 30–50° and 20–30° respectively (Palastanga, Field and Soames, 1989). Marked variations occur both between individuals and following injury, and normal foot function can be achieved with as little as 20° of plantarflexion and 10° of dorsiflexion (McPoil and Brocato, 1990). Greater amounts of dorsiflexion are required as running speed or stride length increase.

The ankle is essentially a hinge, externally rotated to between 20–25° with the malleoli (Fig. 9.1). In the neutral position, with the foot perpendicular to the lower leg, there is very little frontal or transverse plane motion. With dorsiflexion, abduction of the foot is possible, and during plantarflexion, adduction can occur. In dorsiflexion the broad anterior part of the talus is forced into the narrower mortice between the tibia and fibula. The interosseous and transverse tibiofibular ligaments are stressed, as the bones

Axis of foot

Ankle joint axis

Malleolar axis (due to outward rotation of lower end of tibia)

Knee joint axis

Axis of femoral neck (anteverted)

Figure 9.1 Relationship between the ankle, knee and hip joint axes. From Palastanga, Field and Soames (1989), with permission.

part slightly, and the joint moves into close pack position.

Plantarflexion sees the narrow posterior part of the trochlear surface of the talus moving into the broader tibio-fibular mortice. Recoil of the above ligaments causes the malleoli to approximate and maintain contact with the talus.

During running, the ankle is dorsiflexed at heel strike, and plantarflexes to bring the forefoot to the ground. Plantarflexion occurs again at push off, and the foot dorsiflexes throughout the swing phase.

Sub-talar joint

The sub-talar joint (STJ) lies between the concave undersurface of the talus and the convex posterior portion of the upper surface of the calcaneum. The STJ is in neutral position when the posterior aspect of the heel lies vertical to the supporting surface of the foot, and parallel to the lower one-third of the leg (Subotnick, 1989). An essential feature of the STJ is its ability to perform tri-plane

motion. This occurs when movement of one joint is in all three body planes, because the joint axis is oblique.

Pronation of the foot is a tri-plane movement of the calcaneum and foot consisting of calcaneal eversion (frontal plane), abduction (transverse plane) and dorsiflexion (sagittal plane). Supination is an opposing movement of calcaneal inversion, adduction and plantarflexion in the same planes. These are both open chain movements in their pure forms. Functionally, the movements occur in closed chain formation with the foot on the ground. Abduction and adduction, and dorsiflexion and plantarflexion will not therefore occur in their pure form. Instead, the talus takes over these movements with supination consisting of calcaneal inversion with adduction and dorsiflexion of the talus, while pronation combines calcaneal eversion with adduction and plantarflexion of the talus (Fig. 9.2).

The foot has two important functions during the gait cycle. The first is to act as a mobile adaptor, adjusting to alterations in the ground surface and reducing the shock travelling up to the other lower limb joints. Secondly, the foot must efficiently transmit force from the muscles of the lower leg to provide propulsion to push off. For this, the foot must change into a rigid lever. These two diametrically opposed functions of mobile adaptor and rigid lever are achieved by changing the bony alignment of the foot joints, and 'locking' or 'unlocking' the foot.

Mid-tarsal joint

The movement of the STJ alters the alignment of the two components of the mid (transverse) tarsal joint (MTJ). These are laterally the calcaneal cuboid joint, and medially the talocalcaneonavicular joint. The mid-tarsal joint has two axes of motion, one oblique, and one longitudinal. The longitudinal axis primarily allows inversion and eversion of the forefoot, while the oblique axis permits adduction/abduction and plan-

Figure 9.2 Weight-bearing motion of the sub-taloid joint. (a) Supination. (b) Neutral position. (c) Pronation. From Gould (1990), with permission.

tarflexion/dorsiflexion. The direction of the motions at the mid-tarsal joint causes the dorsiflexion force created by weight-bearing to lock the forefoot against the rearfoot.

The position of the STJ alters the neutral alignment of the mid-tarsal joint axes (Fig. 9.3b). Supination of the STJ causes the axes to become more oblique (Fig. 9.3c), and less motion can take place. The foot is said to be locked, and acts as a rigid lever ideal for propulsion. Pronation of the STJ causes the mid-tarsal joint axes to become more parallel (Fig. 9.3a), and therefore more mobile. Now the foot is unlocked, and acts as a mobile adaptor capable of accommodating to changes in the ground surface.

First ray complex

The first ray is a functional unit consisting of the first metatarsal and the first cuneiform. Its axis is at 45° to the sagittal and frontal planes. The joint does have tri-plane motion, but little abduction and adduction occur functionally. Dorsiflexion of the first ray is accompanied by inversion, and plantarflexion is combined with eversion.

The gait cycle

The gait cycle can be conveniently divided into two phases. The stance phase occurs when the foot is on the floor, supporting the body weight. Closed chain motion occurs in the lower limb, as it decelerates. The swing phase takes place as the foot comes off the ground and open chain motion follows. This time the limb is accelerating.

The foot moves through four positions in three phases during stance. Initially, the heel strikes the ground (contact phase) and as the body weight moves forwards, the foot flattens (mid-stance). Forward movement continues and the heel lifts off the ground,

Figure 9.3 Position of mid-tarsal joint axes. (a) Pronation, axes parallel increasing mobility. (b) Neutral. (c) Supination, axes oblique reducing mobility. From Gould (1990), with permission.

finally the toes push off (propulsion) and the leg moves into the swing phase.

At the start of the swing phase the limb is accelerating. In the mid-swing position the speed is constant, and finally the leg decelerates, and is lowered to the ground where heel strike again occurs and the cycle is repeated (Fig. 9.4).

The stance phase in walking is approximately 60% of the total gait cycle while the swing phase is 40%. Walking at a normal rate of 120 steps/min the total cycle takes 1 s, so stance occurs for 0.6 s while swing takes only 0.4 s. With running, the movements occur more rapidly, and the stance phase occupies less of the total cycle time. A runner with a pace of 6 min/mile has a total cycle time of only 0.6 s. The stance phase would last for 0.2 s, and so events occurring within this phase are performed three times faster.

During the walking gait cycle, overlap of the stance phases of both legs occurs so that for a short period both feet are on the ground at the same time (double leg support). As walking speed increases, the double leg support period reduces. When the stance leg 'toes-off' before the swinging leg contacts the ground, double leg support is eliminated and an airborne period is created. Walking has now progressed to running.

Stance phase

During the stance phase, the forces taken by the various areas of the foot will vary from a peak at the heel during the contact phase, to a more gradual and later occurring force curve at the first metatarsophalangeal region at toe-off (Fig. 9.5).

Figure 9.4 (a) The walk cycle, and (b) the run cycle. Subotnick (1989).

Figure 9.5   Force acting through the foot during walking. From Reid (1992).

Contact

With the contact phase, the lateral aspect of the calcaneum strikes the ground. The ankle joint is close to its neutral (90°) position, and the subtalar joint is slightly supinated. The hip is flexed to about 30°. The pelvis and the body's centre of gravity are moving laterally over the weight-bearing leg, producing closed chain adduction of the hip. Total lateral motion of the trunk is 4–5 cm (Whittle, 1996).

The STJ starts to pronate, and the mobility of the mid-tarsal joint is increased. The ankle begins to plantarflex to bring the foot flat onto the ground for mid-stance. Pronation causes the tibia to internally rotate, and this in turn unlocks the knee allowing it to flex to about 20°, in a movement opposite to the screw home effect. The hip begins to extend and internally rotate and this continues until heel raise.

The anterior tibials contract eccentrically to stop the foot slapping at heel strike, and the posterior tibials decelerate pronation. The quadriceps work eccentrically to allow the knee to bend, and the hamstrings prevent trunk flexion at the hip. Later, the hamstrings work concentrically to extend the hip (closed chain extension). The hamstrings are used in favour of the gluteals here possibly because they have been pre-stretched. When the knee bends, the hamstrings can no longer produce hip extension, and the gluteals take over.

The hip abductors work eccentrically to control lateral movement over the supporting leg and then concentrically to pull the body weight back again in preparation for the next cycle.

Mid-stance

In mid-stance, the transition of the foot from mobile adaptor to rigid lever occurs. The STJ starts to supinate, reducing mid-tarsal mobility and locking the foot. When hip adduction is completed, closed chain abduction occurs for the rest of the stance phase.

The action of the calf is eccentric to control dorsiflexion and with it forward motion of the body, and the posterior tibials contract concentrically to supinate the foot.

Propulsion

The heel rises with plantarflexion at the ankle and the propulsion phase begins, the knee reaching its point of maximal extension. At toe-off, dorsiflexion again occurs at the ankle to prevent toe drag, and the hip begins to flex. The calf now works concentrically to actively plantarflex the ankle, and the peroneus longus and brevis are eccentric to control supination. The peroneus longus also stabilizes the first ray. The quadriceps work eccentrically to control the knee.

Swing phase

During the swing phase, the maximally supinated STJ moves back to its position of slight supination just before heel strike. The knee continues to flex during the acceleration position of the swing phase, and starts to extend again before heel strike. The hip continues to flex, until it has reached its 30° position to begin the cycle again. The quadriceps continue to contract eccentrically to stop the knee 'snapping' back, and the hip flexors are concentric to accelerate the leg forwards. Phasic muscle action during running is summarized in Fig. 9.6.

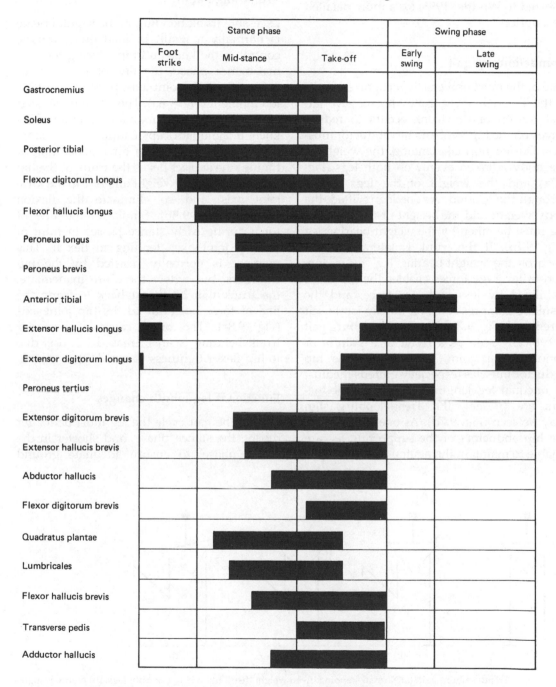

Figure 9.6 Phasic muscular activity during normal ambulation. From McGlamry (1987), with permission.

Abnormal gait patterns

Several abnormalities of gait are commonly seen in clinical practice, and the reader is referred to Whittle (1996) for a more detailed description.

Trendelenburg gait

One of the most universally recognized faults is the Trendelenburg gait. An excessive lateral flexion of the trunk occurs to reduce forces on the hip joint and hip abductor muscles. During normal standing, the weight of the body is taken evenly on both legs (Fig. 9.7a) and the weight of the legs passes through the ground. As one leg is lifted, the body weight and the weight of the opposite leg must be taken by the weight-bearing leg (Fig. 9.7b). If the trunk is laterally flexed towards the weight-bearing leg, the reduction in leverage forces enables the hip to be stabilized by less abductor force, and the resultant compression over the hip joint itself is reduced (Fig. 9.7c). The Trendelenburg gait is typically seen as a result of a painful or abnormal hip joint, weakness of the hip abductor muscles (especially gluteus medius) or unequal leg length. Where weak abductors are present, the Trendelenburg sign may be seen (Fig. 9.7d). As one leg is lifted, the hip abductors of the supporting leg are unable to maintain the neutral position of the pelvis. As a result, the pelvis dips towards the lifted leg.

Trunk angulation

Excessive trunk bending in the sagittal plane is normally a result of inadequate muscle control in the knee and hip. During the normal stance phase, the line of force passes behind the knee joint axis, producing a flexion moment (Fig. 9.8a). This must be resisted by the quadriceps to maintain stability of the knee. If the quadriceps contraction is inadequate (either in terms of force generation or timing) the subject flexes the trunk at the hip to move the body weight anterior to the knee joint axis, and so eliminate the flexion moment (Fig. 9.8b). Similarly, the line of force during early stance passes in front of the hip joint axis, tending to flex it. This moment is normally resisted by the hip extensors, but where these are inadequate, the trunk will be thrust back to bring the line of force posterior to the hip joint axis (Fig. 9.8c). The other cause of posterior trunk bending is an increased lordosis due to hip flexor tightness (see p. 162).

Functional leg length changes

During the gait cycle the leg must be longer during the stance phase, and shorter in the swing phase, to ensure adequate ground

Figure 9.7 Trendelenburg gait. (a) Normal standing. Even weight distribution between both legs. (b) Normal single-leg standing. (c) Trunk lateral flexion eliminating lever arm. (d) Weak hip abductors allow pelvis to dip.

Figure 9.8 Trunk angulation during gait. (a) Normal stance phase. Knee joint axis in front of force line, hip joint axis behind. (b) Flexing the trunk brings the force line anterior to the knee axis. (c) Extending the trunk moves the force line posterior to the hip axis. Modified from Whittle (1996).

clearance. Functional lengthening is achieved by extending the hip and knee and plantarflexing the ankle. Conversely, shortening is brought about by flexing the hip and knee and dorsiflexing the ankle. Where range of motion is reduced or stability/strength is poor, the leg length may not be changed adequately, and the body must compensate by altering the gait cycle.

Four gait changes may occur (Whittle, 1996). Circumduction, hip hiking, and steppage are all modifications of the swing phase. Vaulting is a modification of the stance phase. Circumduction involves swinging the leg out to the side to clear the ground, and is best noticed by viewing the subject from behind. Where weakness of the hip flexors is present, circumduction will move the leg forwards via action of the hip abductors. Hip hitching (hiking) achieves ground clearance by lifting the pelvis on the side of the moving leg (the opposite of the Trendelenburg gait). Often, this pelvic lift is accompanied by excessive pelvic rotation to thrust the leg forwards. Steppage (high stepping) is an increase in both knee and hip flexion to exaggerate the ground clearance.

This is especially common in patients with foot drop. Finally, vaulting increases ground clearance by lifting onto the toes of the support leg, and therefore increasing the vertical displacement of the body.

Abnormal biomechanics of the foot

Excessive pronation/supination

These conditions occur if the normal pronation and supination periods of the gait cycle are extended, or when there is a change in the angulation of the foot segments. Causes may be extrinsic, such as tight muscles or abnormal lower leg rotation, or intrinsic, as occurs with fixed deformities of the STJ and MTJ.

Severe pronation causes foot flattening. The range of motion at the STJ is increased, making the mid-tarsal joint axes more parallel and unlocking the foot. The foot can then remain pronated and mobile after the stance phase, hence the terms 'hypermobile' or 'weak' foot.

With excessive supination the MTJ is locked, the foot is more rigid, and the arch higher (cavus). In time the plantar fascia and intrinsic foot muscles become tight, reducing the capacity of the foot to dissipate shock.

Rearfoot varus

With this condition, the calcaneus appears inverted when the foot is examined in the neutral position. Left uncompensated (Fig. 9.9) the forefoot would invert and leave the medial side of the foot off the ground. To compensate, the STJ pronates excessively on ground contact. This deformity has been associated with an increased number of lateral ankle sprains (Weil, 1979).

Rearfoot varus is usually a result of developmental abnormality. From the eight to twelfth fetal week the calcaneum lies at the side of the talus. As the fetus develops the calcaneum rotates to a more plantar position,

Figure 9.9   Rearfoot varus (posterior view). (a) Uncompensated—both rearfoot and forefoot are inverted. (b) Compensated—the talus is abducted and plantarflexed to bring the calcaneus to a vertical position. From Gould (1990), with permission.

Figure 9.10   Forefoot varus (anterior view). (a) Uncompensated. (b) Compensated—the talus adducts and plantarflexes (arrow). The calcaneus everts. From Gould (1990), with permission.

so that it lies below the talus. However, the calcaneus may not be completely perpendicular to the ground until the child is 6 years old, and in some cases the rotation is never complete. In addition to the subtalar deformity, the condition is also associated with tibial varum.

Rearfoot valgus

This unusual condition can occur if the calcaneum rotates excessively in its development, or following a Pott's fracture. The posterior surface of the calcaneum will appear everted, and the foot will hyperpronate giving a severe flatfoot.

Forefoot varus

In this deformity (Fig. 9.10), the forefoot is inverted in respect to the rearfoot, when the STJ is in a neutral position. To compensate, and bring the forefoot to the ground, the STJ everts and the entire plantar surface of the foot becomes weight-bearing, flattening the medial longitudinal arch. The head of the talus bulges proximally to the tuberosity of navicular. Plantar callouses are apparent over the second and third metatarsal heads, and an associated hallux valgus deformity may be present.

If the STJ is unable to pronate sufficiently, the entire plantar surface of the foot will be unable to touch the ground. Weight-bearing will therefore be lateral, with callus formation this time over the fourth and fifth metatarsal heads.

Abnormal pronation continues into the propulsive phases of the gait cycle, and the foot tries to push off without becoming a rigid lever. This instability causes shearing forces between the metatarsal heads giving rise to associated pathologies. Interdigital neuroma, postural fatigue, fasciitis, chondromalacia and shin pain have all been described as resultant to this deformity (McPoil and Brocato, 1990).

Forefoot valgus

Here, there is an eversion of the forefoot in relation to the rearfoot, a situation exactly opposite to that above (Fig. 9.11). The medial foot structures are in contact with the ground while the lateral side is suspended. Deformities greater than 6° (McPoil and Brocato, 1990) will require STJ and MTJ compensations. To place the foot flat on the ground, the calcaneus will invert pulling the talus into an abducted-dorsiflexed position. During the contact phase of gait, the foot will pronate more than normal, and remain pronated and therefore mobile into

Figure 9.11 Forefoot valgus (anterior view). (a) Uncompensated. (b) Compensated—the talus abducts and dorsiflexes (arrow). The calcaneus inverts. From Gould (1990), with permission.

the propulsive phase. Symptoms associated with hypermobility of the metatarsophalangeal and interphalangeal joints occur.

Plantarflexed first ray

This condition is present when the first metatarsal lies below the level of the other metatarsals in neutral position, causing the forefoot to appear slightly everted relative to the rearfoot. When forefoot eversion continues, a forefoot valgus is present.

Various conditions may give rise to this problem. If the first metatarsal phalangeal (MP) joint is rigid (hallux rigidus, see p. 320) the foot is forced rapidly into supination (a supinatory rock) to allow the lateral side of the foot to bear weight. In so doing, the fifth metatarsal head strikes the ground rapidly (Wernick and Langer, 1985). In addition, weakness of the tibialis anterior will allow the peroneus longus to pull the first ray into plantarflexion unopposed. Deformity occurs over time, and is particularly exaggerated in certain neuromuscular diseases.

Biomechanical examination and treatment

Examination of the lower limb may reveal problems with the spine, pelvis, hip or knee. The aim of this section, however, is to deal with the examination of the limb in relation to foot problems, assessment procedures for the other body parts being covered in the sections describing injuries to these areas. Equally, foot examination in isolation is not enough. Forces acting through the kinetic chain, and referral of pain from other structures, make holistic evaluation of lower limb function essential.

Subjective examination and inspection of the lower limb will act as pointers to further assessment, and give clues about any additional tests which may be required.

Objective examination is made both with the athlete weight-bearing and then non-weight-bearing. Positions include standing, sitting, walking and then running. With walking and running, video analysis is often used to slow the motion down and aid in the identification of faults. In each case the examination may be carried out with the athlete in shorts and bare feet, and then while wearing their normal training shoes. The wear pattern of the shoes (Fig. 9.12) is often a useful general guide to the existence of underlying biomechanical faults.

In standing, the alignment of the various body segments is assessed. Starting from the top of the body and working down, viewed from behind, the head and shoulder positions are noted, as is the symmetry of the spine. Shoulder and pelvic levels are assessed. Buttock and knee creases are examined for equal level. Knee position gives a clue to the presence of coxa valga/vara and genu vara/valga (Fig. 9.13).

Tibial vara can be measured in standing by comparing the line of the distal third of the leg to a line perpendicular to the supporting surface which passes through the posterior contact point of the calcaneus (Fig. 9.14)

From the front, similar comparisons of shoulder, pelvic, spinal and leg alignments are made. The position of the patella relative to the foot will suggest any tibial torsion. Tibial torsion can be further assessed with the patient in sitting with the knee flexed to

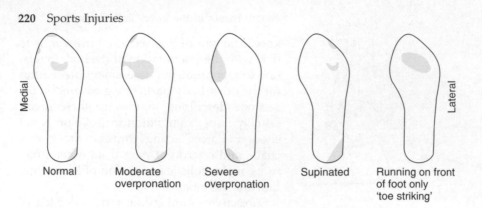

Normal | Moderate overpronation | Severe overpronation | Supinated | Running on front of foot only 'toe striking'

Medial | Lateral

Figure 9.12   Wear patterns on sports shoes. From Reid (1992).

Coxa valgum

Coxa vara

Genu vara

Genu val

Figure 9.13   Femoral and tibial alignment. From Subotnick (1989), with permission.

Line perpendicular to supporting surface

Line of tibia

Figure 9.14   Tibia vara measurement made from standing position.

90° over the end of the couch. The examiner places his thumbs over the patient's malleoli and compares an imaginary line connecting these two points with the knee axis.

In supine lying, active and passive range of movement at the knee and hip and measured and any asymmetry or alteration in normal end feel is noted. Resisted strength is measured and limb girths measured. The distribution of any pain or alteration in sensation is mapped. The appearance of the foot is observed and any skin abnormalities noted. In prone lying, range of movement of the foot is measured and compared to normal values.

Calcaneal inversion and eversion are measured by marking a line bisecting the back of the calcaneus and comparing this to a line bisecting the calf and achilles. Forefoot position is assessed by placing the foot in its neutral position (Table 9.1). This is achieved by inverting and everting the foot (with the ankle in neutral), palpating the head of the talus and placing the STJ in its mid-position (see below).

A goniometer is placed over the metatarsal heads, and its line compared to one perpendicular to the line of calcaneal bisection. Alternatively, a forefoot measuring device (FMD) may be used. This has a slit which is placed over the line of calcaneal bisection, the plateaux on the front of the FMD is placed over the plantar surface of the foot in line with the met heads, and a value for forefoot–rearfoot alignment read from the scale. Using both goniometry and the FMD the most common forefoot–rearfoot relationship is one of varus, with average values

Table 9.1   Neutral position of the foot

(i)	Mid-position (90°) at the ankle joint
(ii)	STJ aligned so that the posterior surface of the heel is vertical to the supporting surface and parallel to the lower leg
(iii)	Maximal pronation of the MTJ, so the line of the metatarsal heads is perpendicular to the line of bisection of the calcaneus, and on the same plane
(iv)	The first ray is in neutral position, neither plantarflexed nor dorsiflexed, and on the same plane as the other metatarsals
(v)	The fifth ray is in mid-position as above and on the same plane as the other metatarsals
(vi)	The second, third and fourth rays are dorsiflexed and the metatarsal heads are approximately at the same level as the other metatarsal heads
(vii)	The first metatarsal phalangeal joint is dorsiflexed to 20–25° relative to the long axis of the first metatarsal in its neutral position
(viii)	The lesser metatarsal phalangeal joints are slightly dorsiflexed

Adapted from Subotnick (1989).

being 7.5° (Garbalosa, Donatelli and Wooden, 1989).

Significant biomechanical faults of the foot can be managed by using a functional orthotic device.

Orthotics

An orthotic device is usually made after taking a plaster impression of the foot in the neutral position. This may be sent to an orthotic laboratory where a device is fabricated according to the practitioner's prescription and laboratory assessment of the cast.

The orthotic aims to alter the mechanical functioning of the foot, and so is more than a simple arch support. When worn, the device changes the foot's alignment to make the lower limb function more normally. There are generally few long-term benefits, and much like with a pair of eye glasses, once the orthotic is removed, the body returns to its previous state.

The most common casting technique is the neutral impression cast or slipper cast, and this will be described. Initially, the line of bisection of the calcaneus is marked on the skin in ink, so that the line will bleed into the cast and act as a reference point.

The patient lies supine on a couch with the lower third of the leg over the couch end. The foot should be vertical, and not allowed to fall to one side; a sand bag can be used to support the leg if necessary. Two strips or more of plaster of Paris are used, each about 13 × 75 cm, folded in half. Each splint is folded over by 1 cm on the upper border to strengthen the edge of the cast.

The first strip is placed over the calcaneus and along the medial and lateral border of the foot to the tips of the toes. The under edge is moulded over the sole of the foot. The second strip is again placed in a U fashion, this time starting over the toes and overlapping the first. The two strips are moulded using a wet finger, into the sole of the foot and together into one unit. When the cast is in place, the foot is placed into a neutral position and the cast kept moulded firmly into the foot until set. When tapped, the plaster should sound hollow.

Neutral position of the foot is obtained by first finding the STJ mid-position. This is done by palpating the head of the talus as it begins to emerge from behind the navicular. The point where it is just palpable is the mid-position. At this point the skin lines above and below the lateral malleolus should be equal. Taut skin indicates the foot is supinated, and excessive skin folding shows a pronated foot position. In addition, the concavities above and below the lateral malleolus should appear equal.

Neutral position is maintained while the cast is setting by locking the MTJ. The practitioner dorsiflexes the foot until slight resistance is felt by pushing the sole of the foot up and slightly outwards (abduction). Pressure is over the fourth and fifth digits, while constantly palpating the head of the talus to ensure neutral STJ position is maintained.

When dry, the cast is removed by grasping it behind the calcaneus and removing the heel first, and then sliding the foot out as though the cast were a slipper. This cast can now act as mould for the foot model.

At the orthotic laboratory, the cast is lined with plaster parting agent and then filled with liquid plaster. Once hardened, the original slipper cast is removed leaving a positive model of the athlete's foot, which is then trimmed and smoothed.

Various substances are used for orthotic fabrication such as acrylics for rigid devices and plastics for semi-rigid orthotics. These materials are vacuum formed over the positive cast. Forefoot and rearfoot posts are added and ground down so that the cast will align with the calcaneal bisection line perpendicular to the supporting surface.

Forefoot posts are needed to ensure that the MTJ will lock to provide a rigid lever during the propulsive gait phase. Rearfoot posts ensure proper STJ alignment at heel contact. As the foot rolls forward into midstance, the rearfoot post must allow adequate motion. This is achieved either by grinding down the distal medial aspect of the post, or by making this part of the post from a compressible material.

In some cases, a temporary orthotic is all that is required. This may be to correct a temporary fault occurring as a result of injury, or to assess whether a permanent (and more expensive) orthotic is justified. In this case, no cast is made, but the practitioner makes a temporary device using his own examination results as a reference. More malleable substances, such as cork or non-compressible foam materials, are used this time.

References

Garbalosa, J.C., Donatelli, R. and Wooden, M.J. (1989) Dysfunction, evaluation and treatment of the foot and ankle. In *Orthopaedic Physical Therapy* (eds R. Donatelli and M.J. Wooden), Churchill Livingstone, London, pp. 533–553

Gould, J.A. (ed.) (1990) *Orthopaedic and Sports Physical Therapy*, 2nd edn, Mosby, St Louis

McGlamry, J.G. (1987) *Fundamentals of Foot Surgery*, Williams and Wilkins, Baltimore

McPoil, T.G. and Brocato, R.S. (1990) The foot and ankle: biomechanical evaluation and treatment. In *Orthopaedic and Sports Physical Therapy*, 2nd edn (ed. J.A. Gould), Mosby, St Louis, pp. 293–321

Reid, D.C. (1992) *Sports Injuries. Assessment and Rehabilitation*, Churchill Livingstone, London

Palastanga, N., Field, D. and Soames, R. (1989) *Anatomy and Human Movement*, Butterworth-Heinemann, Oxford

Subotnick, S.I. (1989) *Sports Medicine of the Lower Extremity*, Churchill Livingstone, London

Weil, L.S. (1979) A biomechanical study of lateral ankle sprains in basketball. *Journal of the American Podiatry Association*, **69**, 687

Wernick, J. and Langer, S. (1985) *A Practical Manual for a Basic Approach to Biomechanics*, Langer Biomechanics Group, Stoke-on-Trent.

Whittle, M.W. (1996) *Gait Analysis*, 2nd edn, Butterworth-Heinemann, Oxford

Section II

10

The hip and thigh

Whereas the gleno-humeral joint functions mainly in a open kinetic chain position, the hip (coxo-femoral) joint functions mainly in a closed chain position. For this reason, its structure is one of stability for weight-bearing. In the standing position, however, the joint is not fully congruent, the anterosuperior portion of the cartilage of the head being exposed. It is only when the joint is taken into a position equivalent to that of the quadruped (90° flexion, 5° abduction, and 10° lateral rotation) that maximum articular contact of the head with the acetabulum occurs (Palastanga et al., 1994).

The femoral neck makes an angle (angle or inclination) with the shaft of 120–130° in the adult, representing the adaptation of the femur to the parallel position of the legs in gait (Fig. 10.1a). This changes from 150° in the newborn to 142° by age 5, 133° by age 15, and 125° in the adult (Reid, 1992; Palastanga et al., 1994). Greater angles than these are termed coxa valga, lesser angles as coxa vara. Similarly, the axis of the femoral head and neck make an angle with the axis of the femoral condyles (Fig. 10.1b). This angle (angle of torsion or angle of anteversion) is normally 10° in the adult, having reduced from 25° in the infant.

In order to take weight most effectively, bony trabeculae line up in the direction of imposed stress. Two major systems exist within the femur (Fig. 10.2). The medial trabecular system travels from the medial cortex of the upper femoral shaft to the superior aspect of the head. This system takes vertically aligned forces created by weight-bearing, and is aligned with the superior aspect of the acetabulum, the main weight-bearing region. The lateral trabecular system begins from the lateral cortex of the upper femoral shaft, crosses the medial system, and terminates in the cortical bone on the inferior aspect of the head. The lateral system is aligned to take oblique forces created by contraction of the hip abductors during gait.

In addition to the medial and lateral trabecular systems, the upper femur is reinforced by medial and lateral accessory systems which take forces created about the trochanters. A zone of weakness is left within the femoral neck which is susceptible to bending forces and is the site of femoral neck fracture (Norkin and Levangie, 1992).

The hip joint is strengthened by three capsular ligaments. The ilio-femoral ligament and the pubo-femoral ligament are on the anterior aspect of the joint, while the ischio-femoral ligament is on the posterior aspect (Fig. 10.3). As the hip is flexed, all three ligaments relax. However, in extension all three ligaments are tight with the inferior band of the ilio-femoral ligament being placed under greatest tension as it runs almost vertically. It is this ligamentous

Figure 10.1 Angulation of the femoral neck. (a) Angle of inclination. (b) Angle of torsion.

Figure 10.2 Bony trabeculae of upper femur. After Norkin and Levangie (1992).

band which limits posterior tilt of the pelvis (Palastanga et al., 1994). During adduction it is the turn of the superior band of the ilio-femoral ligament to become tighter while the pubo-femoral ligament and ischio-femoral ligament relax. In abduction the opposite occurs. In lateral rotation both the ilio-femoral ligament and pubo-femoral ligament are taut while in medial rotation the ischio-femoral ligament tightens.

Screening examination

Hip conditions may refer pain anywhere within the L3 dermatome, over the front of the thigh and down to the knee. Initial observation includes resting position, muscle wasting, leg length and gait. Examination for range of motion may be carried out in a supine position for flexion, abduction and adduction and both rotations. Medial and lateral rotation are best compared between the affected and unaffected hip in a prone position with the knees flexed to 90°. Resisted abduction is better tested in a side-lying position with the affected joint uppermost.

Compression of the joint through the flexed knee and circumduction with compression to 'scour' the femoral head into the acetabulum is an important assessment for arthritic changes. Both the lumbar spine and sacroiliac joints must be examined to eliminate them as a potential cause of pain referral. The straight leg raise and slump test

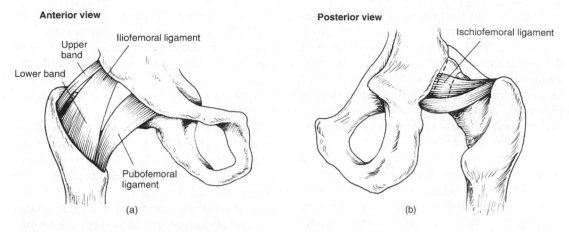

Anterior view

Upper band
Lower band
Iliofemoral ligament
Pubofemoral ligament

(a)

Posterior view

Ischiofemoral ligament

(b)

Figure 10.3   Capsular ligaments of the hip joint. After Palastanga et al. (1994).

should be tested to eliminate the possible involvement of neural tissue. Cyriax (1982) warned that serious pathology may be present if the sign of the buttock is positive. Here, hip flexion with the knee bent is more painful and more limited that straight leg raising. A non-capsular limitation is present, and pain may make the end feel empty. As straight leg raising is full the sciatic nerve is unimpinged, and the non-capsular limitation precludes the hip joint. Possibilities include an inflammatory disease state, neoplasm and fracture.

Muscle tests for the hip region, including the Thomas test and the Ober manoeuvre, are described on p. 156.

Muscle injuries

Quadriceps

On the whole, strains occur mostly in two-joint muscles, due to the more complex coordination involved in controlling movement of two body segments simultaneously. Direct trauma, however, can be imposed on any muscle. In the hip region, this means that the rectus femoris, hamstrings and gracilis muscles tend to suffer strain. The more anterior position of the quadriceps, however, exposes these muscles to risk during contact

sports, and to blunt trauma through collision with sports apparatus. A quadriceps contusion is often referred to colloquially as a 'dead leg' or 'charley horse'.

Initially, there is local swelling over the front of the thigh, with some superficial bruising appearing later, often tracking down to the knee. The main danger with this injury is the development of myositis ossificans traumatica (MOT, see pp. 53). Thigh contusions may be rated as grade one (mild), in which knee flexion beyond 90° is possible, grade two (moderate), in which motion is restricted to 45–90° or grade three (severe), in which swelling and pain limit movement to less than 45°. This grading system can be an accurate predictor of the likelihood of MOT development. Jackson and Feagin (1973) assessed quadriceps contusions in 65 subjects, and found that none of the subjects with grade one injuries had developed MOT. However, 13 out of 18 subjects who had been graded two or three later went on to develop the condition, so the amount of movement present in the initial stages is an important indicator of the severity of the lesion, and the prognosis.

It is important to limit movement in grade one and two injuries, and to discourage the use of massage, vigorous stretching or exercise, and ultrasound, as these are contraindicated in the early post-injury stage. The RICE protocol is used to limit the tissue damage. Ice is applied with compression with the knee and hip flexed as far as is comfortable. Internal compression is therefore applied by fascial tightening (Reid, 1992) while external compression comes from the elastic bandage.

The athlete resuming contact sports should wear padding over the damaged area. In cases of MOT, calcification is slow, with fibroblasts beginning to differentiate into osteoblasts about 1 week after injury. Radiographic evidence of bone formation is usually visible after 3 weeks, and by 6–7 weeks after injury, the calcified mass generally stops growing. Total reabsorption may occur with minor lesions, but more major conditions may continue to show remnants of the mass. The mass rarely interferes with muscle contraction, so excision is not normally required (Estwanik and McAlister, 1990).

Rectus femoris

The rectus femoris is frequently injured by a mistimed kicking action. On examination, pain is usually apparent to resisted knee extension and hip flexion. Passive stretch into knee flexion coupled with hip extension and adduction is also painful. Injury is usually to either the upper insertion or the mid-belly. Upper insertion injuries are palpated with the patient half-lying to relax the muscle. The area of injury is usually the musculotendinous junction approximately four finger widths below the anterior superior iliac spine.

Mid-belly tears are less common and are usually sited within the middle third of the thigh. Here, the muscle is subcutaneous and any swelling is immediately apparent. The athlete should flex the hip and knee to 45° against resistance, and as the muscle stands out any abnormality will become apparent.

The rectus femoris can be worked concentrically by flexing the hip against a resistance supplied by a weight bag attached to the knee. Two-joint action of the muscle can be worked with the athlete in supine with the injured leg over the couch side, flexed at both the knee and hip. Manual resistance is applied to the foot of the athlete as he or she extends the knee and flexes the hip simultaneously (Fig. 10.4a).

Stretching must involve both knee flexion and hip extension and can be carried out in a side-lying position by the athlete, or by the therapist. When performing a rectus femoris stretch in standing (Fig. 10.4b), the abdominal muscles must be tightened to stabilize the pelvis before the hip stretch is applied. Failure to do so will increase the apparent range of motion by anterior tilt of the pelvis

(a)   (i)   (ii)   (c)
             (b)

Figure 10.4 (a) Rectus femoris strengthening combining hip flexion and knee extension against elastic band resistance. (b) Rectus stretch (i) correct with pelvis fixed. (ii) Incorrect, anterior pelvic tilt throws stress on lumbar spine. (c) Alternate leg lunge. Front leg stresses quadriceps and gluteals, rear leg stresses hip flexors and knee extensors.

with stress thrown on the lumbar spine. Lunging actions are also useful, for both general flexibility and eccentric control (Fig. 10.4c).

Sartorius

Injury to the sartorius is usually an avulsion from the anterior superior iliac spine. There is usually immediate pain, often radiating into the anterior thigh. Swelling and bruising is seen over the iliac crest, often tracking down the thigh. Flexion/adduction of the hip with flexion of the knee causes pain. Displacement of the bone fragment may be from a few mm to 3 cm, but although surgical re-attachment of the bone fragment has been described (Veselko and Smrkolj, 1994), conservative treatment normally suffices. The athlete should be non-weight-bearing initially, followed by partial weight-bearing ambulation for 3–6 weeks, depending on the intensity of pain. Full strength and flexibility must be regained before competitive sport is resumed.

The hamstrings

The hamstrings may be injured either at their attachment to the ischial tuberosity or within their mid-bellies and, less commonly, at the knee (see below). The hamstring pull is the classic sprinting injury, with the athlete spectacularly pulling up in mid-flight with obvious pain.

Pain is apparent on straight leg raising and resisted knee flexion. Resisted flexion and tibial rotation will determine whether the biceps femoris or semi-membranosus and semi-tendinosus is affected.

To palpation, the structure of the muscles differentiates them. The semi-tendinosus and long head of biceps have a combined attachment on the lower medial facet of the ischial tuberosity, the two muscles travelling together for a short distance until they form fusiform muscle bellies. The semi-tendinosus almost instantly forms into a long slender

tendon, and travels around the medial condyle of the tibia to attach to the medial surface of the tibia below gracilis. The biceps has two proximal attachments; the long head, as described, and the short head from the lower linea aspera. The muscle swings downwards and laterally across the posterior aspect of the thigh and around the lateral ligament to insert into the head of the fibula. The biceps has a dual innervation and asynchronous stimulation of the two heads has been described as a factor in injury (Burkett, 1975). The semi-membranosus comes from the lateral facet of the ischial tuberosity and travels down and medially becoming flattened and broader as it does so. The semi-membranosus is deep to both the semi-tendinosus and biceps, and divides into five components when it reaches the knee (p. 282). The principal insertion is to the posterior aspect of the medial tibial tubercle.

Biomechanics and hamstring injury

During the running cycle (p. 212) the hamstrings contract eccentrically to decelerate the leg in late forward swing. This action also helps to stabilize the knee. During the support phase, the hamstrings act concentrically to extend the hip and continue to stabilize the knee by preventing knee extension. During push-off the hamstrings and gastrocnemius, both two-joint muscles, paradoxically extend the knee (see p. 17, action of two-joint muscles). This action is necessary because the mechanical efficiency of the quadriceps is reducing at this point (Sutton, 1984).

The ratio of the strength of the hamstrings to that of the quadriceps muscles (HQ ratio) is important. Normally, the quadriceps is the stronger of the two muscle groups (Table 10.1), as demonstrated by its greater volume. However, any disturbance to this natural balance may leave the weaker muscle group open to injury. The optimum value of the HQ ratio varies from 50% to 80% (Kannus, 1989), with average values in the

Table 10.1   Percentage of strength relative to quadriceps at 100%

Hamstrings	50–60%
Adductors	90%
Abductors	60%
Hip flexors	55%

From Reid (1992).

region of 60%. After knee injury, quadriceps wasting may result in the two muscle groups producing the same power giving an HQ ratio of 100% (Burnie and Brodie, 1986a).

Strength measures comparing quadriceps to hamstrings are traditionally carried out with an isometric dynamometer. However, the disadvantages of joint specificity and lack of movement make isokinetic testing more desirable. During isokinetic testing the speed of movement should match the speed of the sport as closely as possible. The speed must be quoted as the absolute value of the HQ ratio increases as velocity of movement increases (Burnie and Brodie, 1986b). Slow speeds ($45°/s$) have been shown to give ratios of 60% and high speeds ($300°/s$) ratios of 80% (Sutton, 1984). Isokinetic testing in the standard sitting position does not allow hip motion, and movement of the limb does not occur in a closed kinetic chain, so testing is not ideal.

Aetiology of hamstring injury

Tears tend to occur when there is a breakdown in the reciprocal action of the quadriceps and hamstrings, and happen at one of two instances in the running cycle. First, during late forward swing as the hamstrings are decelerating the limb, and the athlete feels the muscle 'stretch', and secondly, during the take off phase as the athlete 'pushes'. Changes in muscle coordination as a result of an alteration in the sensitivity of muscle spindles have been cited as a contributory factor to injury. It has been suggested (Sutton, 1984) that when an athlete is fatigued he or she unconsciously increases the sensitivity of his muscle spindles, which respond to stretch with an exaggerated contraction, and this in turn causes injury.

Lack of flexibility may predispose to hamstring injury, and may be assessed with the athlete lying supine with one hip flexed to $90°$. Maintaining this position by gripping the leg with the hands, the athlete attempts to straighten the leg with quadriceps power only. Adequate flexibility is indicated by an ability to lock the leg out while maintaining $90°$ hip flexion (see also p. 157). Alterations in the normal 60% strength ratio between the quadriceps and hamstrings and a deficit greater than 10% between the two sets of hamstrings has also been cited as a predisposing factor (Burkett, 1970).

Many hamstring injuries tend to recur, and lack of full rehabilitation may be one cause. After injury, athletes are usually aware of lack of mobility in the hamstrings and are often conscientious about stretching exercises. However, muscle wasting is not so obvious in the hamstrings as it is in the quadriceps, and so many athletes forget to spend time regaining hamstring strength. In addition, using eccentric exercises as part of a general leg conditioning programme may strengthen the series elastic components within the hamstrings making them better equipped to withstand loading at heel strike (Stanton and Purdam, 1989). The inclusion of plyometric training in late stage rehabilitation of hamstring injury is therefore essential.

Exercise therapy following hamstring injury

Exercise therapy aims to progressively increase the function of all the fitness components relevant to hamstring function (see p. 111). Strength restoration begins with isometric contractions within the pain-free range to facilitate muscle broadening and reduce adhesion formation. Concentric strength is later introduced against limb resistance initially followed by therapist resistance and later light-weight resistance.

Knee flexion may be used in both lying and standing. Hip extension (from outer to inner range) is used in prone lying and also standing. The two may be worked in PNF patterns using hip extension, abduction and external rotation combined with knee extension, and the reverse using hip flexion, adduction and internal rotation combined with knee flexion. Both patterns are used initially against controlled therapist resistance but may be later usefully modified against elastic band or pulley resistance.

Where isokinetics are available, a variation of speeds is important. Slow speeds of 60° and 120°/s may be used to begin with, progressing to 240° and 300°/s as pain allows.

Hamstring isolation exercises, such as leg curls in lying and standing (Fig. 10.5), have their place in initial rehabilitation to ensure maximal muscle broadening, but have distinct limitations which must be recognized. First, these exercises work only the knee flexion function of the hamstrings, with little activity over the hip. Secondly, the action is open chain only when the predominant function of the hamstrings occurs in closed chain format. Thirdly, the exercises are often performed with the emphasis placed on inner range contraction, which may tend to shorten the muscle (see p. 148). However, these muscles are unlikely to be posturally lengthened so that they require shortening.

It is more likely that the muscles will already lack flexibility so full range resisted work is preferable.

Closed chain exercises may be performed by modifying many common exercises. Leg rowing (Fig. 10.6a) is a useful exercise. The athlete sits on a towel (on a wooden floor) or plastic tray (on a carpeted floor) with the feet fixed. The action is to pull the body forwards by hamstring action, mimicking a rowing position. Sitting astride a gym bench or 'form' (Fig. 10.6b) the athlete digs his or her heels into the ground and again pulls the body forwards using leg strength alone. Both of these actions may be performed unilaterally or bilaterally. The popular slide trainer may also be used for sagittal leg pumping actions with the knees straight or bent (Fig. 10.6c). The sitting leg press weight training apparatus may be used for the sprint kick exercise (Fig. 10.6d). Instead of sitting on the bench, the athlete turns around and places his or her shoulder against the chair back, and the ball of the foot on the machine pedal. The action is to press the machine

Figure 10.6 Hamstring exercises in closed kinetic chain. (a) Athlete sits on a towel on a wooden floor with feet fixed. Pull body forwards by flexing the knees and hips. (b) Sitting astride a gym bench, grip the feet against the floor and pull the body forwards. (c) Using a commercial slide trainer, straight leg hip flexion and extension is performed. (d) Kneeling on a seated leg press machine, hip and knee extension is performed.

Figure 10.5 Hamstring isolation exercises. (a) Standing leg curl, (b) lying leg curl. These are non-functional movements which must be used with caution.

pedal with a combined hip and knee extension action.

Speed and power (see p. 11) are worked using plyometric activity. Stepping, jumping, lunging and hopping actions are all useful and are progressed for range and speed against body weight resistance and for power against weight resistance. For this later aspect, a weighted jacket is easier (and safer) than holding weights.

Flexibility exercises for the hamstrings must take account of pelvic action and the action of the two-joint muscle. In addition, relative flexibility (p. 145) may dictate that the majority of the stretching force is imposed on the lumbar spine in toe-touching type movements (Fig. 10.7a).

Flexibility may begin with active knee extension (Fig. 10.7b). The advantage of this movement is the reciprocal innervation gained from quadriceps action, and the control that the athlete has over the movement. In addition, the back is supported throughout the action. The tripod stretch (Fig. 10.7c) is also a useful exercise which requires a combination of pelvic stability with hamstring flexibility.

Adductor strain

Variously called groin strain and rider's strain, a tear of the adductor muscles gives pain to resisted adduction, and abduction stretch. Damage is usually to the musculo-tendinous junction about 5 cm from the pubis, or more rarely the teno-osseous junction, giving pain directly over the pubic tubercle (adductor longus) or body of the pubis.

The condition is more common in sports requiring a rapid change of direction, and where the adductors are used for propulsion. Pain is often experienced with sprinting, lunging, and twisting on the straight leg.

Ultrasound must be used with caution because of the proximity of this area to the genitalia. Isometric contractions may be carried out by gripping a foam pillow between the knees. During the sub-acute phase transverse frictions may be applied with the athlete in a supine position, with the affected leg abducted and the knee flexed and supported on a pillow.

The adductor muscles are often neglected with respect to strengthening and flexibility, particularly in the male athlete. Sagittal plane leg movements are common in weight training, and although frontal plane actions are possible, they are infrequently used.

Treatment for the condition must therefore involve stretching and strengthening the adductors. Initially, strength exercises such as side-lying (injured limb down), hip adduction with a weight bag over the knee (early) or ankle (more advanced) are useful. Later, adduction may be performed using a weight and pulley apparatus (Fig. 10.8). Power training may be carried out by flicking a medicine ball with the foot with an adduction action.

(a) (b) (c)

Figure 10.7 Hamstring flexibility exercise. (a) Tight hamstrings limit anterior pelvic tilt, throwing stress onto the less flexible thoraco-lumbar junction. (b) Active knee extension. (c) Tripod stretch.

Figure 10.8 Hip adductor strethening. (a) Unilateral weight-training. (b) Bilateral weight-training approach. (c) Weight bag. (d) Resistance tubing.

Swimming exercises, such a breast stroke, and hip adduction with a paddle secured to the lower leg are also of benefit. Closed kinetic chain actions using running, side stepping, jumping and hopping are included during late stage rehabilitation.

Adductor stretching may be used for both the short adductors with the knee bent, and gracilis with the knee straight. One common exercise is the 'taylor position' stretch (Fig. 10.9a) where the soles of the feet are together and the knees are pressed down with the hands or elbows. Although a useful movement, athletes often allow the pelvis to posteriorly tilt flexing the lumbar spine (Fig. 10.9b). The posterior tilt of the pelvis pushes the pubic bone forwards allowing a greater apparent range of motion and the knee to drop down further. A neutral pelvic position may be maintained by sitting on a wedge (Fig. 10.9c), or alterna-

tively placing a rolled towel beneath the ischial tuberosities. As the knees are pressed down, the spine should be lengthened ('stretch the top of your head to the ceiling'). The gracilis may be stretched in the stride sitting position with the leg straight, the same cautions concerning pelvic tilt applying. A more advanced gracilis stretch can be performed against a wall (Fig. 10.9d). The hips are flexed to 90° and the legs straight. Contract release stretching (p. 120) is performed by closing the legs (adduction resisted by limb weight) and then relaxing them into abduction.

One complication of the disorder is the formation of myositis ossificans traumatica within the adductor origin. This is usually a consequence of inadequate rest during the acute stage of the condition. This condition is often described, somewhat inaccurately, under the general term 'osteitis pubis'.

Figure 10.9 Adductor stretching. (a) Common adductor stretch. (b) Allowing the pelvis to posteriorly tilt pushes the pubis forwards. (c) Sitting on a wedge maintains the neutral lordosis. (d) Long adductor stretch.

Osteitis pubis

True osteitis pubis is a condition affecting the pubic symphysis rather than the pubis itself, although the two conditions often coalesce. Shearing stress is placed on the pubic symphysis during mid-stance as the non-weight-bearing hip drops, tilting the pelvis. With distance runners, and particularly after pregnancy when the pubic symphysis is still mobile, this repetitive stress may inflame the pubic symphysis, a condition known as pubis stress symphysitis (Rold and Rold, 1986).

With osteitis pubis no instability of the pubic symphysis occurs, but there is tenderness over the area with rarefaction of the pubic bones and widening of the symphysis pubis apparent on X-ray. The athlete often has a waddling gait, and may describe occasional crepitus. Severe cases may progress to sclerosis and eventual narrowing of the symphysial joint space requiring wedge resection (Grace, Shives and Coventry, 1989). Differential diagnosis between the various persistent groin conditions calls for radiographic investigation and, possibly, bone scan.

Bursitis

The main sites of bursitis around the hip are the trochanteric bursa, and, to a lesser extent, the ischial bursa and psoas bursa (Fig. 10.10).

Trochanteric bursitis

The trochanteric bursa lies between gluteus maximus and the posterolateral surface of the greater trochanter. Bursitis may arise if flexibility of the ilio-tibial band (ITB) is reduced. Normally, the ITB moves forwards with flexion and backwards with extension of the hip. The bursa may be irritated if the

Figure 10.10 Common sites for bursitis around the hip.

movement of the ITB is limited, a cause of 'snapping hip syndrome' (see below). Biomechanical faults in running which tax the gluteus maximus or alter pelvic tilt in the frontal plane are also a causal factor. Running on a banked surface with one foot lower than the other, and excessive posterolateral heel wear, which increases supination at heel strike, will increase pressure on the bursa via the ITB. Muscle imbalance between the adductors and abductors, especially in an athlete with a wide pelvis, or, in young athletes with a tendency to run with the feet crossing, may also be a contributory factor.

Pain often comes on gradually over the lateral aspect of the hip, in some cases radiating down to the knee. It may be aggravated by crossing the legs, climbing stairs and getting into and out of a car. Pain may be elicited by passively flexing, adducting, and medially rotating the affected hip, and with resisted hip abduction allowing muscle tension to compress the bursa beneath the gluteus maximus. Palpation for tenderness is carried out in a side-lying position, with the injured limb uppermost and slightly flexed. The patient can often feel the injury while lying in this position because of the hip adduction involved. Pressure for palpation should be directed behind, rather than on top of, the trochanter. The Ober manoeuvre (p. 157) is often positive.

Treatment aimed at reducing pain and inflammation must be linked to a removal of the cause, be it training or biomechanically related. Phonophoresis with hydrocortisone gel may be useful as the bursa is fairly superficial. If the ITB is shortened (the Ober manoeuvre will confirm this) stretching is obviously called for.

In patients where pain is referred and point tenderness is not present, trochanteric bursitis may be differentiated from arthritis by the absence of a capsular pattern.

Ischial and psoas bursitis

Psoas bursitis usually occurs as a result of excessive activity. Pain is reproduced by passive hip flexion and adduction. In addition, slight pain can occur on contraction of the psoas in a position of maximal hip flexion. Palpation over the lesser trochanter is made easier by flexing the hip and knee to 45°, and externally rotating the hip. The limb is supported on a pillow.

Ischial bursitis (Weavers' bottom) gives pain after prolonged sitting, and may be set off by direct trauma, such as a fall onto the backside when ice skating. There is pain on palpation of the bursa between the ischial tuberosity and the gluteus maximus. This condition may be mistaken for a hamstring pull but is differentiated by the absence of pain to resisted knee flexion. The condition is aggravated by tight hamstrings, speed work, and excessive hill running.

Neural structures and posterior thigh pain

Discal involvement

The hip is an L3 structure and so can refer pain down the front of the thigh. However, posterior thigh pain frequently accompanies low back pain and may be a result of nerve entrapment in the absence of accompanying symptoms in the back. Distinguishing between sciatic impingement and hamstring injury is not always straightforward. A history of trauma is important, and if straight leg raising causes pain but resisted knee flexion does not, the spine should be examined further. Weakness on resisted knee flexion could be through intramuscular trauma, pain inhibition, or impaired neural conduction. Laseague's sign will cause pain from sciatic and hamstring stretch, but adding neck flexion will not affect the hamstrings but will stretch the dural covering of the cord and nerve roots. Pain of discal origin will therefore be worse and that of hamstring origin unchanged.

The slump test is helpful both diagnostically and therapeutically (see p. 350), and is used to assess tension in the pain-sensitive structures around the vertebral canal and/or intervertebral foramen. During the slump test, a hamstring tear will give pain as the leg is straightened, but will not be made worse by slumping the spine, providing the pelvis does not tilt.

Kornberg and Lew (1989) assessed athletes with grade I hamstring tears using the slump test. Where positive, they used the slump therapeutically as a stretching exercise, and found that the addition of the slump procedure to standard physiotherapy management of the injuries (which had included stretching exercises) was significantly more effective in returning a player to full function. They argued that abnormal neural tension had produced symptoms which mimicked hamstring injury. In addition, they made the point that increased tension in the neural structures could elevate the resting tone of the hamstrings predisposing them to intrinsic injury.

Piriformis syndrome

The piriformis muscle (Fig. 10.11) attaches from the front of the second to fourth sacral segments, the gluteal surface of the ileum and the sacrotuberous ligament. It then travels through the greater sciatic notch to attach to the upper medial side of the greater trochanter. Its position is such that the sciatic nerve rests directly on the muscle, and in 15% of the population (Calliet, 1983) the muscle is divided into two with the sciatic nerve passing between the two bellies.

Piriformis syndrome occurs in women more frequently than men (ratio 6:1). If the muscle is inflamed, shortened, or in spasm it will impinge on the sciatic nerve giving pain and tingling in the posterior thigh and buttock. Pain is deep and localized and examination of the lumbar spine and sacro-iliac joints is unrevealing. Palpation of the muscle may be carried out with the patient prone in

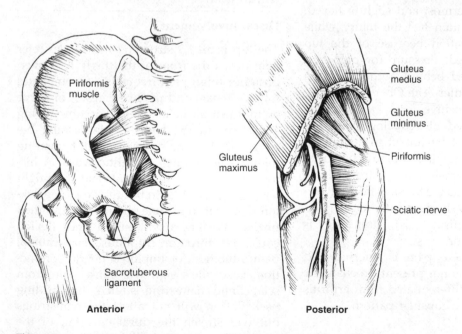

Figure 10.11   Position of the piriformis muscle.

the frog position (hip flexed and abducted bringing knee to chest), or rectally. Resisted lateral rotation of the affected hip gives pain, and passive stretch into internal rotation is painful and may be limited.

Management involves pain relieving modalities and stretching the external rotators of the hip. A simple self-stretch can be taught to the patient. If the right hip is affected, the left hip is flexed to 90° and the right foot is placed on the left knee. The right hip is pushed gently into abduction and external rotation (Fig. 10.12).

Hamstring syndrome

Puranen and Orava (1988) described athletes with gluteal pain radiating into the posterior thigh who had no history of trauma. Pain occurred most often in the sitting position, and when stretching the hamstrings. Local tenderness was evident to the ischial tuberosity, neurological examination was normal, and extensive physiotherapy, including electrical modalities stretching and strengthening (no specific details given), failed to remove the symptoms.

At operation, tight fibrotic bands were found from the semi-tendinosus and biceps femoris, with the thickest actually within the bulk of the biceps. These were located close to the sciatic nerve and in some cases actually adhered to it.

Release of the tight bands gave symptomatic relief to 52 of the 59 patients treated. The authors proposed that excessive stretching may have led to hypercompensation within the muscles, particularly in sprinters and hurdlers.

Figure 10.12 Gluteal stretch.

Hip pain and the young athlete

Pain and limitation of movement in the hip in children should always be treated with caution. The extreme forces placed on the hip by weight-bearing, combined with osseous and vascular changes occurring about the joint during adolescence, can lead to a variety of serious orthopaedic conditions.

The blood supply to the femoral head may be compromised in the very young. From birth until the age of 4 years blood reaches the femoral head via the metaphysis. From the age of 8 years, vessels through the ligamentum teres supply the head. Between these two periods the lateral epiphyseal vessels are the only source of blood to the femoral head (Cyriax, 1982). In addition, the upper femoral epiphysis does not fuse with the shaft until about 20 years of age.

Persistent hip or groin pain and/or a limp in young males (4–12 years) may be the result of Perthes' disease, an avascular necrosis (osteochondrosis) of the femoral head. The bony nucleus of the epiphysis becomes necrosed. The upper surface of the femoral head flattens and the epiphyseal line widens, altering the biomechanical alignment of the joint. When the bone is revascularized it hardens again, leaving a permanent deformity. Objective examination often reveals slight limitation of all hip movements with protective spasm. The condition may be precipitated by joint effusion at the hip following trauma, or a non-specific synovitis (Apley and Solomon, 1989).

Trauma, or more usually simply weight-bearing, in the young athlete (10–20 years) may result in slipping of the upper femoral epiphysis. Pain is usually felt in the hip or knee. The epiphyseal junction may soften and with weight-bearing or trauma may cause the head of the femur to slip on the neck, usually downwards and backwards. If left, the epiphyses will fuse to the femoral neck in the abnormal position. Objective examination often reveals limitation of flexion, abduction and medial rotation with the limb often lying in lateral rotation. Leg short-ening up to 2 cm is common, and radio-graphs reveal widening and a 'woolly' appearance of the epiphyseal plate. On the X-ray, a line traced along the superior aspect of the femoral neck will reveal a step defor-mity (Fig. 10.13). The line remains superior to the head rather than passing directly through it (Trethowan's sign).

Capsular tightening

Inflammation within the hip joint leads to the characteristic capsular pattern of marked limitation of flexion and medial rotation with some limitation of abduction. Ad-duction and lateral rotation are generally full (Cyriax and Cyriax, 1983). Initially, the synovium becomes inflamed giving synovi-tis. Pain is from chemical stimulation of sen-sory nerve endings within the synovium and is often dull and throbbing in nature, being worse at night and at rest. If the synovitis does not resolve, swelling causes capsular pain by mechanically stretching nerve end-ings between the collagen fibres of the cap-sule. Eventually, secondary capsular fibrosis occurs leading to capsular tightening and deformity. When pain and inflammation abate, the capsular tightening and associated

Figure 10.13 Slipped upper femoral epiphysis. The step deformity is apparent on X-ray.

loss of muscle stretch and strength leave the patient with hip dysfunction.

Capsular tightening will respond to mobi-lization procedures and later to stretching exercises. Longitudinal mobilizations, fol-lowed by full hip traction, may be used, with the hip in its open pack position (30° flexion, 30° abduction and slight external rotation). A belt is used to stop the patient from sliding on the couch. Hip flexion may be stretched using the Thomas test as an exercise (see p. 156). The patient lies supine with the popliteal area of the knees over the couch end. The unaffected leg is straight and hangs below couch level, while the knee and hip of the affected side are flexed to chest level. Hip extension may be promoted with the modified lunge described above.

Hip pointer

The relatively unprotected iliac crest is vul-nerable to direct blows from any hard object, be it a hockey ball, boot or another player's head. Contusion is often persistent, espe-cially if the periosteum is affected, and the condition is described as a 'hip pointer'. The pain from the injury is so severe that the trunk is flexed to the affected side. The athlete is often unable to take a breath and may panic.

Following reassurance, the iliac crest is examined and usually reveals dramatic pain but little bruising or swelling. The abdominal muscles are often rigid and the hips pulled into flexion. After 24–48 hours more extensive bruising appears and local tenderness may last for weeks. A raised area may persist for many months. Ice may be used initially to relieve pain, and the area padded when the athlete resumes sport.

Clicking hip syndrome

Clicking or snapping hip can occur to repeated flexion and extension movements.

The condition is common in dancers and young athletes, and is usually painless. However, it is of obvious concern to the athlete as in some cases the sound is loud enough for others to hear.

There are two main types of clicking hip, internal and external (Reid, 1992). Although there have been many proposed causes of this condition one of the most common causes of internal clicking hip is the suction phenomenon. This can occur during exercises such as sit-ups and requires reassurance rather than treatment. Alternative causes include tight ligaments and tendons passing over bony prominences. External clicking hip is usually a result of the gluteus maximus tendon clicking over the greater trochanter, or the ilio-tibial band clicking over the greater trochanter.

Sometimes the click can be reproduced during examination by flexing and extending the hip in adduction, in which case tight abductors are a contributory factor. The Ober manoeuvre is often positive in these cases.

If the condition is painful, treatment designed to reduce local inflammation may be required. In painless instances, stretching of the ITB and hip abductors can help. The athlete begins in a side-lying position with the affected leg upper most. The upper leg is abducted, and hip hitching is performed to shorten the leg (lateral tilt of the pelvis). The pelvic fixation is maintained as the upper leg is lowered into adduction (Fig. 7.17 p. 157).

References

Apley, A.G. and Solomon, L. (1989) *Concise System of Orthopaedics and Fractures*, Butterworth-Heinemann, Oxford

Burkett, L.N. (1970) Causative factors in hamstring strains. *Medicine and Science in Sports and Exercise*, **2**, 39–42

Burkett, L.N. (1975) Investigation into hamstring strains: the case of the hybrid muscle. *American Journal of Sports Medicine*, **3**, 228–231

Burnie, J. and Brodie, D.A. (1986a) Isokinetic measurement in preadolescent males. *International Journal of Sports Medicine*, **7**, 205–209.

Burnie, J. and Brodie, D.A. (1986b) Isokinetics in the assessment of rehabilitation: a case report. *Clinical Biomechanics*, **1**, 140–146

Cailliet, R. (1983) *Soft Tissue Pain and Disability*, F.A. Davis, Philadelphia

Cyriax, J. (1982) *Textbook of Orthopaedic Medicine*, Vol. 1, 8th edn, Baillière Tindall, London

Cyriax, J.H. and Cyriax, P.J. (1983) *Illustrated Manual of Orthopaedic Medicine*, Butterworth-Heinemann, London

Estwanik, J.J. and McAlister, J.A. (1990) Contusions and the formation of myositis ossificans. *Physician and Sports Medicine*. **18**(4), 52–64

Grace, J.N., Shives, T.C. and Coventry, M.B. (1989) Wedge resection of the symphysis pubis for the treatment of osteitis pubis. *Journal of Bone and Joint Surgery*, **71A**, 358–364

Jackson, D.W. and Feagin, J.A. (1973) Quadriceps contusions in young athletes. Relation of severity of injury to treatment and prognosis. *Journal of Bone and Joint Surgery*, **55A**(1), 95–105

Kannus, P. (1989) Hamstring/quadriceps strength ratios in knees with medial collateral ligament insufficiency. *Journal of Sports Medicine and Physical Fitness*, **29**(2), 194–198

Kornberg, C. and Lew, P. (1989) The effect of stretching neural structures on grade one hamstring injuries. *Journal of Orthopaedic and Sports Physical Therapy*, June, 481–487

Maitland, G.D. (1986) *Vertebral Manipulation*, 5th edn, Butterworth, London

Norkin, C.C. and Levangie, P.K. (1992) *Joint Structure and Function*, 2nd edn, F.A. Davis, Philadelphia

Palastanga, N., Field, D. and Soames, R. (1994) *Anatomy and Human Movement*, 2nd edn, Butterworth-Heinemann, Oxford

Puranen, J. and Orava, S. (1988) The hamstring syndrome. A new diagnosis of gluteal sciatic pain. *American Journal of Sports Medicine*, **16**(5), 517–521

Reid, D.C. (1992) *Sports Injury Assessment and Rehabilitation*, Churchill Livingstone, London

Rold, J.F. and Rold, B.A. (1986) Pubis stress symphysitis in a female distance runner. *Physician and Sports Medicine*, June, **14**, 61–65

Stanton, P. and Purdam, C. (1989) Hamstring injuries in sprinting – The role of eccentric exercise. *Journal of Orthopaedic and Sports Physical Therapy*, **10**(9), 343–349

Sutton, G. (1984) Hamstrung by hamstring strains: a review of the literature. *Journal of Orthopaedic and Sports Physical Therapy*, **5**(4), 184–195

Veselko, M. and Smrkolj, V. (1994) Avulsion of the anterior superior iliac spine in athletes: case reports. *Journal of Trauma*, **36**, 444–446

11

The knee

Biomechanics of the extensor mechanism

The patella is the largest sesamoid bone in the body. It is attached above to the quadriceps tendon, below to the patellar tendon, and medially and laterally to the patellar retinacula. The breadth of the pelvis and close proximity of the knee creates a valgus angulation to the femur. Coupled with this, the direction of pull of the quadriceps is along the shaft of the femur and that of the patellar tendon is almost vertical (Fig. 11.1). The difference between the two lines of pull is known as the Q angle and is an important determinant of knee health. Normal values for the Q angle are in the region of 15–20°, and knees with an angle greater or less than this can be considered malaligned.

As the knee flexes and extends, the patella should travel in line with the long axis of the femur. However, the horizontal force vector created as a result of the Q angle tends to pull the patella laterally, a movement which is resisted by the horizontal pull of the lower fibres of vastus medialis. These lower fibres can be considered as a functionally separate muscle, the vastus medialis oblique (VMO) (Speakman and Weisberg, 1977). The quadriceps as a whole have been shown to undergo reflex inhibition as the knee swells (de Andrade, Grant and Dixon, 1965; Stokes and Young, 1984). However, the VMO can be inhibited by as little as 10 ml effusion while the vastus lateralis and rectus femoris require as much as 60 ml (Arno, 1990). Minimal effusion occurs frequently with minor trauma and may go unnoticed by the athlete. However, this will be enough to weaken the VMO and alter the biomechanics of the patella.

In full extension the patella does not contact the femur, but lies in a lateral position. As flexion progresses, the patella should move medially. If it moves laterally it will butt against the prominent lateral femoral condyle, and the lateral edge of the patellar groove of the femur. As flexion progresses different areas of the patella's undersurface are compressed onto the femur. At 20° flexion the inferior pole of the patella is compressed and by 45° the middle section is affected. At 90° flexion, compression has moved to the superior aspect of the knee. In a full squatting position, with the knee reaching 135° flexion, only the medial and lateral areas of the patella are compressed (Fig. 11.2). Compression tests of the patella to examine its posterior surface must therefore be performed with the knee flexed to different angles.

Patello-femoral loads may be as high as three or four times body weight as the knee flexes in walking, and nine times body weight when descending stairs (Cox, 1990). While the posterior surface of the patella is

Figure 11.1 The Q angle.

Figure 11.2 Contact areas of the patella at different angles of flexion.

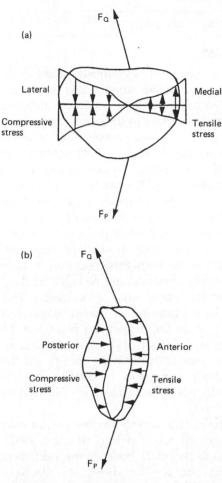

Figure 11.3 Patellar stress. (a) The Q angle causes the lateral edge of the patellar cartilage to be compressed, while the medial aspect is subjected to tensile stress. (b) The posterior surface of the patella is compressed. F_Q, quadriceps pull; F_P, patellar tendon. From Cox (1990), with permission.

compressed, the anterior aspect receives a tensile force when seen in the sagittal plane (Fig. 11.3b). The effect of the Q angle is to create both horizontal and vertical force vectors which tend to compress the lateral aspect of the patella but submit the medial aspect to tensile stress (Fig. 11.3a). Clearly, alterations in Q angle will change the pattern of stress experienced by the patellar cartilage.

Knee angles in the stance phase of walking or running will be altered by foot and hip mechanics through the closed kinetic chain. Excessive foot pronation and hip internal rotation and adduction (causing a 'knock-knee' posture) have been linked to anterior knee pain (see below).

Anterior knee pain

Pathology

Anterior knee pain is variously called chondromalacia patellae and patella malalignment syndrome. It is a condition affecting the posterior surface of the patella sometimes attributed to cartilage damage and on occasion incorrectly seen as a direct precursor to osteoarthritis. Since hyaline cartilage is aneural, changes in the patellar cartilage surface itself would not result in anterior knee pain. Furthermore, at arthroscopy cartilage changes are often seen in patients who have no anterior knee pain. If cartilage degeneration does occur with this condition, it is to the ground substance and collagen at deep levels on the lateral edge of the patella. This results in a blistering of the cartilage as it separates from the underlying bone, but the cartilage surface itself is still smooth (Gruber, 1979). In osteoarthritis (OA) (see p. 48) the initial changes occur to the cartilage surface of the odd facet (medial) and are followed by fibrillation.

The retinacula supporting the patella may be a major source of pain (Fulkerson, 1982), or the sub-chondral bone of the odd facet (Hertling and Kessler, 1990). As we have seen, the odd facet is only occasionally compressed in a full squatting position, and so its sub-chondral bone is less dense and weaker. Lateral movement of the loaded patella could pull the odd facet into rapid contact with the patellar surface of the femur causing pain.

The complex mechanical relations of the patella make biomechanical assessment of the lower limb a necessity in the treatment of anterior knee pain, and static and dynamic posture should be analysed.

Muscular factors

Flexibility and strength of the knee tissues and muscles will often reveal asymmetry. The relationship between the hamstrings and quadriceps (HQ ratio) is particularly important and may require isokinetic assessment of peak torque values (see p. 25). Isokinetic testing also demonstrates characteristic changes in the anterior knee pain patient (Fig. 11.4). Eccentric torque production during knee extension is often poor (Bennett and Stauber, 1986) and the torque curve may be irregular (Hoke, Howell and Stack, 1983). Both changes have been suggested to represent a deficiency in motor control, which would explain the often rapid response to quadriceps training that is achieved in these patients. One possibility is that malalignment and patello-femoral (PF) pressure alterations may result partly from subtle shifts in the timing or amount of VMO activity in particular parts of the movement range (Reid, 1992). The aim of rehabilitation is therefore more a case of motor skill acquisition than pure strength training.

Weakness or malfunction in the VMO will allow the patella to drift laterally as the quadriceps contract. Normally the ratio of VMO to vastus lateralis (VL) is 1:1, and VMO activity is that of a stabilizing muscle (see p. 144) in that it is tonic (Reynolds et al., 1983). In the anterior knee pain patient the VMO to VL ratio is less than one as the VMO weakens. In addition, its contractile nature becomes phasic, as its endurance capacity is reduced.

Strengthening has traditionally been achieved by the use of short-range quadriceps exercises and straight leg raising exercises. However, these are both open chain movements and as the knee is in closed chain motion during the stance phase of gait, closed chain actions are more likely to carry over into functional activities.

Closed chain VMO re-education may be carried out by performing limited range squats ($\frac{1}{4}$ squat exercise) or lunges moving the knee from 20–30° flexion to full extension. Step downs from a single stair are useful as they can retrain correct knee motion. The patient should be instructed to keep the

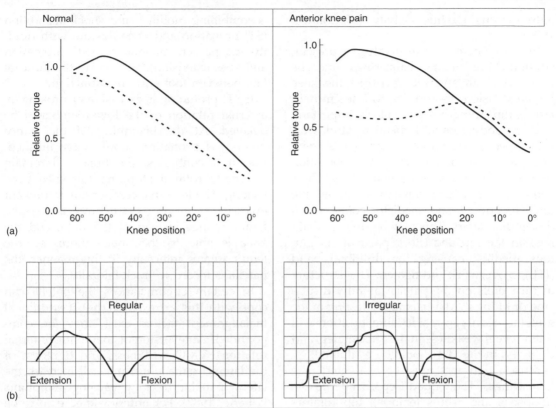

(a)

(b)

Figure 11.4   Characteristic changes in isokinetic evaluation with anterior knee pain. (a) Relative torque. (b) Shape of torque curve.

knee over the centre of the foot (avoiding adduction and medial rotation) throughout the movement. The use of surface electromyography (sEMG) can help with re-education. The sEMG electrode is placed over the VMO and the patient is taught to activate the muscle in standing and then to maintain this activation throughout the $\frac{1}{4}$ squat exercise. The full motor pattern is of foot supination, slight hip abduction and external rotation while maintaining VMO contraction. This may be achieved by standing side on to a wall with the injured leg on the outside (Fig. 11.5). The inner knee and hip are flexed to 45° and this knee presses against the wall enabling the athlete to hold the trunk vertical while standing on one leg. This body position places significant loading on the gluteus

medius of the outer leg to maintain the horizontal pelvic alignment. The foot is supinated, leg turned out and knee slightly flexed to 20°. EMG biofeedback is used over the VMO, and palpation is used to facil-

Figure 11.5   Closed chain patellar stability re-education.

itate gluteus medius activity (McConnell, 1994).

In cases where genu recurvatum is present, strengthening of the hamstrings may be required in an attempt to correct the knee hyperextension. In addition to knee musculature, hip strength is particularly important. The hip abductors and lateral rotators warrant special attention as weakness here has been associated with this condition (Beckman, Craig and Lehman, 1989). It is common for young athletes to allow the knee to adduct and medially rotate when descending stairs. This may be due to weakness in the hip abductors, particularly gluteus medius, causing the ilio-tibial band (ITB) to overwork and tighten. This structure in turn pulls on the patella laterally displacing or tilting it. Manual muscle testing of the gluteus medius in a side-lying position will often reveal weakness in the affected leg, and tightness in the ITB should be evaluated.

Muscle tightness must be evaluated. The hamstrings, ITB, quadriceps, hip flexors (iliopsoas and rectus femoris), hip rotators and gastrocnemius should all be addressed. Tests, which may also be used as stretching exercises, are shown with average values in Table 11.1. ITB tightness may pull the patella laterally during flexion, while tight hamstrings could result in increased knee flexion and a resultant increase in patello-femoral compression forces. A tight gastrocnemius, in addition to increasing or prolonging knee flexion during gait, will also cause compensatory sub-talar pronation.

Foot biomechanics

During normal running gait (see Chapter 9) the sub-taloid joint (STJ) is slightly supinated at heel strike. As the foot moves into ground contact, the joint pronates pulling the lower limb into internal rotation, and unlocking the knee. As the gait cycle progresses, the STJ moves into supination externally rotating the leg as the knee extends (locks) to push the body forward. This biomechanical action is combining mobility and shock absorbtion (STJ pronation and knee flexion) with rigidity and power transmission (STJ supination and knee extension), and shows the intricate link between foot and knee function.

If STJ pronation is excessive or prolonged, external rotation of the lower limb will be delayed. At the beginning of the stance phase, STJ pronation should have finished. But, if it continues, the tibia will remain externally rotated stopping the knee from locking. The leg must compensate to prevent excessive strain on its structures, and so the femur rotates instead of the tibia, and the knee is able to lock once more. As the femur rotates internally in this manner, the patella is forced to track laterally.

In certain circumstances the patella can cope with this extra stress, but if additional malalignment factors exist, they are compounded. Anteversion of the femur (internal rotation), VMO weakness, and tightness of the lateral retinaculum may all increase the lateral patellar tracking causing symptoms (Tiberio, 1987). For anterior knee pain to be treated effectively therefore, a biomechanical assessment of the lower limb is mandatory. If hyperpronation is present, it must be corrected. This will involve assessment of sports footwear, patient education and orthotic prescription.

Patella position

A number of forces are imposed on the patella as a result of active and passive structures (Fig. 11.6). The vastus lateralis pulls at 12–15° to the long axis of the femur while the vastus medialis longus pulls at 15–18°, and the VMO at 50–55° (Lieb and Perry, 1968). The medial and lateral retinacula, if tight, may tilt the patella (Norkin and Levangie, 1992). The ITB attaches to the patella via a small slip from its lower end, called the iliopatellar band (Terry, Hughston and Norwook, 1986). The ITB has a connection

Table 11.1   Flexibility tests/exercises used in the management of anterior knee pain

Hamstrings 70–80°

Iliopsoas—femur horizontal
Rectus femori—tibial vertical

Quadriceps—knee < 10 cm from buttock

Hip rotators—45° to vertical

ITB—upper leg below horizontal

Hip adductors—knees 10–15 cm from floor

Gastrocnemius—45° dorsiflexion

(Average values quoted)

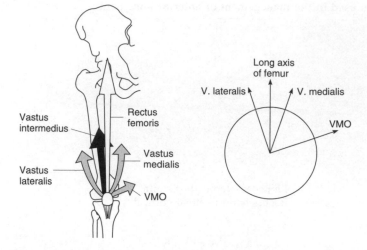

Figure 11.6   Angle of pull of quadriceps onto patella.

to the biceps femoris through the lateral intermuscular septum.

Quantifying the position of the patella is important because, as we have seen above, excessive pressure on the odd facet may result if the patella position is at fault. McConnell (1986) described four different patellar position faults which could be assessed with the patient in the supine position with the quadriceps relaxed. By using the patellar poles as landmarks and comparing their position to the planes of the femur any malalignment becomes evident. In addition, accessory patellar movements can be assessed with particular emphasis on medial and lateral gliding.

Patellar glide occurs when the patella moves from a neutral position. The distance from the centre of the patella to the medial and lateral femoral condyles is assessed. A difference in the medial distance compared to the lateral of greater than 0.5 cm is significant (Fig. 11.7a). Tightness in the lateral retinaculum, a frequent occurrence in anterior knee pain sufferers, will cause lateralization of the patella. Patellar tilt evaluates the position of the medial and lateral facets of the patella, with PF pain patients frequently showing a more prominent medial facet

with difficulty actually palpating the lateral and posterior edge of the patella (Fig. 11.7b). Patellar rotation occurs when the inferior pole of the patella deviates from a neutral position. Medial (internal) rotation occurs when the inferior pole of the patella lies med-

Figure 11.7   Patellar position. (a) Medial and lateral glide. (b) Medial and lateral tilt. (c) Rotation—M: medial, L: lateral. (d) Antero-posterior tilt.

ial to the long axis of the femur. Lateral (external) rotation is present when the inferior pole of the patella lies lateral to the long axis of the femur (Fig. 11.7c). Anteroposterior (AP) tilt exists when both the superior and inferior poles are not clear to palpate, indicating that one is lower into the surrounding soft tissue (Fig. 11.7d).

Arno (1990) attempted to quantify the patellar position with a description of the A angle. This relates patellar orientation to that of the tibial tubercle. The poles of the patella are palpated and a line is drawn bisecting the patella. Another line is drawn from the tibial tubercle to the apex of the inferior pole of the patella and the angle of intersection forms the A angle (Fig. 11.8). The same author argued that an A angle greater than 35° constituted malalignment when the Q angle remained constant.

Pain relief may often be provided by temporarily correcting any underlying fault in patella position through taping. Exercising with this taping in place may re-educate correct muscle sequencing to improve patellar alignment (McConnell, 1994). Initially, open web adhesive taping is applied to protect the skin against excessive tape drag. The pull of the final taping is applied using 5-cm zinc-oxide tape. Decreased medial glide is corrected by pulling a piece of tape from the lateral border of the patella (Fig. 11.9a). The

Figure 11.8 The A angle. From Arno (1990).

soft tissue over the medial femoral condyle is lifted towards the patella to give a skin bunching appearance. Lateral tilt is corrected again by a medially orientated tape. This time however, the tape covers only the medial half of the patellar face, and again the medial soft tissue is lifted towards the patella (Fig. 11.9b). Rotation is corrected by pulling the patella around its central axis. Internal rotation is corrected by attaching the tape to the upper inner quadrant of the patella. The tape is pulled down medially to rotate the patella clockwise (Fig. 11.9c). External rotation is corrected by placing the tape over the lower inner quadrant of the patella and pulling anti-clockwise. A posterior tilt of the inferior pole should be corrected first to elevate the pole away from the fat pad. The tape is placed over the upper pole of the patella and the patella is taped medially (Fig. 11.9d).

Surgery

Before surgery is considered, conservative management must be attempted. Indeed, Insall (1979) stated that surgery was only indicated when continuous pain limited normal activities for at least six months and the condition had not responded to conservative management. The complex aetiology of the condition has led to a number of different surgical procedures (Fig. 11.10).

Release of tight lateral retinaculum is performed through a small incision or arthroscopy to divide the retinaculum from the lower fibres of the vastus lateralis. Patellar debridement/shaving has been carried out to remove degenerate articular cartilage on the patella undersurface. Small areas of cartilage may be removed *en bloc* or larger areas shaved (chondroplasty).

Realignment procedures involve structural transfer to reduce or alter compression forces on the patella. The Maquet operation elevates the tibial tubercle to reduce patella reaction forces and the Hauser manoeuvre uses distal and medial transfer to reduce

Figure 11.9 Correction of patellar position using tape. After McConnell (1992).

Figure 11.10 Surgical procedures used in anterior knee pain treatment. (a) Excision of diseased area (chrondoplasty). (b) Shaving (debridement). (c) Lateral release. (d) Lateral release and medial reefing. (e) Release and transfer of part of tendon (Goldthwait). (f) Release and transfer of entire extensor insertion (Hauser). (g) Tibial tubercle elevation (Maquet). (h) Patellectomy. From Apley and Solomon (1993).

the valgus vector acting on the patello-femoral joint. The Goldthwait procedure involves release and transfer of part of the patellar tendon. Proximal realignment, by moving the attachment of the vastus media-lis, aims at increasing the mechanical advan-tage of the VMO. This technique is used in the young where alteration of the tibial tuberosity will detrimentally affect the apophysis. Facetectomy involves excision of all or part of a single patellar facet, and patellectomy entails excision of the whole patella.

Patellar fracture

Patellar fractures in sport occur most frequently in adolescent athletes, usually as a result of jumping. Fracture may occur at the pole of the patella, or as transverse, vertical, or comminuted injuries. In the young, the bony fragment may pull off a substantial amount of articular cartilage from the patella undersurface, giving a 'sleeve' fracture. Stress fracture at the distal third of the patella has been reported after sprinting (Jerosch, Castro and Jantea, 1989). Conservative treatment, consisting of immobilizing the limb in a cast for two to three weeks, is sufficient in 50–60% of cases (Exler, 1991). Surgical treatment involves internal fixation of the patellar fragments, and hemipatellectomy or total patellectomy in the case of comminuted injuries, combined with immobilization in a cast.

Following immobilization, mobility exercises and quadriceps strengthening is started. Strengthening begins with quadriceps setting (QS) exercises and straight leg raising (see p. 250). An extension lag is common in these patients. The leg is locked from a long sitting position, and as it is raised, the tibia falls 2–3 cm as the patient is unable to maintain locking. Re-education of the knee-locking mechanism may be achieved in a side-lying (gravity eliminated) position. This is followed by knee bracing with a rolled towel under the knee, the patient being instructed to 'push down' on the towel with the back of the knee and at the same time to lift the heel from the couch surface. Short range movements over a knee block using a weight bag is the next progression. When 60–90° knee flexion is achieved, light weight training on a universal machine with a relaxation stop,

or isokinetic training, is used before closed chain activities.

Patellar dislocation

Patellar dislocation may occur traumatically with any athlete, but is more frequently seen in children between the ages of 8–15 years and middle-aged women who are overweight and have poor muscular development of the quadriceps. Biomechanically, the individual is more susceptible to this condition if they demonstrate genu valgum, femoral anteversion or external rotation of the tibia, and if the VMO is weak.

The injury usually occurs when the knee is externally rotated and straightened at the same time, such as when the athlete turns to the left while pushing off from the right foot. In this position the tibial attachment of the quadriceps moves laterally in relation to the femur, increasing the lateral force component as the muscle group contracts. The patella almost always dislocates laterally and is accompanied by a ripping sensation and excruciating pain, causing the knee to give way. As the knee straightens, the patella may reduce spontaneously with an audible click.

Swelling is rapid due to the haemarthrosis, causing the skin to become taught and shiny. Bruising forms over the medial retinaculum, and the athlete is normally completely disabled by pain and quadriceps spasm. On occasion the VMO may avulse from the patella, revealing a hollow, and little tissue resistance to palpation, along the medial edge of the patello-femoral joint.

Initial treatment is to immobilize the knee completely and apply the RICE protocol. Aspiration may be required if pain is intense, but usually swelling abates with non-invasive management. Quadriceps re-education plays an important part in the rehabilitation process, with VMO strengthening being particularly important. The medial retinaculum must be allowed to heal fully, and it is a mistake to allow these athletes to mobilize unprotected too soon. Only when 90° knee flexion is achieved and the patient is able to perform a straight leg lift with 30–50% of the power of the uninjured leg are they ready to walk without support.

Early quadriceps exercises

The question of which quadriceps exercise to use at the beginning of rehabilitation is one of considerable debate within physiotherapy. The decision depends on a number of factors including PF reaction forces, the efficiency of an exercise to emphasize the VMO, and the relevance of an exercise movement to functional requirements (see Training specificity, p. 112).

The choice is often between open and closed chain movements, and bracing or lifting leg actions. In the gait cycle, the quadriceps are active during leg loading as the opposite leg moves into the swing phase, and to a lesser extent at the beginning of toe-off. In jumping, these muscles create very large concentric and eccentric forces in closed chain format. In a fast kicking action they work in an open chain action, but most of the work is from the two-joint rectus femoris (Richardson and Bullock, 1986). Both open chain and closed chain actions are important, but for early stage rehabilitation closed chain action emphasizing stability is more appropriate.

Comparing the leg extension with the leg press, Steinkamp et al. (1993) found PF joint stress, PF reaction force, and quadriceps force to be significantly greater in a leg extension exercise from 0–30° but significantly greater in a leg press action from 60–90°. These authors concluded that the leg press was more appropriate because is placed minimal stress on the PF joint in the functional range of motion and simulated normal movement patterns.

It is often argued that QS with isometric hip adduction will increase the recruitment of the VMO because some of the VMO fibres originate from adductor magnus (Reid, 1992). However, Karst and Jewett (1993) compared quadriceps setting (QS), straight leg raising (SLR), SLR with the hip laterally rotated, and SLR with isometric hip adduction with resistance equivalent to 5% body weight. These authors found that QS elicited a greater degree of activity than SLR. In addition, SLR with either hip adduction or lateral rotation failed to increase emphasis on the VMO over that of the rest of the quadriceps.

ITB friction syndrome

The ITB is a non-elastic collagen cord stretching from the pelvis to below the knee. At the top it is attached to the iliac crest where it blends with the gluteus maximus and tensor fascia lata. As the tract descends down the lateral side of the thigh its deep fibres attach to the linea aspera of the femur. The superficial fibres continue downwards to attach to the lateral femoral condyle, lateral patellar retinaculum and anterolateral aspect of the tibial condyle (Gerdy's tubercle).

In standing, the ITB lies posterior to the hip axis and anterior to the knee axis and therefore helps to maintain hip and knee extension, reducing the muscle work required to sustain an upright stance. As the knee flexes to 30° the ITB passes posterior to the knee joint axis, in so doing it glides over the lateral femoral condyle. In running, during the swing phase the ITB lies anterior to the greater trochanter and hip flexion/extension axis, reducing the workload required for hip flexion.

Aetiology

Tightness of the ITB can occur in a number of patient groups. The tall, lanky teenager who has recently undergone the adolescent growth spurt may experience pain if soft tissue elongation lags behind long bone development. Tightness in adolescent females is a consistent factor in anterior knee pain, although the relationship between the ITB and the patella has been debated by some authors (Rouse, 1996). The second major group of sufferers are adult athletes, particularly distance runners. A number of factors can contribute to problems within this group. Running on cambered roads and using shoes worn on their lateral edge will increase varus knee angulation and may overstretch a tight ITB. Rapid increases in speed or hill work can place excessive stress on the structure. In addition, imbalances of muscle strength and flexibility around the knee and hip may lead to the gradual onset of symptoms.

Pain normally occurs either over the trochanteric bursa or the lateral femoral condyle (Fig. 11.11). Pain is experienced to palpation, but also to limited range squats or lunges on the affected leg. As the knee flexes and the ITB passes over the lateral femoral condyle, friction may occur causing pain of increasing intensity. Flexibility tests, particularly the Ober manoeuvre and Thomas test often reveal pain and a lack of flexibility. In addition, compressing the ITB over the proximal part of the lateral femoral condyle with the knee flexing and extending to 30° may elicit pain (Noble, 1980).

Management

The initial inflammation of this condition responds to anti-inflammatory modalities, but the underlying cause must be addressed. Modifications include alterations of running surface and footwear, and changes to training intensity, frequency, duration and content. Where limited range motion is identified, stretching procedures are called for. Hip flexor and extensor flexibility is regained by using exercises previously described, and the ITB itself is stretched using an adaptation of the Ober manoeuvre.

The ITB insertion at the knee is first heated with hot packs or diathermy. The pelvis is stabilized by the patient flexing and holding the lower knee. The affected upper leg is initially abducted and extended at the hip and flexed at the knee. From this position, hip extension is maintained and the leg is pushed downwards into adduction, and held for 30–60 seconds, with the stretch being repeated four or five times. As adduction commences, the patient's pelvis will tend to tilt and an assistant should press down on the rim of the ilium to stabilize the pelvis and increase the stretch (see p. 157).

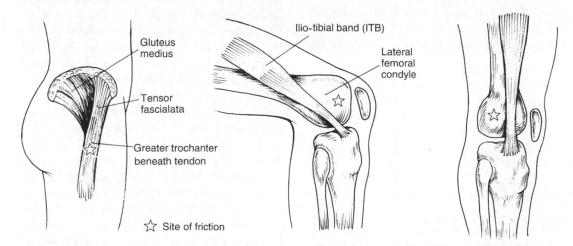

Gluteus medius

Tensor fascialata

Greater trochanter beneath tendon

Ilio-tibial band (ITB)

Lateral femoral condyle

☆ Site of friction

Figure 11.11 Ilio-tibial band friction syndrome.

Between treatment sessions the patient should attempt this procedure at home. The weight of the leg may be used to press it into adduction, and a weight bag on the knee will assist this. In addition, a training partner or family member can be taught to help maintain lumbo-pelvic stability.

Weakness in the hip abductors may allow the pelvis to tilt or 'dip' during the stance phase of walking or running. This often gives the impression of a mild Trendelenberg gait, and may be habitual following lower limb injury. Gait re-education and abductor strengthening are called for. The abductors may be strengthened from an open chain or more functional closed chain starting position. Open chain strengthening is performed using a weight bag in a side-lying hip abduction exercise. Closed chain strengthening is carried out with the athlete standing on the affected leg, and keeping it locked. The unaffected leg is flexed at the knee. From this position the pelvis is allowed to drop towards the unsupported side and pulled back to the horizontal position by hip abductor action (Fig. 11.12).

Collateral ligament injuries

The medial collateral ligament (MCL) is a broad flat band about 8 or 9 cm in length. It travels downwards and forwards from the medial epicondyle of the femur to the

(a)   (b)

Figure 11.12   Hip abductor strengthening. (a) Athlete stands on affected leg. (b) Allowing the opposite hip to drop and then pulling it up works the abductors of the weight-bearing limb.

medial condyle and upper medial shaft of the tibia. The ligament has both deep and superficial fibres, with the deep fibres attaching to the medial meniscus, and the superficial fibres extending below the level of the tibial tuberosity. The superficial fibres have anterior, middle and posterior portions.

When the knee is in full extension, it is in close pack formation. The medial femoral condyle is pushed backwards, and the medial epicondyle lifts away from the tibial plateaux, tightening the posterior part of the MCL. As the knee is flexed, the posterior part of the ligament relaxes, but the anterior and middle parts remain tight. By 80–90° flexion, the middle of the ligament is still tight, but the anterior and posterior portions are lax. In this way, the strong middle section of the ligament remains tight for most of the range of movement. The changing distribution of tension strain in the ligament means that the section which is affected through injury will depend on the knee joint angle when the injury occurred, so an accurate history is extremely helpful.

The lateral collateral ligament (LCL) is a round cord about 5 cm long, which stands clear of the joint capsule. It travels from the lateral epicondyle of the femur to the lateral surface of the head of the fibula. The ligament splits the tendon of biceps femoris, and is separated from the joint capsule by the popliteus muscle, and the lateral genicular vessels and nerve (Palastanga, Field and Soames, 1989). The lower end of the lateral ligament is pulled back in extension and forwards in flexion of the knee.

Damage to the MCL can result from excessive valgus angulation of the knee coupled with external rotation, while LCL damage is normally through varus strains coupled with internal rotation. MCL damage usually gives pain over the medial epicondyle of the femur, the middle third of the joint line, or the tibial insertion of the ligament. With LCL damage, pain is normally over the head of the fibula or lateral femoral epicondyle.

Palpation of the medial aspect of the knee is made easier by dividing the area into thirds (Fig. 11.13). The anterior third comprises the edge of the patellar tendon and extensor retinaculum and the superficial border of the MCL. Inferior and medial to the tibial tubercle are the insertions of semi-tendinosus, sartorius and gracilis (pes anserine structures). The middle third comprises the MCL and the coronary ligaments. The posterior third comprises the deep part of the MCL and the diverse expansion from the semi-membranosus. Palpation of the lateral aspect of the knee may be similarly divided into thirds (Fig. 11.14). The anterior third consists of the lateral edge of the patellar tendon and the lateral retinaculum. The middle third is dominated by the ITB and the posterior third consists of the fibular collateral ligament, the tendon of biceps femoris, the lateral head of gastrocnemius and popliteus.

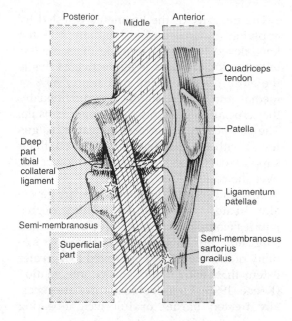

Figure 11.13   Palpation of medial knee structures.

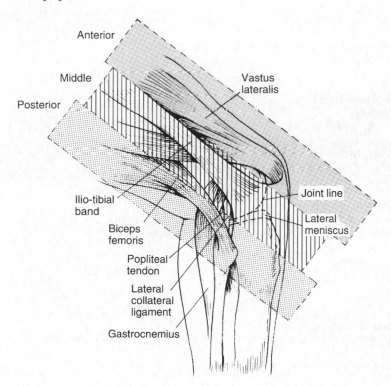

Figure 11.14   Palpation of lateral knee structures. Adapted from Reid (1992).

The integrity of the ligaments is tested by applying a varus and valgus stress to the knee flexed to 30°. Performing the same test with the knee locked is ineffective as this is the close pack position, and nearly 50% of medial and lateral stability is provided by the cruciate ligaments and joint capsule. The easiest way to perform the varus/valgus test is with the patient's hip abducted, thigh supported on the couch and the lower leg over the couch side.

First and second degree injuries are generally treated conservatively. Third degree injuries (complete rupture) have been treated surgically, but some authors argue that stability of the knee is not improved to a greater extent than with non-operative intervention (Keene, 1990). First degree injuries are generally treated partial or full weight-bearing with the ligament supported by strapping. Second and third degree injuries are managed non-weight-bearing.

Initially, the aim is pain relief, swelling reduction and the start of mobile scar formation. Isometric quadriceps drill is begun and modalities used to reduce pain and swelling (Table 11.2). At night a knee brace may be used to protect the ligament. By the third or fourth day after injury (sometimes earlier with a first degree and later with a third degree injury) gentle mobility exercises are begun either in a side-lying starting position or in the pool. Gentle transverse frictions are used to encourage mobile scar formation. The sweep should be quite broad and a large section of the ligament treated. Free, or light resisted exercises are begun to the knee, hip and calf musculature within the

Table 11.2   Guidelines for medial collateral ligament rehabilitation

Phase one (0–7 days)
Immediate post-injury care
   RICE protocol
   Knee immobilizer (grade II/III injuries) or knee sleeve (grade I injury)
   Modalities to reduce pain and inflammation

2–7 days
   Active knee mobility exercises within pain-free range
   Progress to static cycle (high saddle)
   Deep transverse frictions at multiple joint angles
   Avoid valgus stress
   Begin hip adductor strengthening with resistance above knee
   Begin quadriceps and hamstring strengthening, open and closed chain

Phase 2 (7–14 days)
   Increase resistance on open chain isotonic exercise
   Progress closed chain exercise to 1/4 squat (partial weight-bearing if still painful)
   Increase range motion using active assisted and automobilization exercises
   Begin proprioceptive work

Phase three (14 days onwards*)
   Progress all strength exercise
   Obtain final degrees of motion range
   Progress proprioceptive work
   Introduce acceleration/deceleration work
   Multi-direction agility skills (sports specific), e.g. zig-zag run, shuttle run, plyometric exercises

(Use aerobic/upper limb activities throughout programme)

*Criterion for progression to phase three: no joint effusion; minimal pain to direct ligament palpation; full or near full painless range of motion; knee stable to hop/hop and turn tests. After Reid (1992).

pain-free range. Isokinetics may be used, with the aim of restoring the HQ ratio to that of the uninjured limb.

When 90° of pain-free movement is obtained (usually 10–14 days after injury with a grade three sprain) the rehabilitation programme can be progressed further to include more vigorous activities, and increased mobility and strength training. An exercise cycle or light jogging may be used, and swimming (not breast stroke) started. Weight training is progressed to use leg machines, and some power training is added. Towards the end of this period, depending on pain levels, shallow jumping, bench stepping, circle running, and zig-zagging in the gym are used to gradually introduce rotation, shear, and valgus stress to the knee. In addition to improving strength and power, these exercises build confidence and provide an assessment of knee stability.

Occasionally, anteroposterior X-ray will show a bony plaque under the femoral attachment of the MCL (Pellegrini–Stieda disease). The attachment of the adductor magnus onto the adductor tubercle may also be partially avulsed. The condition is normally due to ossification of the haematoma formed at the time of injury (Apley and Solomon, 1993), although infrequently it may occur in the absence of apparent trauma. The condition is normally painless, but where it is a source of pain, surgical removal is required.

Cruciate ligaments

The cruciate ligaments are strong rounded cords within the knee joint capsule, but outside its synovial cavity. The ligament fibres are 90% collagen and 10% elastic, arranged in two types of fasciculi. The first group travels directly between the femur and tibia as would be expected, but the second set spiral around the length of the ligament. This structure enables the ligament to increase its resistance to tension when loaded. Under light loads only a few of the fasciculi are under tension, but as the load increases, the spiral fibres unwind bringing more fasciculi into play and effectively increasing the ligament strength.

The anterior cruciate ligament (ACL) is attached from the tibia, anterior to the tibial spine. Here, it blends with the anterior horn of the lateral meniscus and passes beneath the transverse ligament. Its direction is posterior, lateral and proximal to attach to the posterior part of the medial surface of the lateral femoral condyle. As it travels from the tibia to the femur, the ligament twists in a medial spiral. The posterolateral part of the ACL is taut in extension and the anteromedial portion is lax. In flexion, all of the fibres except the anteromedial portion are lax.

The posterior cruciate ligament (PCL) arises from the posterior intercondylar area of the tibia and travels anteriorly, medially, and proximally passing medial to the ACL to insert into the anterior portion of the lateral surface of the medial femoral condyle. The majority of the PCL fibres are taut in flexion, with only the posterior portion being lax, and in extension the posterior fibres are tight but the rest of the ligament is lax.

The ACL provides 86% of the resistance to anterior displacement and 30% to medial displacement, while the PCL provides 94% of the restraint to posterior displacement and 36% to lateral stresses (Palastanga, Field and Soames, 1989).

Of the two ligaments the ACL is far more commonly injured in sport, with over 70% of knee injuries with acute haemarthrosis involving ACL damage (Noyes, Bassett and Grood, 1980). The athlete has often participated in either a running/jumping activity or skiing. The history is usually of a non-contact movement such as rapid deceleration, a 'cutting' action in football, or a twisting fall. The combination is frequently one of rotation and abduction, a similar action to that which causes MCL or medial meniscus damage, and the three injuries often coalesce to form an 'unhappy triad'.

Most ligament tests assess instability in only one plane (see below), but various combinations of instability exist in two or more planes (Fig. 11.15). The two most common instabilities are anteromedial, in which the medial tibial plateau moves anteriorly on the femur, and anterolateral, where the lateral tibial plateau moves anteriorly. Movement of the lateral tibial plateau posteriorly (posterolateral instability) or the medial tibial plateau posteriorly (posteromedial instability) may also occur. In addition, combined instabilities are seen in cases of severe trauma.

Following injury, swelling is usually immediate as a result of haemarthrosis, leaving a hot, tense, inflamed knee within one or two hours after injury. This contrasts with simple effusion which may take many hours to form (normally overnight). In addition, the athlete often describes 'something going', 'popping' or 'ripping' inside the knee as it gave way. Rapid swelling, a feeling

of internal tearing and giving way are essential elements of the history of injury with this condition. The classic anterior draw test is often negative at this stage due to hamstring muscle spasm and effusion. The high strain rates encountered in sports situations cause the majority of injuries to occur to the ligament substance rather than the osseous junction and so X-ray is usually unrevealing.

Diagnosis relies heavily on clinical history and tests for instability, the latter being the subject of some debate. The two most common tests are the anterior drawer test and modifications of this, and the pivot shift.

The classic anterior drawer test (Fig. 11.16) involves flexing the patient's knee to 90° and stabilizing the foot with the examiner's body weight. The proximal tibia is pulled anteriorly and the amount of movement compared to the 'normal' value of the uninjured leg. Various grades of movement may be assessed, grade one being up to 5 mm of anterior glide, grade two, 5–10 mm and grade three over 30 mm. The test can, however, give false negatives if haemarthrosis prevents the knee being flexed to 90°. Movement can also be limited by protective hamstring spasm or if the posterior horn of the medial meniscus wedges against the medial femoral condyle.

The Lachman test, a modification of the anterior draw, has been shown to be highly reliable (Donaldson, Warren and

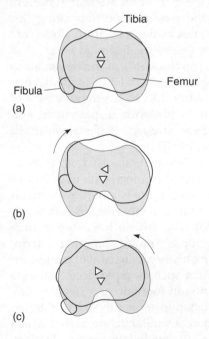

(a)

(b)

(c)

Figure 11.15 Combined instabilities of the knee.
(a) Normal alignment. (b) Antero-lateral instability.
(c) Antero-medial instability.

Figure 11.16 Anterior draw test.

Wickiewicz, 1985). The test is performed with the patient lying supine. The examiner holds the patient's knee in 20° flexion, minimizing the effect of hamstring spasm and reducing the likelihood of meniscal wedging. The reduced angle of flexion compared with the anterior draw test is less painful for the patient, and comfort can be further enhanced by placing the knee over a pillow. One hand stabilizes the femur and the other applies an anterior shearing force to the proximal tibia, avoiding medial rotation (Fig. 11.17a). Clinically, the test may be modified in a number of ways to avoid holding the weight of the whole leg. The therapist may place his

Figure 11.17 The Lachman test and modifications. (a) Standard test. (b) Patient's leg supported over therapist's knee. (c) Patient's leg over couch end and supported by a strap.

or her flexed knee on the couch and rest the patient's leg over it (Fig. 11.17b). Alternatively the patient's femur may be supported on the couch with the tibia over the couch end. The femur is stabilized with a strap, leaving both of the therapist's hands free to shift the tibia (Fig. 11.17c). If anterior translation of the tibia is felt, the test is positive. The movement is compared to the uninjured knee, both for range and end feel, an ACL tear giving a characteristically soft end feel. The same grading system is used as with the anterior draw test.

Another frequently used test is the pivot shift, and its adaptations (Galway, Beaupre and MacIntosh, 1973). These work on the basis that the ACL-deficient knee will allow the lateral tibial plateau to sublux anteriorly. By applying forces to enforce this and then moving the knee, the tibia can be made to reduce rapidly causing a 'thud'. The pivot shift test starts with the affected leg in full extension. The examiner grasps the ankle of this leg with his or her distal hand and the outside of the ipsilateral knee with his or her proximal hand. The ankle and tibia is forced into maximum internal rotation, subluxing the lateral tibial plateau anteriorly. The knee is slowly flexed as the proximal hand applies a valgus stress. If the test is positive, tension in the ITB will reduce the tibia at 30–40° causing a sudden backward 'shift'. The major disadvantage with this test is that the patient must be relaxed throughout the manoeuvre, a situation often not possible because of pain. Donaldson, Warren and Wickiewicz (1985) tested over 100 ACL-deficient knees pre-operatively and found the pivot shift test to be positive in only 35% of cases. The same examination carried out under anaesthesia (muscles completely relaxed) gave 98% positive results.

This test is reversed in the Jerk test (Table 11.3), while the flexion rotation drawer (FRD) test eliminates the need for a valgus force by using gravity to sublux the tibia. A reliability of 62% has been reported for the

Table 11.3   Manual laxity tests of the knee

Anterior draw	Knee flexed to 90°, foot stabilized, tibia drawn forwards
Lachman	Knee flexed to 20°, femur stabilized, tibia drawn forwards
Pivot shift (MacIntosh)	Knee extended, foot/tibia internally rotated, valgus strain on knee as it is flexed
Jerk (reverse pivot shift)	Knee flexed to 90°, valgus stress on knee, internally rotate tibia and extend knee
Flexion/rotation drawer	Leg held by tibia only, knee in 20° flexion posterior force on tibia, then flex knee
Slocum	Patient on uninjured side, pelvis rotated posteriorly. Ankle on couch. Knee flexed to 10°, apply valgus stress and push further into flexion
Losee	Knee flexed to 45°, tibia externally rotated. Knee extended, and valgus force applied, allowing tibia to internally rotate

Adapted from Jensen (1990).

FRD, rising to 89% with the anaesthetized patient (Jensen, 1990). The Slocum test (Slocum, James and Larson, 1976) uses a side-lying position to perform a pivot shift and is particularly suitable for heavier patients.

Since the ACL has two functionally separate portions (see above), depending on the knee angle at the time of injury, only one portion may be damaged resulting in a partial ligament tear. If the anteromedial band is damaged but the posterolateral portion is intact, the Lachman test may be negative, but the anterior draw positive. This is because the anteromedial portion is tightened as the knee flexes, and so will be tighter (and therefore instability will be more apparent) with the 90° knee angle of the anterior draw. Similarly, if the posterolateral band is disrupted (the more usual situation) the anterior draw may be negative but the Lachman positive, as this portion of the ligament becomes tighter as the knee approaches extension.

Partial tears usually remain intact and show good long-term results. However, Noyes et al. (1989) argued that progression to complete deficiency, although unlikely in knees which have sustained injury to one quarter of the ligament, may be expected in 50% of knees with half ligament tears and 86% of those with three-quarter tears.

Arthrometer testing

An arthrometer measures joint motion. The most commonly reported arthometer in the literature, for assessing knee joint motion, is the KT-1000 (Med Metrics Corp. Inc., San Diego, California, USA). To perform anteroposterior testing, patients are placed in the Lachman test position (see above) with the knee flexed to 30°. In this position the patella is engaged in the trochlea, so that it does not move during assessment of tibial movement relative to the femur. The arthrometer unit is placed on the anterior tibia and held in place with velcro straps around the calf. Leg rotation is avoided by supporting the heel in a shallow rubber cup on the couch.

The arthrometer handle applies a force to the tibia usually of 67 N (15 lb) and 89 N (20 lb). The difference in anterior displacement between the two forces is called the 'compliance index' and is a frequently quoted measure of knee joint stability. Alternatively, maximal manual force may be used and the injured and non-injured legs compared (side-to-side measurement). Tibial translation (to the nearest 0.5 mm) is measured by the change in relative alignment of pads placed on the tibial tuberosity and patella. However, the translation values seen with arthrometry do not represent actual bony motion specifically. When arthrometer readings are compared with stress radiographs, different values are obtained (Staubli and Jakob, 1991), suggesting than an amount of tissue compression is occurring.

Arthrometer measurement has been found to be consistently accurate. Using maximal manual testing and side-to-side measurement, 90% of conscious and 100% of anaesthetized patients with acute ACL tears had measurements greater than 3 mm (Daniel et al., 1985). Using 141 uninjured subjects, Bach et al. (1990) showed 99% to have side-to-side measurements less than 3 mm using a force of 89 N.

A number of factors can influence measurement consistency and accuracy. First, muscle relaxation must be obtained. Comparing conscious and anaesthetized patients at force values of 67 N and 136 N, Highgenboten, Jackson and Meske (1989) found side-to-side differences greater than 2 mm in 64% and 81% in conscious patients, but 72% and 83% in anaesthetized patients, respectively. Greater muscle relaxation can be obtained as patients become familiar with the testing procedure, and repeated measurements have certainly been shown to be more effective than isolated tests (Wroble et al., 1990). In addition, arthrometer measurement has been found to be operator dependent (Forster and Warren-Smith, 1989). Consistently accurate results will only be obtained with trained testors who have gained significant expertise. Larger testing forces tend to produce better reproducibility, with maximal manual testing giving the most accurate results with all instruments (Torzilli, 1991; Anderson et al., 1992).

Management

First and second degree injuries may be immobilized initially and then subjected to intense rehabilitation to re-strengthen the supporting knee musculature. A de-rotation brace may be used to protect the knee until muscle strength is sufficient. Third degree injuries, with marked instability, may be treated surgically, although some authors argue that rehabilitation alone is the better solution (Garrick and Webb, 1990).

General guidelines of indications for surgery include combined injuries (ACL, MCL and/or meniscus), and high degrees of anterior shear (Feagin et al., 1995). Isolated injuries treated conservatively seem to remain functional. Jackson et al. (1980) reported a retrospective study with a mean follow-up of ten years. Of those patients treated non-operatively, 80% of isolated ACL injuries had no functional deficit, compared to only 10% of those with combined injuries. In a later study (Jackson, Peters and Marczyk, 1994), 90% of those with isolated injuries who were treated non-operatively reported that they were satisfied with the result compared to 60% for those with combined injuries.

Patients treated non-operatively are often presumed to be at risk of developing meniscal injury and joint degeneration (Kannus and Jarvinen, 1989). However, X-ray examination and bone scan of patients treated both operatively and non-operatively has shown an increased incidence of degenerative joint disease in the surgically treated group. However, the explanation for this finding is the subject of debate (Woo et al., 1994).

Surgery involves repair and reconstruction, most authors agreeing that the later is more appropriate. Reconstruction techniques may be either extracapsular, intracapsular, or a combination of the two.

Extracapsular reconstruction has been described using the MacIntosh procedure (Wilson, Lewis and Scranton, 1990). A 10 × 1 cm strip of the ITB is passed beneath the fibular collateral ligament, under the lateral attachment of the gastrocnemius and then looped back on itself. The knee is flexed to 60° and the leg externally rotated before the ITB is pulled tight and secured with sutures.

Alternatively, a graft may be cut from the middle third of the patellar tendon, to include both non-articular patellar and tibial tubercle bone. This has the advantage that it leaves other structures around the knee intact. Tunnels are then drilled in the tibia and femur travelling through the attachments of the ACL. The graft is passed through the bone tunnel and attached to the lateral aspect of the lateral femoral condyle and the tibial tubercle. The graft is secured with cancellous screws and sutures. This procedure gives a very strong graft, but may have the complication of patellar pain following surgery. Flexion contraction of 5° or more may be present in almost one quarter of these patients (Sachs et al., 1989), and PF irritability can result. Where contracture is a likelihood, rehabilitation should place a greater emphasis on maintaining full knee extension. A similar technique has been described by Wilson and co-workers (1990) using the semi-tendinosus tendon instead of the patellar tendon, to avoid patellar complications.

Several structures may be used for grafts, and Noyes, Butler and Grood (1984) showed the patellar tendon graft to have a strength of 168% of the ACL while the semi-tendinosus had only 70%, gracilis 49% and the quadriceps/patellar retinaculum only 21%. Synthetic tissues, such as polytetrafluoroethylene (PTFE), are now used more frequently, and mobility may be attained more rapidly following surgery using these materials. However, synthetics are generally only used where intra-articular reconstructions have failed. Bovine substances have been used, but problems have been caused by reactive synovitis following these operations. Allogenic tendon grafts from cadavers and amputation specimens have been used to good effect with patients suffering chronic ACL insufficiency (Shino et al., 1986).

Guidelines for rehabilitation following ACL reconstruction

Rehabilitation will depend very much on the particular surgical procedure which has been performed. As synthetic grafts do not need to re-develop a blood supply, they can be rehabilitated more quickly than autogenous grafts. Intra-articular repairs weaken with revascularization, so the repairing ligament will reach only 25–50% of its ultimate strength by 6–12 weeks following surgery. In contrast, extra-articular grafts regain approximately 75% of their original strength in the same time (Reid, 1992). Tendon grafts often suffer less complications and the patello-femoral joint remains mobile, while extracapsular grafts require more restraint on movement. Patellar tendon reconstructions tend to the strongest grafts but cause greater morbidity due to the anterior surgical approach (Briggs, Sandor and Kenihan, 1995). Arthroscopic repairs will recover more quickly than open repairs as the knee joint is less affected. There is less swelling and a reduced likelihood of complications.

The dichotomy is that immobilization is thought desirable for healing of the graft, but early mobility is required to avoid cartilage degeneration, soft tissue contracture and muscle atrophy. To overcome the combined problem of healing and mobility, the patient is mobilized early, providing the movement used does not overly stress the graft.

The range of motion possible, without placing undue tension on the graft, must be established, and a protective brace may be used to limit undesirable movements. Sandberg, Nilsson and Westlin (1987) showed the time needed to return to sport to be five weeks shorter and range of motion significantly better following the use of a hinged cast allowing knee flexion from 20° to 70°. Noyes, Mangine and Barber (1987) mobilized patients on the second day after surgery and found no adverse effects on the ligament reconstruction. Some authors even begin weight bearing immediately (Shelbourne and Nitz, 1990).

Early rehabilitation (up to 4 days following surgery) focuses on avoiding the standard complications following general surgery, and reducing pain (Table 11.4). Simultaneous contraction of the hamstrings and

Table 11.4   Guidelines for ACL rehabilitation After Reid (1992).

Initial stage (0–4 days)
Modalities to reduce pain/inflammation, and facilitate healing
Co-contractions of quadriceps and hamstrings
Prone leg hanging
Patellar mobilizations

Intermediate stage (5–14 days)
Standing single-leg bracing (partial weight-bearing)
Add trunk flexion to above to increase hamstring work
Wall and floor heel slide (ROM)
Shuttle exercise on smooth floor or gym bench
Upper body work for cardiopulmonary fitness
Ensure terminal extension gained
Proprioceptive work (static joint repositioning)
Proprioceptive work (joint stability)
— single-leg standing
— single-leg stand on trampette
Passive (auto-assisted) flexion work

Late stage (15 days–6 weeks)
Static cycle and step machine (holding hand rail)
Leg press
1/4 squat (partial weight-bearing initially)
Restore muscle balance (Q/H ratio)
Proprioceptive work (joint stability)
— uneven surface walking
— balance board
— single-leg standing on trampette, simultaneous arm and contralateral leg actions
— slide trainer
Hop and hold exercises
Speed walking, flat, incline, uneven (not decline)
Step up (not down)
Side step, backward walk, grapevine speed walk
Flexion mobility exercises

Late stage (6–12 weeks)
Speed walk on varying terrain
Progress weight training
Jogging
— flat ground
— figure of eight
— shuttle run
— zig-zag (slow)
— cutting (slow)
— backward running
Box jump (up, not down)
Controlled hopping
Stair running (up, not down)
Controlled single hop down (50 cm box) progressing to repetitions
As above with twist
As above with eyes closed
Progress to full range flexion

Pre-competition testing
Run and sudden stop
Sudden directional change
Downhill running
Descending stairs (fast walk)
Repeated jump down from low (50 cm) box
Sports-specific skills, e.g. dribbling, tackling

quadriceps are used to aid the leg muscle pump, but isolated quadriceps exercises and straight leg raising is avoided. Isolated quadriceps bracing has been shown to place considerable stress on the ACL whereas isolated hamstring actions actually reduce strain (Renstrom, Arms and Stanwick, 1986). Prone-lying leg hanging (Fig. 11.18a) is a useful exercise for regaining terminal extension while placing minimal stress on the healing tissues. The patient lies prone, with the thigh supported on a folded towel, leaving the anterior knee free. The weight of the tibia presses the knee into extension. Resistance may be supplied by a small weight bag attached to the heel. The patient then performs eccentric hamstring actions, allowing the tibia to lower as far as pain will allow. A wedge may be used below the tibia as a relaxation stop.

From 5 to 14 days following surgery co-contraction activities of the quadriceps and hamstrings are performed by using simple closed chain actions. Co-contraction of the hamstrings and quadriceps has been shown to place 15% of the quadriceps tension on the ACL at 5° knee flexion. By the time flexion had increased to a mean angle of 7.4° this force is reduced to zero. As the angle of flexion increases still further a pos-terior draw force is imposed (Yasuda and Sasaki, 1987).

Closed chain terminal leg extension is a useful exercise for co-contraction of the quadriceps and hamstrings (Fig. 11.18b). The athlete stands predominantly on the unaffected leg, placing sufficient weight on the injured leg to prevent the foot from moving. An elastic resistance band attached to a wallbar is placed around the mid thigh, and the action is to extend the hip and knee simultaneously. Adding trunk flexion (Fig. 11.18c) has been shown to increase hamstring activity on surface EMG (Ohkoshi et al., 1991).

The heel slide against a wall or on the floor is useful at this stage (Fig. 11.19a). This exercise may be progressed by performing it against isometric resistance using a large diameter swiss ball or isotonic resistance against rubber tubing. Shuttle exercises may be used on a sliding platform or low friction surface. A declined bench is useful and a linoleum surface or the 'slide trainer' used in popular exercise classes, both provide suitable low friction surfaces. Static cycles and step machines provide useful closed kinetic chain actions in a partial weight-bearing starting position, and will also improve cardiopulmonary fitness.

(a)   (b)   (c)

Figure 11.18 Stage ACL exeercises. (a) Prone leg hang—to regain terminal extension while working the hamstring muscles. (b) Closed chain co-contraction of quadriceps and hamstrings. (c) Adding trunk flexion increases hamstring muscle work.

Figure 11.19 Closed kinetic chain actions following ACL repair. (a) Floor slide. (b) Slide against resistance tubing. (c) Wall slide. (d) Shuttle. (e) Declined bench. (f) Gym ball pass.

Muscle imbalance and proprioception in the ACL deficient knee

Excessive hypertrophy of the quadriceps relative to the hamstrings will lead to a muscle imbalance which will alter ACL loading (Fig. 11.20). The normal even distribution of pressure on the femoral articular surface seen with balanced musculature has been shown to change to a focused high pressure point in the absence of opposing hamstring co-activation (Barratta et al., 1988).

However, functional return is not related directly to hamstring strength, but rather to reflex contraction (Seto, Orofino and Morrissey, 1988). Co-contraction of the ago-

Figure 11.20 Articular surface pressure distribution with muscle co-activation. A, Focused high pressure point at the anterior articular surface in the absence of opposing hamstring co-activation. B, Low, evenly distributed articular surface pressure with hamstring co-activation. After Baratta et al. (1988).

nist and antagonist muscles of a joint will enhance stability. As the knee extends, the muscle spindles in the hamstrings will be stretched, leading to mild hamstring contraction (Solomonow, Barratta and D'Ambrosia, 1989). In addition, mechanical stress on the ACL has an inhibitory effect on the quadriceps, but will simultaneously excite the hamstrings (Barratta et al., 1988). A reflex arc from the ACL mechanoreceptors may allow dynamic torque regulation during ligament loading, and mechanoreceptor stimulation from muscles and the joint capsule causes hamstring stimulation to stabilize the knee (Reid, 1992).

Both tension and mechanoreceptors are present in the ACL. Failure of the feedback system from these structures can result in a loss of reflex muscular splinting and the increased likelihood of re-injury (Kennedy et al., 1982). Normally there is a minimal, 2%, variation in the threshold to detection of passive movement (TTDPM, see p. 172) between the two knees. With ACL-deficient knees variation values as high as 25% have been found (Kennedy, Alexander and Hayes, 1982). The proprioceptive deficit seems to be increased at near terminal range of motion.

Lephart and Fu (1995) reported longer TTDPM in the involved knee tested at 15° knee flexion, but no significant difference when tested at 45°.

Hamstring contraction of ACL-deficient patients occurs earlier in the gait cycle and is of longer duration (Kalund et al., 1990; Sinkjaer and Arendt-Nielsen, 1991). Clinically, ACL deficient patients have an increased hamstring contraction latency, the time interval between displacement of the tibia and reflex reaction of the hamstrings (Fig. 11.21). ACL-deficient patients have been found to have a mean contraction latency of 90.4 ms compared to the normal uninjured knee with a mean latency of 49.1 ms (Beard et al., 1994).

Quadriceps exercises using short range (from 45° to full extension) should be preceded by isometric hip extension to facilitate hamstring contraction (Seto, Brewster and Lombardo, 1989). Indeed, the use of a standard leg extension regime using a sitting position has been severely criticized (Palmitier et al., 1991). Contraction of the quadriceps from this open chain position places considerable anterior shear on the knee and may stretch the ACL. When performing leg extension on an isokinetic dynamometer, an anti-shear device will greatly reduce shear forces generated with the exercise (Malone, 1986; Timm, 1986). When using weight training, however, closed chain motions such as the squat or leg press movement are more appropriate as they produce co-contraction of the quadriceps and hamstrings to reduce shear.

Proprioceptive exercises for the knee include three components. First, sudden alterations in joint position are employed to retrain reflex stabilization. Secondly, general posture and balance activities are used. Finally, joint positioning skills form the basis of retraining for automatic motor control.

Single-leg standing activities begin the training, progressing from positions with the eyes open to those with eyes closed.

Figure 11.21   Reflex hamstring contraction latency is the time interval between the initial tibial displacement and the first measureable reaction of the hamstrings. A: reflex hamstring contraction latency. B: first recorded displacement of the tibia (accelerometer). C: first reflex reaction of the hamstrings (EMG). Adapted from Beard et al. (1994).

These activities may be performed on an uneven surface (thick mat and then mini trampette) and later in combination with trunk and upper limb movements. Reflex hamstring contraction may be performed in crook sitting (Fig. 11.22a). A towel is placed under the patient's heel, and he or she must hold the towel in place with a sudden downward pressure (hip extension and knee flexion) as the therapist pulls on the towel suddenly. Similar actions may be performed on a low stool (Fig. 11.22b). The patient stands on the affected leg only, with his eyes closed. The therapist produces a very small but sudden displacement of the stool. Partner activities include single leg standing (eyes closed) with a partner suddenly pushing on the patient's shoulders from any direction. Again, the movement, while rapid, is of small amplitude.

Posture and coordination activities include backward walking, zig-zags, crossover drills of varying complexity and figure-of-eight running. Running on uneven surfaces and lateral step-ups are useful as is speed walk-ing and uphill walking. Multi-directional running skills based on the functional tests used for the knee (p. 269) also form part of the rehabilitation at this stage.

Accurate static joint re-positioning uses cognitive skills and is helpful at various stages of rehabilitation. This may be per-formed by passive movement on a one-to-one basis with the therapist, or on a dynam-ometer which shows a display for range of motion. In each case, the patient is encour-aged to re-position the joint exactly in the range that the limb rested in before move-ment began.

A variety of apparatus is useful for pro-prioceptive rehabilitation. Standard rocker boards and wobble boards, used so fre-quently for ankle re-education, are also of use for the knee. The 'slide trainer' (Forza Fitness Equipment, London) or 'fitter' machine (Fitter International, Calgary, Canada) is also helpful.

The early stages of rehabilitation empha-sized hamstring activity to reduce shear forces imposed on the knee. Now, any imbal-

Figure 11.22   Rehabilitation of reflex hamstring contraction. (a) Therapist pulls towel suddenly, athlete must rapidly flex knee to stop movement. (b) Therapist minimally displaces stool suddenly, athlete must maintain balance.

ance between the quadriceps and hamstring muscle groups must be corrected with both concentric and eccentric quadriceps training. Again, the emphasis is on closed chain activity, but limited open chain activity may be introduced. With all activities the shearing stress placed on the knee must be considered (Fig. 11.23), noting that downhill running and resisted isometric quadriceps activity at 20° flexion, for example, produce the greatest ACL elongation (Henning, Lynch and Glick, 1985).

It must be remembered that following knee injury there is a selective atrophy of type I muscle fibres (see p. 145), so endurance ability must be regained to ensure joint stabilization. Patients have been shown to be able to restore quadriceps strength 6 weeks after surgery (on a leg extension bench) but to still have a 20% deficit in endurance capacity (Costill, Fink and Habansky, 1977).

The squat exercise in knee rehabilitation

The squat is a controversial exercise in both rehabilitation and general training. Gen-

erally, the parallel squat (to a point where the femur is horizontal) rather than the full squat (buttock to heel) is recommended (Baechle, 1994), as it is claimed that less stress is placed on the knee using the reduced range of motion. When performing this exercise, less skilled individuals have been shown to produce a large initial drop velocity, to bounce in the low position, and to lean the trunk forwards while pushing the hips back (McLaughlin, Lardner and Dillman, 1979). This trunk angulation increases the leverage forces imposed on the lower back (Norris, 1993). The more skilled individual, by limiting trunk extension, places more stress on the quadriceps and reduces the leverage effect on the lower spine.

The squat has the advantage of being a closed chain activity, but is often said to 'over stretch the knee ligaments' and so is frequently derided. The squat has been shown to work the quadriceps, but significant co-contraction of the hamstrings has been questioned (Gryzlo et al., 1994). Heavy resistance squatting (130–200% body weight) used over a 21-week training period has not been shown to increase knee laxity

Figure 11.23 ACL elongation relative to Lachman test (using an 80 lb pull). After Henning (1988).

(Panariello, Backus and Parker, 1994). Ligament stability was assessed in 32 professional football players using an arthrometer at 30° and 90° flexion after 12 and 21 weeks.

Knee stiffness

Knee stiffness is a common problem following ACL surgery. There are a variety of possible causes including adhesions within the suprapatellar pouch and/or patello-femoral joint, quadriceps contracture and retraction of the alar folds (Reid, 1992). Furthermore, patients have been described with an involvement of the infra-patellar fat pads (p. 284) producing infra-patellar contracture syndrome (Paulos, Rosenberg and Drawbert, 1987).

Initially, stiffness begins with inflammation, immobility and quadriceps weakness. Patients are unable to gain full extension and may complain of excessive pain. Patellar glide is restricted and pain may be located around the patello-femoral joint. Later, fat pad involvement may be noted and the patellar tendon may become rigid. Patellar mobility is virtually eliminated and both active and passive knee motion is severely restricted. Flexion contracture is often present by this time and the patient walks with an apparent 'short leg'.

If progress in regaining knee mobility begins to slow, this must be recognized immediately and acted upon. Intense rehabilitation is the key to preventing development of this condition. Patello-femoral joint mobilization and the restoration of full knee extension is vital.

Posterior cruciate damage

The PCL is the strongest ligament in the knee (Baylis and Rzonca, 1988) and much less frequently damaged in sport than the ACL. When an injury does occur it may be the result of a posteriorly directed force onto a flexed knee (typically a road traffic accident), forced hyperextension, or forced flexion where the athlete falls into a kneeling position pressing the ankle into plantarflexion (Keene, 1990). Unlike ACL injury, the athlete with a damaged PCL can usually continue playing and may only notice minimal swelling, but there is marked pain on the posterior aspect of the knee.

Posterior subluxation of the tibia may be seen from the side if the knee is flexed to 90° (Fig. 11.24). This may be accentuated if the patient contracts their quadriceps against a resistance provided by the examiner. The patient is asked to 'slide the foot down the couch' (Daniel et al., 1988), as the examiner stabilizes the ankle. If not viewed from the side, the subluxation may be missed, and the injury wrongly diagnosed as an ACL tear, the tibia moving forwards to reduce and mimicking an anterior drawer sign.

The posterior shift of the tibia moves the patellar tendon closer to the axis of rotation of the knee, reducing the mechanical advantage of the quadriceps (Fig. 11.25). The change in quadriceps muscle efficiency is reflected in the gait cycle. With the PCL deficient knee, athletes demonstrate quadriceps activity before heel strike, in contrast to normal individuals who show this contraction after heel strike (Reid, 1992).

As with ACL damage, conservative treatment involving intensive muscle strengthening is tried first. Isolated hamstring contractions will cause posterior shear of the tibia on the femur and so should be avoided. In addition, excessive external rotation of the tibia as the knee approaches full extension will stress the repaired tissue. As with ACL rehabilitation, co-contraction exercises should be favoured.

(a)   (b)

Figure 11.25   Alteration in mechanical advantage of the knee following PCL rupture. (a) Normal knee: axis of rotation to patellar tendon distance gives mechanical advantage. (b) PCL deficient knee: tibial shift gives reduced mechanical advantage.

The PCL is contained within a synovial sheath which enhances its ability to heal in continuity (Fowler and Messieh, 1987). Reconstruction may be attempted using a similar patellar tendon graft to that described above. This time, the graft is positioned lateral to the tibial attachment of the PCL and travels through the femur at the junction of the medial condyle and the intercondylar notch.

The knee with isolated PCL insufficiency producing unidirectional instability generally does well when treated conservatively, but, when PCL damage is associated with additional tissue damage which results in multi-directional instability, surgery should be considered (Torg, 1989). In a study investigating the long-term effects of non-operative management of PCL damage, Parolie and Bergfeld (1986) assessed 25 athletes on average 6.2 years after injury. Of these 84% had returned to their previous sport. Importantly, those who were not satisfied with their knee had less than 100% strength compared to the undamaged knee (measured as mean torque on an isokinetic dynamometer at varying angular velocities), and those who were satisfied had strength values greater than 100%. The importance of maintaining superior muscle strength following PCL injuries is therefore clear.

Infra patellar dip

Figure 11.24   Posterior sag with PCL deficient knee.

Of those patients who are symptomatic enough to seek treatment, damage to the medial compartment is more common with chronic injuries, and to the lateral compartment with acute injuries (Geissler and Whipple, 1993). Damage includes meniscal tears and articular cartilage defects.

Functional testing of the cruciate ligament deficient knee

Functional testing may be used to assess stability, pain and confidence in the knee. Tests normally aim to reproduce some key aspect of a sport to enhance specificity. In each case the injured and uninjured sides of the body are compared.

For the crossover test the athlete stands on the affected leg and uses the unaffected leg to step in front and behind the injured one, imparting multi-plane stress on the knee (Fig. 11.26). The test may also be performed with the injured leg on a small stool to increase flexion stress on the knee.

The single-leg hop test measures the distance obtained on the injured side and divides this figure by that obtained for the uninjured side to obtain a 'hop ratio' which

Figure 11.26 Functional testing of the knee. (a) Crossover, (b) crossover on box, (c) zig-zag, (d) figure-of-eight, (e) single leg hop, (f) slope running, (g) ascending and descending stairs.

may be recorded throughout treatment (Reid, 1992). Combining straight hopping with hop-and-turn activities increases and varies the stress imposed on the knee, as does hopping down or up from a low stool.

Figure-of-eight, slalom, and slope/stair running circuits are also useful. The figure-of-eight may be performed with a gradual curve or a sharp one to impose more or less stress on the knee. The knee on the outside of the circle is exposed to a varus stress as the body leans inwards. The slalom or 'zig-zag' run imposes sudden direction changes and shear on the knee. This test is particularly suitable for assessing function in sports which involve 'cutting' actions. Slope/stair running may be performed on an inclined or declined surface, or on a camber. In each case repetitive shearing stress is imposed on the knee.

The menisci

The menisci are fibrocartilage structures which rest on the tibial condyles. They are crescent-shaped when viewed from above,

but triangular in cross-section. Their peripheral border is formed from fibrous tissue and attached to the deep surface of the joint capsule. These same fibres attach the menisci to the tibial surface forming the coronary ligaments. Anteriorly, the two menisci are joined by the transverse ligament, a posterior transverse ligament being present in 20% of the population (Palastanga, Field and Soames, 1989).

The medial meniscus is the larger of the two, semi-circular in shape, and broader posteriorly. Its anterior horn is attached to the front of the intercondylar area of the tibia in front of the ACL. The posterior horn attaches to the posterior intercondylar area between the PCL and the lateral meniscus. It has an attachment to the MCL, and the oblique popliteal ligament coming from semi-membranosus (Fig. 11.27a). The upper part of the meniscus is firmly attached to the MCL, the fibres here forming the medial menisco-femoral ligament (Fig. 11.27b). The lower part, attached to the coronary ligament, is more lax. This has important functional consequences because the medial meniscus is anchored more firmly to the

(a)   (b)

Figure 11.27   Attachments of the medial menisces.

femur than to the tibia. In flexion/extension the femur is thus able to glide on the tibia, while in rotation, the meniscus can slide over the tibial plateau (Evans, 1986).

The lateral meniscus is more circular, and has a uniform breadth. Its two horns are attached close together, the anterior horn blending with the attachment of the ACL. The posterior horn attaches just anterior to the posterior horn of the medial meniscus. The meniscus has a postero-lateral groove which receives the popliteus tendon, and a few fibres from this muscle attach to the meniscus itself. In addition, the tendon of popliteus partially separates the lateral meniscus from the joint capsule, a configuration which makes the lateral meniscus more mobile than its medial counterpart. The posterior part of the lateral meniscus has two ligamentous attachments, the anterior and posterior menisco-femoral ligaments (Fig. 11.28). These divide around the PCL, and in extreme flexion, as the PCL tightens, so do the anterior and posterior menisco-femoral ligaments. The lateral meniscus is thus pulled back and medially.

The menisci receive blood flow from the inferior genicular arteries which supply the perimeniscal plexus (Fig. 11.29). Small pene-

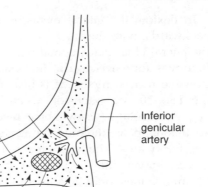

Figure 11.29 Perimeniscal plexus. After Reid (1992).

trating branches from this plexus enter the meniscus via the coronary ligaments. Up until the age of about 11 years, the whole meniscus has a blood supply, but in the adult only 10–25% of the periphery of the meniscus is vascular. The anterior and posterior horns are covered by vascular synovium and have a good blood supply (Arnoczky and Warren, 1983). The peripheral vessels are within the deeper cartilage substance, the surface receiving its main nutrition via diffusion from the synovial fluid. A few myelinated and non-myelinated nerve fibres are found in the outer third of the menisci, but no nerve endings.

Because the menisci are held more firmly centrally, they are able to alter their shape and move forwards and backwards over the tibial plateau. The lateral meniscus has a greater amount of movement, and is often 'pulled away from trouble' leaving the medial meniscus to be more commonly injured in association with the MCL and ACL to which it has attachments.

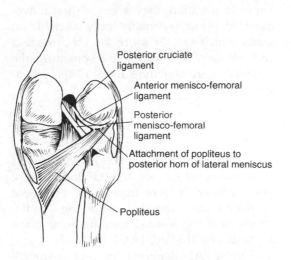

Figure 11.28 Posterior aspect of left knee.

In flexion, the lateral meniscus is carried backwards, onto the steep posterior slope of the lateral tibial plateau, and with extension, it moves forwards again. In flexion/extension the medial meniscus is held firm until the last 20° of extension when the knee begins to rotate (screw home mechanism). As this happens, the medial meniscus is carried backwards. The lateral meniscus has the greater movement, therefore, approximately 11 mm versus only 5 mm for the medial (Reid, 1992). In extension, the menisci are squeezed and elongated in an antero-posterior direction, and in flexion, they become wider (Fig. 11.30).

The menisci enlarge the tibio-femoral contact area, thus spreading the pressure taken by the sub-chondral bone (Fig. 11.31). It has been estimated that the menisci disperse between 30% and 55% of the load across the knee (Kelley, 1990). When only a portion of the meniscus is removed, the joint surface contact forces may increase by 350% (Seedhom and Hargreaves, 1979). The menisci contribute substantially to knee stability. In the ACL deficient knee, the anterior

Figure 11.31   The effect of cartilage removal (meniscectomy) on the knee. (a) Forces on the normal knee. (b) Menisci removed. The bones take more jarring strain.

drawer test may be positive in only 35% of knees with an intact medial meniscus, but in 83% when the meniscus is removed (Levy, Torzilli and Warren, 1982). The menisci limit sagittal gliding of the femur over the tibial plateau, a movement greatly increased in patients who have undergone meniscectomy. In addition, they allow a dual movement to occur, normally only possible in joints which are far more lax. The menisci also aid joint lubrication by spreading the synovial fluid over the surface of the articular cartilage.

Injury

It has been estimated that meniscal injury has a frequency of 61 per 100 000 individuals. The condition is three times more prevalent in males than females, with the medial meniscus being injured four times as often as the lateral (Kelley, 1990).

With ageing, degeneration and asymptomatic tearing occurs. Noble and Hamblen

Figure 11.30   Movement of the menisci with flexion and extension of the knee.

(1975) examined 400 cadaveric menisci and found 29% to have horizontal cleavage tears, and 60% to have a significant meniscal lesion of some sort.

In the active athlete, the history of injury is usually one which combines twisting on a semi-flexed knee with the foot fixed on the ground. The onset is sudden, and pain is felt deep within the knee, the patient often saying they 'felt something go'. Effusion may be extensive after injury, and haemarthrosis may result if the injury occurs in combination with ACL or MCL damage. Tears may be to the periphery or body of the meniscus, running horizontally or vertically (Fig. 11.32). A longitudinal tear (bucket handle) of the medial meniscus may allow its lateral portion to slip over the dome of the medial femoral condyle causing blocked extension (true

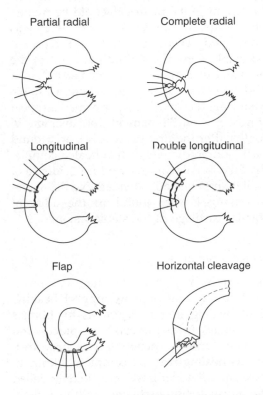

Figure 11.32 Common meniscal tears. The longitudinal tear may extend anteriorly to form a bucket handle tear. From Zuluaga et al. (1995).

locking). Shakespeare and Rigby (1983) reviewed 272 patients found to have bucket handle tears at operation. Of these, 43% presented with true locking. When the knee unlocks, either spontaneously or through manipulation, anterior extension of the bucket handle tear, rather than meniscal relocation, may occur (Reid, 1992).

On examination effusion is apparent and tenderness is often found over the joint line, most usually medially. A capsular pattern may be noticeable (Table 2.3, p. 50), and terminal extension is often blocked with a springy end feel if muscle spasm is not present. Various tests are used to assess the problem, of which the two most common are McMurray's and Apley's.

McMurray's test (Fig. 11.33a) requires full flexion of the knee and so is not suitable for the acute joint. The medial joint line is palpated and from the fully flexed position the knee is externally rotated and extended, as a slight varus strain is applied. If positive, a painful click or thud is felt over the medial meniscus. The lateral meniscus can be similarly tested by extending the knee with internal rotation and a valgus strain, although the value of lateral testing in this way is questionable (see below). In each case only the middle and posterior portion of the meniscus is tested, and so a negative McMurray's sign does not preclude meniscal damage, but when positive the test is clinically revealing.

The McMurray's test has been shown to be useful only with medial meniscal tears (Evans, Bell and Frank, 1993). In this evaluation the authors found that a thud elicited on the medial joint line was the only significant sign to correlate with meniscal injury. They showed the test to have a positive predictive value of 83% and a specificity of 98%.

Apley's grinding test (Fig. 11.33b) involves placing the patient in a prone-lying position, flexing the knee to 90°, rotating the tibia and compressing it against the femur in an attempt to elicit a popping or snapping sensation. It is important not to force the movements too far, as this may further tear the

Figure 11.33 (a) Apley grinding test. (b) McMurray's test.

already damaged meniscus (Garrick and Webb, 1990). The intention with this test is to help differentiate between meniscal and MCL damage at the joint line. Symptoms will be present as the knee is compressed when the meniscus is damaged, but not if the MCL alone is injured, because this structure will be relaxed by the compression force (Apley and Solomon, 1989). Conversely, a

distraction force stretches the ligament but disengages the meniscus, so giving pain where MCL damage has occurred in isolation.

The results of meniscal tests combined with the clinical history will indicate if damage is likely, in which case arthroscopy is called for to confirm the findings.

Management

If a meniscal tear is present, the choice is either non-operative management or surgical intervention involving removal or repair of the injured meniscus.

Non-operative management

Henning (1988) argued that meniscal tears of less than 10 mm in length, and partial thickness injuries involving 50% or less of the vertical height of the meniscus could be treated non-operatively, providing the ACL was undamaged. Weiss et al. (1989) reported that stable vertical longitudinal tears in the vascular outer area of the meniscus had a good potential for healing, where as stable radial tears did not. They performed a repeat arthroscopy on 32 patients (on average 26 months after the first procedure), and found that 17 longitudinal tears had healed completely. Five radial tears showed no evidence of healing and one had extended. No degenerative changes were found in the adjacent articular cartilage of the stable lesions.

Meniscal repair

The peripheral part of the meniscus has a blood supply sufficient to support healing. Initial healing in this region is by fibrosis with vessels from the capillary plexus and synovial fringe penetrating the area. Fibrous healing may be complete within 10 weeks, and the scar tissue can be remodelled into normal fibrocartilage within several months (Hammesfahr, 1989). The mid-portion of the meniscus is avascular and has been traditionally thought not to heal. However, Arnoczky and Warren (1983) demonstrated healing in canine tissue by cutting an access channel from the peripheral region to the mid-point of the meniscus. The peripheral vessels proliferated through the channel into the lesion giving fibrovascular scarring throughout both areas.

The peripheral tear may be sutured, and healing improved by abrading the parameniscal synovium. Henning (1988) argued that healing may be further enhanced by injecting an exogenous blood clot into the injury site. Results are good when repair is limited to the vascular area of the meniscus and to vertical tears (Ryu and Dunbar, 1988). Weight-bearing or full range motion will deform the menisci and so pull on the scar site. For this reason rehabilitation of the repaired meniscus is much less intense than that of a patient who has undergone meniscectomy. General recommendations for rehabilitation (DeHaven and Bronstein, 1995) include the restriction of weight-bearing for 6 weeks, with no flexion allowed for the first 2 weeks. After 2 weeks, 20–70° flexion is allowed, with free motion allowed 4 weeks after surgery. Full weight-bearing is allowed, and resistance exercises are progressed. Return to full sports is not permitted for 6 weeks.

For successful repair, DeHaven and Bronstein (1995) produced a number of recommendations. First, that the tear should lie within 3 mm of the menisco-synovial junction and that the overall contour of the meniscus should be normal. In addition, these authors stated that the tear should be at least 7 mm long and making the meniscus unstable. For tears further than 4 mm from the menisco-synovial junction and those with deformity, healing enhancement using fibrin clot was recommended.

DeHaven, Black and Griffiths (1989) reported follow-up results on 80 repaired menisci on average 4.6 years after surgery. Of these, 11% had torn again (only three at the repair zone), and these authors recom-

mended meniscal repair in view of the degenerative changes following meniscectomy.

Meniscectomy

The preceding descriptions of non-operative management and meniscal repair make it apparent that meniscectomy is not the first choice in many cases of meniscal tearing.

Degenerative changes which have been described after total meniscectomy include joint narrowing, ridging and flattening (Fairbank, 1948). Follow up after meniscectomy (Jorgensen et al., 1987) has shown patients to be increasingly dissatisfied with the knee. Incidence of complaint grew from 53% after 4.5 years to 67% after 14.5 years. A positive anterior draw sign was demonstrated in 10% after 4.5 years and 36% after 14.5 years with 34% of the latter group giving up sport as a result of knee symptoms (Table 11.5).

Where the meniscus is grossly damaged, and the knee is unstable, however, a partial or total meniscectomy may be required. The minimum amount of tissue should be removed to reduce the biomechanical impairment to the joint.

The traditional method for meniscectomy (O'Donoghue, 1976) is with the patient supine, knee flexed to 90° over the table end. For a medial meniscectomy a straight incision is often used, starting proximal to the lower pole of the patella and medial to the patellar tendon, and stretching parallel to the tendon. The retinaculum is split and the joint washed out (lavaged) with warm saline to remove any blood. The whole cartilage may be visible if the knee can be sprung open medially, but usually only palpation with forceps is possible. The bony attachment of the meniscus is dissected and the meniscus itself removed.

Arthroscopic removal of all, or part, of the meniscus is commonplace nowadays. An antero-lateral or antero-medial approach may be taken depending in which compartment of the knee the lesion lies. The knee is

Table 11.5 Follow-up after complete meniscectomy

	4.5 years (n = 131) %	14.5 years (n = 101) %
Symptoms		
Swelling	19	29
Pain		
Weight-bearing	38	30
On stairs	15	23
When first walking	–	23
At rest	12	13
Sensation of instability	20	21
Signs		
Crepitus	18	38
Quadriceps wasting	7	12
Positive anterior drawer	10	36
Joint line tenderness	10	12
Activity		
Unchanged	53	19
Reduced because of knee	12	12
No sport because of knee	15	34

After Jorgensen et al. (1987).

held in 10° flexion and the joint is gapped by applying a valgus or varus stress. The joint is distended with fluid to allow easier inspection of the tissue surfaces. An initial incision is made into the anterior part of the meniscus, and the incision is then extended into the middle and posterior segments. The posterior horn is released, followed by the anterior horn and the meniscus is removed. In cases where only part of the meniscus is removed, the edge of the remaining tissue is trimmed.

Arthroscopy, although commonplace, is not without risk of complication. The Committee on Complications of Arthroscopy of North America (1985) found a 0.8% complication rate in over 100 000 procedures, while Sherman et al. (1986) reported a complication rate of 8.2%. Neurological injury, poor wound healing, instrument breakage, intra-articular infection, knee ligament injury and pulmonary embolism resulting in death have all occurred. The patient's age and the length of time that a tourniquet is used have been found to be the most significant factors in predicting problems (Sherman et al., 1986).

The use of arthroscopy with local anaesthesia is steadily increasing (Ngo et al., 1985; Besser and Stahl, 1986; Buckley, Hood and Macrae, 1989), and obviously removes the risk inherent in any procedure involving a general anaesthetic. The skin puncture sites are injected with lignocaine or similar, and the joint is distended with saline and anaesthetic solution. Arthroscopic surgery of this type allows the patient to be discharged significantly earlier than when general anaesthesia is used.

Following meniscectomy of any type, the initial aim is to limit effusion and pain (Table 11.6). As this is achieved, the leg musculature is progressively built up. Initially, open chain movements are used within the pain-free range, to protect the joint from excessive loading. Range of motion is gradually increased, and as this is achieved, closed chain movements are introduced. Functional activities and power training are used in late

Table 11.6   Guidelines for post-meniscectomy rehabilitation

Initial stage (0–2 weeks)
Quadriceps setting (ensure no extensor lag)
Straight leg raise over block
Standing knee brace (partial weight-bearing)
Ankle exercise
Hip exercise (all ranges)
Begin walking re-education
Active and assisted knee flexion within pain-free range
Cardiopulmonary upper body work
Ensure passive range to patello-femoral joint
Modalities to reduce pain and inflammation

Intermediate stage (2–4 weeks)
Static cycle (high seat)
Aquajogger
General lower limb hydrotherapy
Increasing range of motion for knee
Resisted quadriceps in sitting (open chain)
Leg press to 90° (closed chain)
1/4 squat (partial weight-bearing)
Single (injured) leg standing on rebounder
As above with contralateral leg movements
Bench stepping—up, down, over, introduce slow twist
Ensure full accessory movements present
Modalities to increase circulation and warm tissue
Speed walking/inclined speed walk

Late stage (4–6 weeks)*
Cycling
Increased resistance on weight training
Final range of motion obtained (physiological and accessory)
Increased closed chain work and proprioceptive work
Running—shuttle, zig-zag, stop/start, figure-of-eight, uneven surface
Plyometric progressions—jumping, hopping, increasing height, jump and twist
Full squat (free)
Full leg press (resisted)
Introduce sports-specific skills, e.g. ball dribbling, kicking

Pre-competition testing
Sports-specific skills to repetition
Advanced plyometrics
Endurance work for leg

*Progress to late stage when no/minimal swelling is present and full range motion obtained. After Zuluaga et al. (1995) and Reid (1992).

stage rehabilitation, with sports specific progressions forming the mainstay of pre-competitive work.

Meniscal cysts and discoid meniscus

The discoid meniscus (Fig. 11.34) is more usually seen on the lateral side than the medial. Even so, the condition is unusual. Smillie (1974) reported a total of 467 discoid lateral menisci (and only 7 medial) in 10 000 meniscectomies. In the fetus the meniscus is disc-shaped rather than semi-lunar. When this shape remains later in life, the discoid meniscus is said to be present. Discoid menisci may be classified as complete, incomplete

Figure 11.34   Meniscal abnormalities. (a) Normal, (b) partial discoid, (c) complete discoid, (d) cyst.

(partial) or Wrisberg type (DeHaven and Bronstein, 1995). In the latter type the posterior osseous attachment of the meniscus is absent, leaving it attached only by the menisco-femoral ligament (Wrisberg's ligament).

The abnormal shape of the meniscus subtlety alters both the contact area between the tibia and femur, and joint mobility. In the young, the discoid meniscus may be asymptomatic, with 65% of those who present with symptoms being over 18 years old (Reid, 1992). A clunk may be felt in the knee at 110° as it is bent, and at 10° as it is straightened again (Apley and Solomon, 1993). Surgical treatment may be by meniscectomy, or repair.

Meniscal cysts (ganglia) are again more common in the lateral meniscus, with the posterior and mid-portion of the meniscus being affected. The cyst is associated with a horizontal tear, and may be the result of infiltration of synovial fluid through the tear, with the edge of the tear acting as a one-way valve (Barrie, 1979). In a series of 18 patients with MRI documented cysts, all were found to have horizontal cleavage tears at arthroscopy (Ryu and Ting, 1993).

The cyst generally begins as a small pedicle and gradually enlarges, the size fluctuating with varying activities. It is more easily seen with the knee flexed to 45°. Arthroscopic repair of the tear site is possible, allowing the cyst to decompress into the joint (DeHaven and Bronstein, 1995). Where no tear is identified, removal of the cyst is attempted. The meniscal rim is scarified and the perimeniscal tissue re-attached, leaving the meniscus proper fully intact. Some cysts respond to direct aspiration (Reid, 1992).

Jumper's knee

Jumper's knee is an anterior knee pain affecting the teno-osseous junctions of the quadriceps tendon as it attaches to the superior pole of the patella, and the patellar tendon as it attaches to the inferior pole of the patella and tibial tuberosity. It is, therefore, an insertional tendonopathy resulting in derangement of the bone–tendon unit (Colosimo and Bassett, 1990).

The injury is often described as patellar or quadriceps tendinitis, although these conditions represent an inflammation of the tendon itself rather than isolated damage to the teno-osseous (T/O) junction. In a strict sense the conditions should be considered separately, but they are generally accepted as a single entity. However, it should be remembered that tendinitis does not necessarily mean that the T/O junction is affected, but when the tendon insertion itself is damaged, the tendon will almost always be inflamed.

Jumper's knee occurs more frequently in athletes who regularly impose rapid eccentric loading (traction) on the extensor mechanism of the knee, especially on hard surfaces.

The condition affects the inferior pole of the patella in 80% of cases and is most common at this site in athletes over 40 years of age. The insertion of the quadriceps is more commonly affected in the over 40s, and the tibial tuberosity is the most common sight for jumper's knee in children (David, 1989).

Repetitive stress on the T/O junction causes microtearing over time, and an insidious onset of pain. The condition progresses in a series of stages. Initially, pain is experienced only after intense activity, as a well-localized dull ache without a history of trauma. With time, pain occurs at the onset of activity, and disappears when the athlete is warmed up, only to reappear when sport has finished. Eventually, pain is constant with consequent impairment of performance, and as a final, but rare, scenario the tendon may rupture completely.

On examination, quadriceps wasting is apparent in long-standing cases, and pain occurs to resisted extension with slight soreness to full passive flexion. Some swelling may be noticed around the patellar tendon in acute cases, with fluctuance present if the condition is severe. A non-capsular pattern is found.

Palpation is performed with the knee in full extension to relax the patellar tendon. Palpation to the lower pole of the patella is best performed by pressing with the flat of the hand onto the upper surface of the patella to tilt it. This brings the lower pole into prominence and enables the practitioner to reach the part of the T/O junction which lies on the undersurface of the angular lower pole.

Radiographic changes are usually apparent where symptoms have been present for more than 6 months (Colosimo and Bassett, 1990). An elongation of the involved pole of the patella may be seen with calcification of the affected tendon matrix. Bone scan has indicated increased blood pooling and concentration of radioactive tracer in the inflamed area (Kahn and Wilson, 1987).

Both intrinsic and extrinsic factors have been implicated as possible causes. Intrinsic factors include biomechanical alterations in the extensor mechanism, such as hypermobility, altered Q angle and genu valgum or genu recurvatum. Changes in the HQ ratio and hamstring flexibility may also have a part to play and should be examined. Muscle imbalance, consisting of weakness of the glutei, hamstrings, and abdominals, combined with hip flexor shortening has been noted (Sommer, 1988). In addition, on landing, players who are susceptible to this condition, have a greater tendency to adduct the knee and internally rotate the leg (knock-knee posture).

Extrinsic factors include frequency and intensity of training, training surface and footwear. Ferretti (1986) showed a correlation between jumper's knee and both hardness of playing surface and training frequency. In his study, 37% of players (matched for sport, playing position, and training type) using cement surfaces suffered from the condition, compared to only 5% of those using softer surfaces (Fig. 11.35a). In addition, the percentage number of players affected by the condition escalated as the number of training sessions per week increased. Only 3.2% of those with the condition trained twice each week, whereas

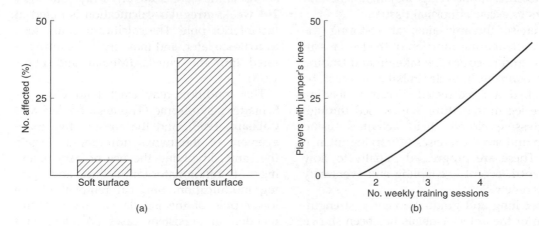

Figure 11.35   Incidence of jumper's knee. Data from Ferretti (1986).

nearly 42% trained four times or over (Fig. 11.35b).

As with any overuse syndrome, part of the management of the condition involves avoidance or modification of training. Athletes should be encouraged to warm-up adequately, and practise flexibility exercises to both the quadriceps and hamstrings. Strength must be developed symmetrically, and footwear should incorporate shock-absorbing materials.

In the early stages of the condition these modifications combined with ice application when pain is acute are usually sufficient. Later, transverse frictional massage is the treatment of choice. Frictions to the T/O junctions attaching to the patella are only effective if the patella is tilted and pressure from the therapist's finger is directed at a 45° angle to the long axis of the femur rather than straight down.

In chronic conditions, where scar tissue has formed at the T/O junctions, limitation in flexion may be apparent. Flexibility exercises will increase the range of movement, but more by stretching the quadriceps than the scar tissue. Where this is the case, a soft tissue manipulation may be required in an attempt to rupture the adherent scarring. If this procedure fails to produce a complete result surgery may be required. Various procedures have been described, some attempting to alter underlying malalignment and others to excise abnormal tissue.

Exercise therapy aims at restoring the shock attenuating function of the leg musculature, and re-educating take-off and landing patterns. Any muscle imbalance must be identified and corrected. Eccentric loading of the leg musculature is increased through progressive closed chain activities, using 'drop and stop' exercises of varying intensities. These are progressed initially to slow concentric-eccentric coupling and eventually to plyometrics.

Stretching and gradual eccentric strengthening of the anterior tibials has been shown to be effective (Reid, 1992). Passive plantar-flexion is performed initially to stretch the musculature. Slow concentric activity is then used as the athlete actively dorsiflexes against manual resistance. Eccentric activity follows as the athlete controls the rate of plantarflexion against therapist resistance. The exact mechanism for the effectiveness of this programme is not known, but both infra-patellar ligament stretching, and quadriceps/foreleg strength ratio changes have been suggested (Reid, 1992).

Sinding–Larsen–Johansson disease

In this condition the secondary ossification centre on the lower border of the patella is affected in adolescents. The epiphysis is tractioned, leading to inflammation and eventual fragmentation. Avascular necrosis is not usually present, but a temporary osteoporosis has been described (Traverso, Baldari and Catalani, 1990) during the adolescent growth spurt. This may weaken the inferior pole of the patella making avulsion more likely.

Sinding–Larsen–Johansson (SLJ) disease can easily be confused with chondromalacia on first inspection as it gives pain to the lower pole of the patella, especially when kneeling. However, on closer examination the differences are soon apparent, and X-ray confirms the bony change. Initially, no abnormalities are seen on X-ray, but after 2–4 weeks irregular calcification is noted at the inferior pole. The calcifications are seen to coalesce later, and may finally be incorporated into the patella (Medlar and Lyne, 1978).

The condition may exist with Osgood–Schlatter's syndrome (Traverso, Baldari and Catalani, 1990), and the conservative management of the two syndromes is largely the same, involving the use of pain relieving/anti-inflammatory modalities, and training modification. Surgical removal of the lower pole of the patella has been recommended in persistent cases (Williams and Sperryn, 1976).

Osgood–Schlatter's syndrome

This condition affects adolescents, especially males. Most often the patient is an active sportsperson who has recently undergone the adolescent growth spurt. With Osgood–Schlatter's syndrome traction is applied to the tibial tubercle, eventually causing the apophysis of the tubercle to separate from the proximal end of the tibia. Initially, fragmentation appears, but with time the fragments coalesce and further ossification leads to an increase in bone. This gives the characteristic prominent tibial 'bump' often noticeable when the knee silhouette is compared to that of the unaffected side.

The infra-patellar tendon shows increased vascularization and, particularly where radiographic changes are not apparent, soft tissue swelling and infra-patellar fat pad involvement is noted. Pain is highly localized to the tibial tubercle and exacerbated by activities such as running, jumping and descending stairs. The condition may coalesce with patellar malalignment faults such as patella infera and patella alta. Patellar tendon avulsion can occur following this condition, and Levi and Coleman (1976) reported 26% of those seen with this type of fracture to have had a previous history of Osgood–Schlatter's disease.

Initial management is by limiting activity. Pain relief and reduction of inflammation may be obtained by using electrotherapy modalities alone or iontophoresis with an anti-inflammatory medication and local anaesthetic (Antich and Brewster, 1985). Injection of the tibial tubercle with hydrocortisone has been described (Grass, 1978). The use of an infra-patellar strap to reduce the pull of the quadriceps onto the tibial tubercle has been used with some success (Levine and Kashyap, 1981).

Assessment of the lower limb musculature often reveals hypertrophy and inflexibility of the quadriceps. When passive knee flexion is tested, intense pain precludes the use of quadriceps stretching. However, when pain has subsided, flexibility of this muscle group must be regained. Where prolonged rest has given rise to muscle atrophy, strengthening exercises are indicated. Ice packs may be used to limit pain or inflammation following activity. Restoration of acceleration/deceleration mechanics in jumping and landing (closed chain) is as for jumper's knee (see above).

Synovial plica

The synovial plica is a remnant of the septum which separates the knee into three chambers until the fourth intrauterine month. Three types of plica are seen. The infra-patellar plica (ligamentum mucosum) lies within the intercondylar notch and runs parallel to the anterior cruciate ligament. The supra-patellar plica is found on the medial aspect of the supra-patellar pouch, lying proximal to the superior pole of the patella. The medio-patellar plica extends from the medial supra-patellar pouch over the medial femoral condyle and onto the synovium covering the infra-patellar fat pad (Fig. 11.36). The

Supra-patellar pouch

Plica

Infra-patellar fat pad

Figure 11.36 The medio-patellar plica. After Reid (1992).

medio-patellar plica is by far the most important in terms of pathology.

A medio-patellar plica may be present in some 20–60% of knees (Amatuzzi, Fazzi and Varella, 1990), but does not necessarily cause symptoms. In a series of 3250 knee disorders, Koshino and Okamoto (1985) found only 32 patients to have the complaint (1%). The structure separates the knee joint into two reservoirs, one above the patella and the other constituting the joint cavity proper. The normal plica is a thin, pink, flexible structure, but when inflamed it becomes thick, fibrosed and swollen, loosing its elasticity and interfering with patello-femoral tracking.

These tissue changes are often initiated by trauma that results in synovitis, and is more common in athletes. Pain is usually intermittent and increases with activity. Discomfort is experienced when descending stairs and may mimic anterior knee pain. However, pain of plical origin normally subsides immediately when the knee is extended. In addition, the 'morning sign' may be present. This is a popping sensation which occurs as the knee is extended, particularly on rising, but disappears throughout the day. The popping may be accompanied by giving way, and is caused by the thickened plica passing over the medial femoral condyle. As the day progresses, joint effusion pushes the plica away from the condyle. This sign may be reproduced with some patients by extending the knee from 90° flexion while internally rotating the tibia and pushing the patella medially. The pop is usually experienced between 45° and 60° flexion.

Conservative treatment has been found to be effective in 60% of cases (Amatuzzi, Fazzi and Varella, 1990) and aims at reducing the compression over the anterior compartment of the knee, by using stretching exercises. The length of the hamstrings, quadriceps and gastocnemius muscles should be assessed, and these muscles stretched if noticeable shortening is found. Where conservative treatment fails, and symptoms limit sport or daily living, surgery may be warranted. Koshino and Okamoto (1985) reported pain and symptom relief in 90% of knees treated surgically by plical resection, but did not quote figures for long-term follow-up.

Tendinitis

Tendinitis around the knee occurs most commonly within the patellar tendon (jumper's knee, see above), the semi-membranosus, and the popliteus.

Semi-membranosus has a complex insertion consisting of five slips onto the proximal tibia (Williams, 1995), making direct palpation of an inflamed area difficult. The five insertions are:

1   into a small tubercle on the posterior aspect of the medial tibial condyle (the tuberculum tendinis)
2   the medial margin of the tibia immediately behind the medial collateral ligament
3   a fibrous expansion to the fascia covering popliteus
4   a cord-like tendon to the inferior lip of the medial tibial condyle below the MCL
5   the oblique popliteal ligament passing upwards and laterally (Fig. 11.37).

Tendinitis of this muscle gives a persistent ache over the posteromedial aspect of the knee. It occurs as the semi-membranosus tendon slides over the medial corner of the medial femoral condyle, and is distinct from semi-membranosus bursitis which affects the area of the medial tibial condyle. Pain may occur within the tendon substance itself, or over the teno-osseous junction, when an insertional tendinitis is present. Increased tracer uptake has been noted on bone scan with this latter condition (Ray, Clancy and Lemon, 1988).

Popliteus tendinitis is related to increased pronation of the STJ and excessive internal rotation of the tibia (Brody, 1980). The

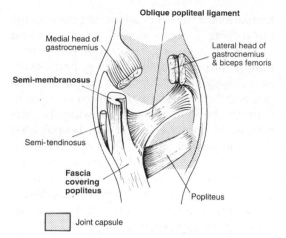

Figure 11.37 Extensive insertion of semi-membranosus.

increased internal rotation causes traction on the popliteus attachment to the lateral femoral condyle. The popliteus acts with the PCL to prevent forward displacement of the femur on the flexed tibia, and so will be overworked with downhill running (Baylis and Rzonca, 1988). On examination, tenderness is revealed over the popliteus just anterior to the fibular collateral ligament. The patient is examined in a supine position with the injured knee in the 'figure of four' posi-tion, that is affected hip flexed, abducted and externally rotated, knee bent to 90° and foot placed on the knee of the contralateral leg. The condition is differentiated from ITB fric-tion syndrome by testing resisted tibial inter-nal rotation with the knee flexed, and palpating the popliteus while internal rota-tion is resisted in extension (Allen and Ray, 1989).

Treatment for tendinitis involves rest, anti-inflammatory modalities, and training modification. Flexibility of the knee muscu-lature and the biomechanics of the lower limb should be assessed and corrected as necessary.

Bursitis

The knee joint has on average 14 bursae (see Table 11.7) in areas where friction is likely to occur, between muscle, tendon, bone and skin. Any of these can become inflamed and give pain when compressed through muscle contraction or direct palpation. Those most commonly injured in sport include the pre-patellar, pes anserine, and semi-membranosus.

Table 11.7 Bursae around the knee

Bursa	Lying between
Subcutaneous pre-patellar	Lower patella/skin
Deep infrapatellar	Upper tibia/patellar ligament
Subcutaneous infrapatellar	Lower tibial tuberosity/skin
Suprapatellar	Lower femur/deep surface of quadriceps (communicates with joint)
No specific name	Lateral head of gastrocnemius/capsule
	Lateral collateral ligament/tendon of biceps femoris
	Lateral collateral ligament/popliteus
	Popliteus tendon/lateral condyle of femur
	Medial head gastrocnemius/capsule
	Medial head of gastrocnemius/semi-membranosus
Pes anserine	Superficial to medial collateral ligament/sartorius, gracilus, semi-tendinosus
No specific name	Deep medial collateral ligament/femur, medial meniscus
Semi-membranosus	Semi-membranosus/medial tibial condyle, gastrocnemius
No specific name	Semi-membranosus/semi-tendinosus

The pre-patellar bursa is usually injured by falling onto the anterior aspect of the knee, or by prolonged kneeling (housemaid's knee). Haemorrhage into the bursa can cause an inflammatory reaction and increased fluid volume. Enlargement is noticeable and the margins of the mass are well defined, differentiating the condition from general knee effusion or subcutaneous haematoma. Knee flexion may be limited, the bursa being compressed as the skin covering the patella tightens.

Septic bursitis may result by secondary infection if the skin over the bursa is broken by laceration or puncture wound. If the condition becomes chronic, the bursa may collapse and the folded walls of the thickened bursal sac appear as small hardened masses on the anterior aspect of the knee. In these cases, erythema and exquisite tenderness is usually present.

Minor cases normally respond to rest and ice, but more marked swelling requires aspiration. Aspiration is carried out under sterile conditions, and a compression bandage applied.

Semi-membranosus bursitis gives rise to pain and swelling over the lower posteromedial aspect of the knee. Pain may be made worse by hamstring or gastrocnemius contraction against resistance, and in activities involving intense action of these muscles, such as sprinting and bounding.

Pes anserine bursitis gives pain and swelling over the metaphyseal area of the tibia, sometimes referred to the medial joint line (Baylis and Rzonca, 1988). The bursa may be injured by direct trauma (hitting the knee on a hurdle) or by overuse of the pes anserine tendons.

With both of the latter causes of bursitis, rest and anti-inflammatory modalities are required. Biomechanical assessment of the lower limb and analysis of the athlete's training regime are called for where there is no history of injury.

One condition often referred to as 'bursitis' is a Baker's cyst. This is actually a posterior herniation of the synovial membrane into the bursa lying between semi-membranosus and the medial head of gastrocnemius. The mass bulges into the popliteal space, and occurs particularly in rheumatoid arthritis. The posterior knee ligaments weaken and fail to support the joint capsule, allowing the herniation to occur. The cyst can be palpated over the medial side of the popliteal space beneath the medial head of gastrocnemius.

When painless, the condition may be managed conservatively, but where the enlargement compromises venous return or causes severe pain, aspiration is called for.

Fat pads

Fat pads consist of fat cells (adipose tissue) packed closely together and separated from other tissues by fibrous septa. They have an abundant blood supply, and are well innervated. Most significant to the knee is the infra-patellar fat pad, lying beneath the patellar tendon, and in front of the femoral condyles. The fat pad is intracapsular but extrasynovial, and a piece of synovial membrane (ligamentum mucosum, see above) may pass from the pad to the intracondylar notch of the femur. When the knee is fully flexed, the infra-patellar fat pad fills the anterior aspect of the intercondylar notch. As the knee extends, the fat pad covers the trochlear surface of the femur within the patellar groove (Hertling and Kessler, 1990).

The usual pathology of the infra-patellar fat pad is an enlargement causing increased pressure with resultant pain (Hoffa's disease). Direct trauma can cause haemorrhage and local oedema, and swelling may also occur as a result of pre-menstrual water retention. Space occupying lesions, such as osteochondrotic fragments, may also cause enlargement, and Smillie (1974) described a case where a displaced bucket handle tear of the medial meniscus was forced into the infra-patellar fat pad of the knee.

Enlargement and entrapment of the patellar fat pad has been described by Finsterbush, Frankl and Mann (1989). The entrapped pad was shown to be in various stages of tissue degeneration, including fat necrosis and replacement of the fatty tissue with fibrinoid material. Complete fibrosis was later seen. Silver and Campbell (1985) described persistent inflammation of the knee fat pads as a cause of delayed recovery in dancers with knee injuries. Surgical removal of the pad resulted in restoration of full range motion at the knee. Tsirbas, Paterson and Keene (1990) described excision of the fat pad tip to relieve patello-femoral pain. Patients presented with a history of pain infero-medial, and sometimes infero-lateral, to the patella. On examination, impingement pain occurred deep to the inferior pole of the patella at 20° flexion with resisted quadriceps contraction.

Relief of mild compression pain may be achieved with taping (McConnell, 1992). Taping begins over the tibial tubercle and extends laterally and medially in a 'V' shape. The tape is placed under traction to lift the patella in a cephalic direction. This effectively forms a sling to prevent the patella pressing into the fat pad (Fig. 11.38).

Skin puckering shows patella lifted

Begin tape over tibial tubercle

Figure 11.38 Fat pad unloading using taping.

References

Allen, M.E. and Ray, G. (1989) Popliteus tendinitis, a new perspective. *Sports Training and Medical Rehabilitation*, **1**, 219–226

Amatuzzi, M.M., Fazzi, A. and Varella, M.H. (1990) Pathologic synovial plica of the knee. *American Journal of Sports Medicine*, **18**(5), 466–469

Anderson, A.F., Snyder, R.B., Federspiel, C.F. and Lipscomb, A.B. (1992) Instrumented evaluation of knee laxity: a comparison of five arthrometers. *American Journal of Sports Medicine*, **20**, 135–140

Antich, T.J. and Brewster, C.E. (1985) Osgood–Schlatter disease: review of literature and physical therapy management. *Journal of Orthopaedic and Sports Physical Therapy*, **7**(1), 5–10

Apley, A.G. and Solomon, L. (1989) *Concise System of Orthopaedics and Fractures*, Butterworth-Heinemann, Oxford

Apley, A.G. and Solomon, L. (1993) *Apley's System of Orthopaedics and Fractures*, 7th edn, Butterworth-Heinemann, Oxford

Arno, S. (1990) The A angle: a quantitative measurement of patella alignment and realignment. *Journal of Orthopaedic and Sports Physical Therapy*, **12**(6), 237–242

Arnoczky, S. and Warren, R. (1983) Microstructure of the human meniscus. *American Journal of Sports Medicine*, **11**(3), 131–140

Bach, B.R., Warren, R.F. and Wickiewicz, T.L. (1990) Arthrometric evaluation of knees that have a torn anterior cruciate ligament. *Journal of Bone and Joint Surgery*, **72A**, 1299

Baechle, T.R. (1994) *Essentials of Strength Training and Conditioning*, Human Kinetics, Champaign, Illinois

Baratta, R., Solomonow, M., Zhou, B.H., Letson, D., Chuinard, R. and D'Ambrosia, R. (1988) Muscular coactivation: the role of the antagonist musculature in maintaining knee stability. *American Journal of Sports Medicine*, **16**, 113–122

Barrie, H.J. (1979) The pathogenesis and significance of meniscal cysts. *Journal of Bone and Joint Surgery*, **61B**, 184

Baylis, W.J. and Rzonca, E.C. (1988) Common sports injuries to the knee. *Clinics in Podiatric Medicine and Surgery*, **5**, 3

Beard, D.J., Kyberd, P.J., O'Connor, J.J., Fergusson, C.M. and Dodd, C.A.F. (1994) Reflex hamstring contraction latency in anterior cruciate ligament deficiency. *Journal of Orthopaedic Research*, **12**(2), 219–227

Beckman, M., Craig, R. and Lehman, R.C. (1989) Rehabilitation of patellofemoral dysfunction in the athlete. *Clinics in Sports Medicine*, **8**(4), 841–860

Bennett, J.G. and Stauber, W.T. (1986) Evaluation of anterior knee pain using eccentric exercise. *Medicine and Science in Sports and Exercise*, **18**, 520

Besser, M.I.B. and Stahl, S. (1986) Arthroscopic surgery performed under local anesthesia as an outpatient procedure. *Archives of Orthopaedic Trauma and Surgery*, **105**, 296–297

Briggs, C., Sandor, S.M. and Kenihan, M.A.R. (1995) The knee. In *Sports Physiotherapy* (ed. M. Zuluaga), Churchill Livingstone, London

Brody, D.M. (1980). Running injuries. *Clinical Symposia*, **32**(4), Ciba Pharmaceutical Company

Buckley, J.R., Hood, G.M. and Macrae, W. (1989) Arthroscopy under local anaesthesia. *Journal of Bone and Joint Surgery*, **71B**, 126–127

Colosimo, A.J. and Bassett, F.H. (1990) Jumper's knee – diagnosis and treatment. *Orthopaedic Review*, **19**, 2

Committee on Complications of Arthroscopy Association of North America (1985) Complications of arthroscopy and arthroscopic surgery: results of a national survey. *Arthroscopy*, **1**, 214–220

Costill, D.L., Fink, W.J. and Habansky, A.J. (1977) Muscle rehabilitation after knee surgery. *Physician and Sports Medine*, **7**, 71

Cox, A.J. (1990) Biomechanics of the patello-femoral joint. *Clinical Biomechanics*, **5**, 123–130

Daniel, D.M., Malcom, L.L. and Losse, G. (1985) Instumented measurement of anterior knee laxity in patients with acute anterior cruciate ligament disruption. *American Journal of Sports Medicine*, **13**, 401

Daniel, D.M., Stone, M.L., Barnett, P. and Sachs, R. (1988) Use of the quadriceps active test to diagnose posterior cruciate ligament disruption and measure posterior laxity of the knee. *Journal of Bone and Joint Surgery*, **70A**, 386–391

David, J.M. (1989) Jumper's knee. *Journal of Orthopaedic and Sports Physical Therapy*, **11**(4), 137–141

de Andrade, J.R., Grant, C. and Dixon, A. (1965) Joint distention and reflex muscle inhibition in the knee. *Journal of Bone and Joint Surgery*, **47A**, 313–322

DeHaven, K.E. and Bronstein, R.D. (1995) Injuries to the menisci of the knee. In *The Lower Extremity and Spine in Sports Medicine*, 2nd edn (eds J.A. Nicholas and E.B. Hershman), C.V. Mosby, St Louis

DeHaven, K.E., Black, K.P. and Griffiths, H.J. (1989) Open meniscus repair: technique and two to nine year results. *American Journal of Sports Medicine*, **17**, 788–795

Donaldson, W.F., Warren, R.F. and Wickiewicz, T. (1985) A comparison of acute anterior cruciate ligament examinations. *American Journal of Sports Medicine*, **13**, 5–10

Evans, P. (1986) *The Knee Joint: A Clinical Guide*, Churchill Livingstone, London

Evans, P.J., Bell, G.D. and Frank, C. (1993) Prospective evaluation of the McMurray test. *American Journal of Sports Medicine*, **21**, 604–608

Exler, Y. (1991) Patella fracture: review of the literature and five case presentations. *Journal of Orthopaedic and Sports Physical Therapy*, **13**, (4) 177–183

Fairbank, T.J. (1948). Knee joint changes after meniscectomy. *Journal of Bone and Joint Surgery*, **30B**(4), 664–670

Feagin, J.A., Levy, A.S., Lintner, S.A. and Zorilla, P.A. (1995) Current concepts in anterior cruciate ligament surgery. *Sports Exercise and Injury*, **1**(4), 176–182

Ferretti, A. (1986) Epidemiology of jumpers knee. *Sports Medicine*, **3**, 289–295

Finsterbush, A., Frankl, U. and Mann, G. (1989) Fat pad adhesion to partially torn anterior cruciate ligament: a cause of knee locking. *American Journal of Sports Medicine*, **17**(1), 62–69

Forster, I.W. and Warren-Smith, C.D. (1989) Is the KT-1000 knee ligament arthrometer reliable? *Journal of Bone and Joint Surgery*, **71B**, 843

Fowler, P.J. and Messieh, S.S. (1987) Isolated posterior cruciate ligament injuries in athletes. *American Journal of Sports Medicine*, **15**, 553–557

Fulkerson, J.P. (1982). Awareness of the retinaculum in evaluating patello-femoral pain. *American Journal of Sports Medicine*, **10**, 147–149

Galway, R.D., Beaupre, A. and MacIntosh, D.L. (1973) Pivot shift: a clinical sign of symptomatic anterior cruciate ligament insufficiency. *Journal of Bone and Joint Surgery*, **54B**, 763

Garrick, J.G. and Webb, D.R. (1990). *Sports Injuries: Diagnosis and Management*, W.B. Saunders, London

Geissler, W.B. and Whipple, T.L. (1993) Intraarticular abnormalities in association with posterior cruciate ligament injuries. *American Journal of Sports Medicine*, **21**, 846–849.

Grass, A.L. (1978) Treatment of Osgood–Schlatter injury. *Journal of the American Medical Association*, **240**, 212–213

Gruber, M.A. (1979) The conservative treatment of chondromalacia patellae. *Orthopedic Clinics of North America*, **10**(1), 105–115.

Gryzlo, S.M., Patek, R.M., Pink, M. and Perry, J. (1994) Electromyographic analysis of knee rehabilitation exercises. *Journal of Orthopaedic and Sports Physical Therapy*, **20**, 36–43

Hammesfahr, R. (1989) Surgery of the knee. In *Orthopaedic Physical Therapy* (eds R. Donatelli and M.J. Wooden), Churchill Livingstone, London

Henning, C.E. (1988) Semilunar cartilage of the knee: function and pathology. *Exercise and Sports Science Review*, **16**, 67–75

Henning, C.E., Lynch, M.A. and Glick, K.R. (1985) An in vivo strain gauge study of elongation of the ACL. *American Journal of Sports Medicine*, **13**, 34–39

Hertling, D. and Kessler, R.M. (1990) *Management of Common Musculoskeletal Disorders*, J.B. Lippincott, Philadelphia.

Highgenboten, C.L., Jackson, A. and Meske, N.B. (1989) Genucom, KT-1000, and Stryker knee laxity measuring device comparisons: device responsibility and interdevice comparison in asymptomatic subjects. *American Journal of Sports Medicine*, **17**, 743

Hoke, B., Howell, D. and Stack, M. (1983) The relationship between isokinetic testing and dynamic patellofemoral compression. *Journal of Orthopaedic and Sports Physical Therapy*, **4**, 150

Insall, J. (1979) Chondromalacia patellae: patellar malalignment syndrome. *Orthopaedic Clinics of North America*, **10**, 117–127

Jackson, R.W., Peters, R.I. and Marczyk, R.I. (1980) Late results of untreated anterior cruciate ligament rupture. *Journal of Bone and Joint Surgery*, **62B**, 127

Jensen, K. (1990) Manual laxity tests for anterior cruciate ligament injuries. *Journal of Orthopaedic and Sports Physical Therapy*, **11**(10), 474–481

Jerosch, J.G., Castro, W.H.M. and Jantea, C. (1989) Stress fracture of the patella. *American Journal of Sports Medicine*, **17**, 4

Jorgensen, U., Sonne-Holm, S. and Lauridsen, E. (1987) Long term follow up of meniscectomy in athletes: a prospective longitudinal study. *Journal of Bone and Joint Surgery*, **69**, 80

Jorgensen, K. and Nicolaisen, T. (1987) Trunk extensor endurance: Determination and relation to low-back trouble. *Ergonomics*, **30** (2), 259–267

Kahn, D. and Wilson, M. (1987) Bone scintigraphic findings in patellar tendinitis. *Journal of Nuclear Medicine*, **28**, 1768–1770

Kalund, S., Sinkjaer, T., Arendt-Nielsen, L. and Simonsen, O. (1990) Altered timing of hamstring muscle action in anterior cruciate ligament deficient patients. *American Journal of Sports Medicine*, **18**, 245–248

Kannus, P. and Jarvinen, M. (1989) Post-traumatic anterior cruciate ligament insufficiency as a cause of osteoarthritis in a knee joint. *Journal of Rheumatology*, **18**, 251–260

Karst, G.M. and Jewett, P.D. (1993) Electromyographic analysis of exercises proposed for differential activation of medial and lateral quadriceps femoris muscle components. *Physical Therapy*, **73**, 286–299

Keene, J.S. (1990) Ligament and muscle tendon unit injuries. In *Orthopaedic and Sports Physical Therapy*, 2nd edn (Ed. J.A. Gould), C.V. Mosby, St Louis, pp. 137–165

Kelley, M.J. (1990) Meniscal trauma (of the knee) and surgical intervention. *Journal of Sports Medicine and Physical Fitness*, **30**(3), 297–306

Kennedy, J.C., Alexander, I.J. and Hayes, K.C. (1982) Nerve supply of the human knee and its functional importance. *American Journal of Sports Medicine*, **10**, 329

Koshino, T. and Okamoto, R. (1985) Resection of painful shelf (Plica synovialis mediopatellaris) under arthroscopy. *Arthroscopy*, **1**, 136–141

Lephart, S.M. and Fu, F.H. (1995) The role of proprioception in the treatment of sports injuries. *Sports Exercise and Injury*, **1**(2), 96–102

Levi, J.H. and Coleman, C.R. (1976) Fractures of the tibial tubercle. *American Journal of Sports Medicine*, **4**, 253–263

Levine, J. and Kashyap, S. (1981). A new conservative treatment of Osgood–Schlatter's disease. *Clinical Orthopaedics and Related Research*, **158**, 126–128

Levy, I.M., Torzilli, P.A. and Warren, R.F. (1982) The effect of medial meniscectomy on anterior-posterior motion of the knee. *Journal of Bone and Joint Surgery*, **64**, 883–888

Lieb, F.J. and Perry, J. (1968) Quadriceps function: An anatomical and mechanical study using amputated limbs. *Journal of Bone and Joint Surgery*, **50A**, 1535–1548

Malone, T. (1986) Clinical use of the Johnson anti-shear device: How and why to use it. *Journal of Orthopaedic and Sports Physical Therapy*, **7**, 304–309

McConnell, J. (1986) The management of chondromalacia patella: a long term solution. *Australian Journal of Physiotherapy*, **31**, 214–223

McConnell, J. (1992) *McConnell Patellofemoral Course*, London

McConnell, J. (1994) *McConnell Patello-femoral Course*, London

McLaughlin, T.M., Lardner, T.J. and Dillman, C.J. (1979) Kinetics of the parallel squat. *Research Quarterly*, **49** (2), 175–189

Medlar, R.C. and Lyne, D. (1978) Sinding-Larsen-Johansson disease: its etiology and natural history. *Journal of Bone and Joint Surgery*, **60A**, 1113

Ngo, I.U., Hamilton, W.G., Wichern, W.A. and Andree, R.A. (1985) Local anesthesia with sedation for arthroscopic surgery of the knee: a report of 100 consecutive cases. *Arthroscopy* **1**, 237–241

Noble, C.A. (1980) Iliotibial band friction syndrome in runners. *American Journal of Sports Medicine*, **9**, 232

Noble, J. and Hamblen, D.L. (1975) The pathology of the degenerate meniscal lesion. *Journal of Bone and Joint Surgery*, **57**, 180

Norkin, C.C. and Levangie, P.K. (1992) *Joint Structure and Function. A Comprehensive Analysis*, 2nd edn, F.A. Davis, Philadelphia

Norris, C.M. (1993) *Weight Training. Principles and Practice*, Black, London

Noyes, F.R., Bassett, R.W. and Grood, E.S. (1980) Arthroscopy in acute traumatic hemarthrosis of the knee. *Journal of Bone and Joint Surgery*, **62A**, 687

Noyes, F.R., Butler, D.L. and Grood, E.S. (1984) Biomechanical analysis of human ligament grafts used in knee ligament repairs and reconstructions. *Journal of Bone and Joint Surgery*, **66A**, 344

Noyes, F.R., Mangine, R.E. and Barber, S. (1987) Early motion after open and arthroscopic anterior cruciate ligament reconstruction. *American Journal of Sports Medicine*, **15**, 149–160

Noyes, F.R., Mooar, L.A., Moorman, C.T. and McGinniss, G.H. (1989) Partial tears of the anterior cruciate ligament: Progression to complete ligament deficiency. *Journal of Bone and Joint Surgery*, **71B**, 825–833

O'Donoghue, D.H. (1976) *Treatment of Injuries to Athletes*, W.B. Saunders, Philadelphia

Ohkoshi, Y., Yasuda, K., Kaneda, K., Wada, T. and Yamanaka, M. (1991) Biomechanical analysis of rehabilitation in the standing position. *American Journal of Sports Medicine*, **19**, 605–611

Palastanga, N., Field, D. and Soames, R. (1989) *Anatomy and Human Movement*, Butterworth-Heinemann, Oxford

Palastanga, N., Field, D. and Soames, R. (1994) *Anatomy and Human Movement*, 2nd edn, Butterworth-Heinemann, Oxford

Palmitier, R.A., An, K., Scott, S.G. and Chao, E.Y.S. (1991) Kinetic chain exercise in knee rehabilitation. *Sports Medicine*, **11**(6), 402–413

Panariello, R.A., Backus, S.I. and Parker, J.W. (1994) The effect of the squat exercise on anterior-posterior knee translation in professional football players. *American Journal of Sports Medicine*, **22**, 768–773

Parolie, J.M. and Bergfeld, J.A. (1986) Long term results of nonoperative treatment of isolated posterior cruciate ligament injuries in the athlete. *American Journal of Sports Medicine*, **14**, 53–58

Paulos, L.E., Rosenberg, T.D. and Drawbert, C.W. (1987) Infrapatellar contraction syndrome: an unrecognised cause of knee stiffness with patellar entrapment and patella infera. *American Journal of Sports Medicine*, **15**, 331

Ray, J.M., Clancy, W.G. and Lemon, R.A. (1988) Semimembranosus tendinitis: an overlooked cause of medial knee pain. *American Journal of Sports Medicine*, **16**, 4

Reid, D.C. (1992) *Sports Injury Assessment and Rehabilitation*, Churchill Livingstone, London

Renstrom, P., Arms, S.W. and Stanwick, R.J. (1986) Strain within the anterior cruciated ligament during hamstring and quadriceps activity. *American Journal of Sports Medicine*, **14**, 83–87

Reynolds, L., Levin, T., Medeiros, J., Adler, N. and Hallum, A. (1983) EMG activity of the vastus medialis oblique and vastus lateralis and their role in patellar alignment. *American Journal of Physical Medicine*, **62**(2), 61–71

Richardson, C. and Bullock, M.I. (1986) Changes in muscle activity during fast, alternating flexion–extension movements of the knee. *Scandinavian Journal of Rehabilitation Medicine*, **18**, 51–58

Rouse, S.J. (1996) The role of the iliotibial tract in patellofemoral pain and iliotibial band friction syndromes. *Physiotherapy* **82**(3), 199–202

Ryu, R.K.N. and Dunbar, W.H. (1988) Arthroscopic meniscal repair with two-year follow-up: a clinical review. *Arthroscopy*, **4**, 168–173

Ryu, R.K.N. and Ting, A.J. (1993) Arthroscopic treatment of meniscal cysts. *Arthroscopy*, **9**, 591–595

Sachs, R.A., Daniel, D.M., Stone, M.L. and Garfein, R.F. (1989). Patellofemoral problems after anterior cruciate ligament reconstruction. *American Journal of Sports Medicine*, **17**, 760–765

Sandberg, R., Nilsson, B. and Westlin, N. (1987) Hinged cast after knee ligament surgery. *American Journal of Sports Medicine*, **15**, 270–274

Saunders, H.D. (1989) *Assessing Flexibility and Strength in Industrial Workers*, Educational Opportunities, Bloomington

Seedhom, B.B. and Hargreaves, D.J. (1979) Transmission of the load in the knee joint with special reference to the role of the menisci. Part II: Experimental results, discussion and conclusions. *Engineering Medicine*, **8**, 220–228

Seto, J.L., Orofino, A.S. and Morrissey, M.C. (1988) Assessment of quadriceps/hamstring strength, knee ligament stability, functional and sports activity levels five years after anterior cruciate ligament reconstruction. *American Journal of Sports Medicine*, **16**, 170–180

Seto, J.L., Brewster, C.E. and Lombardo, J. (1989) Rehabilitation of the knee after anterior cruciate ligament reconstruction. *Journal of Orthopaedic and Sports Physical Therapy*, **10**, 8

Shakespeare, D.T. and Rigby, H.S. (1983) The bucket handle tear of the meniscus: a clinical and arthrographic study. *Journal of Bone and Joint Surgery*, **65**, 383

Sherman, O.H., Fox, J.M., Snyder, S.J., Pizzo, W.D., Friedman, M.J., Ferkel, R.D. and Lawley, M.J. (1986) Arthroscopy – 'No problem surgery'. An analysis of complications in two thousand six hundred and forty cases. *Journal of Bone and Joint Surgery*, **68A**, 256–265

Shino, K., Kimura, T., Hirose, H., Inoue, M. and Ono, K. (1986) Reconstruction of the anterior cruciate ligament by allogenic tendon graft: an operation for chronic ligamentous insufficiency. *Journal of Bone and Joint Surgery*, **68B**, 739–746

Silver, D.M. and Campbell, P. (1985) Arthroscopic assessment and treatment of dancer's knee injuries. *Physician and Sports Medicine*, **13**, (11) 74–82

Sinkjaer, T. and Arendt-Nielsen, L. (1991) Knee stability and muscle coordination in patients with anterior cruciate ligament injuries: an electromyographic approach. *Journal of Electromyography and Kinesiology*, **1**, 209–217

Slocum, D.B., James, S.L. and Larson, R.L. (1976) Clinical test for anteriolateral rotatory instability of the knee. *Clinical Orthopaedics and Related Research*, **118**, 63

Smillie, I.S. (1974) *Diseases of the Knee Joint*, Churchill Livingstone, London

Solomonow, M., Barratta, R. and D'Ambrosia, R. (1989) The role of the hamstrings in the rehabilitation of the anterior cruciate ligament deficient knee in athletes. *Sports Medicine*, **7**, 42

Sommer, H.M. (1988) Patellar chondropathy and apicitis and muscle imbalances of the lower extremities in competative sports. *Sports Medicine*, **5**, 386

Speakman, H.G.B. and Weisberg, J. (1977) The vastus medialis controversy. *Physiotherapy*, **63**(8), 249–254

Staubli, H-U. and Jakob, R.P. (1991) Anterior knee motion analysis: measurement and simultaneous radiography. *American Journal of Sports Medicine*, **19**, 172

Steinkamp, L.A., Dillingham, M.F., Markel, M.D., Hill, J.A. and Kaufman, K.R. (1993) Biomechanical considerations in patellofemoral joint rehabilitation. *American Journal of Sports Medicine*, **21**, 438–444

Stokes, M. and Young, A. (1984) The contribution of reflex inhibition to arthrogenous muscle weakness. *Clinical Science*, **67**, 7–14

Terry, G.C., Hughston, J.C. and Norwook, L.A. (1986) Anatomy of the iliopatellar band and iliotibial tract. *American Journal of Sports Medicine*, **14**, 39–45

Tiberio, D. (1987) The effect of excessive subtalar joint pronation on patellofemoral mechanics: a theoretical model. *Journal of Orthopaedic and Sports Physical Therapy*, **9**, 4

Timm, K.E. (1986) Validation of the Johnson anti-shear accessory as an accurate and effective clinical isokinetic instrument. *Journal of Orthopaedic and Sports Physical Therapy*, **7**, 298–303

Torg, J.S. (1989) In *Year Book of Sports Medicine* (eds R.J. Shephard, J.L. Anderson, E.R. Eichner et al.), Yearbook Medical Publishers, Chicago, p. 186

Torzilli, P.A. (1991) Measurement reproducibility of two commercial knee test devices. *Journal of Orthopaedic Research*, **9**, 730

Traverso, A., Baldari, A. and Catalani, F. (1990) The coexistence of Osgood–Schlatter's disease with Sinding-Larsen-Johansson's disease. *Journal of Sports Medicine and Physical Fitness*, **30**(3), 331–333

Tsirbas, A., Paterson, R.S. and Keene, G.C.R. (1990) Fat pad impingement: a missed cause of patello-femoral pain? *Australian Journal of Science and Medicine in Sport*, December, 24–26

Weiss, C.B., Lundberg, M., Hamberg, P., DeHaven, K.E. and Gillquist, J. (1989) Non-operative treatment of meniscal tears. *Journal of Bone and Joint Surgery*, **71A**, 811–822

Williams, J.G.P. and Sperryn, P.N. (1976) *Sports Medicine*, Edward Arnold, London

Williams, P.L. (1995) *Gray's Anatomy*, 38th edn, Churchill Livingstone, Edinburgh

Wilson, W.J., Lewis, F. and Scranton, P.E. (1990) Combined reconstruction of the anterior cruciate ligament in competitive athletes. *Journal of Bone and Joint Surgery*, **72A**(5), 742–748

Woo, S.L-Y., Ohno, K., Weaver, C.M., Pomaybo, A.S. and Xerogeanes, J.W. (1994) Non-operative treatment of knee ligament injuries. *Sports Exercise and Injury*, **1** (1), 2–13

Wroble, R.R., Van Ginkel, L.A., Grood, E.S. et al. (1990) Repeatability of the KT-1000 arthrometer in a normal population. *American Journal of Sports Medicine*, **18**, 396

Yasuda, K. and Sasaki, T. (1987) Muscle exercise after anterior cruciate ligament reconstruction: biomechanics of the simultaneous isometric contraction method of the quadriceps and hamstrings. *Clinical Orthopaedics and Related Research*, **220**, 266–274

Zuluaga, M., Briggs, C. and Carlisle, J. (1995) *Sports Physiotherapy*, Churchill Livingstone, Edinburgh

12

The shin

The term 'shin splints' is often used as a blanket description of any persistent pain occurring between the knee and ankle in an athlete. A more accurate description comes with the various 'compartment syndromes' which identify the anatomical structures affected. The anterior compartment contains the tibialis anterior, extensor hallucis longus, extensor digitorum longus, and the anterior tibial artery and vein. The lateral compartment contains the peronei, and the superficial peroneal nerve. The superficial posterior compartment contains the gastrocnemius and soleus and the deep posterior compartment contains the tibialis posterior, flexor digitorum longus, flexor hallucis longus, the peroneal artery and vein, and the posterior tibial artery and vein (Fig. 12.1). The deep and superficial posterior compartments are separated by the deep transverse fascia of the leg.

Anterior compartment syndrome

Anterior compartment syndrome involves pain in the anterior lower leg (Fig. 12.2a), which is increased in resisted dorsiflexion. There is usually a history of a sudden increase in training intensity, frequently involving jumping or running on a hard surface. The anterior compartment muscles swell, and in some cases hypertrophy occurs.

The fascia covering the muscles may be too tight and inflexible to accommodate the increase in size. As a consequence, when the muscles relax, their intramuscular pressure remains high and fresh blood is unable to perfuse the tissues freely. This decrease in blood flow leads to ischaemia with associated pain and impairment of muscle function.

Usually, when a muscle contracts, its blood flow is temporarily stopped. Arterial inflow occurs once more between the muscle contractions as the intramuscular pressure falls. Normal resting pressure within the tibialis anterior in the supine subject is about 5–10 mmHg, increasing to as much as 150–250 mmHg with muscle contraction. Muscle relaxation pressure, that which occurs between repeated contractions, is between 15–25 mmHg in the normal subject, but in athletes with anterior compartment syndrome pressures may rise to 30–35 mmHg and take up to 15 minutes to return to normal values (Styf, 1989).

The exact cause of the condition is not known. Hypertrophy may be one factor, as the condition occurs frequently when training intensity is increased. However, bodybuilders rarely suffer from the condition so the rate rather than the amount of muscle hypertrophy may be important. Microtrauma and excessive stress to the blood capillaries and lymphatics may give rise to

Figure 12.1   Compartments of the lower leg.

Figure 12.2   (a) Anterior compartment syndrome. Pain on the antero-lateral aspect of the lower leg. (b) Deep posterior compartment syndrome (medial tibial stress syndrome). Pain over distal third of tibia (see also Fig. 12.3). (c) Superficial posterior compartment syndrome. Pain within the calf bulk. (d) Lateral compartment syndrome. Loss of sensation over the dorsum of foot.

inflammation and in some cases myositis in the area (Styf, 1989).

Lateral compartment and superficial peroneal nerve

This is an unusual cause of shin pain and occurs when the peronei muscles are affected, usually by hyperpronation (Brody, 1980). The condition may have existed for some time but is brought to the fore when running begins. Again, there is ischaemia and pain, but in addition the superficial peroneal nerve may be compressed as it emerges from the lateral compartment.

The nerve lies deep to the peroneus longus and then passes forwards and downwards between the peronei and the extensor digitorum longus. It pierces the fascia in the distal third of the leg where it divides into medial and lateral branches to enter the foot. Entrapment may occur if muscle herniation or fascial defect exist. In addition, ankle sprain, fasciotomy, and an anomalous course of the nerve have been suggested as contributory factors (Styf, 1989). Clinically, the patient presents with loss of sensation over the dorsum of the foot, especially the second to fourth toes (Fig. 12.2d). Certain resting positions may compress the nerve and bring on the symptoms. To test the nerve, it is compressed over the anterior intermuscular septum 8–15 cm proximal to the lateral malleolus while the patient actively dorsiflexes and everts the foot. Tinel's sign, involving local percussion over the compression site, may be positive.

Posterior compartment

The superficial compartment contains the soleus and gastrocnemius. These muscles are usually affected by trauma rather than ischaemia, and are dealt with separately below. Pain occurs within the calf bulk (Fig. 12.2c) and is increased with resisted plantarflexion.

The deep posterior compartment contains tibialis posterior, flexor digitorum longus and flexor hallucis longus, and is the most common site for shin pain. Pain in this region is usually experienced over the distal third of the medial tibia (Fig. 12.2b) and represents 'medial tibial stress syndrome' (Mubarak et al., 1982). The exact site of pain will vary depending on the specific structures affected, and Detmer (1986) described a system of classification involving three types of chronic condition (Fig. 12.3).

Type I involves microfractures or stress fracture of the bone itself. The patient is usually a runner who has recently increased his or her mileage. The stress imposed by the sport exceeds the ability of the bone to adapt and remodel. The condition may present as a stress fracture showing a concentrated positive uptake in a single area on bone scan and point tenderness to palpation (type IA), or as a diffuse area along the medial edge of the tibia giving more generalized pain (type IB). In chronic conditions which have existed for some time, the tibial edge may be uneven due to new bone formation.

Type II medial tibial stress syndrome involves the junction of the periosteum and fascia, and occurs particularly in sprinters, and those involved in jumping activities. Pain is maximal just posterior to the bone, and has often persisted for a number of years. Initially, pain occurs only with activity, but as the condition progresses discomfort is felt with walking and even at rest. In this condition compartment pressures may not be elevated, and the periosteum is unchanged. One explanation is that the periosteum is traumatically avulsed from the bone by the action of soleus through its attachment to the fascia. During the chronic stage of this condition, adipose tissue has been found, during surgery, between the periosteum and underlying bone (Detmer, 1986). In the early stages of the condition the periosteum may heal back with rest, but

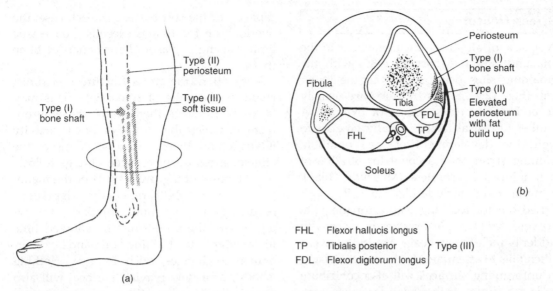

Figure 12.3 Medial tibial stress syndrome. (a) Painful areas of palpation. (b) Cross-section of structures affected. After Detmer (1986).

when the condition becomes chronic, it is unable to heal, and continues to cause pain when stressed by activity.

The type III condition involves ischaemia of the distal deep posterior compartment, and presents as a dull aching over the posterior soft tissues brought on by exercise. Intramuscular pressures are elevated as with anterior compartment syndrome (see above), and remain elevated after exercise.

Management

Initial management of shin pain involves a reduction of the stresses which caused the condition in the first place. This involves accurately identifying the structures affected and taking a thorough history of causal factors, particularly stresses imposed during training. Biomechanical assessment of the lower limb is mandatory and prescription of orthotics should be made where necessary. Initially, rest and anti-inflammatory modalities are used to allow the acute

inflammation to settle, but external compression and elevation of the limb may exacerbate the problem (Di Manna and Buck, 1990). If training stresses can be modified and the condition has been identified early enough this may be all that is required.

In chronic conditions in which conservative management has failed, decompression by fasiotomy may be called for. Here, the fascia of the affected compartment is surgically split along its length. The procedure is often performed on an out-patient basis, with two incisions being made, at the junction of the proximal and middle third of the leg and the middle and distal third. Athletes mobilize early and are often able to resume running after three weeks.

If fasciotomy is not successful, it may be the case that the epimysium over the tibialis posterior has been missed at surgery. Hannaford (1988) argued that the tibialis posterior should be classified as a condition independent from that affecting the other deep posterior muscles.

Stress fractures

Over 50% of all stress fractures occur to the tibia and fibula (McBryde, 1985) with the remaining sites being mostly to the lower limb (Fig. 12.4). Stress fractures are usually the end point in a sequence of overuse. A number of causal factors usually co-exist to begin the development of the condition. Training errors may account for 60–75% of such injuries in runners (McBryde, 1985). Common faults include high intensity work carried out for too long with an inadequate recovery, for example a distance runner who suddenly increases mileage. Faulty footwear which fails to attenuate shock, and exercising on unforgiving surfaces will also contribute to lower limb pathology. These factors, coupled with an underlying malalignment problem of the lower limb (or biomechanical faults in technique of upper limb actions, see p. 405), will exacerbate the problem. With novice runners, an additional factor is muscular weakness in the lower extremity leading to a reduction in shock-absorbing

capacity of the soft tissues. In each case, the overload on the tissues exceeds their elastic limit causing a plastic deformation of bone (p. 8).

Very often, the stress fracture is a direct result of a change of some type. This may be of the athletes themselves, the environment in which they train, or of the activity (Garrick and Webb, 1990). In terms of the athlete, stress fractures often emerge following the onset of a growth spurt or the menopause due to the large body adaptations occurring at these times. Similarly, following illness, the body must be allowed time to re-adapt to training demands. Environmental changes, such as new clothing (shoes), or a new playing surface, will also require time to allow tissue adaptation, failure to do so may lead to tissue breakdown of which stress fractures are one. Finally, alterations in the quality or quantity of a training programme itself will require a period of adaptation.

Far from being inert, bone is a dynamic tissue which is continually remodelling in

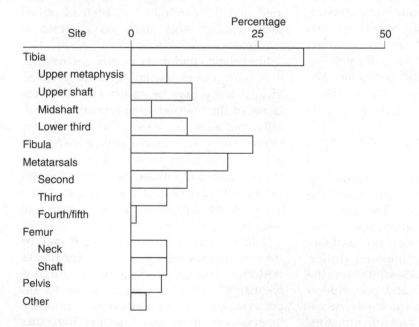

Figure 12.4   Distribution of stress fractures. After McBryde (1985).

response to mechanical stress. A balance usually exists between bone proliferation and reabsorption, which maintains the bone integrity. The result of athletic activity is normally that bone strengthens, but if unbalanced stresses cause bone reabsorption to exceed proliferation, the bone weakens. Examining excessive running and jumping in rabbits, Li et al. (1985) demonstrated that osteoblastic activity occurred from seven to nine days later than osteoclastic activity. Remodelling began on day two, with the haversian blood vessels dilating, and by day seven osteoclastic activity was noted in the bone cortex. New bone formation began in the periosteum by the 14th day of excessive stress. The adaptation to this excessive stress was reabsorption which occurred for some time before the formation of new cortical bone, thus weakening the bone structure. Abnormal X-rays were not found until day 21 after the stress was imposed.

Angular stresses, in particular, may cause failure of the bone with a resultant stress fracture. Two theories are generally accepted for the mechanisms by which stress affects bone. The first (fatigue) proposes that training which is too intense causes the muscles to fatigue so that they are no longer able to support the skeleton and absorb shock. The strain passes to the bone causing the fracture. The second theory (overload) suggests that when certain muscles contract, they cause the bones to bend slightly. Training which is too intense will exceed the capacity of the bone to recover from this stress.

The main symptom of a stress fracture is pain. This has been categorized into four types, depending on its characteristic (Puffer and Zachazewski, 1988). With type I pain, the athlete only feels discomfort after activity. With type II and III pain, discomfort is felt while training, but with type II this does not restrict activity. Type IV pain is chronic and unremitting in nature. Further symptoms include warmth and tenderness over the injured area, made worse with sporting activity and better with rest.

Swelling may be evident in the later stages of the condition if the bony surface is superficial. Accuracy of palpation when assessing bone pain is vital. The tenderness of a stress fracture is usually well localized, whereas that of compartment syndrome is more diffuse. Initially radiographs are usually negative, it taking at least two weeks for X-ray changes to be apparent (Li et al., 1985; Rzonca and Baylis, 1988). Local periosteal reaction and new bone growth may be seen after 6 weeks in long bone (Markey, 1987) and compressive stress fractures in cancellous bone are sometimes visible after 24 hours (Puddu et al., 1994). Taunton and Clement (1981) found radiographs to be positive in only 47.2% of their cases, while bone scan was accurate in 95.8%. Bone scan is normally revealing at the onset of symptoms and is generally more reliable. Phosphate labelled with technetium-99m is incorporated into osteoblasts and a hot spot appears over the active area, 6–72 hours after the onset of pain (Puddu et al., 1994).

Pain may be produced over the superficial fracture site by vibration. This may be produced from a tuning fork or ultrasound unit (Lowden, 1986), and is generally of more use in low risk areas, such as the foot and shin. Where there is a risk of complication through displacement (such as in the neck of the femur, see p. 226) bone scan with possible surgical intervention may be more appropriate.

Treatment of a stress fracture is primarily that of rest. As a general guide, with type I or II pain the workload should be reduced by 25% and 50%, respectively. Total rest is called for where type III pain is experienced, and type IV pain requires immediate medical investigation (Table 12.1). In the more severe conditions, rest should be total, because even allowing an athlete to train his upper body will often result in him 'just trying the leg out' in the gym. Training should not resume until the athlete has been totally pain free for 10 days. It should be emphasized to the athlete that this means at the end of each day,

Table 12.1   Pain classification

Classification	Characteristics	Action
Type I	Pain only after activity	↓ workload by 25%
Type II	Pain during activity but not restricting performance	↓ workload by 50%
Type III	Pain during activity restricting performance	Total rest
Type IV	Chronic unremitting pain at rest	Splint/cast Medical investigation

After Puffer and Zachazewshi (1988).

they should go to bed having felt no pain over the injured area in that day.

The timescale of healing will vary depending on the site of injury. With reduced activity, fibular stress fractures will normally heal in 4–6 weeks, tibial stress fractures in 8–10 weeks and femoral neck stress fractures in 12–16 weeks (Reid, 1992).

When activity is resumed, the athlete should be closely monitored, and activities stopped if any pain occurs. Return to sport should be progressive and varied. Different speed, running surfaces, and activities should all be used to spread the emphasis of training. Alternative training should be used, to reduce the weight-bearing on the limb. Swimming and cycling may be utilized to restore cardiopulmonary fitness for example.

Tennis leg

Of the sural muscles, it is the gastrocnemius which is usually injured. The soleus is infrequently affected by trauma being a single-joint muscle, but is more usually the victim of temporary ischaemia, giving rise to superficial posterior compartment syndrome.

Tennis leg is a strain of the gastrocnemius, normally involving the medial head at its musculo-tendinous junction with the Achilles tendon. The history of injury is usually a sudden propulsive action, such as a lunge or jump as the athlete pushes off from the mark. Women are more commonly affected, and the athlete is usually over 30 years of age (Garrick and Webb, 1990). The condition is often described as a rupture of the plantaris, more by tradition than anything else, because this muscle is rarely the cause of symptoms.

The athlete often feels something 'go' in the back of the leg as though he were hit from behind. Pain and spasm occur rapidly, preventing the athlete from putting his or her heel to the ground. Later, swelling and bruising develop distal to the injury site peaking at 48 hours after injury. There is local tenderness over the medial head of gastrocnemius at the junction between the middle and proximal third of the calf. Pain to passive stretch is worse with the knee straight than with it flexed.

Initial treatment is to immobilize the calf to prevent further tissue damage. Some authorities recommend a plantarflexed position with a 2–4 cm heel lift (Cyriax, 1982), while others claim that a 90° neutral ankle position gives a better result by preventing contraction and tightening the fascia to limit the spread of bruising (Garrick and Webb, 1990). Pain and the amount of tissue damage is usually the deciding factor. Partial ruptures are best immobilized non-weight-bearing in plantarflexion to approximate the tissue, whereas less serious injuries can be prevented from shortening by adopting a neutral resting position.

Compression from an elastic bandage limits the formation of swelling, and strength and flexibility is maintained by starting rehabilitation early. Massage involving calf kneading and transverse frictions ensures adequate broadening of the muscle fibres. Stretching to the gastrocnemius begins in the long sitting position. A towel or band is placed over the foot and the athlete gently pulls the foot into dorsiflexion. Stretching with the toes on a block in a partial, and later full weight-bearing position is the exercise progression. Strength is regained by utilizing a comparable long sitting position but substituting an elastic band for the strap. The foot is pressed into plantarflexion against the resistance of the band. Heel raises are performed in a standing position, initially from the floor and later with the heel on a 2–3 cm block.

Gait re-education is used to encourage equal stride length and the adoption of a normal heel–toe rhythm avoiding external rotation of the leg. When the calf is pain free, strength activities give way to power movements, to build up the fast twitch nature of the muscle (Ng and Richardson, 1990). Gentle jogging, jumping and skipping are used and progressed to plyometrics. The athlete should be instructed to jump and land correctly. The toes should be the last point to leave the floor in a jump and the first to contact the floor on landing. Toe contact is followed by progressive lowering through the foot with the knee and hip flexing as the heal touches the floor to minimize shock. Flat foot landing and remaining on the toes must be avoided (Fig. 12.5). Slow squats raising up onto the toes at the top point, give way to toe springing actions with and without weight resistance (dumb-bells or a weighted jacket). Leg drives from a mark, are useful, as are 'side hops' and 'hop and twist' actions over a bar.

(a)   (b)   (c)   (d)

Figure 12.5   Correct landing action from a jump. (a) Toe contacts floor first. (b) Foot flexes to absorb shock. (c, d) Knee and hip flex ('give') as heel touches ground.

Achilles tendon

Achilles tendon pain (achillodynia) is a common condition in sport, with the incidence in runners being as high as 9% (Lysholm and Wiklander, 1987). Interestingly, the condition was relatively uncommon until the 1950s and is still very rarely seen in China (40 Achilles tendon ruptures among 2.5 million people over a 5-year period) (Jozsa, Kvist and Balint, 1989). The increased incidence of Achilles tendon rupture may be a result of the increasingly sedentary lifestyles seen in the Western industrialized countries (Kvist, 1994).

The Achilles tendon is the largest tendon in the body, being some 15 cm long and about 2 cm thick. It originates from the musculo-tendinous junction of the calf muscles, the soleus inserting lower down on the deep surface of the tendon. The Achilles tendon gradually becomes more rounded as it travels distally, and flares out to insert into the posterior aspect of the calcaneum. The tendon is separated from the calcaneum by the retrocalcaneal bursa and from the skin by the subcutaneous calcaneal bursa.

The force from the Achilles tendon is delivered not through its insertion into the calcaneum, but via the point of contact on the posterior aspect of the calcaneum over the retrocalcaneal bursa (Reid, 1992). With increasing plantarflexion, the tendon 'unrolls' in such a way that this contact point moves lower down. In this way, the lever arm is maintained throughout the range of motion (Fig. 12.6).

The whole tendon rotates through 90° as it descends, so that the medial fibres become posterior by the time the tendon attaches to the calcaneum. This rotation is thought in part to account for the elastic properties of the tendon, giving it an elastic recoil when stretched. In the running action, as the lower limb moves from heel strike to mid-stance, the Achilles tendon is stretched, storing elastic energy. At toe off, the tendon recoils, releasing its stored energy and reducing the work required from the calf muscles to propel the body forwards.

The Achilles tendon is surrounded by a soft membranous paratenon which is continuous proximally with the muscle fascia and distally with the calcaneal periosteum. On the medial and lateral aspects of the dorsal surface there are thin spaces between the tendon and skin. These spaces are filled with thin gliding membranes covered in lubricating mucopolysaccharides. The membranes move freely over each other and greatly reduce friction. On the ventral side of the tendon there is fatty areolar tissue and connective tissue containing blood vessels.

The blood supply to the tendon is from either end and from the paratenon itself, but a relatively avascular zone exists between 2 and 6 cm proximal to the tendon insertion. Under normal circumstances, blood vessels do not travel from the paratenon to the tendon substance, and removal of the paratenon does not seem to compromise the blood supply (Williams, 1986). Tendon tissue in general has a low metabolic rate, and this coupled with the poor blood supply to the tendon means that the structure has a slow rate of healing.

Injuries to the Achilles tendon fall broadly into one of two categories. First, those which affect the tendon substance (partial or complete rupture), and, secondly, injury to the surface of the tendon and its covering (tendinitis or peritendinitis).

Tendinitis

Tendinitis presents as a swelling of the Achilles tendon of gradual onset. The main change is a disruption of the ground substance causing the tendon fibres to separate, which in turn leads to degeneration.

In peritendinitis the paratenon is inflamed and thickened, and there is local oedema and crepitus. Kager's triangle (the space between the inner surface of the Achilles tendon, the deep flexors and the calcaneus) is obliterated. Hard scarred bands appear within the paratenon and adhesions develop between the Achilles tendon and surrounding tissue. Kvist et al. (1988) showed that the fatty tissue surrounding the tendon was still thickened and swollen, after nearly two years in subjects with paratenonitis (peritendinitis). Connective tissue had increased, and local blood vessels had degenerated or been obliterated, suggesting the presence of immature scar tissue.

Initial management of tendinitis or peritendinitis aims at reducing local oedema. Rest and ice are used in conjunction with electro-

(a)   (b)

Figure 12.6 Contact point of Achilles tendon moves downwards as plantarflexion increases.

therapy modalities aimed at reducing pain and resolving inflammation. Transverse friction massage has been used extensively (Cyriax and Cyriax, 1983), for both the teno-osseous (T/O) junction and tendon itself. The T/O junction may be frictioned with the patient prone and the foot plantarflexed (Fig. 12.7a). The therapist uses the side of his flexed forefingers to impart the friction, pulling the hands distally against the curved insertion of the Achilles tendon into the calcaneum. The musculotendinous junction is frictioned with the foot dorsiflexed, and the tendon gripped from above between the finger and thumb. The movement is perpendicular to the tendon fibres (Fig. 12.7b). The tendon sheath may be treated by placing the length of the finger alongside the tendon and pressing inwards. The forearm is pronated/supinated to impart the friction (Fig. 12.7c).

A heel raise is used to reduce the stretch on the tendon, and the calf may be strapped in plantarflexion (Fig. 5.3, p. 106). If pain is intense the patient should initially be non-weight-bearing.

Tendon substance

Focal degeneration may occur in the tendon with athletes in their early 30s. The onset is usually gradual, giving highly localized pain. Microscopically there is proliferation of capil-

Figure 12.7 Transverse frictional massage for the Achilles tendon. (a) Teno-osseous junction. (b) Musculo-tendinous junction. (c) Tendon sheath/underside.

lary cells and lacunae along the tendon fibres giving a loss of the normal wavy alignment of collagen.

Tendon rupture generally occurs later in an athlete's life, being more common from the late 30s to mid-40s. With partial rupture, a few fibres or nearly all of the tendon may be affected. The characteristic history is one of sudden onset. There is swelling, pain on resisted movement, and the patient is unable to support his weight through the toes of the affected foot.

In complete rupture there is usually a single incident where the patient feels a sudden sharp 'give' in the tendon as though he or she had been struck from behind. Immediately afterwards there may be little pain but gross weakness. The patient is again unable to take his or her weight through the toes. Active plantarflexion is minimal, being accomplished by the peronei and posterior tibial muscles only. With the patient in a prone position, Simmond's test may be performed. The calf is squeezed, and the foot fails to plantarflex. Closer examination reveals a depression (the Toygar angle) visible in the normal smooth contour of the Achilles tendon. If the athlete is not seen for a number of days, this hollow will have been bridged by haematoma and scar tissue, giving a raised fibrous area unless the tendon ends have retracted. Without surgery, the tendon will heal, but very slowly. Granulation tissue forms poorly, partly due to repeated use, and partly as a result of the anticoagulant effect of synovial fluid contained by the unruptured paratenon (Williams, 1986).

Lesions of the tendon may be differentiated from those of the paratenon by using the 'painful arc' sign (Williams, 1986). The point of maximum tenderness is palpated as the foot is dorsiflexed and plantarflexed. When the tendon alone is affected, the painful area will move up and down as the tendon moves. However, when the paratenon is affected, as the tendon slides within its sheath, the area of maximum pain remains fixed (Fig. 12.8).

When examining the patient it must be remembered that the Achilles tendon is painful to palpation normally, so the intensity of discomfort must always be compared with that of the contra-lateral limb.

Surgical management of Achilles tendon injuries carries a high rate of complication. Williams (1986) described complications in 64 out of 461 surgical procedures (13.9%). These included mainly wound dehiscence (bursting), scar hypertrophy, and wound infection. Surgery may be called for where conservative management has failed and symptoms have persisted for more than 3 months.

Achilles tendon repair is the subject of considerable debate. Many authors claim that conservative treatment does not allow direct realignment of the torn tendon fibres and so the repair is less secure. In addition, they claim that re-rupture of surgically treated injuries is less likely (Turco and Spinella, 1987). Others argue that the risk of surgical complications is too great, and that the sophistication of rehabilitation is as important to the eventual outcome of the condition as whether the surgical or non-surgical route was chosen (Garrick and Webb, 1990). A number of repair methods have been described, including direct suture, reinforcement with plantaris or peroneus brevis ten-

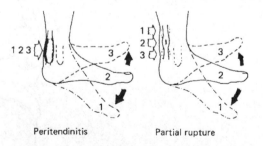

Peritendinitis   Partial rupture

Figure 12.8 The 'painful arc' in diagnosis of Achilles tendon pain. If the lesion is in the tendon, the point of maximum tenderness moves with excursion into dorsi- or plantarflexion. In peritendinitis it remains fixed. From Williams (1986), with permission.

don, and reconstruction using carbon fibre or polypropylene mesh.

Whatever the surgical method used, following immobilization the main problem is initially lack of flexibility, to the Achilles tendon, ankle, and sub-taloid joint in particular. Intense rehabilitation of the foot, ankle and leg is needed to regain full function.

Rehabilitation following surgery

Early mobility following Achilles tendon repair is a vital factor to the success of the procedure. A typical rehabilitation period normally includes an equinus plaster for 8 weeks followed by a heel raise for a further 6 weeks (Apley and Solomon, 1993). However, Saw et al. (1993) showed improved mobility and strength and a reduction in complications using total immobilization in an equinus plaster for 1 week only. Following this, the plaster was removed and active dorsiflexion was practised in sitting. The plaster was replaced between therapy sessions. Sutures were removed after 2 weeks and the foot placed in a lower leg walker. Solveborn and Moberg (1994) showed similar results using a patellar tendon bearing cast with a metal frame attached for 6 weeks. The cast allowed pain-free motion of the foot while taking full body weight for walking. No complications were seen, with a reduction of skin/tendon adhesions and a rapid return to normal strength values.

On removal of the cast, stretching procedures are begun non-weight-bearing. Hooking a towel over the forefoot and gently pulling into dorsiflexion being sufficient. Partial weight-bearing activities in sitting are used to begin the closed kinetic chain exercises, with the athlete gently pressing into dorsiflexion using varying foot angles. The same starting positions are chosen for early static and later dynamic strength training using straps and elastic bands. Isokinetics is used for the calf specifically and the lower limb in general.

Walking re-education using parallel bars or sticks introduces functional movements and introduces skill work. When full weight-bearing activities are begun the flexibility and strength work is progressed and augmented with skill training involving balance and coordination exercises (see ankle rehabilitation, p. 310) and further walking re-education.

Both static and dynamic flexibility training is used from the earliest stages, and eccentric actions are begun as soon as possible (often in the pool to limit weight-bearing) to mimic the true function of the Achilles tendon. When function has improved sufficiently, walking pace is increased and speed walking introduced, followed by on-the-spot and, later, small-step jogging. Straight running, zig-zags, and circle running are all used. Thick-heeled training shoes are used, and gradually the heel is lowered. Toe walking progresses to jogging on the toes.

General fitness is maintained throughout the programme by cardiopulmonary activities in the pool (assuming good healing of the scar) and, later, static cycle riding, until the intensity of rehabilitation itself is sufficient to challenge aerobic fitness. Pain is the rate limiting factor for both exercise intensity and progression.

Assuming the surgery has been totally successful, the final stages of training must include the use of plyometric exercise to develop elastic strength. Poor results can be expected if the rehabilitation programme is stopped at the stage of heavy isotonic exercise and not progressed in terms of speed. Hopping and jumping actions are used on forgiving surfaces with progression to bounding.

Aetiology

A number of factors may combine to cause Achilles tendon pain, including training alterations, footwear and flexibility. Alterations in training type or intensity, such as a sudden increase in the distance run over a holiday period, or more intensive training in the lead up to a competition, can both produce problems. Only in recreational athletes is trauma the predominant cause. In the competitive athlete, as many as 90% of Achilles tendon injuries result from overuse in the form of microtrauma established over months, or, in some cases, many years (Kvist, 1994).

Footwear is an important factor to the development of this condition. Inadequate shock-absorbing properties stress the Achilles tendon during eccentric loading, a situation aggravated when an athlete has a rigid cavus foot. Good shock absorption of the shoe heel is important for athletes who exercise on a hard surface. In addition to reducing the impact at heel strike, the height of the heel will also reduce the stretch on the Achilles tendon. A rigid sole lengthens the ankle to forefoot lever arm, affecting Achilles tendon mechanics, but may be necessary to protect the first toe (see below). If the heel counter of a sports shoe is hard, it can abrade the Achilles tendon as the foot plantarflexes at toe off. A negative heel counter, or a soft tab, is to be encouraged.

Lack of flexibility in the calf and Achilles tendon may contribute greatly to injury. When flexibility is limited, the tendon loses some of its elastic recoil making it more susceptible to damage through rapid eccentric loading of the calf in mid-stance. Flexibility exercises should be used for prevention and management of the sub-acute injury. Stretching may be performed with the forefoot on an angled block. The heel is kept on the ground and the hip is pressed forward bringing the knee over the forefoot and increasing dorsiflexion. The exercise is first performed with the knee locked to stretch the gastrocnemius, and then with the knee flexed to 20° to stress the Achilles tendon and soleus. A static stretch is used and held for 20–30 seconds. The range of motion is generally greater when the tendon

is warm, after a hot shower or bath for example.   ·

Malalignment of the lower limb is probably a contributory factor to Achilles tendon pain, although as these faults have generally been present for some time before the Achilles tendon condition started they are unlikely to be the sole cause. Increased pronation of the foot stresses the medial aspect of the Achilles tendon. A 30° increase in rearfoot position has been shown to lengthen these fibres by 10% (Nichols, 1989). In addition, excessive tibial rotation caused by hyperpronation will twist the Achilles tendon fibres together 'wringing them out'. This will close any blood vessels between the tendon fibres, temporarily reducing an already poor blood supply. In an interesting survey of 109 runners with Achilles tendon problems, Clement, Taunton and Smart (1984) found 75% showed training errors, 56% demonstrated hyperpronation, 39% suffered inflexibility of the calf and 10% wore improper footwear.

The effect of corticosteroids on ligament failure has been discussed on p. 51. Inhibition of collagen synthesis, reduction in the speed of tendon repair, lower elastic limit, and fatty degeneration have all been described (Nichols, 1989). Various studies have shown an increased likelihood of Achilles tendon rupture after injection (Chechick et al., 1982; Kleinman and Gross, 1983; Urban, 1989). Cyriax (1982) argued that Achilles tendon rupture only occurred when an incorrect injection technique was used, the corticosteroid being introduced into the tendon substance rather than along its surface. However, Williams (1986) claimed that both techniques had been shown to precipitate rupture, and further argued that the benefits of such injections were relatively short-lived. In addition, he contested that in acute peritendinitis, similar results could be obtained using a local anaesthetic and hyaluronidase.

Retrocalcaneal pain

Sever's disease

Calcaneal apophysitis (Sever's disease) may occur in adolescents during the rapid growth spurt, sometimes in association with Achilles tendon pain itself. The condition is more common in boys than girls, and occurs between the ages of 11 and 15 years. The posterior aspect of the calcaneum develops independently of the main body and is separated by an epiphyseal plate. The plate lies vertically and is therefore subjected to shearing stress from the pull of the Achilles tendon and through jarring stress in jumping. Pain frequently occurs during deceleration from running as well as take off and landing from a jump. Sever's is inappropriately named as it is not a true disease entity, but rather a traction injury similar in many respects to Osgood–Schlatter's disease in the adolescent knee.

On examination, there is tenderness to medial and lateral heel compression, but no noticeable skin changes. Radiographically, sclerosis and irregularity of the calcaneal apophysis is seen as a result of avascular necrosis (Caspi, Ezra and Horoszowski, 1989). Associated Achilles tendon tightness has been described, with the affected side showing 4–5° less passive dorsiflexion than the unaffected side (Mitcheli and Ireland, 1987). In addition, excessive foot pronation is also common in this patient group.

Initially, total rest is called for to allow the condition to settle. Later, any sporting activity which exacerbates the pain is avoided, and shock-absorbing heel pads are used in all shoes. Achilles tendon stretching is taught to restore dorsiflexion range, and foot position is corrected.

Haglund's syndrome

Haglund's syndrome is present when an exostosis is found over the posterior lateral aspect of the calcaneum. Radiographically, a spur of bone is seen coming from the calcaneal insertion of the Achilles tendon, showing as a prominence of the posterior superior calcaneal angle (Wooten and Chandler, 1990). Assessment of radiographs may be made by comparing 'parallel pitch lines' (Pavlov et al., 1982). The first line joins the anterior and posterior calcaneal tubercles. A second line is drawn parallel to the first, but this time starting from the posterior lip of the talar articulation (Fig. 12.9). If the posterior superior calcaneal angle stands prominent to this second line, the diagnosis is positive.

In addition to the bony changes, a painful soft tissue swelling (pump bump) is noted at the insertion of the Achilles tendon. This swelling can vary in size and shape depending on the stage of the condition. Haglund's syndrome commonly exists in association with retrocalcaneal bursitis, the inflamed bursa becoming visible on X-ray when low penetrating radiation is used (Rossi et al., 1987).

Contributing factors to the formation of Haglund's syndrome include a hard edge to the posterior aspect of the shoe (heel tab) and a rearfoot varus. As the foot is plantarflexed, the hard heel tab will abrade the posterior aspect of the calcaneum. If a rearfoot varus exists, compensatory pronation will cause the heel to twist in the shoe and soft tissue pressure occurs over the posterior calcaneum. Although soft tissue changes could be expected from abrasion of this type, bony changes are less likely. The bony change itself could be the result of a secondary ossification centre in the calcaneus (Horn and Subotnick, 1989).

Management of retrocalcaneal pain is by pain relief until the condition settles. A horseshoe pad made from non-compressible rubber is placed over the painful calcaneal area, and held in place by an ankle sock. A heel raise may be used to reduce stress through the tendon onto the calcaneus, and gentle tendon stretching is taught.

Figure 12.9 Parallel pitch lines to determine the position of the posterior superior calcaneal angle. A, posterior lip of talar articulation; B, posterior superior calcaneal angle; C, posterior calcaneal tuberosity; D, medial calcaneal tuberosity; E, anterior calcaneal tuberosity. After Rossi et al. (1987).

Electrotherapy modalities are used to alleviate pain and reduce inflammation.

Surgery includes bursectomy and resection of the superoposterior portion of the calcaneus, as far as the insertion of the Achilles tendon. Return to sport is relatively protracted, with athletes taking 3–5 months to begin full competition (Ghiggio, Nobile and Bronzo, 1993). With restoration of sport, athletes should still be advised to wear soft-back shoes to avoid local abrasion.

References

Apley, A.G. and Solomon, L. (1993) *Apley's System of Orthopaedics and Fractures*. 7th edn, Butterworth-Heinemann, Oxford

Brody, D.M. (1980) Running injuries. *Clinical Symposia*, **32**(4), Ciba Pharmaceutical Company, New Jersey

Caspi, I., Ezra, E. and Horoszowski, H. (1989) Partial apophysectomy in Sever's disease. *Journal of Orthopaedic and Sports Physical Therapy*, **10**(9), 370–373

Chechick, A., Amit, Y., Israli, A. and Horoszowki, H. (1982) Recurrent rupture of the achilles tendon induced by corticosteroid injection. *British Journal of Sports Medicine*, **16**, 89–90

Clement, D.B., Taunton, J.E. and Smart, G.W. (1981) A survey of overuse running injuries. *Physician and Sports Medicine*, **9**, 47

Clement, D.B., Taunton, J.E. and Smart, G.W. (1984) Achilles tendinitis and peritendinitis: aetiology and treatment. *American Journal of Sports Medicine*, **12**(3), 179–184

Cyriax, J. (1982) *Textbook of Orthopaedic Medicine*, Vol. 1, 8th edn, Baillière Tindall, London

Cyriax, J.H. and Cyriax, P.J. (1983) *Illustrated Manual of Orthopaedic Medicine*, Butterworth, London

Detmer, D.E. (1986) Chronic shin splints: classification and management of medial tibial stress syndrome. *Sports Medicine*, **3**, 436–446

Di Manna, D.L. and Buck, P.G. (1990) Chronic compartment syndrome in athletes: recognition and treatment. *Athletic training*, **25**, 1

Garrick, J.G. and Webb, D.R. (1990) *Sports Injuries: Diagnosis and Management*, W.B. Saunders, Philadelphia

Ghiggio, P., Nobile, G. and Bronzo, P. (1993) Haglund's disease in athletes. *Journal of Sports Traumatology*, **15**, 89–96

Hannaford, P.G.H. (1988) Shin splints re-visited. *Excel*, **4**(4), 16–19

Horn, L.M. and Subotnick, S.I. (1989) Surgical intervention. In *Sports Medicine of the Lower Extremity* (ed. S.I. Subotnick), Churchill Livingstone, Edinburgh, pp. 461–566

Jozsa, L., Kvist, M. and Balint, B.J. (1989) The role of recreational sports activity in Achilles tendon rupture. A clinical, pathoanatomical, and sociological study of 292 cases. *American Journal of Sports Medicine*, **17**, 338–343

Kleinman, M. and Gross, A.E. (1983) Achilles tendon rupture following steroid injection: report of three cases. *Journal of Bone and Joint Surgery*, **65A**, 1345–1346

Kvist, M. (1994) Achilles tendon injuries in athletes. *Sports Medicine*, **18**, 173–201

Kvist, M.H., Lehto, M.U.K., Jozsa, L., Jarvinen, M. and Kvist, H.T. (1988) Chronic achilles paratenonitis. *American Journal of Sports Medicine*, **16**(6), 616–622

Kvist, M (1994) Achilles tendon injuries in athletes. *Sports Medicine*, **18**, 173-201.

Li, G., Zhang, S., Chen, G., Chen, H. and Wang, A. (1985) Radiographic and histological analysis of stress fracture in rabbit tibias. *American Journal of Sports Medicine*, **13**, 285–294

Lowden, A. (1986) Application of ultrasound to assess stress fractures. *Physiotherapy*, **72**(3), 160–161

Lysholm, J. and Wiklander, J. (1987) Injuries in runners. *American Journal of Sports Medicine*, **15**, 168–171

Markey, K.L. (1987) Stress fractures. *Clinics in Sports Medicine*, **6**, 405–425

McBryde, A.M. (1985) Stress fractures in runners. *Clinics in Sports Medicine*, **4**(4), October, 737–752

Micheli, L.J. and Ireland, M.L. (1987) Prevention and management of calcaneal apophysitis in children: an overuse syndrome. *Journal of Paediatric Orthopaedics*, **7**, 34–38

Mubarak, S.J., Gould, R.N., Lee, Y.F. and Schmidt, D.A. (1982) The medial tibial stress syndrome. *American Journal of Sports Medicine*, **10**, 201–205

Ng, G. and Richardson, C.A. (1990) The effects of training triceps surae using progressive speed loading. *Physiotherapy Practice*, **6**, 77–84

Nichols, A.W. (1989) Achilles tendinitis in running athletes. *Journal of the American Board of Family Practice*, **2**(3), 196–203

Pavlov, H., Henegan, M., Hersch, A., Goldman, A. and Vigorita, V. (1982) The Haglund syndrome: initial and differential diagnosis. *Radiology*, **144**, 83–88

Puddu, G., Cerullo, G., Selvanetti, A. and De Paulis, F. (1994) Stress fractures. In *Oxford Textbook of Sports Medicine* (eds M. Harries, C. Williams, W.D. Stanish and L.J. Micheli), Oxford University Press, Oxford

Puffer, J.C. and Zachazewski, J.E. (1988) Management of overuse injuries. *American Family Physician*, **38**(3), 225–232

Reid, D.C. (1992) *Sports Injury Assessment and Rehabilitation*, Churchill Livingstone, London

Rossi, F., La Cava, F., Amato, F. and Pincelli, G. (1987) The Haglund syndrome: clinical and radiological features and sports medicine aspects. *Journal of Sports Medicine*, **27**, 258–265

Rzonca, E.C. and Baylis, W. J. (1988) Common sports injuries to the foot and leg. *Clinics in Paediatric Medicine and Surgery*, **5**(3), July

Saw, Y., Baltzopoulos, V., Lim, A., Rostron, P.K.M., Bolton-Maggs, B.G. and Calver, R.F. (1993) Early mobilisation after operative repair of ruptured achilles tendon. *Injury*, **24**, 479–484

Solveborn, S-A., and Moberg, A. (1994) Immediate free ankle motion after repair of acute achilles tendon ruptures. *American Journal of Sports Medicine*, **22**, 607–610

Styf, J. (1989) Chronic exercise-induced pain in the anterior aspect of the lower leg. *Sports Medicine*, **7**, 331–339

Taunton, J.E., and Clement, D.B. (1981) Lower extremity stress fractures in athletes. *Physician and Sports Medicine*, **9**, 77–86

Turco, V.J. and Spinella, A.J. (1987) Achilles tendon ruptures: Peroneus brevis transfer. *Foot and Ankle*, **7**, 253–259

Urban, K. (1989) Partial rupture of the achilles tendon in athletes. *Acta Chirurgiae Orthopaedicae et Traumatologiae Cechoslovaca*, **56**(1), 30–38

Williams, J.G.P. (1986) Achilles tendon lesions in sport. *Sports Medicine*, **3**, 114–135

Wooten, B. and Chandler, J. (1990) Use of an orthotic device in the treatment of posterior heel pain. *Journal of Orthopaedic and Sports Physical Therapy*, **11**(9), 410–413

13

The ankle

Approximately 14% of all sports injuries are sprains to the ankle, representing one ankle injury each season for every 17 participants. In high risk sports, such as jumping and running, this percentage is even higher, at 25% of all lost-time injuries (Reid, 1992). Ankle sprain has been shown to be 2.4 times more common in the dominant leg, and to have a high (73.5%) prevalence of recurrence (Yeung et al., 1994).

The joint mechanics of the ankle and foot have been described in Chapter 9. The ankle joint is the articulation between the trochlear surface of the talus and the distal ends of the tibia and fibula. The fibula may support 15–20% of the body weight (Lambert, 1971), with the fibula moving downwards and laterally during the stance phase of running to deepen the ankle mortice and enhance stability. This fibular motion creates tension in the interosseous membrane and tibio-fibular ligament to provide some shock attenuation. Loss of this mechanism through tibio-fibular disruption greatly affects the ankle joint, with a 1–2 mm lateral shift of the fibula increasing joint forces by as much as 40% (Reid, 1992).

The ankle is subjected to considerable compression forces during sport (Fig. 13.1). Compression forces as high as five times body weight have been calculated during walking and up to 13 times body weight during running (Burdett, 1982).

Collateral ligaments

The joint is strengthened by a variety of ligaments, the collaterals being the most important from the point of view of injury. Both medial and lateral collateral ligaments travel from the malleoli, and have bands attaching to the calcaneus and talus.

The medial (deltoid) ligament (Fig. 13.2a) is triangular in shape. Its deep portion may be divided into anterior and posterior tibiotalar bands. The more superficial part is split into tibionavicular and tibiocalcaneal portions, which attach in turn to the spring ligament. The lateral ligament (Fig. 13.2b) is composed of three separate components, and is somewhat weaker than its medial counterpart. The anterior talofibular (ATF) ligament is a flat band 2–5 mm thick and 10–12 mm long, which travels from the anterior tip of the lateral malleolus to the neck of the talus, and may be considered the primary stabilizer of the ankle joint (Palastanga, Field and Soames, 1989). The posterior talofibular (PTF) ligament travels almost horizontally from the fossa on the bottom of the lateral malleolus to the posterior surface of the talus. Lying between the ATF and PTF ligaments is the calcaneofibular ligament, arising from the front of the lateral malleolus to pass down and back to attach onto the lateral surface of the calcaneum. The role of the collateral lig-

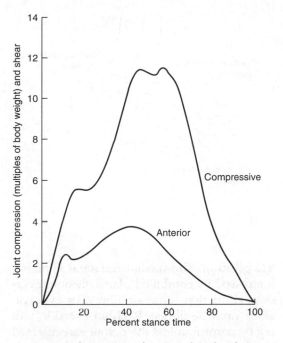

Figure 13.1 Compression forces on the talus during running. From Burdett (1982).

ments in maintaining talocural stability is summarized in Table 13.1.

Injury

The most common injury to the ankle is damage to the ATF ligament with or without involvement of the peroneus brevis. The sub-taloid and mid-tarsal joints may be involved, but will be dealt with separately for clarity. The typical history of ankle injury is one of inversion, sometimes coupled with plantar-flexion. The athlete 'goes over' on the ankle, usually on an uneven surface. One of three grades of ligament injury may occur (p. 51).

There is usually an egg-shaped swelling in front of, and around, the lateral malleolus. When viewed from behind, the definition of the Achilles tendon is a good indicator of severity of injury (Reid, 1992). With more severe injuries (grade III) the definition of the Achilles tendon is lost due to excessive bleeding into the joint (Fig. 13.3).

The lateral malleolus should be gently pal-pated to assess if bone pain is present; if it is, an X-ray may be required. If palpation reveals tenderness below, rather than over, the lateral malleolus and the athlete is able to bear weight, there is a 97% probability of soft tissue injury alone (Vargish and Clarke, 1983). Any fracture that is missed by this type of close palpation is likely to be an avul-sion or non-displaced hairline type that will respond favourably to management as a sprain (Garrick and Webb, 1990).

Stress tests to the ankle are useful to assess the degree of instability in the sub-acute phase, and to give a differential diagnosis. Acute injuries may be exacerbated by full range motion with overpressure. The capsule of the ankle joint itself is assessed by passive dorsiflexion and plantarflexion only, the cap-sular pattern presenting as a greater limita-tion of plantarflexion. However, as the ankle ligaments span the sub-taloid and mid-tarsal joints, inversion/eversion and adduction/ abduction are also included in ankle joint examination.

Table 13.1 Role of the collateral ligaments in ankle stability

Movement	Controlled by
Abduction of talus	Tibiocalcaneal and tibionavicular bands
Adduction of talus	Calcaneofibular ligament
Plantarflexion	ATF ligament and anterior tibiotalar band
Dorsiflexion	Posterior tibiotalar band and PTF ligament
External rotation of talus	Anterior tibiotalar and tibionavicular bands
Internal rotation of talus	As above with ATF ligament

Adapted from Palastanga, Field and Soames (1989).

Figure 13.2   The ankle ligaments. (a) Deltoid (medial). (b) Lateral.

Figure 13.3   Assessing severity of ankle injury from swelling. (a) Normal joint. Contour of Achilles tendon well defined. (b) Grade I/II injury. Clear swelling but Achilles tendon outline still visible. (c) Grade III injury. Profuse swelling obscures outline of Achilles tendon.

The ATF ligament is placed on maximum stretch by passive inversion, plantarflexion, and adduction. The heel is held with the cupped hand and the sub-taloid joint inverted. The opposite hand grasps the forefoot from above and swings it into plantarflexion and adduction. In addition, anterior glide of the talus on the tibia should be assessed with the foot in a neutral position. The heel is again held in the cupped hand, but this time the palm of the opposite hand is over the anterior aspect of the lower tibia. The calcaneus and talus are pulled forward as the tibia is pushed back. Movements are compared with that of the uninjured side for range and quality.

The calcaneocuboid ligament is stressed by combined supination/adduction and the calcaneofibular ligament by inversion in a neutral position. The medial collateral ligament is stressed by combined plantarflexion/eversion/abduction (anterior fibres) or eversion alone (middle fibres). Resisted eversion will not be painful unless the peronei are affected (see below).

Following severe ankle sprain or fracture, a bony link may form between the tibia and fibula (tibiofibular synostosis). Typically, pain occurs after an injury, and increases during vigorous activity, mimicking stress fracture. Pain is most severe during the push-off action of running and jumping, and dorsiflexion is often limited to 90°, mimicking impingement pain (see below). The synostosis is revealed by X-ray and removed surgically (Flandry and Sanders, 1987).

Management of an ankle sprain

Immediate management consists of the RICE protocol, with electrotherapy modalities as appropriate. Intermittent pneumatic compression (IPC) used in conjunction with cooling is effective. In the sub-acute phase, massage, especially finger kneading around the malleolus is of value in preventing the development of pitting oedema. Transverse frictions may be used to encourage the development of a mobile scar, and as a prelude to manipulation for scar tissue rupture in a chronic injury. Grade II and III injuries present with marked swelling and are protected non-weight-bearing (severe injury) or preferably partial weight-bearing with a compression bandage. Where minimal swelling indicates a grade I injury, an eversion strapping may be applied to protect the ligament from inversion stresses and to shorten it. A felt wedge is used beneath the heel to evert the sub-taloid joint, and a U-shaped pad is placed over the sub-malleolar depressions to prevent pockets of oedema forming and to apply even compression when the ankle is strapped. Adhesive strapping is applied after skin preparation or underwrap, initially to lock the sub-taloid joint and then to passively evert the foot. The athlete can then walk partial weight-bearing in a well-supporting shoe.

Early mobility is essential to increase ligament strength and restore function. For grade I and II injuries, early mobilization has been shown to be more effective than immobilization. In a group of 82 patients with these grades of injury, 87% who were immobilized with a plastercast for 10 days still had pain after 3 weeks. This compared to 57% of those who received early mobilization in the form of an elastic strap for 2 days followed by a functional brace for 8 days (Eiff, Smith and Smith, 1994).

Non-weight-bearing ankle exercise is instigated within the pain-free range, and fitness is maintained by general exercise. Strapping is replaced by a tubular elastic bandage as pain subsides.

Rehabilitation of the injured ankle

As with any joint, rehabilitation of the ankle aims at restoring mobility, strength and function (Table 13.2). With the ankle, however, of particular concern is the restoration of normal proprioception.

Resisted exercise using rubber power-bands is used for inversion, eversion, dorsi-flexion and plantarflexion, together with combinations of these movements. Maximum repetitions are used to restore muscle endurance, while strength is developed using maximal resistance. Eversion movements are performed with the band placed over both forefeet. For other movements, one end of the band is placed around a table leg, and the other over the foot. Various thicknesses of band are used as the exercises are progressed.

Static stretching exercises include calf and Achilles tendon stretching (see above), and inversion/eversion movements applied manually by the athlete. The starting position for these latter movements is sitting with the injured leg crossed over the contralateral limb. The exercise mimics the stability test for the ligaments outlined above.

Partial and then full, weight-bearing exercises are used to develop strength in a closed kinetic chain position and to restore proprioception. In single leg standing (wall-bar support) trunk movements are performed to throw stress onto the ankle, in addition, exercises such as heel raising, toe lifts, and inversion/eversion are performed. A balance beam (flamingo balance) is used, and again trunk and hip movements of the contralateral limb throw stress onto the injured ankle. The foot may be placed along the beam, or with the beam travelling transversely and only the toes supported. Intense muscle activity is seen around the ankle as the athlete attempts to maintain his or her balance. By varying the athlete's footwear, and performing the exercises in bare feet the stresses imposed are altered.

A balance board with a single transverse rib is used for sagittal movements, and a longitudinal rib for frontal plane actions. A board with a domed central raise (wobble board or ankle disc) is used to combine movements for circumduction. In addition to trunk movements, actions such as throwing and catching while standing on the balance board are helpful as these take the athlete's attention away from the ankle, and

Table 13.2   Guidelines for rehabilitation of ankle sprain

Immediate post-injury management
RICE protocol
Consider use of intermittent pneumatic compression (IPC) with ice
Other modalities to reduce pain and inflammation
Careful assessment of possible bony injury
Athlete non-weight-bearing

Initial rehabilitation (2–5 days after injury)
Massage, especially finger kneading around malleolus
Range of motion exercise, inversion to pain tolerance only
Transverse frictions to encourage mobile scar formation
Partial weight-bearing with eversion taping and felt padding or ankle orthosis
Walking re-education
Begin resisted exercise (elastic bands)
Active stretch into inversion and plantarflexion
Begin accessory mobilizations of surrounding joints

Intermediate rehabilitation (6–14 days)
Progress resisted exercise of ankle in all directions
Passive stretching into inversion and plantarflexion
Proprioceptive work (single-leg standing, eyes closed)
Gradually introduce balance board and trampette work
Ensure full range dorsiflexion
Uphill treadmill work progressing to speed walk and slow run
Side step and zig-zag speed walking—building endurance
Introduce varied terrain—slopes, rough ground, sand
Ensure cuboid mobility

Final rehabilitation (2–6 weeks)
Build to maximum resisted eversion
General weight training for lower limb
Running drills—figure-of-eight, circle run, zig-zag
Introduce low hop and progress to hop and hold, side hop, and hop and twist—building power
  and speed
Sport specific work including ball kicking and varying terrain

so are a progression in terms of skill. Performing balance board exercises blindfolded, and therefore eliminating visual input, has been shown to be effective at improving proprioception in the ankle (De Carlo and Talbot, 1986).

Running, hopping and jumping activities are all used, on varying surfaces including sand, grass, and a mini-trampoline. Hopping direction is varied to alter the stress on the joint. Straight line hopping places an anteroposterior stress on the joint while lateral hopping imposes a mediolateral stress. Combined directions, diagonal hopping, and twisting when hopping are all used to imposed multiple stresses on the joint (Fig. 13.4). Running in a circle, figure-of-eight and on hills/cambers all change the stress on the ankle, and hopping and jumping develop power rather than strength.

The importance of proprioceptive training to prevent the development of chronic instability (giving way in normal usage) is of great importance. Freeman, Dean and Hanham (1965) compared ligament injuries to the foot and ankle treated by immobilization, 'conventional' physiotherapy, and proprioceptive training, which consisted of balance board exercises. After treatment, 7% of the proprioceptive group showed instabil-

Straight line   Lateral   Combined   Diagonal   Twisting

Figure 13.4 Hopping patterns in ankle rehabilitation.

ity compared to 46% of those treated by other means. Balance ability was measured using a modified Rhomberg test, which assesses the ability to maintain single leg standing while the eyes are closed. Lentell, Katzman and Walters (1990) assessed the strength of the ankle musculature in 33 subjects with instability and found that there was no significant difference between the injured and uninjured sides. However, when balance ability was measured the majority of subjects exhibited a deficit between the two extremities. Konradsen and Ravn (1990) measured the time taken for peroneal contraction to occur in response to a sudden inversion stress, in chronically unstable ankles. Their results showed the peroneal reaction time to be prolonged in unstable ankles, indicating a proprioceptive deficit.

As the ankle ligaments and capsule are torn, articular nerve fibres are also likely to be damaged, leading to a partial de-afferentiation of the joint. This, in turn, will decrease the athlete's motor control and inhibit reflex stabilisation of the foot and ankle. Proprioceptive training should, therefore, be incorporated into general rehabilitation training. Where chronic instability is seen, the modified Rhomberg test should be used to assess the degree of proprioceptive deficit.

Ankle taping

Reduction of excessive inversion–eversion stress in the previously injured athlete, or as a preventive measure is widely used, more so in the USA than in Europe. Taping has traditionally been used, but semi-rigid orthoses are becoming increasingly popular. These allow dorsiflexion–plantarflexion but limit inversion–eversion and so should have a less detrimental effect on overall lower limb mechanics.

Orthoses have been shown to be as effective as taping at reducing inversion–eversion movement, but have the advantage that this support is more effectively maintained throughout training. Greene and Hillman (1990) compared several ankle orthotics with taping and found that after 20 minutes of exercise the taping revealed maximal losses of restriction while the orthoses demonstrated no mechanical failure. Rovere et al. (1988) showed ankle stabilizers to be more effective than taping at reducing ankle injuries. Surve et al. (1994) showed a lower incidence of ankle sprain and a reduced severity of injury in soccer players with a previous history of ankle injury who wore a semi-rigid ankle orthosis. No change in incidence of injury was seen in those without a previous history of injury.

In addition to support characteristics, the effect on lower limb mechanics is important. Taping has been shown to throw stress onto the forefoot as the foot compensates for the reduction of dorsiflexion in mid-stance in walking subjects (Carmines, Nunley and McElhaney, 1988). Where an ankle orthosis allows normal dorsiflexion, the forefoot is likely to receive less compensatory stress.

The combination of forefoot stress and loss of restriction capabilities may make the use of ankle orthoses preferable to taping in certain circumstances. The contribution of taping to proprioception, providing an increased skin stimulation to movement may also be of importance. Restoration of full ankle function with a combination of strength and balance activities must always be the main consideration, with ankle supports used as an interim measure wherever possible.

Impingement syndromes

Repeated forced dorsiflexion, such as occurs with dismounts in gymnastics, may cause anterior impingement of the talus on the tibia. The synovium may be repeatedly trapped, becoming chronically swollen and hypertrophied. Pain occurs over the front of the ankle, and is exacerbated by dorsiflexion with overpressure. Radiographs may reveal talar osteophytes, but these do not usually contribute to the impingement. Forced plantarflexion, for example repeated karate kicks or football, may cause posterior impingement giving pain over the back of the ankle without tenderness to the Achilles tendon.

Both conditions show slight swelling, and represent a repeated impaction of the joint surfaces leading to compression of the articular cartilage and sub-chondral bone. These structures do not show great sensitivity, and will not be the primary source of pain. Instead, pain must come either from the periosteum, joint capsule, or more likely from chemical irritation and mechanical stress caused by the inflammatory response itself. Impingement syndromes respond to rest, anti-inflammatory modalities and training modification.

If the impingement force persists, an exostosis may form, on the back or front of the lower tibia depending on the type of stress involved. The exostosis may be up to 1 cm long in some cases (O'Donoghue, 1976), and should this break off it will float in the joint as a loose body. In cases where the exostosis

causes symptoms, it should be surgically removed.

Rapid, forceful dorsiflexion, such as may occur in a fall onto the feet, can force the talus up with enough force to stress the distal tibiofibular ligament. The joint is tender to palpation within the sulcus between the tibia and fibula, and pain is elicited to passive dorsiflexion but not inversion or eversion. Treatment involves strapping the foot to limit dorsiflexion, and using a heel raise.

On the posterior aspect of the talus the flexor hallucis longus travels in a small groove. If the bone lateral to this point is extended, it is called Stieda's process. When this piece occurs as a separate bone (ossicle) attached to the talus by fibrous tissue, it is known as the os trigonum. Between 8 and 13% of the population have one of these bony configurations (Brodsky and Khalil, 1987) (Fig. 13.5). Three mechanisms have been proposed for the development of the os trigonum (Reid, 1992). The secondary ossification centre in the region may fail to fuse, or repeated trauma (impingement) may cause a stress fracture. An acute fracture may also ensue following forced plantarflexion with or without avulsion of the posterior band of the lateral ligament (Cedell, 1974).

Figure 13.5 Lateral view of the ankle, showing the os trigonum and Stieda's process. From Brodsky and Khalil (1987), with permission.

Repeated plantarflexion may compress the os trigonum and give impingement pain, palpable over the posterolateral talus between the Achilles tendon and the peroneal tendons. If symptoms fail to settle with conservative management, surgical removal of the ossicle may be called for. This is often performed with release of the adjacent tendon sheath of flexor hallucis longus.

Tendinitis in association with the malleoli

The tendons of peroneus longus and brevis pass around the lateral malleolus, while those of tibialis posterior, flexor digitorum longus, and flexor hallucis longus pass around the medial malleolus (Fig. 13.6). Any of the tendons, their sheaths, or their retaining retinacula may be inflamed or injured.

One complication of ankle sprain is a strain or avulsion of the peroneus brevis as it attaches to the base of the fifth metatarsal. There may be local bruising, and pain is reproduced by resisted eversion. Point tenderness, proximal to the base of the fifth metatarsal, indicates the tendon, while bone pain may indicate avulsion. Radiographs are required to differentiate avulsion from a fracture to the fifth metatarsal itself (Jones' fracture). Treatment is similar to that of an ankle injury, with frictions performed to the ten-

Figure 13.6 Tendons near the malleoli. (a) Lateral view, (b) medial view.

don while the foot is inverted, and exercises to restore strength and flexibility of the peroneus brevis.

Peroneal tendon dislocation may occur if the tip of the lateral malleolus is fractured with forced dorsiflexion (skiing) or a direct blow (soccer). Occasionally, severe inversion injury may rupture the peroneal retinaculum and allow the tendons to sublux or dislocate forwards over the fibula with resisted dorsiflexion and eversion. Local pain is present, and a 'snapping' sensation is felt as the tendons move over the bone. Surgical management is required with several procedures being performed to re-establish the anatomy of the region. Re-attachment of the retinaculum, deepening of the peroneal groove, and placing the peroneal tendons under the calcaneofibular ligament have been variously described (Martens, Noyez and Mulier, 1986; Apley and Solomon, 1993).

The flexor hallucis longus (FHL) passes behind the medial malleolus in a separate tendon sheath, which runs along the anterior aspect of the talus. The sheath passes between the medial and lateral tubercles of the talus, under the sustentaculum tali, and beneath the flexor retinaculum. The fibroosseous tunnel so formed predisposes the tendon to mechanical irritation.

Pain may occur to resisted hallux flexion, with tenderness lying medial to the Achilles tendon. Pain is usually noticeable during the push-off phase of walking and running. A fusiform swelling and thickening of the tendon may occur in dancers with repeated point work. Eventually, the thickening may interfere with the movement of the tendon within its sheath giving rise to 'trigger toe' (Sammarco and Miller, 1979).

The tibialis posterior tendon passes in a groove around and beneath the medial malleolus, the latter structure acting as a pulley. During pronation, the tendon is pressed onto the underlying bone of the groove, and in athletes who hyperpronate during the stance phase, tendon or tendon sheath pathology may occur. Tenderness, swelling and/or cre-

pitus is noted in the local area along the tendon sheath. Resisted plantarflexion and inversion may cause pain and will cause the tendon to stand out making palpation easier.

Subtaloid joint

The sub-taloid joint (STJ) (Fig. 13.7) has a thin capsule strengthened by the medial, posterior and lateral talocalcaneal ligaments. The joint cavity is isolated from that of the ankle and mid-tarsal joints, and its stability is largely maintained by the interosseous talocalcanean ligament running from the sinus tarsi to the talus.

Sub-taloid mobility is often reduced following ankle sprain or fracture of the calcaneus from a fall onto the heel. Movement may also be reduced by impaction when jumping on a hard surface in inadequate footwear. The lack of mobiliy sometimes goes unnoticed, unless the patient is assessed by a physiotherapist.

Figure 13.7 The sub-taloid and mid-tarsal joints. (a) From above, (b) lateral view.

Manual assessment and mobilization of accessory movements may be performed with the patient in a supine-lying position, with the heel over the couch end. Initially, the therapist grips around the distal part of the patient's leg with one hand pressing the leg onto the couch. His or her forefingers grip the talus and the calcaneum is cupped in the opposite hand (Fig. 13.8a). The calcaneum is then moved on the fixed talus. Releasing the talus, both talus and calcaneum are moved together on the fixed lower leg. Gross sub-taloid joint movement may be performed by cupping the heel in both hands and performing forceful inversion/eversion actions (Fig. 13.8b).

Some distraction may be given to the STJ in supine with one hand cupping the calcaneum laterally and applying a caudal force while the other hand stabilizes the dorsomedial aspect of the mid-foot (Fig. 13.8c). In the prone position, with the patient's foot slightly plantarflexed, and the toes over the couch end, a distraction force may be imparted by pushing caudally with the heel of the hand onto the posterior aspect of the calcaneus near the Achilles tendon insertion (Fig. 13.8d). Following injury, rear-

Figure 13.8 Manual therapy of the sub-taloid joint. (a) Stabilize lower leg and move talus. (b) Gross sub-talar movement. (c and d) Distraction and gliding.

foot position should be assessed as posting may be required.

Mid-tarsal joint

The mid-tarsal joint (Fig. 13.7) is composed of the calcaneal cuboid joint (lateral), and the talocalcaneonavicular joint (medial). Four ligaments are important from the perspective of sports injuries. The plantar calcaneonavicular (spring) ligament is a dense fibro-elastic structure running from the sustentaculum tali to the navicular behind its tuberosity. The plantar calcaneocuboid ligament passes from the anterior inferior aspect of the calcaneus to the plantar surface of cuboid behind the peroneal groove. The long plantar ligament stretches the whole length of the lateral aspect of the foot. It arises from between the tubercles of the calcaneus and passes forwards giving off a short attachment to the cuboid, and so forming a roof over the tendon of peroneus longus. The ligament then attaches to the bases of the lateral four metatarsal bones. The bifurcate ligament is in two parts, and travels from a deep hollow on the upper surface of the calcaneus to the cuboid and navicular.

The calcaneocuboid joint takes the full body weight as it forms part of the lateral longitudinal arch of the foot. Stability is provided by the plantar calcaneocuboid and long plantar ligaments, reinforced by the tendon of peroneus longus. The talocalcaneonavicular joint is stabilized by the plantar calcaneonavicular and bifurcate ligaments together with the tendon of tibialis posterior.

The calcaneocuboid ligament may be injured at the same time as the ATF. Pain is reproduced by fixing the rearfoot in dorsiflexion and eversion, and inverting and adducting the forefoot. Often the condition goes unnoticed at the time of injury as the AFT sprain is the dominant pain. Chronic pain results, and transverse frictions and scar tissue rupture may be required, with

temporary forefoot posting. Mobilization of the cuboid or navicular may be called for (see p. 325).

References

Apley, A.G. and Solomon, L. (1993) *Apley's System of Orthopaedics and Fractures*, 7th edn, Butterworth-Heinemann, Oxford

Brodsky, A.E. and Khalil, M.A. (1987) Talar compression syndrome. *Foot and Ankle*, **7**, 338–344

Burdett, R.G. (1982) Forces predicted at the ankle during running. *Medicine and Science in Sports and Exercise*, **14**, 308

Carmines, D.V., Nunley, J.A. and McElhaney, J.H. (1988) Effects of ankle taping on the motion and loading pattern of the foot for walking subjects. *Journal of Orthopaedic Research*, **6**, 223–229

Cedell, C.A. (1974) Rupture of the posterior talotibial ligament with avulsion of a bone fragment from the talus. *Acta Orthopaedica Scandinavica*, **45**, 454

De Carlo, M.S. and Talbot, R.W. (1986) Evaluation of ankle joint proprioception following injection of the anterior talofibular ligament. *Journal of Orthopaedic and Sports Physical Therapy*, **8**(2), 70–76

Eiff, M.P., Smith, A.T. and Smith, G.E. (1994) Early mobilisation versus immobilisation in the treatment of lateral ankle sprains. *American Journal of Sports Medicine*, **22**, 83–88

Flandry, F. and Sanders, R.A. (1987) Tibiofibular synostosis: An unusual cause of shin splint-like pain. *American Journal of Sports Medicine*, **15**, 280–284

Freeman, M.A.R., Dean, M.R.E. and Hanham, I.W.F. (1965) The etiology and prevention of functional instability of the foot. *Journal of Bone and Joint Surgery*, **47B**(4), 678–685

Garrick, J.G. and Webb, D.R. (1990) *Sports Injuries: Diagnosis and Management*, W.B. Saunders, London

Greene, T.A. and Hillman, S.K. (1990) Comparison of support provided by a semirigid orthosis and adhesive ankle taping before, during, and after exercise. *American Journal of Sports Medicine*, **18**(5), 498–506

Konradsen, L. and Ravn, J.B. (1990) Ankle instability caused by prolonged peroneal reaction time. *Acta Orthopaedica Scaninavica*, **61**(5), 388–390

Lambert, K. (1971) The weight bearing function of the fibula. *Journal of Bone and Joint Surgery*, **53A**, 507

Lentell, G.L., Katzman, L.L. and Walters, M.R. (1990) The relationship between muscle function and ankle stability. *Journal of Orthopaedic and Sports Physical Therapy*, **11**(12), 605–611

Martens, M.A., Noyez, J.F. and Mulier, J.C. (1986) Recurrent dislocation of the peroneal tendons: results of rerouting the tendons under the calcaneofibular ligament. *American Journal of Sports Medicine*, **14**, 148–150

O'Donoghue, D.H. (1976) *Treatment of Injuries to Athletes*, W.B. Saunders, Philadelphia

Palastanga, N. Field, D. and Soames, R. (1989) *Anatomy and Human Movement*, Heinemann Medical, Oxford

Reid, D.C. (1992) *Sports Injury Assessment and Rehabilitation*, Churchill Livingstone, London

Rovere, G.D., Clarke, T.J., Yates, C.S. and Burley, K. (1988) Retrospective comparison of taping and ankle stabilizers in preventing ankle injuries. *American Journal of Sports Medicine*, **16**, 228–233

Sammarco, G.J. and Miller, E.H. (1979) Partial rupture of the flexor hallucis longus in classical ballet dancers. *Journal of Bone and Joint Surgery*, **61A**, 440

Surve, I., Schwellnus, M.P., Noakes, T. and Lombard, C. (1994) A fivefold reduction in the incidence of recurrent ankle sprains in soccer players using the sport-stirrup orthosis. *American Journal of Sports Medicine*, **22**, 601–606

Vargish, T. and Clarke, W.R. (1983) The ankle injury—Indications for the selective use of X-rays. *Injury*, **14**, 507-512

Yeung, M.S., Chan, K-M., MPhil, C.H.S. and Yuan, W.Y (1994) An epidemiological survey on ankle sprain. *British Journal of Sports Medicine*, **28**, 112-116

14

The foot

The foot is the athlete's main contact area with the ground, an obvious point, but one which helps account for the very high number of conditions affecting this area in sport. An athlete's foot may have to withstand forces two or three times greater than body weight, and this may be repeated more than 5000 times every hour when running. Most sports involve some sort of running or jumping, and so the foot is continually called upon to provide both stability and shock attenuation.

The first metatarsophalangeal joint

The first metatarsal bone joins proximally to the first cuneiform to form the first ray complex. Distally, the bone forms the first metatarsophalangeal (MP) joint with the proximal phalanx of the hallux. The first MP joint is reinforced over its plantar aspect by an area of fibrocartilage known as the volar plate (plantar accessory ligament). This is formed from the deep transverse metatarsal ligament, and the tendons of flexor hallucis brevis, adductor hallucis, and abductor hallucis. It has within it two sesamoid bones which serve as weight-bearing points for the metatarsal head (Fig. 14.1).

Movement of the joint is carried out by flexor hallucis longus, flexor hallucis brevis, extensor hallucis longus, the medial tendon of extensor digitorum brevis, and abductor and adductor hallucis. This fairly complex structure is often taken for granted but does give rise to a number of important conditions.

Turf toe

Turf toe is a sprain involving the plantar aspect of the capsule of the first MP joint. It is most often seen in athletes who play regularly on synthetic surfaces, and results from forced hyperextension (dorsiflexion) of the first MP joint. Normally this joint has a range of 50–60°, but with trauma the range may be forced to over 100°. The condition is quite common, with studies of American football players showing that 45% of athletes had suffered from turf toe at some stage (Rodeo et al., 1989).

Forced hyperextension of the first MP joint causes capsular tearing, collateral ligament damage and damage to the plantar accessory ligament. Sometimes force is so great that disruption of the medial sesamoid occurs (Fig. 14.2). Examination reveals a hyperaemic swollen joint with tenderness over the plantar surface of the metatarsal head. Local bruising may develop within 24 hours. Differential diagnosis must be made from sesamoid stress fracture (insidious onset) and metatarsal or phalangeal fractures (site of pain and radiograph).

Figure 14.3   Turf toe taping.

Figure 14.1   Structure of the first metatarsophalangeal joint.

Figure 14.2   Forced hyperextension causes soft tissue damage and possible sesamoid disruption—'turf toe'.

Treatment aims at reducing pain and inflammation and supporting the joint by taping (Fig. 14.3). An oval piece of felt or foam with a hole in the middle is placed beneath the toe, the hole corresponding to the metatarsal head. The first MP joint is held in neutral position and anchors are applied around the first phalanx and mid-foot. Strips of 2.5 cm inelastic tape are applied as stirrups between the anchors on the dorsal and plantar aspects of the toe. In each case the tape starts at the toe and is pulled towards the mid-foot, covering the first MP joint. The mid-foot and phalanx strips are finished with fixing strips.

A number of factors may predispose the athlete to turf toe. The condition is more common with artificial playing surfaces than with grass (Bowers and Martin, 1976). Artificial turf is less shock-absorbing, and so transmits more force directly to the first MP joint. Sports shoes also have an important part to play. Lighter shoes tend to be used with artificial playing surfaces. These shoes are more flexible around the distal forefoot, and allow the MP joint to hyperextend. In addition, shoes which are fitted by length size alone, rather than width, may cause problems for athletes with wider feet. This person must buy shoes which are too long to accommodate his or her foot width. Such a shoe increases the leverage forces acting on the toe joints and allows the foot to slide forwards in the shoe increasing the speed of movement at the joint.

Preventive measures include wearing shoes with more rigid soles, to avoid hyper-extension of the injured joint. In addition, semi-rigid (spring steel or heat-sensitive plastic) insoles may be used. Some authors recommend the use of rigid insoles as a preventive measure when playing on all-weather surfaces, for all athletes with less than 60° dorsiflexion at the first MP joint (Clanton, Butler and Eggert, 1986). An increased range of ankle dorsiflexion has been suggested as a risk factor which may predispose an athlete to turf toe (Rodeo et al., 1989). However, in walking subjects, when the ankle is strapped to reduce dorsiflexion, the heel actually lifts up earlier in the gait cycle, causing the range of motion at the metatarsal heads to increase (Carmines, Nunley and McElhaney, 1988). This increased range may once again predispose the athlete to turf toe (George, 1989), so the amount of dorsiflexion per se may not be that important. If injury has recently changed the range, the athlete may not have had time to fully adapt to the altered movement pattern, and the altered foot/ankle mechanics in total may be the problem.

As with many soft tissue injuries, if incorrectly managed the condition may predispose the athlete to arthritic changes in later life. In the case of turf toe, this may occur as calcification of the soft tissues around the injury site, presenting as hallux valgus or hallux rigidus.

Hallus valgus

Hallux valgus usually occurs when the first MP joint is hypermobile, and the first ray is shorter than the second (Morton foot structure). When this is the case, the second metatarsal head takes more pressure than in a non-Morton foot (Rodgers and Cavanagh, 1989) (Fig. 14.4). In addition, hallux valgus is more common in athletes who hyperpronate. As the first MP joint dorsiflexes during the propulsive phase of running, the instability allows the hallux to deviate from its normal plane. Adduction and axial rotation occur, and the long flexors which normally stabilize the joint, now themselves become

Figure 14.4 Pressure distribution in (a) Morton and (b) non-Morton feet. From Rodgers and Cavanagh (1989), with permission.

deforming influences. As the first metatarsal head adducts, the sesamoids sublux and eventually erode the plantar aspect of the first metatarsal head—this is one source of pain. Compensatory stress is placed on the joints proximal and distal to the first MP and further pain arises through synovial inflammation and capsular distraction. Eventually, secondary osteoarthritis occurs in the first MP joint and sesamoids. Bunion formation to the side of the first metatarsal head is common.

Management of this condition is initially to stabilize the first MP joint by correcting faulty foot mechanics (especially hyperpronation) and advising on correct athletic footwear. If conservative management fails, surgery may be required. If the deformity is purely soft tissue in nature, the bunion may be removed, and the dynamic structures around the first toe realigned. If bony deformity is present, osteotomy or arthroplasty may be necessary.

Hallux limitus/rigidus

A reduction in movement of the first MP joint, hallus limitus, may progress to complete immobility or hallux rigidus. The condition is more common when the first metatarsal is longer than the second. Pain is generally worse during sporting activities, and occurs especially when pushing off. On examination, the joint end feel is usually firm, and limitation of movement is noted to dorsiflexion. To differentiate between a tight flexor hallucis longus and joint structures, the foot is assessed both with the foot dorsiflexed and everted (tendon on stretch) and then plantarflexed and inverted (tendon relaxed). Limitation of motion through muscle tightness responds well to stretching procedures, while joint limitation which is soft tissue in nature is treated by joint mobilization. Distal distraction, and gliding mobilizations with the metatarsal head stabilized are particularly useful (Cibulka, 1990). Where bony deformity is present, surgery is indicated.

A number of surgical procedures are available for hallux conditions, and the interested reader is referred to Horn and Subotnick (1989) for an excellent review.

Plantar fasciitis

The plantar fascia (plantar aponeurosis) is the thickest fascia in the body. It attaches from a point just behind the medial tubercle of calcaneus and runs anteriorly as five slips. As the slips approach the metatarsal heads, they split into superficial and deep layers (Fig. 14.5a). The superficial layer attaches to superficial fascia beneath the skin, while the deep layer divides into medial and lateral portions to allow the passage of the flexor tendons. Each of the five portions attaches to the base of a proximal phalanx and to the deep transverse ligament. As the toes dorsiflex the fascia is wound around the metatarsal head (windlass effect). In so doing the fascia is tightened and the longitudinal arch elevated (Fig. 14.5b).

Inflammation of the plantar fascia is common in sports which involve repeated jumping, and with hill running. Overuse may cause microtears and inflammation of the fascial insertion, and nodules from the fascial granuloma can occasionally be felt (Tanner and Harvey, 1988).

(a)

Longitudinal arch elevated

(b)   Fascia tightened

Figure 14.5 Plantar fascia structure and action. (a) Normal tension in fascia. (b) Raising on to the toes tightens the plantar fascia and raises the longitudinal arch.

Normally, during mid-stance, the foot is flattened, stretching the plantar fascia and enabling it to store elastic energy to be released at toe off. However, a variety of malalignment faults may increase stress on the fascia. Excessive rearfoot pronation will lower the arch and overstretch the fascia, and a reduction in mobility of the first metatarsal may also contribute to the condition (Creighton and Olson, 1987). In addition, weak peronei, often the result of incomplete rehabilitation following ankle sprains, will reduce the support on the arch thus stressing the plantar fascia. Congenital problems such as pes cavus will also leave an athlete more susceptible to plantar fasciitis.

As the foot is plantarflexed with the toes on the ground, the fascia is stretched over the metatarsal heads, raising the longitudinal arch and making the foot more rigid. Plantar fasciitis is therefore exacerbated if the Achilles tendon is tight, or if high-heeled shoes are worn. Pain is often worse when taking the first few steps in the morning until the Achilles tendon is stretched.

Sports shoes play an important part in the course of this condition. Inadequate rearfoot control may fail to eliminate hyperpronation, and a poorly fitting heel counter will allow the calcaneal fat pad to spread at heel strike, transmitting extra impact force to the calcaneus and plantar fascia. On a hard surface, the shock-absorbing qualities of the shoe are important, and a patient's footwear should always be examined.

Pain is usually over the calcaneal attachment of the fascia or its medial edge. Pain may be localized to the heel as though the athlete is 'stepping on a stone', or may present as a burning pain over the arch. The problem must be differentiated from rheumatoid conditions which often give bilateral pain, and Sever's disease which gives pain to the insertion of the Achilles tendon.

Taping the foot (Fig. 14.6) may often give surprisingly rapid relief. The foot is locked in neutral position (pp. 221) and an anchor strap placed just behind the metatarsal heads. Three strips of tape (medial, lateral and central) are then passed from the anchor over the heel to stop on the posterior aspect of the calcaneum. A horseshoe-shaped fixing strip secures the tape behind the heel. Additional strips may be placed transversely across the foot from the metatarsal heads to the calcaneal tubercle.

More permanent management may require rearfoot posting to control excessive pronation. In addition, strengthening the intrinsic foot musculature is important. Although the plantar fascia is inert, stress on the structure may be increased when the intrinsic foot musculature is weak. The role of foot strengthening, including actively increasing the arch height, and 'gripping'

1. Anchor
2/3/4. Reins

Figure 14.6   Plantar fascia taping.

the floor with the toes, may have a re-education effect on plantar proprioception.

Heel pad

The calcaneus is covered by elastic adipose tissue in the same way as the finger tips. The fat cells are arranged in columns made from fibrous septa which lie vertically. As weight is taken, the walls of the columns bulge and spring back as the weight is released. With age the septa loose elasticity and the thickness of the heel pad reduces.

Athletes who wear poorly padded sports shoes and those who land heavily on the heel when jumping, may bruise this area. In more severe cases rupture of the fibrous septa may occur causing spillage of the enclosed fat cells (Reid, 1992). In turn, the loss of the heel pad shock-absorbing mechanism places excessive compression stress onto the calcaneum.

Pain is increased when walking bare foot. Typically, athletes complain of pain first thing in the morning when getting out of bed. The first few steps are exquisitely tender, later subsiding to a dull ache. Pain is brought on by prolonged standing and walking.

Management is by additional padding, and preventing the heel pad from spreading. Non-bottoming shock-absorbing materials are useful, and taping to surround the heel and prevent spread of the pad is effective in the short term (Fig. 14.7). Activity modification is required during the acute stage of the condition.

Morton's neuroma

Morton's neuroma affects the plantar interdigital nerve between the third and fourth metatarsal heads. Symptoms may occur spontaneously and are often described as feeling like 'electric shocks' along the sensory nerve distribution. The condition is more common with runners (particularly when sprinting and running uphill) and dancers, and is often aggravated by wearing narrow

high-heeled shoes. The sustained dorsiflexed position of these activities stretches the digital nerve causing inflammation. Once swollen, the nerve is open to entrapment between the metatarsal heads, and eventually the nerve is scarred and permanently enlarged to form a neuroma.

The patient's pain may be reproduced by direct pressure over the neuroma while compressing the forefoot medially and laterally. If the condition is caught in its oedematous stage, alteration of footwear (larger toe box and lower heel), ice application and ultrasound are effective. Injection with corticosteroid and local anaesthetic is also used. Padding the area with orthopaedic felt (Fig. 14.8) to take some of the body weight off the neuroma can give temporary relief. The arms of the pad rest on the adjacent metatarsals, leaving the area of the neuroma free.

Once the neuroma has formed, surgical excision under local anaesthesia is frequently required, with studies showing improvement in 80% of patients (Mann and Reynolds, 1983). There may be a permanent loss of sen-

Figure 14.8   Padding for interdigital neuroma.

Figure 14.7   Taping for heel pad.

sation over the plantar aspect of the foot supplied by the digital nerve, but in some cases regeneration occurs between 8 and 12 months after surgery.

Metatarsalgia

The term 'metatarsalgia' is often used to describe any pain in the forefoot. Such pain may come from a variety of conditions, including those affecting the hallux, a digital neuroma, or even stress fractures. However, in this description, we will limit the term to 'functional metatarsalgia', where altered foot function causes abnormal mechanical stress in the forefoot, which is symptomatic.

The transverse arch of the foot is supported at the level of the cuneiforms by peroneus longus, which pulls the medial and lateral edges of the foot together (Palastanga, Field and Soames, 1989). More distally, the arch is formed by the metatarsal heads, the highest point or 'keystone' being the second metatarsal. In mid-stance, the arch flattens and the five metatarsal heads come to lie in the same transverse plane to take the body weight. The first metatarsal takes weight through its sesamoid bones, and it and the fifth metatarsal are more mobile than the other three. Stability to the metatarsal heads is provided both passively by the transverse metatarsal ligament, and actively by adductor hallucis, and to a lesser extent, the intrinsics. Normally, these structures keep the metatarsals together. However, in cases of hypermobility such as excessive pronation or hallux valgus, the metatarsal heads may splay apart, effectively increasing the width of the forefoot, and allowing the central metatarsal heads to take too much weight.

Hypermobility may cause abnormal shearing forces, especially in an ill-fitting shoe, giving plantar keratosis. As the metatarsal heads splay, the transverse ligament and intrinsic muscles are subjected to tensile stress giving pain. Rigidity of the foot may

also cause problems. If any of the metatarsals are fixed, or if the toes are 'clawed', plantar compression will occur, again giving keratoma (Neale and Adams, 1989).

Clearly, successful management of the condition relies to a large extent on the identification of any underlying biomechanical abnormality in the foot. Short-term relief may be obtained by using anti-inflammatory modalities, and padding and strapping to relieve the stress on the forefoot tissues. An adhesive plantar metatarsal pad (PMP), made from orthopaedic felt, is contoured to cover the heads and upper shafts of the three central metatarsals, lifting them above ground level on weight-bearing (Fig. 14.9). The pad is cut around the head of the first metatarsal to avoid excessive pressure at this point. To prevent metatarsal splaying, inelastic strapping is placed around the forefoot, encircling the metatarsals just beneath the first and fifth metatarsal heads. If the metatarsals are immobile, a metatarsal bar may be built into the shoe. This has the effect of transferring the body weight to the metatarsal shafts and away from the painful metatarsal head.

Coupled with strapping and padding, strengthening the intrinsic muscles is essential. Simple exercises, such as 'gripping the floor' with the toes in bare feet, are effective at building isometric strength and endurance of the intrinsics. Eccentric strength is simi-

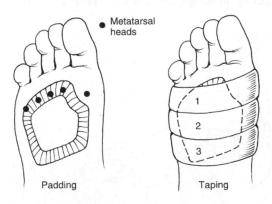

Figure 14.9 Metatarsal padding and tape.

larly developed by initially tensing the intrinsic muscles of the foot and increasing the arch with the leg non-weight-bearing. The body weight is then taken onto the foot and gradually the arch is allowed to flatten under control.

Cuboid syndrome

Pain over the lateral aspect of the foot may represent subluxation of the cuboid. This is more common in dancers, where 17% of foot and ankle injuries have been found to be cuboid-related (Marshall and Hamilton, 1992). The condition is also seen following ankle sprain. At the time of injury, the ligamentous support of the calcaneocuboid joint and the metatarsal cuboid joint may be disrupted. When this occurs in an athlete with a markedly pronated foot, the peroneus longus, travelling through the groove of the cuboid, may pull the medial edge of the cuboid down.

Dull pain is experienced over the lateral aspect of the foot and along the course of peroneus longus tendon. Pain is increased with prolonged standing and exercise on unforgiving surfaces and/or in poor athletic footwear. Typically, the pain is worse for the first few steps in the morning and is lessened when non-weight-bearing, and when walking on the toes (foot supinated).

The subluxation may be reduced by manual therapy. Two methods are typically used (Marshall and Hamilton, 1992). In the first, the patient is supine and the therapist distracts the cuboid fourth metatarsal joint by placing traction through the fourth metatarsal shaft. At the same time the foot is plantarflexed and relocation of the cuboid is spontaneous. Where this technique fails, manipulation may succeed. The patient is prone and the therapist grasps the patient's foot placing his thumbs over the plantar surface of the cuboid. A high velocity low amplitude thrust is then performed forcing the foot into plantarflexion, while the reduc-tion pressure is maintained over the base of the cuboid. Once reduced, the cuboid position is maintained with a felt pad and tape.

Accessory movements of the foot

In many conditions affecting the foot and ankle, accessory movements of the joints of the mid-foot and forefoot may be reduced. Mobilization procedures require accurate fixation of one segment while mobilization of an adjacent segment is carried out. Kaltenborn (1989) described a logical series of movements of use for examination and manual treatment.

On the lateral side of the foot a number of movements focus on the cuboid. Initially, the cuboid is moved on the fixed calcaneum. The navicular and lateral cuneiform are fixed and the cuboid is then moved upon them. Finally the cuboid itself is fixed and the fourth and fifth metatarsals are moved.

On the medial side of the foot, movements are around the navicular and cuneiforms. The navicular is fixed and the cuboid and then the cuneiforms are moved. The navicular itself is moved on the talus. Finally, the cuneiforms are fixed and the second and third metatarsals moved (Fig. 14.10).

Skin and nail lesions

Subungual haematoma

In this condition, a haematoma forms directly below the nail plate as a result of direct trauma. Pressure builds up in the space between the nail and nail bed, causing acute pain and throbbing. In some cases the pressure may be great enough to loosen the nail from its bed. Subungual haematoma is often referred to as 'black toe' or 'runner's toe'. Ill-fitting shoes are a common cause, if the toe box is too small the nail may rub, especially when running downhill.

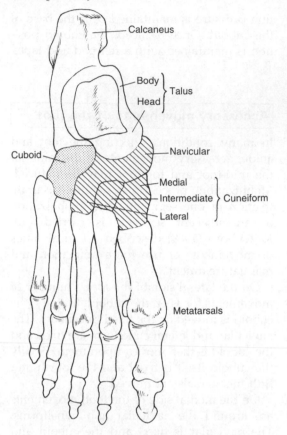

Figure 14.10 The lateral side of the foot is moved around the cuboid. The medial side around the navicular and cuneiforms.

When the problem is acute, the haematoma is often decompressed by the athlete penetrating the nail with a red-hot needle or paperclip to release the blood (Subotnick, 1989). A less hazardous approach is for the therapist to use a sterile needle. The best treatment for chronic haemorrhage is to remove the cause, and buy shoes which allow enough room for the toes to spread on weight-bearing and expand with warmth. When standing, a sports shoe should allow one thumb's breadth between the end of the shoe and the athlete's longest toe.

Onychocryptosis

Onychocryptosis, or ingrown toe-nail, is particularly common in the hallux of athletes, especially males. It may occur secondarily to ill-fitting sports shoes, or to incorrect toenail cutting. Shoes are often too narrow, leading to lateral pressure on the hallux, and athletes often cut the toe nails too short causing the underlying soft tissues to protrude. Cutting across the corners of the nail is another common fault in footcare, allowing the nail to embed itself into the nail grooves. Frequently, excessive sweating (hyperhidrosis) causes skin softening, a condition exacerbated by prolonged hot bathing.

A splinter of nail grows into the subcutaneous tissue, and with time, acute inflammation occurs possibly with infection (paronychia). The skin becomes red, tight and shiny, and the toe swells. There is throbbing pain and acute tenderness to palpation. Normal healing will not take place as long as the nail splinter remains, and so hypergranulation occurs. The combination of granulation tissue and the swollen nail-fold overlaps the nail plate itself.

When the condition occurs without infection, the nail splinter may be removed with a scalpel (size 15), avoiding further damage to the sulcus. The edge of the nail is smoothed and the area washed with saline. The nail edge is then packed with cotton wool allowing some to rest under the nail plate itself. The area is protected with a sterile dressing, and regularly inspected.

When the condition is accompanied by infection, a local anaesthetic is used, injecting at the base of the toe away from the infected area. Oral antibiotics may be used and/or an antiseptic dressing applied. Hypergranulation tissue is excised. If this procedure is ineffective, nail surgery involving partial or complete nail avulsion is required (Neale and Adams, 1989).

Prevention of the problem relies on the use of correctly fitting sports shoes, and on cutting the nails to the shape of the end of the toe, while avoiding splintering the nail sides. It is good practice to address basic footcare at the beginning of the season, especially with athletes new to the squad.

Blisters

Blisters occur as a result of compression or shearing on the skin. A narrow toe box may cause blisters over the medial aspect of the fifth toe, and between the first and second toes in the case of hallux valgus. Blisters over the plantar aspect of the foot are common when sports shoes are loose. Shoes should be fitted correctly and friction reduced wherever possible. Petroleum jelly, or plastic backed moist gel squares used between the toes is helpful. Proper foot hygiene which may include powder or astringents to dry the foot should be observed.

Acute blisters may be drained through a puncture hole. A sterile needle is used and enters the blister at the side, the needle being held parallel to the skin. This will leave a skin flap intact for protection. The underlying cause of the blister should be addressed.

Athlete's foot

Tinea pedis or 'athlete's foot' is the most common fungal infection of the feet, and is particularly rampant in communal washing areas within sport, and where standards of hygiene are poor. Sports shoes create moisture and warmth between the toes, conditions in which the complaint thrives. Three types of tinea pedis are generally seen. First, the lateral toe spaces become macerated, due to three organisms, *Trichophyton rubrum*, *Trichophyton interdigitale* and *Epidermophyton floccosum*. Secondly, the condition may spread to the soles of the feet where vesiculation occurs as a result of *T. interdigitale* and *E. floccosum*, and finally a diffuse 'moccasin type' scaling appears usually due to *T. rubrum*. The condition may also spread to the nails, and hands in some cases.

Treatment is initially aimed at removing the scaling tissue by the application of surgical spirit. When the scaling has cleared, antifungal dusting powders, such as tolnaftate, are used. Sprays containing clotrimazole,

and dusting powders are used by the athlete, and socks and footwear should be changed daily and preferably disinfected. While the infection remains, athletes should not go barefoot in public areas (changing rooms and swimming baths), and should not share towels, socks or footwear.

Hyperkeratosis

Keratinization is a normal physiological process which turns the stratum corneum of the skin into a hard protective cover. The process becomes overactive if the skin is continually subjected to mechanical stress, for example on the hands of heavy manual workers, or the feet of athletes. Hyperaemia occurs, stimulating a proliferation of epidermal cells, and at the same time the rate of desquamation reduces. This type of keratoma or callus on the foot has a protective function, and providing it is asymptomatic it should be left in place. However, when the bulk of such tissues becomes excessive and causes pain or deformity, treatment is required.

The size and shape of the hyperkeratosis is largely dictated by the stress imposed on the skin. A callus is a diffuse area of thickened skin resulting from stress over a fairly wide area, while a corn is a smaller concentrated area which has formed into a nucleus. Corns typically seen in sports medicine are either soft or hard, although vascular and neurovascular types do exist. Soft corns are common in the cleft between the fourth and fifth toes, and appear macerated due to sweat retention. The corn nucleus is generally ring-shaped and the centre of the lesion is very thin. Hard corns occur on the plantar aspect of the foot beneath the metatarsal heads, or on the dorsum of the interphalangeal joints. They develop because of concentrated pressure due to body weight and ground reaction forces. The corn nucleus is often associated with surrounding callus due to shearing stress.

The corn or callus may be removed with a scalpel by a therapist and the corn nucleus eradicated. Antiseptic agents such as cetrimide and chlorhexidine are then applied. Moist skin is treated with salicylic acid or aluminium chlorohydrate, and excessively dry skin managed with an emollient containing urea, or soft white paraffin. It is important to remove the underlying cause of the keratoma so that it does not simply return. Examination of foot biomechanics and sports footwear is therefore essential.

Verruca

Verruca pedis is a lesion caused by one of the human papilloma viruses (HPV), of which about 15 have been identified. A benign epithelial tumour, which is self-limiting, is produced in the plantar skin. The wart is covered by hyperkeratotic tissue, and contains brown or black specks caused by intravascular thromboses within its dilated capillaries. Where the wart is over a weight-bearing site, it is forced into the dermis leaving just the hyperkeratotic area on the surface. For this reason athletes often assume a verruca is simply a corn or callus. However, close inspection will usually reveal the papillary appearance of the verruca. A number of other factors differentiate the two. A wart has a far more rapid onset than an area of callus, and may occur in an area of skin not associated with mechanical stress. In addition, bleeding can occur if the verruca is cut because of capillary dilatation, whereas a callus is avascular.

The virus normally enters the body through broken skin in the foot, especially if the foot has been wet and the skin macerated. Unfortunately, the virus spreads quickly through a population before the plantar wart becomes obvious. The aim of treatment is to destroy all the cells within the lesion by chemical cautery or cryosurgery. Various preparations are used. The skin surrounding the area is protected, and a liquid or paste of salicylic acid (or monochloroacetic acid) is applied. An aseptic necrosis is produced, and destroyed tissue is removed one week later.

Cryosurgery aims at freezing the verruca, with carbon dioxide snow, nitrous oxide, or liquid nitrogen applied through a probe. Tissue necrosis with blister formation occurs when the skin is cooled to $-20°C$ and bluish coloration results. The rapid cooling causes ice crystals to form in the body cells and interstitial fluids, which in turn ruptures the cells. Liquid nitrogen is perhaps the most common of the cryosurgery techniques, applied by dipping a cotton-tipped stick into the liquid. This is applied to the verruca for about 30–60 seconds. The lesion is protected by a cavity pad if it is over a weight-bearing area.

If the verruca is not painful, treatment may not be required as the lesion will regress naturally in some months (Neale and Adams, 1989). However, cross-infection must still be guarded against by the use of plastic waterproof socks in public areas.

The sports shoe

The design of sports shoes has received a great deal of attention over the last two decades. This interest has to a large extent been market-led due to the massive increase in the number of people jogging. Manufacturers vie with each other to produce a shoe feature which can act as a 'unique selling point' to give them an increased market share.

There is little doubt that shoe design has improved, and that athletes have benefited from this. However, many developments are simply variations on the same theme and give little substantial improvement to overall shoe design. In addition, the mounting cost of sports shoes makes it imperative that athletes receive the right advice concerning the shoe which will best suit their foot and be appropriate to their sport.

As most sports involve running, more emphasis will be given to the features of running shoes, as many of these features are carried over into other sports footwear.

Forces acting on the foot

During the stance phase of running, the foot must accommodate to three phases, heel strike, mid-stance and toe off, during which the biomechanics of the foot changes considerably. At heel strike the single force of the foot moving downwards and forwards may be resolved into two components. The first, is an impact stress acting vertically, and the second a horizontal shearing force, creating friction. Not all athletes strike the ground with the heel when running. For some 80% the initial contact point is at the heel (Frederick et al., 1984). The ground reaction force curve in this case shows an initial (passive) peak at heel strike of about half body weight, occurring 20–30 ms after heel strike. A secondary (active) peak occurs approximately 100 ms after heel contact as the centre of pressure

moves over the ball of the foot prior to toe off (Fig. 14.11).

Other runners show a centre of pressure over the mid-foot or rearfoot (Fig. 14.12). The magnitude of the force acting on the foot can be as much as three times body weight.

The rearfoot runner strikes the ground with his knee locked, and consequently will require more shock attenuation from the sports shoe. The mid-foot or forefoot striker has his knee slightly flexed, and so part of the contact shock is absorbed by the elasticity of the knee structures. In some cases, the heel does not touch the ground at all, leaving the stance phase under the control of the posterior leg muscles. With this type of runner, the shock-absorbing function of a heel wedge will be under-utilized.

During midstance there can be 5° of abduction of the foot, causing friction between the shoe and running surface. This creates a torsion force which tends to rotate the upper part of the shoe in relation to the sole (Cavanagh, 1989).

Figure 14.11 Ground reaction forces in rearfoot and mid-foot runners. From Segesser and Pforringer (1989), with permission.

Figure 14.12   Force vector curves for rearfoot and mid-foot runners. From Segesser and Pforringer (1989), with permission.

Components of a running shoe

The outer sole (Fig. 14.13) of a shoe is generally a carbon rubber material with treads or studs cut in. The outer sole must provide a combination of four features: grip (traction), durability, flexibility and light weight. Studs provide better cross-country grip while bars are more durable on hard surfaces and so

better suited to road shoes. However, the thicker studs or cleats of a cross-country or fell-running shoe will also add weight, so faster road-racing shoes tend to have thin, smoother soles.

Beneath the sole is the midsole, extending the full length of the shoe, and the wedge which begins behind the metatarsal heads and extends back to the heal. These take the place of the wooden 'shank' of the traditional street shoe. Both the midsole and wedge are designed for cushioning, giving good elastic recoil, but they must also maintain good foot control. They are usually two or three layers of different foam materials, such as ethyl vinyl acetate (EVA), or more expensive polyurethane. Thicker materials tend to give better cushioning, but they will also raise the foot off the ground creating greater leverage forces if the foot contacts the ground at the side of the sole.

On top of the midsole is the insole board, again running the whole length of the shoe. This semi-rigid board stops the foot from twisting and so provides stability. The edge of the shoe upper is usually fastened below the insole board, and the board itself may be chemically treated to resist deterioration from moisture or micro-organism growth.

The heel counter provides rearfoot stability, helping to prevent over pronation and

Figure 14.13   Parts of the sports shoe.

is usually a hard thermoplastic, which will keep its rigidity. Poorer quality shoes may have cardboard heel counters which will feel stiff when the shoe is new, but quickly soften and allow excessive rearfoot motion. Often the heel counter itself will have an additional support.

The shoe upper is contoured to the foot, and made from three sections. The 'vamp' covers the forefoot, and the mid-foot and hindfoot are covered by the medial and lateral quarters, respectively. The nylon upper provides lightness and breathability, and is supported by the eyestay and arch bandage. The eyestay will normally have eyelets for lacing, and the arch bandage is positioned at the highest point of the longitudinal arch of the foot.

The foot rests within the shoe, directly on top of the sock liner. This should be removable for washing and can also have further padding, such as gel or air sacks incorporated into it. The liner is designed primarily to reduce friction and absorb sweat, and may be removed when an orthotic device is placed into the shoe.

The ankle collar should be heavily padded and soft, and the heel tab (pull tab) should be notched to prevent friction on the Achilles tendon during toe off. Some older designs of sports shoes still have so-called 'Achilles tendon protectors'. Unfortunately, the effect of these is usually to injure rather than protect. As the foot is plantarflexed, the Achilles tendon tab will press onto the Achilles tendon causing friction, one cause of Haglund's syndrome (see p. 303). Shoes of this type may be modified by cutting a slot down each side of the tab or simply cutting the tab off, providing neither or these solutions interferes with the overall shoe structure.

Many shoes have variable lacing systems to accommodate different foot widths and ensure that the shoe fits the foot snugly. With reference to shoe width, it is important to encourage athletes to stand and walk around/jog in sports shoes before they buy them. Obviously the foot spreads with weight-bearing, so if the shoe is tried on when sitting it will not give an accurate impression of fit.

Shoe function

Cushioning effects of shoes have been shown to reduce initial impact at heel strike by as much as 50% (Light, McLellan and Klenerman, 1980; Subotnick, 1989). The aim is to reduce or 'attenuate' the peak forces to levels which are well tolerated by the human body, and which do not result either in trauma or overuse injury. At the same time, the forces produced at toe off have to be conserved to maintain running efficiency.

Heel materials which are too soft will compress or 'bottom out', while those which are too hard reduce cushioning. In addition, the construction of the shoe will also affect shock absorption. A stiff insole board for example, cemented to a soft mid-sole will give the shoe a functional hardness usually found only with much firmer mid-sole materials (Frederick, 1989).

The overhand or 'flare' of the sole of a running shoe creates leverage force which exaggerates pronation and foot slap (Fig. 14.14). When running barefoot, the sub-talar joint axis lies over the ground contact point as does the ankle joint axis (Fig. 14.14a). Wearing a typical running shoe, the leverage force created by the heel flare places the ground contact point further away from the sub-talar joint axis, thus increasing the leverage effect by a factor of three (Fig. 14.14b). In the sagittal plane, the heel flare moves the ground contact point back, further from the ankle joint, thus increasing the leverage effect. To compensate, the anterior tibial muscles have to work harder. By altering the heel to a more rounded design, and using a shoe with a dual density mid-sole, over-pronation can be limited.

The sole of a sports shoe should bend at a point just proximal to the metatarsal heads, to an angle of about 30°. Bending a stiffer

Figure 14.14   Effect of leverage in running shoes. (a) Running barefoot, the sub-talar joint axis lies over the ground contact point, as does the ankle joint. (b) The 'overhang' of the shoes moves the ground contact point further from the sub-taloid and ankle joints, increasing the leverage effect. Muscle action is required to compensate. From Subotnick (1989), with permission.

sole may increase energy expenditure, and could therefore lead to local muscle fatigue. A lighter shoe is more energy conserving. Frederick (1985) showed that carrying 100 g excess weight on the foot increased energy expenditure by 1%; enough, he claimed, to add 1 or 2 minutes onto the time of a competitive marathon runner. Similarly, softer soled shoes are more energy conserving. The same author showed a 2.8% reduction in energy expenditure for subjects wearing soft-soled shoes while running a marathon.

The ideal combination of features in a running shoe is unfortunately not possible. There is always a compromise because many of the attributes are contradictory. Cushioning conflicts with qualities of stability and flexibility. Decreasing the hardness of the sole can increase pronation, so to get adequate cushioning, a thicker more shock-absorbing sole is chosen rather than a softer one.

By combining data from various sources, Frederick (1989) analysed the relationship between heel height, maximum pronation, and hardness of a sole to find an 'ideal' combination. He concluded that optimum cushioning and rearfoot control are obtained in a shoe with a heel height of 25–35 mm with cushioning values of 40–55 shore A. Hardness is quantified by measuring the resistance of a material to the penetration of a defined object. The shore A scale runs from 0 (softest) to 100 (hardest).

This combination would, however, give a reduction in sole flexibility, as highly flexible soles are usually soft and thin. Fig. 14.15 demonstrates the stresses produced when a sole is bent. The top of the sole is compressed, and the bottom tensioned. To

Figure 14.15 Stresses produced when the sole is flexed. The bottom layers are in tension, while the top layers are compressed. From Segesser and Pforringer (1989), with permission.

make the sole more flexible, while still maintaining its cushioning effect, a bar of softer material is placed in the top layer of the sole just behind the metatarsal heads. In addition, grooves are cut in the bottom of the sole at the point of bending.

Is a running shoe necessary?

Robbins and Hanna (1987) argued that habitually unshod humans are not susceptible to chronic overloading of the foot. Locomotion in barefoot adapted subjects (those who regularly run unshod) differs considerably from that of normal shod subjects. When walking, unshod subjects attempt to grip the ground with their toes, and when running the medial longitudinal arch flattens completely during mid-stance. Foot flattening when running unshod is probably a result of eccentric muscle action and elastic deformation of the intrinsic foot musculature and plantar fascia. Robbins and Gouw (1990) claimed that this response is behaviourly induced in the barefoot adapted runner. They argued that the subject was attempting to minimize discomfort by transferring forefoot load from the metatarsal phalangeal joints to the distal digits. This process, they claimed, results in hypertrophy of the intrinsic musculature, and relaxes the plantar fascia (Fig. 14.16).

Robbins and Gouw (1990) argued that this shock moderating behaviour of the foot is related to plantar sensibility. The subject attempts to minimize discomfort by increasing the activity of the intrinsic muscles. However, a running shoe with a thick soft sole, will mask sensation to the plantar surface of the foot, and so the subject will not use the intrinsic muscles to their full extent.

The above authors therefore recommend that runners run barefoot, after a progressive period of adaptation. Where a runner is not able to do this each day, or where safety factors prevent it, Robbins and Gouw advised a less yielding shoe which provides adequate sensory feedback.

Figure 14.16 Function of intrinsic musculature in the (a) unshod and (b) shod foot. From Robbins and Gouw (1990), with permission.

When assessing proprioceptive function of the foot, foot position error has been shown to be 107.5% poorer with subjects wearing athletic footwear than those who were barefoot. In addition, those who wore footwear were unable to distinguish between a flat surface and a 20° slope angle when blindfolded (Robbins, Waked and Rappel, 1995). These authors argued that the use of footwear was largely responsible for ankle injury, in that it reduced the input from plantar cutaneous mechanoreceptors.

Athletic footwear has also been shown to contribute to falling frequency (Robbins et al., 1994). Using balance beam walking, these authors found that mid-sole hardness was positively related to stability, while mid-sole thickness was negatively related. The authors concluded that shoes with thick, soft soles acted to destabilize an individual whereas thin, hard-soled shoes provided superior stability.

The above mentioned papers raise a number of interesting points. First, they illustrate the importance of the active shock-absorbing mechanisms of the foot, rather than viewing the foot simply as a 'passive falling object'. Secondly, the often forgotten significance of sensory feedback from the plantar surface of the foot is stressed.

The court shoe

In running, foot movements occur cyclically, but in court games such as tennis, squash and badminton, the movements are more varied both in direction, and speed. The casual tennis player makes contact mostly with the heel, and less with the ball of the foot. However, when a player is under pressure the situation is reversed. Now, contact is more frequently made with the ball of the foot than the heel, and contact with the medial and lateral edges of the foot is increased (Nigg, Luthi and Bahlsen, 1989).

Movement most commonly occurs in the forward direction, but when under pressure the tennis player moves laterally more frequently. This movement is often combined with contact on the forefoot.

A court shoe must allow all of these movements. The same heel–toe mechanism found in a running shoe is required, but in addition, force attenuation from forefoot contact is needed. The frictional characteristics of the shoe to surface are important. Both translational and rotational movements are needed, translation less so in surfaces which permit some degree of sliding, such as indoor courts or sand/granules.

Because the demands placed on the foot when playing court games are so different to those encountered in road running, athletes must be discouraged from wearing the same shoes for both sports unless they use specifically designed 'cross training' footwear. During lateral movements in particular, the leverage involved with the higher (flared) heel of the running shoe makes injury much more likely. Similarly, tennis shoes do not give adequate rearfoot control or shock attenuation for running.

The soccer boot

In football, the ball may reach velocities of 140 km/h (Masson and Hess, 1989). This speed combined with the weight of the ball, especially when wet, leads to deformation of both the boot and foot with kicking. Forces generated may lead to microtrauma to the foot and ankle. Soccer footwear must therefore be as light as possible to minimize any excessive forces created by kicking. At the same time, the shoe must provide both support and protection for the foot.

Combinations of rotation and flexion with the foot fixed to the ground are particularly taxing on the knee structures. Most boots unfortunately compound this problem by the use of cleats or studs, which although improving grip on a wet surface, will also increase rotation forces by reducing 'give'. Indoor surfaces in some cases offer greater grip with similar problems, and shoes need a sole with a greater number of smaller studs to compensate for this.

Shoes must allow the increased range of movement required in soccer, and be flexible enough to accommodate forefoot rocking. Any studs must be placed to avoid pressure irritation to the plantar aspect of the foot. Studs on the heel are placed towards the outside of the shoe to avoid rocking or buckling on weight-bearing.

The sports surface

Ground reaction forces may be resolved into both horizontal and vertical components. The vertical component occurs because of gravity, and the horizontal component is a result of friction. The hardness (ability to withstand distortion) of the ground surface or the sports shoe greatly influences the vertical component of the reaction force on landing (impact force). The playing surface will distort in one of two ways, known as point elasticity and area elasticity (Fig. 14.17). Point elasticity refers to a surface's ability to compress under weight, while area elasticity is a measure of its ability to flex as a whole.

Frictional characteristics occur as a result of the interaction between the shoe and playing surface. The friction that occurs will be influenced by moisture and floor treatments, and surfaces with different frictional proper-

Point elasticity   Area elasticity

Figure 14.17   Distortion of a playing surface.

ties will impose different loads on the body. As a consequence, performance characteristics such as energy expenditure and muscle work will change with different sports surfaces, and so will the type and frequency of injury. High amounts of friction may produce excessive forces on the knees and ankles (Ekstrand and Nigg, 1989) while too little friction can cause slipping which could result in trauma. Both translational (straight line) and rotational (twisting) friction are important. Translational friction is needed for athletes to stop and start, but as it increases so does the possibility for abrasion injuries. Higher levels of rotational friction may increase the likelihood of injury when a player is tackled with his weight-bearing leg fixed to the ground. Clearly, there are optimal levels for both types of friction, and simply increasing the amount of friction by changing the shoe or sports surface to give the player 'more grip' is not satisfactory. Frictional characteristics may also be important for the development of arthritis in later life. In one study (quoted in Nigg and Segresser, 1988) from a group of individuals suffering hip arthritis, a greater number were found to be athletes, and 70% of these had participated on surfaces where the foot was 'locked' to the surface.

While the number of non-severe injuries, such as abrasions, seen on artificial surfaces is increased, the frequency of severe injuries remains about the same. Importantly, the number of abrasions suffered on an artificial surface can be reduced by accustomizing players to the new surface (Nigg and Segesser, 1988; Ekstrand and Nigg, 1989). In addition, because artificial surfaces have different frictional characteristics to grass surfaces, the footwear worn by athletes must also be different. Torg and Quedenfeld (1971) showed both frequency and severity of injury to be greater when athletes used conventional shoes using seven cleats (19 mm) than when they used shoes with 14 smaller (9.5 mm) cleats on an artificial playing surface.

Surface construction

Sports were traditionally performed on grass playing-fields outside, and wooden floors indoors. Later, sprung wooden flooring became the norm for indoor surfaces, while cinder became increasingly popular outdoors. The 1960s saw the development of synthetic resins which could be produced and applied on site at ambient temperatures, to create a playing surface. These new artificial playing surfaces had the advantage of much lower operating and maintenance costs. The maintenance costs of an artificial playing surface for soccer for example is 15% of the cost for a traditional grass surface (Ekstrand and Nigg, 1989).

Outdoor surfaces are most commonly of single layer or sandwich construction, with a variety of porous and non-porous materials being used. Indoor surfaces include spring boards mounted crosswise over wooden slats (area elastic), and elastic base layers with a PVC covering (point elastic).

References

Bowers, K.D. and Martin, R.B. (1976) Turf toe: a shoe-surface related football injury. *Medicine and Science in Sports and Exercise*, **8**, 81–83

Carmines, D.V., Nunley, J.A. and McElhaney, J.H. (1988) Effects of ankle taping on the motion and loading pattern of the foot for walking subjects. *Journal of Orthopaedic Research*, **6**, 223–229

Cavanagh, P.R. (1989) The biomechanics of running and running shoe problems. In *The Shoe in Sport* (eds B. Segesser and W. Pforringer), Year Book Medical Publishers, Wolfe, London

Cibulka, M.T. (1990) Management of a patient with forefoot pain: a case report. *Physical Therapy*, **70**(1), 55–58

Clanton, T.O., Butler, J.E. and Eggert, A. (1986) Injuries to the metatarsophalangeal joints in athletes. *Foot and Ankle*, **7**, 162–176

Creighton, D.S. and Olson, V.L. (1987). Evaluation of range of motion of the first metatarsophalangeal joint in runners with plantar fasciitis. *Journal of Orthopaedic and Sports Physical Therapy*, **8**, 357–361

Ekstrand, J. and Nigg, B.M. (1989) Surface-related injuries in soccer. *Sports Medicine*, **8**(1), 56–62

Frederick, E.C. (1985) The energy cost of load carriage on the feet during running. In *Biomechanics IX* (eds D.A. Winter et al.), Human Kinetics Publishers, Champaign, Illinois

Frederick, E.C. (1989) The running shoe: dilemmas and dichotomies in design. In *The Shoe in Sport* (eds B. Segesser and W. Pforringer), Year Book Medical Publishers, Wolfe, London

Frederick, E.C., Clarke, T.E. and Hamill, C.L. (1984) The effect of running shoe design on shock attenuation. In *Sports Shoes and Playing Surfaces* (ed. E.C. Frederick), Human Kinetics Publishers, Champaign, Illinois, pp. 190–198

George, F.J. (1989). In *Year Book of Sports Medicine* (ed. R.J. Shephard), Year Book Medical Publishers, Chicago, pp. 75

Hertling, D. and Kessler, R.M. (1990) *Management of Common Musculoskeletal Disorders*, J.B. Lippincott, Philadelphia

Horn, L.M. and Subotnick, S.I. (1989) Surgical intervention. In *Sports Medicine of the Lower Extremity* (ed. S.I. Subotnick), Churchill Livingstone, London

Kaltenborn, F.M. (1989) *Manual Mobilisation of the Extremity Joints*, 4th edn, Olaf Norlis Bokhandel, Norway

Light, L.H., McLellan, G.E. and Klenerman K (1980) Skeletal transients on heel strike in normal walking with different footwear. *Journal of Biomechanics*, **13**, 477

Mann, R.A. and Reynolds, J.C. (1983) Interdigital neuroma: a critical analysis. *Journal of Foot and Ankle Surgery*, **3**, 238

Marshal, P. and Hamilton, W.G. (1992) Cuboid subluxation in ballet dancers. *American Journal of Sports Medicine*, **20**, 169–175

Masson, M. and Hess, H. (1989) Typical soccer injuries—their effects on the design of the athletic shoe. In *The Shoe in Sport* (eds B. Segesser and W. Pforringer), Year Book Medical Publishers, Wolfe, London

Neale, D. and Adams, I.M. (1989) *Common Foot Disorders*, Churchill Livingstone, London

Nigg, B.M. and Segesser, B. (1988) The influence of playing surfaces on the load on the locomotor system and on football and tennis injuries. *Sports Medicine*, **5**, 375–385

Nigg, B.M., Luthi, S.M. and Bahlsen, H.A. (1989) The tennis shoe—biomechanical design criteria. In *The Shoe in Sport* (eds B. Segesser and W. Pforringer), Year Book Medical Publishers, Wolfe, London

Palastanga, N., Field, D. and Soames, R. (1989) *Anatomy and Human Movement*, Heinemann Medical, Oxford

Reid, D.C. (1992) *Sports Injury Assessment and Rehabilitation*, Churchill Livingstone, London

Robbins, S.E. and Gouw, G.J. (1990) Athletic footwear and chronic overloading. *Sports Medicine*, **9**(2), 76–85

Robbins, S.E. and Hanna, A.M. (1987) Running related injury prevention through barefoot adaptations. *Medicine and Science in Sports and Exercise*, **19**, 148–156

Robbins, S., Waked, E., Gouw, G.J. and McClaran, J. (1994) Athletic footwear affects balance in men. *British Journal of Sports Medicine*, **28**, 117–122

Robbins, S., Waked, E. and Rappel, R. (1995) Ankle taping improves proprioception before and after exercise in young men. *British Journal of Sports Medicine*, **29**(4), 242–247

Rodeo, S.A., O'Brian, S.J. and Warren, R.F. (1989) Turf toe: an analysis of metatarsophalangeal joint sprains in professional football players. *American Journal of Sports Medicine*, **17**(4), 125–131

Rodeo, S.A., O'Brian, S.J., Warren, R.F., Barnes, R. and Wickiewicz, T.L. (1989) Turf toe: diagnosis and treatment *Physician and Sports Medicine*, **17**(4), 132–147

Rodgers, M.M. and Cavanagh, P.R. (1989) Pressure distribution in Morton's foot structure. *Medicine and Science in Sports and Exercise*, **21**, 23–28

Segesser, B. and Pforringer, W. (eds) *The Shoe in Sport*, Wolfe, London

Subotnick, S.I (1989) *Sports Medicine of the Lower Extremity*, Churchill Livingstone, London

Tanner, S.M. and Harvey, J.S. (1988) How we manage plantar fasciitis. *Physician and Sports Medicine*, **16**(8), 39-47

Torg, J.S. and Quedenfeld, T. (1971) Effect of shoe type and cleat length on incidence and severity of knee injuries among high school football players. *Research Quarterly* **42**, 203–211

15

The lumbar spine

Spinal problems are amongst the most common conditions encountered by the physiotherapist or physical medicine practitioner. More working days are lost because of back pain than any other single condition, and sport does not escape this epidemic. It is estimated that 80% of the population will suffer at least one disabling episode of low back pain during their lives, and at any one time as many as 35% of people will be suffering from backache of some sort (Fryomoyer and Cats-Baril, 1991).

Although an in-depth study of back pain is outside the scope of this book, it is necessary to look at a number of features of spinal injury which are important within the context of sport. Much of the material for the initial parts of this section is modified from Norris (1995), and the reader is referred to this article series for a more in-depth review.

The spinal disc

There are 24 intervertebral discs lying between successive vertebrae, making the spine an alternatively rigid then elastic column. The amount of flexibility present in a particular spinal segment will be determined by the size and shape of the disc, and the resistance to motion of the soft tissue support to the spinal joints. The discs increase in size as they descend the column, the lumbar discs having an average thickness of 10 mm, twice that of the cervical discs. The disc shapes are accommodated to the curvatures of the spine, and the shapes of the vertebrae. The greater anterior widths of the discs in the cervical and lumbar regions reflect the curvatures of these areas. Each disc is made up of three closely related components, the annulus fibrosis, nucleus pulposus and cartilage end plates.

The annulus is composed of layers of fibrous tissue arranged in concentric bands (Fig. 15.1). Each band has fibres arranged in parallel, and the various bands are in turn angled at 45° to each other. The bands are more closely packed anteriorly and posteriorly than they are laterally, and those innermost are the thinnest. Each disc has about 20 bands in all, and fibre orientation, although partially determined at birth, is influenced by torsional stresses in the adult (Palastanga, Field and Soames, 1989). The posterolateral regions have a more irregular make-up, and this may be one reason why they become weaker with age, predisposing them to injury.

The annular fibres pass over the edge of the cartilage end plate of the disc, and are anchored to the bony rim of the vertebra and to its periosteum and body. The attaching fibres are actually interwoven with the fibres of the bony trabeculae of the vertebral

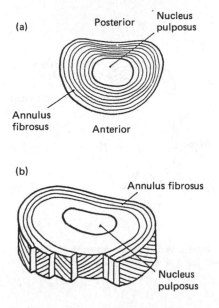

(a)

Posterior   Nucleus pulposus

Annulus fibrosus   Anterior

(b)

Annulus fibrosus

Nucleus pulposus

Figure 15.1 (a) Concentric band of annular fibres. (b) Horizontal section through a disc. From Oliver and Middleditch (1991), with permission.

body. The outer layer of fibres blend with the posterior longitudinal ligament, but the anterior longitudinal ligament has no such attachment (Vernon-Roberts, 1987).

The hyaline cartilage end plate rests on the surface of the vertebra. This is approximately 1 mm thick at its outer edge and becomes thinner towards its centre. The central portion of the end plate acts as a semi-permeable membrane to facilitate fluid exchange between the vertebral body and disc. In addition, it protects the body from excessive pressure. In early life the end plate is penetrated by canals from the vertebral body, but these disappear after the age of 20–30 years. After this period the end plate starts to ossify and become more brittle, the central portion thinning and in some cases being completely destroyed.

The nucleus pulposus is a soft hydrophilic (water attracting) substance taking up about 25% of the total disc area. It is continuous with the annulus, but the nuclear fibres are far less dense. The spaces between the collagen fibres are filled with proteoglycan, giving the nucleus its water-retaining capacity, and making it a mechanically plastic material. The area between the nucleus and annulus is metabolically very active and sensitive to physical force and chemical and hormonal influence (Palastanga, Field and Soames, 1989). The proteoglycan content of the nucleus decreases with age, but the collagen volume remains unchanged. As a consequence, the water content of the nucleus reduces. In early life the water content may be as high as 80–90%, but this decreases to about 70% by middle age.

The lumbar discs are the largest avascular structures in the body. The nucleus itself is dependent upon fluid exchange by passive diffusion from the margins of the vertebral body and across the cartilage end plate. Diffusion takes place particularly across the centre of the cartilage end plate which is more permeable than the periphery. There is intense anaerobic activity within the nucleus (Holm et al., 1981), which could lead to lactate build up and a low oxygen tension, placing the nuclear cells at risk. Inadequate adenosine triphosphate (ATP) supplies could lead to cell death.

The zygapophyseal (facet) joint

The zygaphophyseal joints are synovial joints formed between the inferior articular process of one vertebra and the superior articular process of its neighbour. As with all typical synovial joints, they have articular cartilage, a synovial membrane and a joint capsule. However, the zygaphophyseal joints do have a number of unique features (Bogduk and Twomey, 1991).

The capsule is a lax structure which enables the joint to hold about 2 ml of fluid. It is replaced anteriorly by the ligamentum flavum, and posteriorly it is reinforced by the deep fibres of multifidus. The joint leaves a small gap at its superior and inferior poles creating the subscapular pockets (Fig.

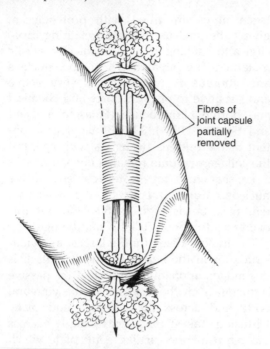

Figure 15.2   Lumbar zygapophyseal joint viewed from behind. Fat in the subcapsular pockets moves through foramina in the superior and inferior capsules. From Bogduk and Twomey (1991).

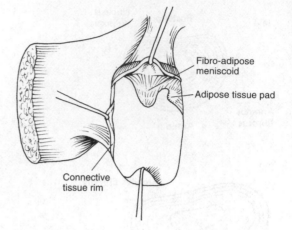

Figure 15.3   Intra-articular structures of the lumbar zygapophyseal joints. From Bodguk and Twomey (1991).

15.2). These are filled with fat, contained within the synovial membrane. Within the subscapular pocket lies a small foramen for passage of the fat in and out of the joint as the spine moves.

Intracapsularly there are three structures of interest (Fig. 15.3). The first is the connective tissue rim, a thickened wedge-shaped area which makes up for the curved shape of the articular cartilage in much the same way as the menisci of the knee do. The second structure is an adipose tissue pad, a 2 mm fold of synovium filled with fat and blood vessels. The third structure is the fibro-adipose meniscoid, a 5 mm leaf-like fold which projects from the inner surfaces of the superior and inferior capsules. These latter two structures have a protective function. During flexion, the movement of the articular facets leaves some of their cartilage exposed. Both the adipose tissue pad and the fibro-adipose menis-coid are able to cover these exposed regions (Bogduk and Engel, 1984).

With ageing, the cartilage of the zygapophyseal joint can split parallel to the joint surface, pulling a portion of joint capsule with it. The split of cartilage with its attached piece of capsule forms a false intra-articular meniscoid (Taylor and Twomey, 1986). Normally, the fibro-adipose meniscus itself is drawn out from the joint on flexion, and should move back in with extension. However, if the meniscoid fails to move back, it will buckle and remain under the capsule causing pain and acute locking (Bogduk and Jull, 1985). A mobilization or manipulation which combines flexion and rotation may allow the meniscoid to reduce and so relieve pain.

The facet has an overlapping neural supply, with ascending, local and descending facet branches coming from the posterior primary ramus. The nerve endings in the facet joint capsules are similar to those in the annulus of the disc, and although the disc is more sensitive, the facet joints can be a source of referred pain to the lower limb (Hirsch, Ingelmark and Miller, 1963), but not neurological deficit (Mooney and Robertson, 1976).

Individual differences in zygapophyseal joint orientation

The shape and orientation of the zygapophyseal joints varies between individuals, and in the same individual, between different spinal levels. Viewed from above the joint surfaces may be flat, slightly curved, or show a more pronounced curvature and be 'C' or 'J' shaped. Curved joint surfaces are more common in the upper lumbar levels (L1–2, L2–3, L3–4) but flat joint surfaces are more often seen at the lower lumbar levels (L4–5, L5–S1) (Horwitz and Smith, 1940).

Where the joint surfaces are flat, the angle that they make with the sagittal plane will determine the amount of resistance offered to both forward displacement and rotation (Fig. 15.4). The more the joint is orientated in the frontal plane, the more it will resist forward displacement, but the less able it is to resist rotation. This orientation is usually seen at the lower two lumbar levels. When the joint surfaces are aligned more sagitally, the resistance offered to rotation is greater, but that to forward displacement is reduced. Where the joint surfaces are curved, the anteromedial portion of the superior facet (which faces backwards) will resist forward displacement.

At birth the lumbar zygapophyseal joints lie in the frontal plane, but their orientation changes and they 'rotate' into the adult position by the age of 11 years. Variations occur in the degree and symmetry of rotation leading to articular tropism. The incidence of tropism is about 20% at all lumbar levels, and as high as 30% at the lumbosacral level (Bogduk and Twomey, 1987). Tropism will alter the resistance to rotation in the lumbar spine, and has an important bearing on injury. Over 80% of unilateral fissures in the lumbar discs occur in spines where zygapophyseal asymmetry exceeds 10°, with the fissure usually occurring on the side of the more obliquely orientated joint (Farfan et al., 1972)

During anterior displacement of the tropic lumbar spine, the upper vertebra of a parti-

Figure 15.4 Zygapophyseal joint orientation. (a) Sagittal plane will resist rotation but not forward displacement. (b) Frontal plane will resist forward displacement but not rotation. (c) Combined plane will resist both movements equally. From Norris (1995).

cular level rotates towards the side of the more frontally orientated zygapophyseal joint. This is because the frontal orientation of the joint provides more resistance to motion causing the vertebra to pivot around this point. This new motion imparts a torsional stress to the annulus of the disc. Over time, the alteration in lumbar mechanics which has occurred can result in an accumulation of stress, and a high number of patients have been shown to report back pain and sciatica on the side of the more obliquely set joint (Farfan and Sullivan, 1967).

Movements of the lumbar spine

Axial compression

Vertebral body

Within the vertebra itself, compressive force is transmitted by both the cancellous bone of the vertebral body and the cortical bone shell. Up to the age of 40 the cancellous bone contributes between 25% and 55% of the strength of the vertebra. After this age the cortical bone shell carries a greater proportion of load as the strength and stiffness of the cancellous bone reduces with decreasing bone density due to ageing (Rockoff et al., 1969). As the vertebral body is compressed, blood flows from it into the subchondral post-capillary venous network (Crock and Yoshizawa, 1976). This process reduces the bone volume and dissipates energy (Roaf, 1960). The blood returns slowly as the force is reduced, leaving a latent period after the initial compression, during which the shock-absorbing properties of the bone will be less effective. Exercises which involve prolonged periods of repeated shock to the spine, such as jumping on a hard surface, are therefore more likely to damage the vertebrae than those which load the spine for short periods and allow recovery of the vertebral blood flow before repeating a movement.

Intervertebral disc

Weight is transmitted between adjacent vertebrae by the lumbar intervertebral disc. The annulus fibrosis of a disc, when healthy, has a certain bulk and will resist buckling. When loads are applied briefly to the spine, even if the nucleus pulposus of a disc has been removed, the annulus alone exhibits a similar load-bearing capacity to that of the fully intact disc (Markolf and Morris, 1974). When exposed to prolonged loading, however, the collagen lamellae of the annulus will eventually buckle.

The application of an axial load will compress the fluid nucleus of the disc causing it to expand laterally. This lateral expansion stretches the annular fibres, preventing them from buckling. A 100 kg axial load has been shown to compress the disc by 1.4 mm and cause a lateral expansion of 0.75 mm (Hirsch and Nachemson, 1954). The stretch in the annular fibres will store energy which is released when the compression stress is removed. The stored energy gives the disc a certain springiness which helps to offset any deformation which occurred in the nucleus. A force applied rapidly will not be lessened by this mechanism, but its rate of application will be slowed, giving the spinal tissues time to adapt.

Deformation of the disc occurs more rapidly at the onset of axial load application. Within 10 minutes of applying an axial load the disc may deform by 1.5 mm. Following this, deformation slows to a rate of 1 mm per hour (Markolf and Morris, 1974) accounting for a subject's loss of height throughout the day. Under constant loading the discs exhibit creep, meaning that they continue to deform even though the load they are exposed to is not increasing. Compression causes a pressure rise leading to fluid loss from both the nucleus and annulus. About 10% of the water within the disc can be squeezed out by this method (Kraemer et al., 1985), the exact amount being dependent on the size of the applied force and the duration of its application. The fluid is absorbed back through pores in the cartilage end plates of the vertebra when the compressive force is reduced.

Exercises which axially load the spine have been shown to result in a reduction in subject height through discal compression. Compression loads of 6–10 times body weight have been shown to occur in the L3–L4 segment during a squat exercise in weight training for example (Cappozzo et al., 1985). Average height losses of 5.4 mm over a 25-minute period of general weight training, and 3.25 mm after a 6 km run have also been shown (Leatt, Reilly and Troup, 1986). Static axial loading of the spine with a 40 kg barbell over a 20-minute period can reduce subject height by as much as 11.2 mm (Tyrrell, Reilly and Troup, 1985). Clearly, exercises which involve this degree of spinal loading are unsuitable for individuals with discal pathology.

The vertebral end plates of the discs are compressed centrally, and are able to undergo less deformation than either the annulus or the cancellous bone. The end plates are, therefore, likely to fail (fracture) under high compression (Norkin and Levangie, 1992). Discs subjected to very high compressive loads show permanent deformation but not herniation (Virgin, 1951; Farfan et al., 1970; Markolf and Morris, 1974). However, such compression forces may lead to Schmorl's node formation (Bernhardt et al., 1992). Bending and torsional stresses on the spine, when combined with compression, are more damaging than compression alone, and degenerated discs are particularly at risk. Average failure torques for normal discs are 25% higher than for degenerative discs (Farfan et al., 1970). Degenerative discs also demonstrate poorer viscoelastic properties and therefore a reduced ability to attenuate shock.

The disc's reaction to a compressive stress changes with age, because the ability of the nucleus to transmit load relies on its high water content. The hydrophilic nature of the nucleus is the result of the proteoglycan it contains, and as this changes from about 65% in early life to 30% by middle age (Bogduk and Twomey, 1987) the nuclear load-bearing capacity of the disc reduces. When the proteoglycan content of the disc is high, up to the age of 30 years in most subjects, the nucleus pulposus acts as a gelatinous mass, producing a uniform fluid pressure. After this age, the lower water content of the disc means that the nucleus is unable to build as much fluid pressure. As a result, less central pressure is produced and the load is distributed more peripherally, even-

tually causing the annular fibres to become fibrillated and to crack (Hirsch and Schajowicz, 1952).

As a result of these age-related changes the disc is more susceptible to injury later in life. This, combined with the reduction in general fitness of an individual, and changes in movement patterns of the trunk related to the activities of daily living, greatly increases the risk of injury to this population. Individuals over the age of 40, if previously inactive, should therefore be encouraged to exercise the trunk under the supervision of a physiotherapist before attending fitness classes run for the general public.

Zygapophyseal joints

The superior/inferior alignment of the zygapophyseal joints in the lumbar spine means that during axial loading in the neutral position the joint surfaces will slide past each other. However, it must be noted that the orientation of the zygapophyseal joints may change from those characteristic of the thoracic spine to those of the lumbar spine, anywhere between T9–T12. Therefore, the level at which particular movements will occur can vary considerably between subjects. During lumbar movements displacement of the zygapophyseal joint surfaces will cause them to impact. Because the sacrum in inclined and the body and disc of L5 is wedge-shaped, during axial loading L5 is subjected to a shearing force. This is resisted by the more anterior orientation of the L5 inferior articular processes. In addition, as the lordosis increases, the anterior longitudinal ligament and the anterior portion of the annulus fibrosis will be stretched giving tension to resist the bending force. Additional stabilization is provided for the L5 vertebra by the iliolumbar ligament, attached to the L5 transverse process. This ligament, together with the zygapophyseal joint capsules, will stretch and resist the distraction force.

Once the axial compression force stops, release of the stored elastic energy in the spinal ligaments will re-establish the neutral lordosis. With compression of the lordotic lumbar spine, or in cases where gross disc narrowing has occurred, the inferior articular processes may impact on the lamina of the vertebra below. In this case the lower joints (L3/4, L4/5, L5/S1) may bear as much as 19% of the compression force while the upper joints (L1/2, L2/3) bear only 11% (Adams and Hutton, 1980).

Flexion and extension

During flexion movements the anterior annulus of the lumbar discs will be compressed while the posterior fibres are stretched. Similarly, the nucleus pulposus of the disc will be compressed anteriorly while pressure is relieved over its posterior surface. As the total volume of the disc remains unchanged, its pressure should not increase. The increases in pressure seen with alteration of posture are therefore due not to the bending motion of the bones within the vertebral joint itself, but to the soft tissue tension created to control the bending. If the pressure at the L3 disc for a 70 kg standing subject is said to be 100%, supine lying reduces this pressure to 25%. The pressure variations increase dramatically as soon as the lumbar spine is flexed and tissue tension increases (Fig. 15.5). The sitting posture increases intradiscal pressure to 140%, while sitting and leaning forward with a 10 kg weight in each hand increases pressure to 275% (Nachemson, 1987). The selection of an appropriate starting position for trunk exercise is therefore of great importance. Superimposing spinal movements from a slumped sitting posture, for example, would place considerably more stress on the spinal discs than the same movement beginning from crook lying.

During flexion the posterior annulus is stretched, and the nucleus is compressed onto the posterior wall. The posterior portion of the annulus is the thinnest part, and the

Figure 15.5 Relative pressure changes in the third lumbar disc. (a) In various positions. (b) In various muscle strengthening exercises. From Nachemson (1976), with permission.

combination of stretch and pressure to this area may result in discal bulging or herniation. Because of the alternating direction of the annular fibres, during rotational movements only half of the fibres will be stretched while half relax. The disc is therefore more easily injured during combined rotation and flexion movements.

As the lumbar spine flexes, the lordosis flattens and then reverses at its upper levels. Reversal of lordosis does not occur at L5–S1 (Pearcy et al., 1984). Flexion of the lumbar spine involves a combination of anterior sagittal rotation and anterior translation. As sagittal rotation occurs, the articular facets move apart, permitting the translation movement to occur. Translation is limited by impaction of the inferior facet of one vertebra on the superior facet of the vertebra below (Fig. 15.6). As flexion increases, or if the spine is angled forward on the hip, the surface of

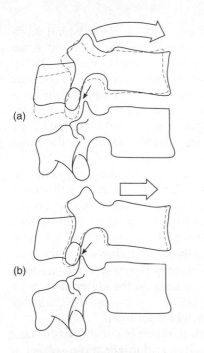

(a)

(b)

Figure 15.6 Vertebral movement during flexion. Flexion of the lumbar spine involves a combination of anterior sagittal rotation and anterior translation. As sagittal rotation occurs, the articular facets move apart (a), permitting the translation movement to occur (b). Translation is limited by impaction of the inferior facet of one vetebra on the superior facet of the vertebra below. From Bogduk and Twomey (1987).

the vertebral body will face more vertically increasing the shearing force due to gravity. The forces involved in facet impaction will therefore increase to limit translation of the vertebra and stabilize the lumbar spine. Because the zygapophyseal joint has a curved articular facet, the load will not be concentrated evenly across the whole surface, but will be focused on the anteromedial portion of the facets.

The sagittal rotation movement of the zygapophyseal joint causes the joint to open and is therefore limited by the stretch of the joint capsule. Additionally, the posteriorly placed spinal ligaments will also be tightened. Analysis of the contribution to limitation of sagittal rotation within the lumbar spine, through mathematical modelling, has shown that the disc limits movement by 29%,

the supraspinous and interspinous ligaments by 19% and the zygapophyseal joint capsules by 39% (Adams et al., 1980).

During extension the anterior structures are under tension while the posterior structures are first unloaded and then compressed, depending on the range of motion. With extension movements the vertebral bodies will be subjected to posterior sagittal rotation. The inferior articular processes move downwards causing them to impact against the lamina of the vertebra below. Once the bony block has occurred, if further load is applied the upper vertebra will axially rotate by pivoting on the impacted inferior articular process. The inferior articular process will move backwards, overstretching, and possibly, damaging the joint capsule (Yang and King, 1984). With repeated movements of this type, eventual erosion of the laminal periosteum may occur (Oliver and Middleditch, 1991). At the site of impaction, the joint capsule may catch between the opposing bones giving another cause of pain (Adams and Hutton, 1983). Structural abnormalities can alter the axis or rotation of the vertebra, so considerable variation between subjects exists (Klein and Hukins, 1983).

Rotation and lateral flexion

During rotation, torsional stiffness is provided by the outer layers of the annulus, the orientation of the zygapophyseal joints and by the cortical bone shell of the vertebral bodies themselves. In rotation movements, the annular fibres of the disc will be stretched according to their direction. As the two alternating sets of fibres are angled obliquely to each other, some of the fibres will be stretched while others relax. A maximum range of 3° of rotation can occur before the annular fibres will be microscopically damaged, and a maximum of 12° before tissue failure (Bogduk and Twomey, 1987). As rotation occurs, the spinous processes separate, stretching the supraspinous and interspinous ligaments. Impaction occurs between the opposing articular facets on one side causing the articular cartilage to compress by 0.5 mm for each 1° of rotation, providing a substantial buffer mechanism (Bogduk and Twomey, 1987). If rotation continues beyond this point, the vertebra pivots around the impacted zygapophyseal joint causing posterior and lateral movement (Fig. 15.7). The combination of movements and forces which occur will stress the impacted zygapophyseal joint by compression, the spinal disc by torsion and shear, and the capsule of the opposite zygapophyseal joint by traction. The disc provides only 35% of the total resistance (Farfan et al., 1970).

When the lumbar spine is laterally flexed, the annular fibres towards the concavity of the curve are compressed and will bulge, while those on the convexity of the curve will be stretched. The contralateral fibres of

the outer annulus and the contralateral intertransverse ligaments help to resist extremes of motion (Norkin and Levangie, 1992). Lateral flexion and rotation occur as coupled movements. Rotation of the upper four lumbar segments is accompanied by lateral flexion to the opposite site. Rotation of the L5–S1 joint occurs with lateral flexion to the same side.

Movement of the zygapophyseal joints on the concavity of lateral flexion is by the inferior facet of the upper vertebra sliding downwards on the superior facet of the vertebra below. The area of the intervertebral foramen on this side is therefore reduced. On the convexity of the laterally flexed spine the inferior facet slides upwards on the superior facet of the vertebra below, increasing the diameter of the intervertebral foramen.

If the trunk is moving slowly, tissue tension will be felt at end range and a subject is able to stop a movement short of full end range and protect the spinal tissues from overstretch. However, rapid movements of the trunk will build up large amounts of momentum. When the subject reaches near end range and tissue tension builds up, the momentum of the rapidly moving trunk will push the spine to full end range stressing the spinal tissues. In many popular sports, exercises often used in a warm-up are rapid and ballistic in nature and performed for high numbers of repetitions. These can lead to excessive flexibility and a reduction in passive stability of the spine.

Figure 15.7 Vertebral movement during rotation. Initially rotation occurs around an axis within the vertebral body (a). The zygapophyseal joints impact and further rotation causes the vertebra to pivot around a new axis at the point of impaction (b). From Bogduk and Twomey (1987).

Discal injury

During flexion, extension, and lateral flexion, one side of the disc is compressed and the other stretched. In flexion, the axis of motion passes through the nucleus, but with extension the axis moves forwards (Klein and Hukins, 1981). This fact, coupled with the increased range of motion during flexion, makes it the more dangerous movement. Combinations of torsion and flexion place the disc at particular risk from plastic deformation, which stretches the annular fibres irreversibly, and may cause fibre damage.

A single movement of flexion will stretch and thin the posterior annulus (Oliver and Middleditch, 1991), but it is repeated flexion, especially under load, which is likely to give the most serious pathological consequences. Discal injury occurs most frequently through repeated flexion movements, and when a flexion/rotation strain is placed on the spine during lifting.

When hyperflexion takes place, the supraspinous and interspinous ligaments will overstretch reducing the support to the lumbar spine. Circumferential tearing will occur to the disc annulus, posterolaterally, usually at the junction between the disc lamina and end plate (Oliver and Middleditch, 1991). The outer annular fibres are innervated, a possible cause of the 'dull ache' in the lumbar spine which often precedes disc prolapse. Rotation strain will increase the likelihood of these injuries. Although rotation is limited in the lumbar spine, it is increased significantly as a result of facet joint degeneration, and during flexion as the facets are separated.

Posterolateral radial fissuring occurs later, and connects the disc nucleus to the circumferential tear, allowing the passage of nuclear material towards the outer edge of the disc. This type of injury has been produced experimentally during discal compression in a combined flexed and laterally flexed posture (Adams and Hutton, 1982). An annular protrusion can occur when the pressure of the displaced nuclear material causes the annulus to bulge. Eventually, nuclear material is extruded (herniated) through the ruptured annular wall (Fig. 15.8).

The discal injury may occur gradually as a result of repeated bending, giving symptoms of gradually worsening pain. Pain occurs initially in the lower back, and with time the symptoms are peripheralized into the buttock and lower limbs. Sudden pain main occur from a seemingly trivial injury which

Figure 15.8 Stages of disc herniation. (a) Normal disc. (b) Nuclear bulge with annulus intact. (c) Ruptured annulus, nuclear protrusion onto nerve root.

acts as the 'last straw' to cause the disc herniation. Loads of sufficient intensity may give rise to an abrupt massive disc herniation. The stress is usually one of weight combined with leverage during a lifting action. Hyperflexion of the spine occurs, due, in part, to overstretching of the posterior lumbar ligaments.

Radiographic investigations of discal movement have been made by inserting metal pins into the lumbar nucleus pulposus and asymmetrically loading the disc (reported in McKenzie, 1990). These have shown that the disc migrates towards the area of least load. When the asymmetrical load was removed, the nucleus remained displaced, but its relocation was accelerated by compression in the opposite direction or by traction.

Spinal ligaments

Six spinal ligaments are of concern to the biomechanics of the lumbar spine, the anterior and posterior longitudinal ligaments, the intertransverse ligament, the ligamentum flavum, the interspinous and supraspinous ligaments, and the capsular ligaments of the facet joint. A general reduction in energy absorption of all the ligaments has been found with age (Tkaczuk, 1968). The stiffest is the posterior longitudinal ligament and the most flexible the supraspinous (Panjabi, Jorneus and Greenstein, 1984). The ligamentum flavum in the lumbar spine is pre-tensioned (resting tension) when the spine is in its neutral position, a situation which compresses the disc. This ligament has the highest percentage of elastic fibres of any tissue in the body (Nachemson and Evans, 1968), and contains nearly twice as much elastin as collagen. The anterior longitudinal ligament and joint capsules have been found to be the strongest, while the interspinous and posterior longitudinal ligaments are the weakest (Panjabi, Hult and White, 1987).

The ligaments act rather like rubber bands resisting tensile forces but buckling under compressive loads (Fig. 15.9). They must allow adequate motion and fixed postures between vertebrae, enabling a minimum amount of muscle energy to be used. In addition, they protect the spine by restricting motion and in particular protect the spinal cord in traumatic situations, where high loads are applied at rapid speeds. In this situation, the ligaments absorb large amounts of energy.

The longitudinal ligaments are viscoelastic materials, being stiffer when loaded rapidly, and they exhibit hysteresis as they do not store the energy used to stretch them. When loaded repeatedly, they become stiffer, and the hysteresis is less marked, making the longitudinal ligaments more prone to fatigue failure (Hukins, 1987). The supraspinous and interspinous ligaments are further from the flexion axis, and therefore need to stretch more than the posterior longitudinal ligament when they resist flexion.

Low back pain

The exact structure which is affected in low back pain is open to discussion, and often it is virtually impossible to identify precisely which tissue is causing a patient's symptoms (Spitzer, LeBlanc and Dupuis, 1987). To a large extent the precise anatomical location becomes irrelevant as long as the patient is made better. The situation is made considerably easier if, instead of focusing attention on the injured structure, we attend to the loss of function and our need to restore this.

To this end, the approach taken by McKenzie (1981) is extremely useful. Back pain may be classified as mechanical, or chemical (non-mechanical) in origin. Mechanical pain is produced by deformation of structures containing nociceptive nerve endings,

Figure 15.9   The spinal segment as a leverage system. From Kapandji (1974), with permission.

and there is a clear correlation between certain body positions and the patient's symptoms.

Non-mechanical pain, on the other hand, is of a constant nature. This may be exacerbated by movement or position, but importantly, no position will be found which completely relieves the symptoms. This category encompasses both inflammatory and infective processes. Inflammation will occur following trauma, and the accumulation of chemical irritant substances will affect the nociceptive fibres and give pain. This type of pain will continue for as long as the nociceptor irritation continues. With rest, irritation will settle and healing progress. Part of this healing process is scar formation, so the type of pain will change from a constant chemical pain to a mechanical pain developed through adaptive shortening of the affected tissues. Non-mechanical conditions also include those which refer pain to the spine, such as vascular or visceral damage and carcinoma. Clearly, it is essential to differentiate between mechanical and non-mechanical pain in the lower back. When no movement can be found which reduces the patient's symptoms and if a period of rest does not allow the symptoms to subside, the patient requires medical investigation.

Screening examination

Examination of the lumbar spine can be very complex, or relatively simple, depending on the approach taken. The reliability and reproducibility of tests for the spine increases when the information to be gained from the tests is kept to a minimum (Nelson et al., 1979). For this reason, the work of Cyriax (1982) and McKenzie (1981) is valuable as it provides enough information to treat the majority of patients. In addition, the tests tell the practitioner when further investigation is necessary.

Observation deals particularly with posture while standing and sitting, and the appearance of the spine at rest. Scoliosis and loss of normal lordosis are of particular note, as is the level of the iliac crests. Flexion, extension and lateral flexion are tested initially as single movements to obtain information about range of motion, end feel and presence of a painful arc. Flexion and extension are then repeated to see if these movements change the intensity or site of pain, bearing in mind the centralization phenomenon and dysfunction stretch (see p. 351). Side-gliding movements are also tested to repetition. Flexion and extension may be further assessed in a lying position to obtain information about nerve root adhesion (flexion) and greater range of extension. This initial examination then indicates whether neurological testing of sensation, power, reflexes and further nerve stretch is required. In addition, the history, signs and symptoms will indicate whether the pelvis and sacro-iliac joints warrant further attention, or if resisted tests should be included.

The straight leg raise

The straight leg raise (SLR) or Laseague's sign is a widely used test to assess the sciatic nerve in cases of back pain. The test also places stretch on the hamstrings, buttock tissues, sacro-iliac joint, posterior lumbar ligaments, and facet joints, in addition to lengthening the spinal canal (Urban, 1986). Confirmation that the nerve root is the source of pain may be made by raising the leg to the point of pain and then lowering it a few degrees. The neuromeningeal structures are then further stretched either from below by dorsiflexing the foot, or applying firm pressure to the popliteal fossa over the posterior tibial nerve. Pressure from above is produced by flexing the cervical spine. When performing the SLR, as the leg is raised, the knee should not be allowed to bend and the pelvis should stay on the couch.

The dura within the spinal canal is firmly attached to the foramen magnum above and the filum terminale below. Trunk flexion causes the spinal canal to lengthen and therefore stretches the dura, whereas extension, by shortening the canal, induces dural relaxation allowing the sheath to fold. The neuromeningeal pathway is elastic, so tension imparted at one point will spread throughout the whole length of the spine. As the SLR is performed, the initial motion is of the nerve at the greater sciatic notch. As hip flexion goes through 35°, movement occurs proximal to the ala of the sacrum, and during the next 35° the movement is at the intervertebral foramen itself. The last degrees of the SLR do not produce further nerve movement, but simply increase the tension over the whole course of the nerve (Grieve, 1970) (Fig. 15.10).

Testing the unaffected leg (crossed SLR or 'well leg' test) may also give symptoms. This manoeuvre pulls the nerve root and dura distally and medially, but increases the pressure on the nerve complex by less than half that of the standard SLR test. When the ipsilateral SLR causes pain, it simply means that one of the tissues connected to the nerve pathway is sensitized. Because the crossed SLR stretches the neural structures less, the resting tension of these tissues must be higher to cause pain. The crossed SLR may therefore be a more reliable predictor of large disc protrusions than the ipsilateral SLR (Urban, 1986).

Slump test

The slump test is used to assess tension in the pain-sensitive structures around the vertebral canal or intervertebral foramen, and to ensure that these structures and able to stretch properly (Maitland, 1986; Butler, 1991). To perform the manoeuvre the patient sits unsupported over the couch side with the knees together and flexed to 90°. The posterior thigh is in contact with the couch. The patient is then instructed to relax the spine completely and 'slump' forward, keeping the cervical spine in its neutral position ('look forwards, not down'). The therapist (standing at the side of the patient) places overpressure onto the patient's shoulders to increase the movement, attempting to bow the spine rather than increase hip flexion (Fig. 15.11a).

From this position the patient is asked to flex the neck ('chin to chest') and then straighten the leg on the unaffected side first (Fig. 15.11b). In each case the examiner places overpressure on the area and assesses the result. The athlete is then asked to dorsiflex the ankle ('pull your toes up'). Neck flexion is slowly released, and the response

Figure 15.10   Effects of straight leg raising. (a) Movement of sciatic nerve begins at the greater sciatic notch. (b) Movement of roots begins at the intervertebral foramen. (c) Minimal movement only, but increase in tension. From Oliver and Middleditch (1991), with permission.

Figure 15.11   The slump test.

monitored. The opposite leg is then tested. A normal test result is one where there is a pain-free lack of knee extension by about 30° and slight central pain over T9/10 (Maitland, 1986).

Mechanical therapy

Three mechanical conditions are recognized in the lower back, the postural syndrome, dysfunction and derangement (McKenzie, 1981). The postural syndrome occurs when certain postures or body positions place soft tissues around the lumbar spine under prolonged stress. Pain is intermittent, and only occurs when the particular posture is taken up, and ceases when the offending posture is changed. This can be frustrating for the patient because they can find nothing wrong. There is no deformity, vigorous activity is frequently painless as the stresses it imposes on the tissues are continually changing. The fault usually lies with poor sitting posture which places the lumbar spine in flexion. After sport, the patient is warm and relaxed and so sits in a slumped position, perhaps in the bar after a game of squash. Discomfort occurs after some time and this gradually changes to pain. The patient often has the idea that sport makes the pain worse, but this is not the case. The poor sitting posture used when relaxing after sport is the true problem.

Pain may also occur in sport from extreme positions. Hyperflexion when lifting a weight from the ground or performing stretching exercises, hyperextension when pressing a weight overhead, or performing a back walkover in gymnastics are common examples.

The most important part of management with the postural syndrome is patient education. To this end, the slouch-overcorrect procedure for correcting sitting posture is useful (McKenzie, 1981). The patient sits on a stool, and is allowed to slouch into an incorrect sitting posture for some time until his back pain ensues. He or she is then taught a position of maximum lordosis, and learns how to change rapidly and at will, from the incorrect slouch to this overcorrect maximum lordosis. Once the patient has seen the relationship between poor sitting posture and pain, he or she is taught a correct sitting posture mid-way between the two extreme movement ranges. The use of a lumbar pad or roll is helpful to maintain the lordosis in sitting.

Where hyperflexion or hyperextension is the cause of postural pain, video is particularly useful in enabling the athlete to appreciate the strain he or she is placing on the lumbar spine. Re-education of movement and skill training, with emphasis on the position of the spine and hips, are helped by video-playback. Body landmarks over the pelvis and spine are marked first using white adhesive dots. Biofeedback is also useful, especially when trying to correct hyperflexion. In its simplest form, strips of pre-stretched elastic tape are placed at either side of the lumbar spine. When the athlete flexes, the tape 'drags' on the skin and reminds him to avoid the flexed position.

Dysfunction pain is caused by overstretching adaptively shortened structures within the lumbar spine. The previously damaged structures have shortened due to prolonged disuse, or scar tissue formation. When the normal range of motion is attempted at the affected segment, the shortened soft tissues are stretched prematurely. The essential feature with dysfunction is pain at the end of movement range which disappears as soon as the end range stretch is released. The position is self-perpetuating because the pain which occurs with stretching causes the patient to avoid the full range motion and so the adaptive shortening is compounded.

Dysfunction may occur secondary to trauma, or as a result of the postural syndrome. Typically, the patient is stiff first thing in the morning and his back 'works loose' through the day, so he is generally better with activity. Loss of extension leads to a reduced lordosis, and loss of flexion becomes apparent when the patient tries to touch his toes. Frequently, he or she will deviate to the side of the dysfunction. Once dysfunction has been detected (static) stretching is required, and/or joint mobilization procedures. Although mobilizations at grades three and four are useful to help restore range of movement, this passive treatment must be coupled with active stretching procedures which the patient can practice at home to help regain lost physiological range. Accessory movements cannot usually be practised by the patient, and are perhaps a more appropriate form of manual therapy where physiological stretching causes excessive pain. It is important that stretching be practised little and often, to allow the patient to recover from the soreness which follows the lengthening of contracted tissues. The patient must be instructed to press gently into the painful end range point in an attempt to increase the range of motion. There is always a tendency to try and avoid the painful position with back pain, but with dysfunction this is precisely the position we want to work in.

The most common dysfunction following low back pain is loss of extension (McKenzie, 1981). The extension loss may be regained by a combination of mobilization, manipulation and mechanical therapy. The classic mechanical therapy procedure is extension in lying (EIL), either with or without belt fixation. The patient lies prone on the treatment Table, with his or her lumbar spine held by a webbing fixation belt. This is placed around both the lower spine and treatment Table at a point just below the spinal segment which is blocked to extension. From this position, the patient performs a modified press-up exercise, trying to fully extend the arms while keeping the hips in contact with the couch surface. At home the patient should continue the exercise at regular intervals throughout the day. Various modifications may be used to apply the pressure—

EIL with the patient lying on a ironing board using a thick belt, or positioning the spine under a low piece of furniture, or manual pressure from a spouse or the weight of a small child.

Loss of flexion may be similarly regained, but this time the mechanical therapy technique is flexion in lying (FIL), or flexion in standing (FIS). Initially the patient uses FIL. The movement begins in a crook-lying position. From this position the patient pulls his knees to his chest. As maximum hip flexion is reached, further movement occurs initially by flexion of the lower lumbar and lumbosacral segments, and then the upper lumbar area. FIS is simply a toe-touching exercise performed very slowly. Gravitation effects place greater stress on the lumbar discs, so the exercise must proceed with caution. The differences between FIS and FIL are twofold. First, with FIS the legs are straight, and so the nerve roots are stretched, a particularly useful effect when dealing with nerve root adhesion. Secondly, the sequence of flexion is reversed, with the upper lumbar areas moving before the lower lumbar and lumbosacral areas. Where there was a deviation in flexion at the initial examination, flexion in step standing may be used. Here, one leg is placed on a stool and the patient pulls his chest downwards onto the flexed knee. In so doing, flexion is combined with slight lateral bending. Other dysfunctions such as loss of lateral flexion, side-gliding, or rotation may occur but they are less common. In addition, it must be remembered when assessing symmetry of bilateral movements that most people are slightly asymmetrical anyway. We must be certain that any asymmetry that exists is relevant to the patient's present symptoms before we spend time correcting it.

Derangement occurs when the nucleus or annulus of the disc is distorted or damaged, altering the normal resting position of two adjacent vertebrae. Pain is usually constant and movement loss is apparent, so much so in some cases that the condition is completely disabling. Derangement of the lumbar disc is a common cause of low back pain, and McKenzie (1981) described seven types, classified according to the site and behaviour of symptoms (Table 15.1), while Cyriax (1982) claimed there are eight ways in which a damaged disc can move, and classified these according to discal position (Table 15.2).

Deformities of scoliosis and kyphosis are common, with local or referred pain over the lumbar and sacral dermatomes depending on the severity of injury. Again, management may be by manual or mechanical therapy or a combination of the two. Mechanical therapy aims at centralizing the pain, and reversing the sequence of pain development which occurred as the disc lesion progressed. The aim is to transfer pain which is felt laterally in the spine or in the leg to a more central position. It is perfectly acceptable for the intensity of the pain to increase providing its position is altered to a more central one.

The movements used are those which reduced the patient's symptoms in the initial examination. Where a scoliosis exists, initially the most effective movement is usually side-gliding in standing (SGIS). The therapist stands at the side of the patient holding his or her hips. The therapist then gently presses the patient's shoulders towards the convexity of the scoliosis aiming to obtain a sliding rather than laterally flexing movement. The patient may continue this by placing his or her hand on a wall (arm abducted to 90°) and shifting his or her hips towards the wall. Once the pain moves into a more central position, the EIL exercise begins with the aim of centralizing the pain further. Although these movements are frequently very effective for postero-lateral protrusions, it must be emphasized that it is the movement which reduces the symptoms which is practised, and this may vary tremendously between patients.

Table 15.1 McKenzie classification of disc derangements

Derangement one
Central or symmetrical pain across L4/5
Rarely buttock or thigh pain
No deformity

Derangement two
Central or symmetrical pain across L4/5
With or without buttock and/or thigh pain
With deformity of lumbar kyphosis

Derangement three
Unilateral or asymmetrical pain across L4/5
With or without buttock and/or thigh pain
No deformity

Derangement four
Unilateral or asymmetrical pain across L4/5
With or without buttock and/or thigh pain
With deformity of lumbar scoliosis

Derangement five
Unilateral or asymmetrical pain across L4/5
With or without buttock and/or thigh pain
With leg pain extending below the knee
No deformity

Derangement six
Unilateral or asymmetrical pain across L4/5
With or without buttock and/or thigh pain
With leg pain extending below the knee
With deformity of sciatic scoliosis

Derangement seven
Symmetrical or asymmetrical pain across L4/5
With or without buttock and/or thigh pain
With deformity of accentuated lumbar lordosis

From McKenzie (1981), with permission.

Manual therapy of the lumbar spine

The point at which manual therapy is used will vary depending on both the condition and the practitioner using the therapy. Some practitioners rarely use manual therapy claiming that to do so could make a patient dependent upon this type of care, while others use only mobilization and manipulation claiming that it gives a more

Table 15.2   Cyriax classification of disc lesions

Gradual small posterior displacement
Pain brought on by stooping or lifting and relieved by standing or resting. Articular signs only, sometimes with painful arc, SLR is full

Swift large posterior displacement
Severe low back pain of traumatic origin, or from overuse following prolonged stooping. Constant ache with intermittent twinges. Articular signs of flexion deformity, dural signs of limited SLR and lumbar pain in full neck flexion

Massive posterior protrusion
Posterior longitudinal ligaments may rupture, compressing sciatic nerve roots and giving sympathetic signs. Perineal pain and bilateral symptoms, limited SLR with root palsy. Saddle analgesia with bladder weakness

Posterolateral protrusion
Previous history of general backache, changing to unilateral pain, pins and needles or numbness, aggravated by coughing. Limitation of trunk flexion and SLR. Pain often increased by neck flexion

Anterior protrusion in the elderly
Backache and/or unilateral pain with pins and needles in the feet, often mimicking claudication. Symptoms are present only when the patient has been upright for some time and relieved by sitting or lying. Flexion reduces symptoms. SLR full, no neurological deficit

Anterior protrusion in adolescents
Osteochondrosis giving pressure erosion of the vertebral body, and kyphotic posture. Associated with excessive weightbearing

Vertical protrusion
Schmorl's node formation. No pain, but radiographic appearance confirms abnormality. T10 most commonly affected. Alternatively, biconcave disc phenomenon with osteoporosis

Circular protrusion
Compression causes uniform discal bulging, with traction to the periosteum and subsequent osteophyte formation. Limited spinal mobility

Adapted from Cyriax (1982).

rapid response. The true picture probably lies somewhere between the two extremes. There are certainly patients for whom mechanical therapy is too painful initially. These usually respond to mobilization to relieve pain and then to increase mobility, and this treatment may be followed by mechanical therapy and exercise therapy at a later date. Equally, there are patients who look upon manual treatment as a panacea which will always cure them, and so they feel they have no need to care for their own spine. For these, clearly mechanical therapy must be emphasized.

Concepts of mobilization and manipulation

Passive movements of a joint may be either physiological, having large ranges of movement measured in degrees, or accessory with small ranges measured in millimetres. When pain and protective spasm limit physiological movement, mobilizing the restricted accessory movements of a joint can provide freedom to the physiological range and reduce pain.

Mobilization techniques (Maitland 1986, 1991) aim to improve joint mobility or reduce pain originating in a joint by using accessory movements of specific grades. If pain is the dominant factor, this is treated first. When stiffness overshadows pain the aim is to increase the patient's range of motion even though some soreness may be produced during and following treatment. Most patients will present with a combination of pain and stiffness, and when there is doubt as to which is the predominant feature, pain is treated first.

When joint movement is limited, the point of limitation falls short of the anatomical range (that which is available to a joint because of its structure). As the joint is mobilized the point of limitation moves closer to the anatomical range. Within a range of movement four grades of mobilization techniques are used (Table 15.3).

Represented diagrammatically (Fig. 15.12) grades I and II do not reach the end range, and are used when pain is the predominant feature. It is thought (Wyke, 1972) that these grades effect pain by stimulating mechanoreceptors and pain receptors within the joint. Grades III and IV are performed to end range movement and are used when stiffness is the main problem. The ratios between the movements remain the same, as the limitation point (L) moves to the right.

A manipulation is a high velocity thrust of small amplitude performed at the end range of motion. The thrust may be accompanied by a pop or click from alteration of gaseous pressure within the synovial fluid when the joint surfaces are tractioned (Unsworth et al., 1971), or a tearing sensation as adhesions are ruptured. Replacing a subluxed joint may also be audible.

Figure 15.12 Grades of joint mobilization. A, Starting point of movement range. B, Anatomical limitation of range. L, Limitation point due to pain or resistance.

Cyriax (1983) claimed that three situations call for manipulation; capsular contraction, joint adhesions, and intra-articular displacement. He described manipulative stretching for capsular contraction as 'a slow steady movement carried out over a number of sessions' a definition more in line with a sustained stretch mobilization within the Maitland definition. Manipulative rupture of adhesions and manipulative reduction is achieved with a high velocity low amplitude movement. Adhesion rupture of superficial ligaments is usually carried out after deep frictional massage, and reduction is achieved during traction using Cyriax methods.

Maitland (1986) used the term manipulation to describe a technique which is carried out at a speed too rapid for a patient to prevent. He stated that the technique is 'often gentle, always small in range, and rarely forceful'. He argued that manipulation is usually a progression of mobilization and is rarely used at the beginning of a treatment and never applied to a very painful joint or one which is protected by muscle spasm. The manipulation used within the Maitland concept is similar in amplitude

Table 15.3   Grades of mobilization procedures

Grade I	Small amplitude movement near the starting position of the range
Grade II	Large amplitude movement occupying any free part of the range
Grade III	Large amplitude movement moving into stiffness
Grade IV	Small amplitude movement at the end of range

After Maitland (1986).

and position in the range of motion to a grade IV mobilization, but performed at a greater velocity.

Techniques for the lumbar spine

For the lumbar spine, there are two techniques (of literally thousands) which are especially valuable and will be briefly described. The first is the rotation movement (Fig. 15.13a). This is performed in the side-lying starting position, with the painful side uppermost, so that the pelvis is rotated away from the painful side. Both knees and hips and bent (crook-side lying) with the upper leg bending slightly more than the lower. The therapist stands behind the patient and imparts a grade I or II mobilization by rhyth-

mically pushing on the patient's pelvis, allowing the thorax to rock freely. With grades III and IV, the patient's underneath arm is pulled through to rotate the thorax so that the chest faces more towards the ceiling. The upper leg bends slightly further so that the knee clears the couch side, and the lower leg is straighter to act as a pivot (increasing the flexion of the lower leg will flex the lumbar spine further). Therapist pressure is now over the pelvis and humeral head. This movement may be taken further to apply a manipulation. A lower couch position is used, and the end range point of spinal rotation is maintained by the therapist pushing down on the patient's pelvis and shoulder through straight arms, and in so doing applying slight traction. As the patient

Grades I and II   Grades III and IV

(a)

(b)

Figure 15.13   Lumbar mobilization. (a) Rotation, (b) extension.

exhales, a high velocity low amplitude thrust is applied. A tremendous number of variations exist to allow for alterations in range of motion, direction of rotation, and combined movements. These procedures are described in detail by Maitland (1986) and Cyriax (1983).

Extension movements in their simplest form may be produced by using postero-anterior pressures and derivatives of this technique (Fig. 15.13b). Postero-anterior central vertebral pressure (Maitland, 1986) may be performed with the patient prone. The pressure may be imparted with the pads of the thumbs, or the ulnar border of the hand (pisiform/hamate) pressing over the spinous processes. Movement is gradually taken up as the therapist moves his weight directly over the patient's spine and an oscillation is begun. Variations include combined movements, unilateral pressures, bilateral pressure over the transverse processes, and the addition of hip extension among others.

Nags and snags

Many patients who have disc lesions seem to respond well to techniques aimed at the facet joints. The connection between these seemingly dissociate conditions is a biomechanical one. As the disc bulges posteriorly, it causes the vertebrae to flex with a loss of lordosis. For this to happen, the facet joints must be mobile enough to open fully. However, in many cases, these joints are far from mobile, and the soft tissue surrounding them is placed on stretch, giving pain, which can be reduced using mobilization procedures.

Mulligan (1989) described a number of procedures which combine manual and mechanical therapy, taking into account the planes of movement at the facet joints. In the lumbar spine, movement may be assisted (snag procedure) by applying therapist pressure over the spinous processes or articular pillars of the lumbar spine as the patient

moves. Flexion, extension or lateral flexion may be used either in sitting or standing. Either pisiform or thumb contact is used, and the direction of pressure is vertical in an attempt to separate, or at least assist separation of the facets.

The starting position is with the patient sitting over the couch side (or standing) with the therapist behind. A belt is placed around the patient's waist over the anterior superior iliac spines (this area may be padded with a towel if necessary). The patient is asked to flex forwards to the point of pain. They then back off slightly and the therapist applies the SNAG as the patient flexes again (Fig. 15.14a). If the correct level has been identified, the movement should be pain-free and of greater range. If pain persists, the level to be treated is changed, or a unilateral SNAG is performed over the articular pillar of the more painful side. For extension, the patient is in the same starting position, but the couch is raised to afford the therapist a better mechanical advantage. The therapist stands slightly to one side so that they are clear of the patient as they extend back. The action must be lumbar extension, with the patient extending over the therapist's hand rather than extension of the whole spine on the hip with the patient pressing their whole body weight against the therapist's hand (Fig. 15.14b). Rotation is performed with the patient stride sitting over the couch to fix the pelvis. The therapist grips around the patient's trunk just above the painful level. Again, the overpressure is given with the ulnar border of the hand in the treatment plane (Fig. 15.14c).

The direction of motion and level of pressure application is decided both by the movement which is limited, and the action which relieves the patient's symptoms. As the patient moves, the vertical pressure is applied until end range is obtained. Pressure is continued until the patient resumes the neutral position once more.

(a)　(b)　(c)

Figure 15.14 'SNAGS' for the lumbar spine. (a) Flexion, (b) extension, (c) rotation.

The sacro-iliac joint

The three bones of the pelvis, the two inno-minates and the sacrum, form a closed ring. Anteriorly, the innominates join together at the pubic symphysis and posteriorly they join the sacrum via the sacro-iliac joints (SIJ). Disorders of the pubic symphysis will often have repercussions on the SIJ, so examination should take place in both joints.

The sacral articular surface is shaped like a letter 'L' lying on its side, and is covered by hyaline cartilage, while the corresponding surface on the ilium is covered by fibrocartilage. The SIJ is a synovial joint, but its posterior surface is firmly secured by the interosseous ligament and so the joint may be considered as fibrous. There is great variation between individuals, in terms of the size, shape and number of articular surfaces, with 30% of subjects having accessory articulations between the sacrum and ilium (Grieve, 1976). With increasing age the joint becomes fibrosed and may eventually show partial bony fusion.

The sacrum is inserted like the keystone of an arch, but seemingly the wrong way round, tending to be displaced rather than forced inwards with pressure. However, as the body weight is taken, the tension developed in the interosseous sacro-iliac ligaments pulls the two halves of the pelvic ring together (Fig. 15.15). In the sagittal plane the body weight falls ventral to the axis of rotation of the SIJ. This alignment would tend to rotate the sacrum forwards, but its lower end is anchored by both the sacrospinous and sacrotuberous ligaments. The sacrotuberous ligament is slack in forward flexion of the trunk without a pelvic tilt (Lee, 1994) and so a stoop lift may dislodge the joint.

The normal SIJ does move. As the trunk is flexed, the sacral base moves forwards between the ilia, and with trunk extension in standing, the sacrum moves back again. The movement is usually only about 5 mm, but ranges up to 26 mm have been recorded (Frigerio, Stowe and Howe, 1974).

Postural asymmetry of the pelvis is common, and is evident when there is torsion of one ilium in relation to the other. On examination, one anterior superior iliac spine may be higher and one posterior superior iliac spine may be lower, for example. Unequal leg lengths, although normally asymptomatic, may cause the SIJ to become 'blocked', with a consequent alteration in gluteal muscle tone (Grieve, 1976). When shortening is more than 1–2 cm, torsion of the pelvis occurs with the ilium and sacral base on the side of the longer leg moving backwards

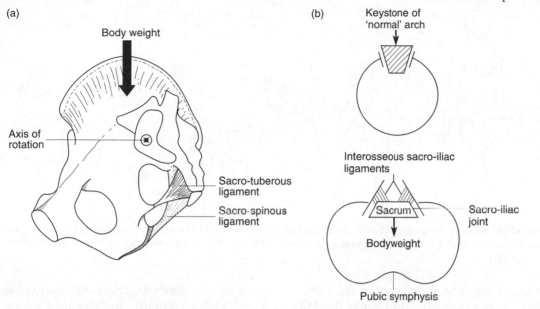

Figure 15.15   The sacro-iliac joint. (a) Position. (b) Action in pelvic arch. After Taylor and Twomey (1994).

and the pubis moving upwards. The degree of postural compensation between individuals will differ and so the pelvic position in reaction to altered leg length is variable.

Hormonal changes in pregnancy and, to a lesser extent, menstruation and menopause will also influence the SIJ. The general softening and relaxation of the pelvis leads to an increased range of motion which may remain for up to 12 weeks following child birth. Local irritation of the SIJ leads to pain on gapping tests and limited hip abduction on the painful side. In addition, the lower PSIS is usually on the painful side.

Subjective examination usually reveals a unilateral distribution of symptoms, perhaps spreading to the buttock, lower abdomen, groin, or thigh, although pain may be referred to the foot. The traumatic history is frequently one of a fall, landing on the ischial tuberosity with patients unable to walk distances without marked pain. The footballer in a mistimed sliding tackle, or the youngster who falls while ice-skating are prime examples. In any sports where the range of motion

required at the hip is great, or repetitive unilateral leg movements are performed, SIJ irritation may be encountered. Tensile forces are increased with jumping activities onto both legs, while shear forces are raised with single leg activities, such as running and hopping. Dancers, gymnasts and high jumpers are particularly prone to SIJ involvement, but any athlete may suffer trauma to the joint leading to local inflammation or mechanical disturbance.

Objective examination of the pelvis and SIJ is made initially with the patient standing. The general bony alignment and muscle contour is noted. The patient may be reluctant to take weight through the affected leg, and might walk with a limp. Loss of gluteal and abdominal muscle bulk has also been reported (Wells, 1986). The level of the gluteal folds and gluteal cleft is noted as is that of the iliac crests and iliac spines.

Two motion tests of the SIJ are particularly useful in sport (Fig. 15.16). The examiner places his or her thumbs over S2/3 and the PSIS. From the standing position the patient

Figure 15.16   Motion tests of the sacro-iliac joints. (a) The right PSIS should move caudally as the leg is lowered back to the ground. (b) Joint assymetry. If one joint is lower, as the patient flexes it will move cephalically (Piedallu's sign).

flexes one hip, and movement of the PSIS is noted. Normally, with hip flexion the PSIS moves caudally and as the leg is brought back to the ground it moves cephalically (Wells, 1986). Both PSISs are palpated as the patient flexes his or her spine. If one joint is markedly restricted, the joint which is lower and more prominent in standing moves higher up as the patient flexes (Piedallu's sign).

Flexibility and power of the hip muscles is tested, and passive movements of the hip joint assessed. Range and end feel are noted, with particular attention being paid to passive flexion adduction (SI ligaments). The FABERE manouevre (Patrick's test) is also used. This involves flexion/abduction/external rotation of the hip with the knee flexed, and lateral malleolus resting above the opposite knee. Pain produced in the groin or anterior thigh with this test indicates hip involvement, while SIJ pain is localized to the joint. Baer's point, one third of the way down a line joining the umbilicus to the ASIS, is often tender.

Iliac gapping and approximation tests will often reproduce SIJ pain, and the apex test is most useful (Fig. 15.17). In a supine-lying, starting position, the therapist places pressure over the anterior superior iliac spines. Initially, his or her arms are crossed and

pressure is directed diagonally outwards (Fig. 15.17a). Secondly, the therapist's forearms are aligned horizontally and the pressure is directed inward against the ASISs (Fig. 15.17b). In crook side-lying (folded towel beneath side of waist) pressure is directed downwards to the opposite trochanter (Fig. 15.17c). In half crook side-lying (upper hip and knee flexed to 90°) pressure may be imparted to the ischial tuberosity and ASIS to place a rotatory strain on the SIJ, especially helpful when pain is associated with a lower PSIS (Fig. 15.17d). With the patient in a prone position, the pelvis rests on the ASIS and the pubis. Firm pressure over the sacrum will shear the SIJs and may reproduce unilateral pain if positive (Fig. 15.17e). The pubic symphysis must be tested as part of the pelvic ring, and pubic pain may be apparent on any of the above tests. For direct testing, in supine lying, the superior portion of the symphysis is palpated with the hypothenar eminence. Pressure is directed from the lower abdomen downwards and then obliquely to each side (Fig. 15.17f).

In each of the tests the aim is to reproduce the patient's symptoms. The movement which achieves this may be used as a technique, at a grade which produces only minimal discomfort (Maitland, 1986). Additional

Figure 15.17   Sacro-iliac stress test – see text.

treatment may include correction of leg length discrepancy, muscle stretching or strengthening, support, and modalities to reduce pain and inflammation.

With persistent bilateral SIJ pain, the possibility of ankylosing spondylitis should be considered. The range of motion, especially lateral flexion, of the lumbar spine is limited, and muscle spasm may be evident. Where costovertebral involvement is present, chest expansion will be affected—often an early sign. The use of radiographs, erythrocyte sedimentation rate (ESR), and the presence of the antigen HLA B27 aid the diagnosis.

Spondylolysis

Spondylolysis is a defect in the neural arch (pars interarticularis), in 90% of cases, between the lamina and pedicle of the fifth lumbar vertebra (Fig. 15.18). It is a fracture of the pars without slippage, and by the age of 7 years is present in 5% of the population

Defect in pars

Spinous process

Pedicle

Transverse process

Pars interarticularis

Lamina

Figure 15.18   Site of defect in spondylolysis. From Gould (1990), with permission.

(Reid, 1992). In athletes, however, the incidence may be as high as 20%, and is often associated with other lumbar anomalies (Hoshina, 1980).

Where symptoms are present but no deformity is detectable on X-ray or bone scan, a pars interarticularis stress reaction has occurred (Weber and Woodall, 1991). At one stage a congenital defect was thought to be present. However, the condition is not present from birth and increases in incidence with age. Furthermore, the ossification centres of the vertebra do not correspond to the position of the defect. Familial tendencies do exist, and racial differences have been described (Colcher and Hursh, 1952).

The most important consideration from the point of view of sport is that of trauma. Direct trauma may result in a non-union of the area or, more likely, a stress fracture forms over a prolonged period, especially as a result of repeated flexion overload, hyperextension, or shearing stress to the lumbar spine. Athletes with hypolordosis in the lumbar spine are at risk from flexion overload whereas those demonstrating

hyperlordosis may suffer the condition as a result of forced rotation causing torsion overload (Farfan, Osteria and Lamy, 1976). The pars interarticularis is positioned as a pivot between the disc and facet joints, and so is subjected to considerable stress. The condition has been described in weight-lifters and oarsmen (Kotanis et al., 1971), hockey players (Letts et al., 1985), gymnasts (Jackson et al., 1981; Weber and Woodall, 1991), and fast bowlers (Williams and Sperryn, 1976).

Repeated stress can lead to microfractures, especially if overtraining has occurred. As these heal they produce an elongated appearance of the bone. Lumbar pain is apparent, which may be unilateral or bilateral, but this is rarely associated with nerve root compression. Pain is experienced first with hyperextension, such as walk-over movements in gymnastics, and increases in intensity. Pain is aggravated by hyperextension or rotation, and may present with paraspinal muscle spasm. Unilateral pain may be reproduced if the athlete performs hyperextension in single-leg standing. It is thought that this movement causes compression on the pars interarticularis (Weber and Woodall, 1991). Flexion is normally painless although pain may occur as the athlete returns to standing. Oblique X-rays give the classic 'terrier dog' appearance (Fig. 15.19) with the dog's collar represented by the pars interarticularis defect, which is bridged by fibrous tissue rather than bone. A nega-

Figure 15.19   An oblique X-ray of the lumbar spine, which has the appearance of a terrier dog. In the lower segment a spondylolysis through the pars interarticularis appears as a collar around the dog's neck. From Corrigan and Maitland (1983), with permission.

tive X-ray does not rule out spondylogenic conditions, and bone scan may be required (Ciullo and Jackson, 1985).

Spondylolisthesis

Spondylolisthesis is an anterior shift of one vertebra on the other, usually L5 on S1. In sport, the condition is usually a progression from spondylolysis, but it may also occur in the elderly as a result of degeneration, or congenitally in association with spina bifida. The first degree injury involves slippage to a distance of one quarter the vertebral diameter, but further movement may occur up to a fourth degree injury which involves a full diameter displacement (Corrigan and Maitland, 1983). The major symptom is of back pain referred to the buttocks, which is aggravated by exercise. Sciatica may be present as the condition is associated with disc protrusion in 5% of cases (Williams and Sperryn, 1976). The alteration in spinal alignment causes dimpling of the skin and extra skin folds above the level of injury. A step deformity to the spinous process at the lower level is normally apparent to palpation. The lordosis is usually increased, and severe spasm of the erector spinae may be present. Lumbar extension is often severely limited, and passive intervertebral pressure over the spinous process at the affected level is painful.

Management of spondylogenic disorders

Treatment aims mainly to eliminate the symptoms of the condition rather than to obtain bony union. Initially, rest is required. This varies from 'active rest' by avoiding painful movements with mild conditions to total bed rest with very severe lesions. Occasionally, braces and casts are used to protect the spine until the acute pain subsides, but the most important component of management is closely supervised exercise therapy. Thorough functional assessment is carried out to investigate strength and flexibility. In addition to absolute values in comparison to norms for a particular athlete population, muscle imbalance is important. Transmission of ground forces to the spine is governed to a large extent by hip and spine musculature, and weakness or asymmetry here must be corrected. Anterior shear forces are compensated by an extension moment created by the abdominal muscles (especially the internal obliques and transversus) and the latissimus dorsi pulling on the thoracolumbar fascia. In addition, the paraspinals counteract shear forces in the lumbar spine (Farfan, Osteria and Lamy, 1976).

The athlete is therefore required to follow an exercise programme to emphasize lumbar stabilization, and re-educate pelvic positioning (Saal and Saal, 1989; Weber and Woodall, 1991).

Spinal stability

When the lumbar spine demonstrates instability, there is an alteration of both the quality and quantity of movement available within a vertebral segment. The unstable segment shows decreased stiffness (resistance to bending) and as a consequence movement is increased even under minor loads. Clinical assessment may reveal a number of physical signs as outlined in Table 15.4.

To maintain spinal stability, three interrelated systems have been proposed (Fig. 15.20). Passive support is provided by inert tissues, while active support is from the contractile tissues. Sensory feedback from both systems provides coordination via the neural control centres (Panjabi, 1992). Importantly, where the stability provided by one system reduces, the other systems may compensate. Thus the proportion of load taken by the active system may increase to minimize stress on the passive system through load-

Table 15.4   Physical signs of instability

Step deformity (spondylolisthesis) or rotation deformity (spondylolisis) on standing which reduces on
  lying
Transverse band of muscle spasm which reduces on lying
Localized muscle twitching while shifting weight from one leg to the other
Juddering or shaking during forward bending
Alteration to passive intervertebral motion testing, suggesting excessive mobility in the sagittal plane

From Paris (1985) and Maitland (1986).

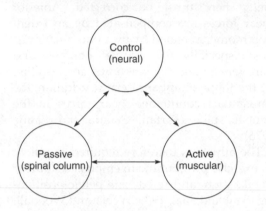

Figure 15.20   The spinal stabilizing system consists of three interrelating sub-systems. From Panjab (1992).

sharing (Tropp, Alaranta and Renstrom, 1993). When this happens, we can view stability as a continuously varying process (Bergmark, 1989). This process is dynamic and quite different to the traditional view of clinical stability being a static mechanical state (stable or unstable).

The concept of a dynamic interrelating system gives the physiotherapist the opportunity to reduce pain and improve function by rehabilitating active or functional lumbar stabilization. Such improvement may be accomplished by augmenting both the active and neural control systems. Simply developing muscle strength is insufficient. Moreover, many popular strength exercises for the trunk actually increase mobility in this region to dangerously high levels (Norris, 1993; 1994). Rather than improving stability, exercises of this type may reduce it and could therefore increase symptoms, especially those associated with inflammation.

Exercise programme to develop active lumbar stability

The active lumbar stabilization (ALS) programme (Richardson and Jull, 1994; Norris, 1995) begins by re-educating the stabilizing muscles of this region. The stabilizers of the lumbo-pelvic region are the deep abdominals, the gluteals, and the intersegmental muscles of the spine, especially multifidus. As described on p. 144, these muscles often function poorly after injury, and may be incorrectly recruited as a result of intense training activities, which lead to muscle imbalance. When this happens the mobilizer muscles of the lumbo-pelvic region (rectus abdominous, hip flexors and hamstrings) often dominate movements with the stabilizers being poorly recruited. The focus of the ALS programme therefore, is to reduce the dominance of the mobilizer muscles and enhance the function of the stabilizers.

The programme essentially consists of three overlapping stages, which parallel to a certain degree the three stages of motor learning (see p. 75). In stage I the therapist helps the patient to gain voluntary control of the stabilizing muscles, and then helps to build up their holding capacity (see p. 149). In stage II dynamic work augments the static activities begun with stage I, and controlled movements are used within mid-range only. In stage III, the speed of muscle contraction is enhanced (through proprioceptive training) in an attempt to redevelop the automatic nature of stabilization.

The process starts with the abdominal hollowing exercise described on p. 152. The patient begins in a prone-kneeling position with the spine in its neutral (mid-range) position (slight lordosis). The action is to pull the abdominal wall in, while breathing normally, without causing spinal flexion (Fig. 15.21a). Once this has been achieved the holding capacity of these muscles is built up until the patient can maintain the contraction for 10 repetitions, each held for 10 seconds (Richardson, 1992). The next exercise is the heel slide (Fig. 15.21b). The patient is in a crook-lying position. They perform the abdominal hollowing action, and while maintaining the neutral lumbar position, one leg is straightened, sliding the heel along the ground. The action of the hip flexors in this case tries to tilt the pelvis forwards (iliacus) and increase the lordosis (psoas). The abdominal muscles must work hard to stabilize the pelvis and lumbar spine against this pull.

Rhythmic stabilization techniques are used to facilitate multifidus contraction together with that of the oblique abdominals. In crook side-lying the therapist pushes forwards onto the subject's pelvis and backwards onto his or her shoulder while the subject resists the action (Fig. 15.21c). The movement direction is then reversed. In a crook-lying position the therapist pushes against the patient's bent knees trying to cause spinal rotation, while the subject resists this movement (Fig. 15.21d).

Gluteal contractions are begun in a prone position to gain voluntary control of the muscle and then quickly progressed to crook-lying bridging actions (Fig. 15.21e). The aim is to perform a co-contraction between the gluteals, spinal extensors, and deep abdominals so that the neutral spinal position is maintained throughout the action (Richardson, Toppenberg and Jull, 1990). The

Figure 15.21 Lumbar stabilization exercise. Stage 1 (a) Abdominal hollowing, (b) heel slide, (c) rhythmic stabilization, (d) developing trunk rotator strength, (e) bridging, (f) single-leg bridge.

exercise progresses to single-leg bridging, maintaining pelvic alignment in the sagittal, frontal and transverse planes (Fig. 15.21f).

A variety of additional movements may be used (Fig. 15.22) with the aim in each case of maintaining correct alignment of the spine and building holding capacity.

During stage II dynamic movements of the spine are used. Now the aim is to maintain both static (neutral position) and dynamic (lumbo-pelvic rhythm) alignment. Actions such as the trunk curl (p. 180) and hip hinge (p. 166) are useful as are more traditional lumbar exercises involving rotation. Resistance training appropriate to individual sporting requirements may be used (Fig. 15.23). The correct relationship between lumbar alignment and pelvic alignment must be

rigorously maintained. A convex contour of the abdominal wall (doming or bow-stringing) indicates that the deep abdominals are failing to maintain stability against the pull of rectus abdominous. A maximally flexed or extended lumbar spine indicates that mid-range (active) stability has been lost and joint approximation and inert tissue stretch are providing passive stability only.

The final stage (stage III) is to increase the speed and complexity of movement so that the athlete is forced to maintain stability automatically. The athlete's attention is fully taken up by focusing on the complexity of the exercise task (see information processing bottleneck, p. 73). Spinal alignment must be maintained in sports-related actions such as cycling, jogging, throwing and plyo-

Figure 15.22 Additional stabilization movements. 1. Straight line arm-spine-leg. 2. Lunging. 3. Prone with double arm lifts. 4. Prone with double leg lifts. 5. Superman. 6. Thoracic bridge. 7. Supine gym ball bridging.

(a)

(b)

(c)

(d)

(e)

(f)

(g)

Figure 15.23 Examples of resistance exercises. Stage II (a) Sitting abdominal curl, (b) reverse crunch, (c) lying cable trunk rotation, (d) heel slide, (e) sitting trunk rotation, (f) prone leg extension, (g) lateral pull down. From Norris (1996).

metric actions. Use of a balance board or balance shoes and swiss gym ball is useful (Irion, 1992; Lester, 1992; Lester and Posner-Mayer, 1993).

References

Adams, M.A. and Hutton, W.C. (1982) Prolapsed intervertebral disc. A hyperflexion injury. *Spine*, **8**(3), 327

Adams, M.A. and Hutton, W.C. (1980) The effect of posture on the role of the apophyseal joints in resisting intervertebral compression force. *Journal of Bone and Joint Surgery (Br)*, **62B**, 358–362

Adams, M.A. and Hutton, W.C. (1983) The mechanical function of the lumbar apophyseal joints. *Spine*, **8**, 327–330

Adams, M.A., Hutton, W.C. and Stott, J.R.R. (1980) The resistance to flexion of the lumbar intervertebral joint. *Spine*, **5**, 245–253

Bergmark, A. (1989) Stability of the lumbar spine. *Acta Orthopaedica Scandinavica Supplementum*, **230**(60), 3–54

Bernhardt, M., White, A.A., Panjabi, M.M. and McGowan, D.P. (1992) Lumbar spine instability. In *The Lumbar Spine and Back Pain* (ed. M.I.V. Jayson), 4th edn, Churchill Livingstone, Edinburgh

Bogduk, N. and Engel, R. (1984) The menisci of the lumbar zygapophyseal joints. A review of their anatomy and clinical significance. *Spine*, **9**, 454–460

Bogduk, N. and Jull, G. (1985) The theoretical pathology of acute locked back: a basis for manipulative therapy. *Manual Medicine*, **1**, 78–82

Bogduk, N. and Twomey, L.T. (1987) *Clinical Anatomy of the Lumbar Spine*. Churchill Livingstone, Edinburgh

Bogduk, N. and Twomey, L.T. (1991) *Clinical Anatomy of the Lumbar Spine*, 2nd edn, Churchill Livingstone, Edinburgh

Butler, D.S. (1991) *Mobilisation of the Nervous System*, Churchill Livingstone, Edinburgh

Cappozzo, A., Felici, F., Figura, F. and Gazzani, F. (1985) Lumbar spine loading during half-squat exercises. *Medicine and Science in Sports and Exercise*, **17**(5), 613–620

Ciullo, J.V. and Jackson, D.W. (1985) Pars interarticularis stress reaction, spondylolysis, and spondylolisthesis in gymnasts. *Clinics in Sports Medicine*, **4**, 95–110

Colcher, A.E. and Hursh, A.M.W. (1952) Pre-employment low back X-ray survey: a review of 1500 cases. *Industrial Medicine and Surgery*, **21**, 319

Corrigan, B. and Maitland, G.D. (1983) *Practical Orthopaedic Medicine*, Butterworth, London

Crock, H.V. and Yoshizawa, H. (1976) The blood supply of the lumbar vertebral column. *Clinical Orthopaedics*, **115**, 6–21

Cyriax, J. (1982) *Textbook of Orthopaedic Medicine*, Vol. 1, 8th edn, Baillière Tindall, London

Cyriax, J.H. and Cyriax, P.J. (1983) *Illustrated Manual of Orthopaedic Medicine*, Butterworth, London

Farfan, H.F. and Sullivan, J.D. (1967) The relation of facet orientation to intervertebral disc failure. *Canadian Journal of Surgery*, **10**, 179–185

Farfan, H.F., Cossette, J.W., Robertson, G.H., Wells, R.V. and Kraus, H. (1970) The effects of torsion on the lumbar intervertebral joints: the role of torsion in the production of disc degeneration. *Journal of Bone and Joint Surgery*, **52A**, 468

Farfan, H.F., Huberdeau, R.M. and Dubow, H.I. (1972) Lumbar intervertebral disc degeneration. The influence of geometrical features on the pattern of disc degeneration – a post mortem study. *Journal of Bone and Joint Surgery (Am)*, **54A**, 492–510

Farfan, H.F., Osteria, V. and Lamy, C. (1976) The mechanical etiology of spondylolysis and spondylolisthesis. *Clinical Orthopaedics and Related Research*, **117**, 40–55

Frigerio, N.A., Stowe, R.R. and Howe, J.W. (1974) Movement of the sacro-iliac joint. *Clinical Orthopaedic and Related Research*, **100**, 370

Fryomoyer, J.W. and Cats-Baril, W.L. (1991) An overview of the incidences and costs of low back pain. *Orthopaedic Clinics of North America*, **22**, 263

Gould, J.A. (ed.) (1989) *Orthopaedic and Sports Physical Therapy*, C.V. Mosby, Baltimore

Grieve, G.P. (1970) Sciatica and the straight leg raising test in manipulative treatment. *Physiotherapy*, **56**, 337

Grieve, G.P. (1976) The sacro-iliac joint. *Physiotherapy*, **62** (12), 384–400

Hirsch, C. and Nachemson, A. (1954) New observations on mechanical behaviour of lumbar discs. *Acta Orthopaedica Scandinavica*, **22**, 184–189

Hirsch, C. and Schajowicz, F. (1952) Studies on structural changes in the lumbar annulus fibrosis. *Acta Orthopaedica Scandinavica*, **22**, 184–189

Hirsch, C., Ingelmark, V.E. and Miller, N. (1963) The anatomic basis for low back pain: studies on the presence of sensory endings in ligamentous capsular and intervertebral disc structures in the human lumbar spine. *Acta Orthopaedica Scandinavia*, **33**, 1–17

Holm, S., Maroudas, A., Urban, J.P.G., Selstam, G. and Nachemson, A. (1981) Nutrition of the intervertebral disc: solute transport and metabolism. *Connective Tissue Research*, **8**, 101–119

Horwitz, T. and Smith, R.M. (1940) An anatomical, pathological and roentgenological study of the intervertebral joints of the lumbar spine and of the sacro-iliac joints. *American Journal of Roentgenology and Radiation Therapy*, **43**, 173–186

Hoshina, H. (1980) Spondylolysis in young athletes. *Physician and Sports Medicine*, **8**, 75–79

Hukins, D.W.L. (1987) Properties of spinal materials. In *The Lumbar Spine and Back Pain* (ed. M.I.V. Jayson), Churchill Livingstone, London

Irion, J.M. (1992) Use of the gym ball in rehabilitation of spinal dysfunction. *Orthopaedic Physical Therapy Clinics of North America*, 375–398

Jull, G.A. and Richardson, C.A. (1994) Rehabilitation of active stabilization of the lumbar spine. In *Physical Therapy of the Low Back* (eds L.T. Twomey and L.T. Taylor), 2nd edn, Churchill Livingstone, Edinburgh

Kapandji, I. (1974) *The Physiology of Joints, Vol. 3, The Spine*, Churchill Livingstone, London

Klein, J.A. and Hukins, D.W.L. (1981) Functional differentiation in the spinal column. *Eng Med*, **12**(2), 83

Klein, J.A. and Hukins, D.W.L. (1983) Relocation of the bending axis during flexion–extension of the lumbar intervertebral discs and its implications for prolapse. *Spine*, **8**, 659–664

Kotanis, P.T., Ichikawa, N., Wakabayashi, W., Yoshii, T. and Koshimune, M. (1971) Studies of spondylolysis found among weight lifters. *British Journal of Sports Medicine*, **6**, 4

Kraemer, J., Kolditz, D. and Gowin, R. (1985) Water and electrolyte content of human intervertebral discs under variable load. *Spine*, **10**, 69–71

Leatt, P., Reilly, T. and Troup, J.G.D. (1986) Spinal loading during circuit weight-training and running. *British Journal of Sports Medicine*, **20**(3), 119–124

Lee, D.G. (1994) Clinical manifestations of pelvic girdle dysfunction. In *Grieve's Modern Manual Therapy*, 2nd edn (eds J.D. Boyling and N. Palastanga), Churchill Livingstone, Edinburgh

Lester, M.N. (1992) Spinal stabilization and compliance utilizing the therapeutic ball. *Proceeding of the International Federation of Orthopaedic Manipulative Therapists*, Vail, Colorado

Lester, M.N. and Posner-Mayer, J. (1993) *Spinal Stabilization: Utilizing the Swiss Ball* (video), Ball Dynamics, Denver

Letts, M., Smallman, T., Afanasiev, R. and Gouw, G. (1985) Fracture of the pars interarticularis in adolescent athletes: a clinical-biomechanical analysis. *Journal of Paediatric Orthopaedics*, **6**, 40–46

Maitland, G.D. (1986) *Vertebral Manipulation*, 5th edn, Butterworth, London

Maitland, G.D. (1991) *Peripheral Manipulation*, 3rd edn, Butterworth-Heinemann, Oxford

Markolf, K.L. and Morris, J.M. (1974) The structural components of the intervertebral disc. *Journal of Bone and Joint Surgery*, **56A**, 675

McKenzie, R.A. (1981) *The Lumbar Spine. Mechanical Diagnosis and Therapy*, Spinal Publications, New Zealand

McKenzie, R.A. (1990) *The Cervical and Thoracic Spine. Mechanical Diagnosis and Therapy*, Spinal Publications, New Zealand

Mooney, V. and Robertson, J. (1976) The facet syndrome. *Clinical Orthopaedics*, **115**, 149–156

Mulligan, B.R. (1989) *Manual Therapy—Nags, Snags, and PRP's etc*, Plane View Services, Wellington, New Zealand

Nachemson, A. (1987) Lumbar intradiscal pressure. In *The Lumbar Spine and Back Pain* (ed. M.I.V. Jayson), Churchill Livingstone, London

Nachemson, A. (1976) The lumbar spine: an orthopaedic challenge. *Spine*, **1**, 59–71

Nachemson, A. and Evans, J. (1968) Some mechanical properties of the third lumbar inter-laminar ligament (ligamentum flavum). *Journal of Biomechanics*, **1**, 211

Nelson, M.A., Allen, P., Clamp, S.E. and De Dombal, F.T. (1979) Reliability and reproducibility of clinical findings in low back pain. *Spine*, **4**, 97–101

Norkin, C.C. and Levangie, P.K. (1992) Joint structure and function. A comprehensive analysis, 2nd edn, F.A. Davis, Philadelphia

Norris, C.M. (1993) Abdominal muscle training in sport. *British Journal of Sports Medicine*, **27**(1), 19–27

Norris, C.M. (1994) Abdominal training. Dangers and exercise modifications. *Physiotherapy in Sport*, **19**(5), 10–14

Norris, C.M. (1995) Spinal stabilisation 2. Limiting factors to end-range motion in the lumbar spine. *Physiotherapy*, **81**(2), 4–12

Norris, C.M. (1996) *Weight training. Physiotools Compatible Computer Programme*. Exercise Association. London

Oliver, J. and Middleditch, A. (1991) *Functional Anatomy of the Spine*, Butterworth-Heinemann, Oxford

Palastanga, N., Field, D. and Soames, R. (1989) *Anatomy and Human Movement*, Butterworth-Heinemann, Oxford

Panjabi, M.M. (1992) The stabilizing system of the spine. Part 1. Function, dysfunction, adaptation, and enhancement. *Journal of Spinal Disorders*, **5**(4), 383–389

Panjabi, M.M., Jorneus, L. and Greenstein, G. (1984) *Lumbar Spine Ligaments: an in vitro Biomechanical Study*, ORS Transactions

Panjabi, M.M., Hult, J.E. and White, A.A. (1987) Biomechanical studies in cadaveric spines. In *The Lumbar Spine and Back Pain* (ed. M.I.V. Jayson), Churchill Livingstone, London

Paris, S.V. (1985) Physical signs of instability. *Spine*, **10** (3), 277–279

Pearcy, P., Portek, I. and Shepherd, J. (1984) Three dimensional X-ray analysis of normal movement in the lumbar spine. *Spine*, **9**, 294–297

Reid, D.C. (1992) *Sports Injury Assessment and Rehabilitation*, Churchill Livingstone, London

Richardson, C.A. (1992) Muscle imbalance: Principles of treatment and assessment. *Proceedings of the New Zealand Society of Physiotherapists Challenges Conference*, Christchurch

Richardson, C.A., and Jull, G.A. (1994) Concepts of assessment and rehabilitation for active lumbar stability. In: *Grieve's Modern Manual Therapy* (eds J.D. Boyling and N. Palastanga). 2nd edn, Churchill Livingstone, Edinburgh

Richardson C., Toppenberg R. and Jull, G. (1990) An initial evaluation of eight abdominal exercises for their ability to provide stabilisation for the lumbar spine. *Australian Journal of Physiotherapy*, **36**, 6–11

Roaf, R. (1960) A study of the mechanics of spinal injuries. *Journal of Bone and Joint Surgery (Br)*, **42B**, 810–823

Rockoff, S.F., Sweet, E. and Bleustein, J. (1969) The relative contribution of trabecular and cortical bone to the strength of human lumbar vertebrae. *Calcified Tissue Research*, **3**, 163–175

Saal, J.A. and Saal, J.S. (1989) Nonoperative treatment of herniated lumbar intervertebral disc with radiculopathy. *Spine*, **14**, 431–437

Spitzer, W.O., LeBlanc, F.E. and Dupuis, M. (1987) Scientific approach to the assessment and management of activity related spinal disorders. A monograph for clinicians. Report of the Quebec Task Force on Spinal Disorders. *Spine*, **12**, 7s

Taylor, J.R. and Twomey, L.T. (1986) Age changes in lumbar zygapophyseal joints. *Spine*, **11**, 739–745

Taylor, J.R. and Twomey, L.T. (1994) The lumbar spine from infancy to old age. In *Physical Therapy of the Low Back*, 2nd edn (eds L.T. Twomey and J.R. Taylor), Churchill Livingstone, London

Tkaczuk, H. (1968) Tensile properties of human lumbar longitudinal ligaments. *Acta Orthopaedica Scandinavica*, **115** (Suppl)

Tropp, H., Alaranta, H. and Renstrom, P.A.F.H. (1993) Proprioception and coordination training in injury prevention. In *Sports Injuries: Basic Principles of Prevention and Care* (ed. P.A.F.H. Renstrom), IOC Medical Commission Publication, Blackwell Scientific Publications, London

Tyrrell, A.R., Reilly, T. and Troup, J.D.G. (1985) Circadian variation in stature and the effects of spinal loading. *Spine*, **10**, 161–164

Unsworth, A., Doverson, D. and Wright, V. (1971) Cracking joints. *Annals of the Rheumatic Diseases*, **30**, 348

Urban, L.M. (1986) The straight-leg raising test: a review. In *Modern Manual Therapy of the Vertebral Column* (ed. G.P. Grieve), Churchill Livingstone, London

Vernon-Roberts, B. (1987) Pathology of intervertebral discs and apophyseal joints. In *The Lumbar Spine and Back Pain* (ed. M.I.V. Jayson), Churchill Livingstone, London

Weber, M.D. and Woodall, W.R. (1991) Spondylogenic disorders in gymnasts. *Journal of Orthopaedic and Sports Physical Therapy*, **14**(1), 6–13

Wells, P (1986) The examination of the pelvic joints. In *Modern Manual Therapy of the Vertebral Column* (ed. G.P. Grieve), Churchill Livingstone, London

Williams, J.G.P. and Sperryn, P.N. (1976) *Sports Medicine*, Edward Arnold, London

Wyke, B. (1972) Articular neurology: a review. *Physiotherapy*, **58**, 94

Yang, K.H. and King, A.I. (1984) Mechanism of facet load transmission as a hypothesis for low-back pain. *Spine*, **9**, 557–565

16

The thorax and thoracic spine

Thoracic spine

The unique feature of the vertebrae in the thoracic region is the presence of facets, both on the sides of the vertebral bodies, and the transverse processes. These are for articulation with the ribs, forming the costo-vertebral and costo-transverse joints (Fig. 16.1). Most of the ribs articulate with two adjacent vertebral bodies and one transverse process. The facets on the head of the ribs articulate in turn with demi-facets on the upper and lower borders of the vertebrae, and the crest on the rib head butts onto the intervertebral disc. The joint capsule is loose and strengthened anteriorly to form the three portions of the radiate ligament. The costo-vertebral joint cavity is divided into two by the intra-articular ligament, except for ribs one, ten, eleven and twelve which articulate with a single vertebra and have a single joint cavity.

The costo-transverse joints are formed only with the upper ten ribs. The joint is made between the articular facet of the transverse process and the oval facet on the rib tubercle. The thin joint capsule is strengthened by the costo-transverse ligaments.

Sternal articulations

The sternocostal joints are formed between the medial end of the costal cartilages of ribs one to seven. The joint between the first rib and the sternum is cartilaginous, but all the others are synovial. Each is surrounded by a capsule and supported by radiate ligaments. The fibres of these ligaments fan out and intertwine with those of the ligaments above and below, and also with those of the opposite sternocostal joints. In addition, the radiate ligament fibres fuse with the tendinous fibres of the pectoralis major. The eighth, ninth, and tenth ribs form interchondral joints between their costal cartilages.

The costo-chondral joints are formed between the end of the rib and the lateral edge of the costal cartilage. The joint formed is cartilaginous, its perichondrium being continuous with the periosteum of the rib itself. Only slight bending and twisting actions are possible at this joint. The manubriosternal articulation is that between the upper part of the sternum and the manubrium. The joint is cartilaginous, with a hollow disc in its centre, and is strengthened by the sterno-costal ligaments and longitudinal fibrous bands. About 7° of movement occurs at the joint in association with breathing.

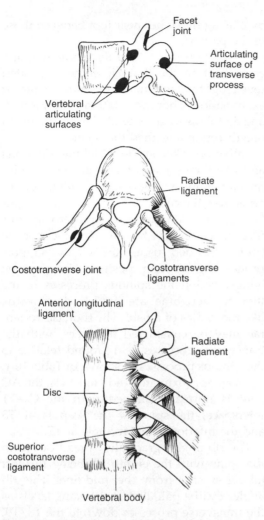

Facet joint

Articulating surface of transverse process

Vertebral articulating surfaces

Radiate ligament

Costotransverse joint

Costotransverse ligaments

Anterior longitudinal ligament

Radiate ligament

Disc

Superior costotransverse ligament

Vertebral body

Figure 16.1 Joints between the ribs and thoracic spine.

Rib movements

Movement of the diaphragm, ribs and sternum increases the volume within the thorax with inspiration. Each ribs acts as a lever, with one axis travelling through the costo-vertebral and sternocostal joints, and another through the costo-vertebral and costo-transverse joints. The two axes permit two types of motion, known as 'pump handle' and 'bucket handle'. In the pump handle action the upper ribs and sternum are raised, increasing the antero-posterior diameter of the thorax. With bucket handle motion the

lower ribs move both up and out, widening the infrasternal angle and increasing the transverse diameter or the thorax. The variation in movement between the upper and lower ribs is due, in part, to the differing structure of their respective costo-transverse joints. The upper joints are cup-shaped permitting mainly rotation (pump handle), while those lower down are flat permitting both rotation and gliding movements (bucket handle).

In addition to respiratory motion, the ribs also move in association with the thoracic spine. With flexion of the spine the ribs move closer together and with extension they are pulled further apart, flattening the rib cage. This latter action in the upper ribs is important for the correct movement of the scapulo-thoracic joint (see p. 167). Lateral flexion causes the ribs on the concave side to move together and those on the convex side to move apart. Rotation gives horizontal gliding of one rib relative to another.

Movement of the thoracic spine

The relative thinness of the discs in the thoracic region, coupled with the presence of the ribs makes movement here more limited than in other spinal areas. Extension is limited to about 30° with slightly more flexion being possible—roughly 40°. Flexion is freer in the lower thoracic region but still restricted by the ribs. Extension is limited by approximation of the facets and spinous processes as well as tissue tension, and causes the thoracic cage to become flatter. Lateral flexion is limited to roughly 25° to each side, a greater range being available in the lower region. Lateral flexion is accompanied by the same amount of rotation, which occurs contralaterally. For example, right lateral flexion is accompanied by right axial rotation, causing the tip of the spinous process to rest to the left of the mid-line. Rib movements accompany lateral flexion, with the ribs on the concave side compressing and those on the side of the convexity being pulled apart.

The range of rotation is larger than other movements, with 35° being possible to either side. However, when the spine is extended, both lateral flexion and rotation are dramatically reduced. As rotation occurs, the inferior facets of the upper vertebra slide laterally with respect to the lower vertebra, towards the direction of the rotation. Movement of the vertebra is accompanied by distortion of the ribs. The rib cage becomes more rounded on the side to which the rotation is occurring, and flattens on the opposite side.

Rotation of the thoracic spine is an important constituent of locomotion. In walking, when the right leg swings forward the lower trunk and the pelvis rotate to the left about the fixed left leg. To keep the head facing forwards the upper spine must rotate to the right pulling the shoulders back into a forward facing direction. As the upper and lower parts of the spine are rotating in opposite directions, there is a point at which the two movements cancel each other out. This point is the intervertebral disc between T7 and T8 which is not subjected to any rotation, while those vertebra immediately above and below rotate maximally, but in opposite directions.

Examination

The screening examination is essentially similar to that of the lumbar spine, except that rotation is the movement most likely to be revealing as this normally has the greatest range. Rotation is performed in a sitting position, with overpressure being given through the shoulders. Resisted flexion and extension may be performed in a lying or a sitting position. Resisted lateral flexion is tested in a standing position with the therapist initially at the patient's side. The patient's near wrist of his or her straight arm is gripped, as is the far shoulder. Stability is improved if the therapist widens his or her base of support by placing his or her near foot between those of the patient.

As rotation and lateral flexion accompany each other in the thoracic spine it is often revealing to combine these movements at examination. Thoracic rotation is performed, and is followed by lateral flexion, firstly in one direction and then the other.

Palpation takes in the vertebrae, rib joints and ribs themselves, and is carried out with the patient in a prone position with his or her arms over the couch side to move the scapulae apart. Alternatively, postero-anterior (PA) pressures may be used with the thoracic spine extended using the elbow support prone-lying starting position. In a prone lying position the spinous processes of the thoracic vertebrae are angled downwards like the 'scales of a fish'. The thoracic vertebrae may be considered in threes, with the transverse processes being found relative to the spinous processes as shown in Table 16.1.

As an approximate guide to levels, the AC joint is normally aligned with the C7–T1 interspace, the spine of the scapula at T3 and the inferior scapular angle at T7.

The rib angles gradually spread out from the spine with the eighth rib being furthest (about 6 cm) from the mid-line. The rib angles can be palpated at the same levels as the transverse processes down to the T8/T9, by pushing the soft tissue to one side. The apophyseal joints lie in the paravertebral sulci, and the transverse processes, which

Table 16.1

T1, 2, 3	— At the same level as spinous process
T4, 5, 6	— Between two successive levels
T7, 8, 9	— Level with spinous process of vertebra below
T10	— Level with vertebra below
T11	— Between two successive levels
T12	— At same level

overlie the costo-transverse joints, are found 3–4 cm from the mid-line.

Modifications to the slump test for the thoracic spine

The slump test was described on p. 350. A variation of this test for the cervical and thoracic spine is to perform it in the long sitting position (Fig. 16.2a). From this position thoracic and lumbar flexion are added followed by cervical flexion (Fig. 16.2b). Altering the order of movement will change the neurodynamic demands (Butler and Slater, 1994) enabling the practitioner to refine the test. For example, performing cervical flexion before lumbar and thoracic flexion will challenge the cervical neural tissues more. The test can be further refined to place emphasis on the sympathetic trunk (Slater, Butler and Shacklock, 1994). This is especially relevant in the presence of sympathetic signs in conditions such as T4 syndrome, thoracic outlet syndrome and Raynaud's syndrome, and in cases where cervico-thoracic conditions mimic cardiac disease. Sympathetic testing is achieved by adding components of lateral flexion and rotation of the thoracic spine and lateral flexion of the cervical spine. Additional stress may be imposed by adding a minimal straight leg raise (SLR).

Injury to the rib cage

Direct trauma to the rib cage can result in damage to the ribs, intercostal muscles or, indirectly, to the rib joints. Deep breathing will usually reproduce the pain of rib or intercostal injury, and palpation can be used to reveal the exact site of injury as these structures are superficial. Trunk extension will open the rib cage and cause pain, and intercostal muscle tearing will generally give pain to resisted trunk flexion. Rib springing at a distance from the point of injury usually produces pain from a rib fracture.

With rib fracture, it is the tearing of the intercostal muscles which gives the pain rather than the fracture itself (Cyriax, 1982). The acute pain may be relieved by local strapping. Pre-stretched elastic adhesive strapping is applied across the area to restrict rib cage expansion and give the athlete a feeling of support. In the sub-acute phase active mobilization is required. If scar tissue formation is excessive and the source of pain, transverse frictions to the intercostal muscles along the line of the ribs are helpful. In addition, holding the rib down with the fingertips and practising deep inspiration will help to stretch the injured area. Exercises to expand the rib cage, such as deep inspiration and overhead reaching, or trunk lateral flexion to the contralateral side with or without rotation is also helpful to stretch the area.

The sternocostal joints may be sprained giving local swelling and tenderness, as

(a)

(b)

Figure 16.2 The slump test (long sitting). (a) Start. (b) Finish. From Butler (1991).

may the costo-chondral joints (Tietze's syndrome). Pressure on the sternum, or applied to the lateral aspect of the thorax, reproduces the pain, and palpation localizes the lesion. The injury can occur when performing exercises which force the arms into extension and abduction. Weight-training movements, such as bench pressing, and gymnastic exercises, such as dips on parallel bars, may both cause problems. Both the costo-vertebral and costo-transverse joints may be subject to sprain, with pain occurring to rib movements and local palpation.

First rib

The first is the shortest and roundest of the ribs. It slopes downwards and forwards, from its attachment to the first thoracic vertebra. It forms attachment for the scalene muscles, serratus anterior, and subclavius. It superior surface bears a deep groove for the subclavian artery (posterior) and the subclavian vein (anterior). The arterial groove is the weakest part of the rib (Gurtler, Pavlov and Torg, 1985).

Fractures of the first rib may either be traumatic or the result of overuse. Overuse injuries have been reported as a result of repeated arm movements, such as heavy lifting and pitching (Bailey, 1985; Lankenner and Micheli, 1985; Gurtler, Pavlov and Torg, 1985). Symptoms are of pain associated with

deep breathing, tenderness in the root of the neck, posterior aspect of the shoulder, or axilla. Often the patient hears or feels a snap in the shoulder as he or she performs a sudden violent movement. Range of shoulder movement will usually be full but painful, especially to extension. Accurate diagnosis by radiographs in traumatic lesions is essential because of the proximity of the major vessels, nerves and the lung. Bailey (1985) recommended serial radiographs for up to 6 months after stress fracture.

Management is by rest from the causal action, with shoulder support in a sling if pain is limiting. Gentle isometric shoulder exercises are used, and the condition usually resolves within 4–6 weeks.

Manual therapy

Joint mobilization

A variety of procedures may be used for the thoracic spine (Fig. 16.3). Postero-anterior central vertebral pressure is the technique normally used first, in the presence of both unilateral and bilateral symptoms (Maitland, 1986). The technique is essentially the same as that described for the cervical spine. In the thoracic spine, however, the spinous processes are larger and so the therapist may use his or her thumbs side by side or one in front of the other. For the upper thoracic

(a)   (b)   (c)

Figure 16.3 Mobilization of the thorax. (a) Costovertebral joint. (b) Thoracic rotation. (c) First rib. After Maitland (1986).

spine the therapist stands at the patient's head, and for the lower regions at the patient's side. The oscillatory motion is given as described for the cervical spine, with the range of movement being particularly great in the middle and lower thoracic areas, but somewhat limited between T1 and T2.

The costo-vertebral and costo-transverse joints are mobilized by springing the rib. The therapist places his or her thumbs, or ulnar border of his or her hand and little finger, along the line of the rib to be mobilized to give a broad (and more comfortable) area of contact. The mobilization must take the patient's respiratory movements into account, pressure for higher grade movements coinciding with expiration.

Antero-posterior movements may be performed on any of the costal joints (costo-chondral, interchondral, sterno-costal). The therapist's thumbs are placed over the joint to be mobilized with his or her fingers fanning out over the patient's chest. The movement may be directed towards the patient's head or feet to reproduce the symptoms, and then continued in this direction at a lesser grade.

Intervertebral rotations may be applied both locally and generally. Local rotation may be carried out using pressure over the transverse processes. The thenar eminence of one hand is placed on the transverse process of one vertebra with the fingers pointing towards the patient's head. The hypothenar eminence of the other hand is placed on the transverse process on the opposing side of the spine either of the same vertebra or that of the vertebra below, with the fingers towards the patient's feet. A number of techniques are used. Rotation may be applied by using alternating pressure from one hand and then the other with the hands over the same spinal level (McKenzie, 1990), or a high velocity low amplitude thrust may be applied as the patient breathes out, with the hands over the transverse processes of two levels (Bourdillon, 1982).

General rotation may be performed with the patient seated over the couch end, with his or her arms folded, with the hands gripping the shoulders, the therapist stands to the side of the patient. The patient rotates as far as is possible away from the therapist, who reaches across the patient's chest and grasps the patient's far shoulder. Overpressure is applied as the therapist pulls the far shoulder towards himself and presses the far scapula away with the flat of his hand. Slight traction may be applied by gripping the far elbow rather than the shoulder. The therapist bends his or her knees before applying the grip and then straightens them as he or she pulls up and round. This technique may be used for mobilization or contract relax stretching.

The close proximity of structures within this area makes it difficult to assess precisely whether a patient's symptoms are coming from the intervertebral joint, the costo-transverse joint, the costo-vertebral joints or a combination of all three. For this reason many of the mobilizations affect all of these joints.

Trunk muscles

The trunk muscles are open to injury in the same way as any other muscle in the body, but muscle conditions are often overlooked in the search for signs of more complex injuries involving the intervertebral joints. Injury to the intercostal muscles has already been mentioned, but the adominal muscles and erector spinae may also give pain from injury or muscle soreness.

The abdominal muscles are tested isometrically to eliminate involvement of the spine. A crook-lying position is preferred, as this partially relaxes the ilio-psoas. Straight flexion taxes the rectus abdominous while flexion-rotation works the oblique abdominals. Pure rotation is tested in a sitting position, while lateral flexion is tested either in a sitting or standing position.

The upper (supra-umbilical) portion of the rectus abdominous is assesed from a sit-up position, while the lower (infra-umbilical) portion is assessed by lowering the straight legs from 90° hip flexion to work the muscle in a reverse origin to insertion fashion. Comparison is made between the right and left sides of the rectus by palpatation, and watching the displacement of the umbilicus which will be pulled to the side of the stronger muscle (Lacote et al., 1987). The oblique abdominals are worked by perfoming a sit-up motion with rotation, for example reaching the right arm towards the left knee. Rotation to the left works the right external oblique and left internal oblique and vice versa. The transversus abdominis acts to support the viscera and is active in forced expiration. It may be tested with the patient in a prone-kneeling position. From this position the subject breathes out against a resistance (balloon or spirometer) and pulls the abdominal wall in.

The erector spinae are tested in a prone-lying position, the subject being asked to extend his or her trunk and lift his or her chest from the couch. Isometric contraction is assessed by having the patient (in a prone-lying position) maintain a horizontal position of the trunk with only the legs supported. Alternatively, the patient should rest his or her chest over the couch end and attempt to straighten the legs to a horizontal position. The quadratus lumborum is tested with the subject prone, leg extended and slightly abducted, to elevate the pelvis laterally. Traction is placed through the elevated leg to oppose the pull of quadratus lumborum (Kendall and McCreary, 1983). Abdominal training in sport is covered on pp. 157–181.

Hernia

A hernia is a protrusion of the contents of a cavity through the cavity wall. Most usually an organ or peritoneum is forced through the muscular layer of the abdominal wall, at sites of natural weakness where nerves and blood vessels leave the abdomen. The most common types are femoral, inguinal and incisional. Less common types include umbilical, epigastric and hiatus herniae.

Inguinal herniae occur as a result of damage or malformation of the structures forming the inguinal canal (Fig. 16.4). The

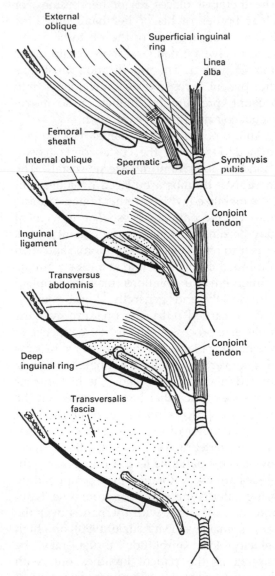

Figure 16.4 Formation of the inguinal canal. From Palastanga et al. (1994).

hernia may be either direct or indirect, and is far more common in men than women. As the testis descends during fetal life, it drags with it a tube-like covering of peritoneum, the processus vaginalis which is usually obliterated. If this tube remains, it constitutes a weakness which may lead to an indirect inguinal hernia. This usually occurs in males and on the right side of the body. Direct inguinal herniae are more common in older men, and rupture through the weak abdominal wall. They are precipitated by obesity, persistent coughing, and straining.

Symptoms of an inguinal hernia are of a dragging sensation in the groin, especially when straining. A swelling may be noticeable over the external ring of the inguinal canal above and medial to the pubic tubercle, the point of attachment of adductor longus. In the case of an indirect hernia, the bulge may be in the upper scrotum. A bulge may be palpated over the hernia when the patient coughs. It is sometimes possible to pass the little finger through the skin of the upper scrotum to the external ring of the inguinal canal, following the line of the spermatic cord. The patient is supine, and the examining finger is directed upwards, backwards and laterally. Again, coughing will produce a bulge when hernia is present.

Groin disruption is a condition which may mimic inguinal hernia in many ways (Gilmore, 1995). It comprises a tearing of the external oblique aponeurosis and the conjoint tendon. There is a dehiscence (separation) between the conjoint tendon and the inguinal ligament but no hernial sac. The condition was originally described in soccer players but may occur in other sports. There is a gradual onset of pain with one-third of the patients reporting a specific injury which may have resulted in tearing. Pain (in the inguinal, adductor or perineal region) is exacerbated by kicking actions and sudden changes in movement direction. The superficial inguinal ring is often dilated to palpation. Treatment is sur-

gical, with repair of the torn conjoined tendon and approximation of the tendon to the inguinal ligament. The external oblique is repaired and the inguinal ring reconstituted.

Both prevention (Gilmore, 1995; Norris, 1995) and successful rehabilitation of this condition rely heavily on correct abdominal training. One of the factors in the development of this condition is the muscle imbalance which is created by sit-up exercises in the athlete. Tightness in the hip flexors, combined with preferential recruitment of the rectus abdominis and poor recruitment of the deep abdominals, leaves the lower abdominal area open to injury. Increasing the training emphasis on abdominal hollowing actions and reducing the emphasis on lumbar flexion actions is a key factor which should be combined with stretching of the tight hip flexors.

A *femoral hernia* is a protrusion of abdominal contents through the femoral ring, which is the point below the inguinal ligament where the blood vessels enter the leg. The condition is more common in women than men. The features are essentially similar to that of the inguinal hernia, except that the femoral hernia is generally smaller and more difficult to detect. An epigastric hernia travels through the linea alba. A small bulge (usually of fat) is found between the two recti above the umbilicus. An umbilical hernia is due to failure of the umbilical ring to close completely. Later in life this may dilate as a result of a rapid increase in intra-abdominal pressure. These hernias may be very large. Incisional hernias occur after abdominal surgery through the weak area created by the incision. A hiatus hernia is a rupture of a portion of the stomach through the oesophageal hiatus in the diaphragm. This type of hernia generally gives no symptoms in itself, but may, in turn, cause reflux and oesophagitis giving heartburn. In addition, reflux of bitter irritating fluid into the pharynx and mouth may occur. Antacids are used to neutralize gastric contents, and weight loss and dietary modification (small frequent meals, avoidance of foods inducing symptoms) are used initially.

Initial management of hernias is conservative, and involves instruction on actions to avoid increasing intra-abdominal pressure. When symptoms persist, surgery is required.

Thoracic outlet syndrome

Thoracic outlet syndrome is a compression of the brachial plexus rather than the nerve roots, and so symptoms appear in the arm instead of the neck. The lower trunk (C8/T1) is most commonly affected, with bilateral tingling appearing over the median or ulnar distributions into the forearm and hand. The anatomy of the region favours compression. The nervous structures travel through the costo-clavicular space, formed by the inner clavicle, first rib and insertions of the scalene muscles. The lower trunk of the brachial plexus and the subclavian artery travel through the outlet formed between the scalenus anterior and scalenus medius to rest on the first rib. The more oblique slope of the first rib in the female changes the costo-scalene angle (Grieve, 1986) and may account for the increased incidence of the condition in females. Lower down, the neurovascular structures pass into the axilla beneath the coracoid process and the tendon of pectoralis minor.

Middle-aged women are more commonly affected, with the typical clinical picture consisting of a round shouldered posture displaying a 'dowager's hump' between C7–T1. The thoracic kyphosis is usually stiff, showing tight pectoral tissues and limited shoulder movements. The thoracic segments and rib angles are often exquisitely tender. The pectoral girdle muscles may have weakened through prolonged disuse, and a 'poking chin' head position is common. This postural complex is summarized in Table 16.2.

Carrying heavy objects or wearing a heavy coat exacerbates the problem, and simply allowing the arm to hang freely by the side can cause aching. The condition is seen commonly as an occupational injury, with the subject often noticing increased pain when he or she reaches overhead. Typically, this pattern also occurs when a middle-aged female takes up exercise in a keep-fit class. When severe, vascular signs such as coldness, blueing or whiteness of the skin may occur if the subclavian artery is affected. Equally, the patient may be woken at night with pain, or can experience numbness first thing in the morning.

Various provocative tests are available which aim to reproduce the patient's symptoms. Sustained scapular elevation, or simply holding the arms overhead may increase the signs. The Adson test examines the radial pulse while the patient breathes in deeply and holds his or her breath, at the same time extending the neck and rotating it towards the affected side (Halbach and Tank, 1990). Abduction of the shoulder to 90° with full external rotation, combined with vigorous hand movements may give rise to symptoms if compression is signifi-

Table 16.2 Postural presentation in thoracic outlet syndrome

Descended scapulae, compressing the subclavian artery and lower trunk of the brachial plexus over the first rib
Possible complication of cervical rib seen on X-ray
Soft tissue contracture limiting range of motion at shoulder joint and girdle
Reduced movement in upper/mid-thoracic region (dowager's hump)
Tenderness to palpation of upper/mid-thoracic segments and costal joints
Head protraction

Adapted from Grieve (1986).

cant. In addition, exaggerating the military posture and at the same time placing longitudinal traction through the arms may limit the costo-clavicular space and reproduce symptoms (Grieve, 1986). Examination of the thoracic spine should also be made to differentiate the condition from T4 syndrome (see below), and the long-sitting slump test (p. 350) and upper limb tension tests (p. 389) should be performed.

Conservative management is to elevate the scapulae in the first instance. Simply strengthening the trapezius may have little effect. First, because the trapezius, as an anti-gravity muscle, is usually very strong, and secondly because the stronger muscle may still not be used correctly. Postural re-education is more successful (Cyriax, 1982), teaching a less depressed shoulder girdle resting position.

Tightness of the scalenes and pectoral muscles demands gentle PNF stretching techniques, while mobilization procedures of the thoracic spine are also helpful. Postural realignment is essential if static scapular position is poor (p. 162). Where neural tension tests are positive, mobilization of the neural tissues is required.

T4 syndrome

The T4 syndrome (Maitland, 1986; McGuckin, 1986) produces vague widespread symptoms of pain and paraesthesia in the upper limbs and head, possibly with autonomic involvement. Any region between T2 and T7 may be affected, but the focus is normally around T4. The distribution of symptoms in the hand is glove-like in contrast to that of thoracic outlet syndrome, but many subjects have sensations extending from the wrist and forearm. Head symptoms appear in a 'skull cap' distribution, and the patient is commonly woken with pain. Onset may be due to unaccustomed activities or trauma (road traffic accident), but in many cases there is no specific history of injury. As with thoracic outlet syndrome, a predisposing factor is postural. Head protraction, shoulder girdle protraction and accentuated thoracic kyphosis are common, and place a stretch on the thoracic tissues.

On examination, movements can be localized by performing rotations and flexion/extension from a slumped sitting starting position. Palpation is carried out with the patient prone, head in mid-position, with the therapist standing at the patient's head. The patient's forearms hang over the couch side and his or her upper arms are abducted to 90° to widen the interscapular space. Signs of joint localization include pain, resistance to passive movement and guarding muscle spasm. Common findings include alteration of the alignment of one spinous process in comparison with its neighbours, with local pain to palpation. Examination must take in the cervical spine and first rib. The first rib is palpated above the centre of the clavicle, with the direction of pressure aimed towards the patient's lower scapula.

Mobilization is used for any joints which exhibited signs at examination, and may be carried out with the patient in a supine position, arms folded across his or her chest, and hands placed over the anterior aspect of the shoulders. The therapist places one hand beneath the patient's thoracic spine with the side of his or her thumb or hand in contact with the area to be mobilized. Downward pressure is exerted through the patient's arms onto the therapist's hand. Postural correction may be carried out as with thoracic outlet syndrome.

Scheuermann's disease

Scheuermann's disease is a condition predominantly affecting the thoracic spine around T9, although the lumbar levels may be involved (Greene, Hensinger and Hunter, 1985). The condition is more common in males, and occurs in about 6% of the adolescent population in the age group 12–18 years

(Corrigan and Maitland, 1983). There is a disturbance of the normal ossification of the vertebra. The vertebrae ossify from three centres, one at the centre of the vertebral body, and two secondary centres (the ring epiphyses) in the cartilage end plates. In Scheuermanns's disease there is an alteration of the normal development of the ring epiphyses, but avascular necrosis does not occur (Gartland, 1987) in contrast to true osteochondrosis. Penetration of discal material is often seen through the cartilage end plate of the disc and into the vertebral body (Schmorl's nodes). The changes are largely developmental, but trauma may play a part in exacerbating the condition. In contrast, when the central bony nucleus is affected Calvé's vertebral osteochondritis is present, a much less common condition affecting a single vertebra.

The changes in Scheuermann's disease are primarily to the anterior margins of the thoracic vertebra as these bear greater weight. The disc narrows anteriorly, and deficient growth of the vertebral body occurs as a result of epiphyseal malformation. The vertebra gradually takes on a wedged formation. Normally, several vertebrae are affected in the thoracic spine. The athlete is usually a skeletally immature adolescent, with a 'rounded back' posture. In the active stage of the condition there may be localized pain, often provoked by repeated thoracic flexion as occurs in certain swimming strokes (Butterflier's back) and aerobic dance classes. Deep notches are visible over the anterior corners of the vertebrae on X-ray, and these appear sclerotic rather than rarefied. The ring epiphyses are irregular, but the erythrocyte sedimentation rate (ESR) is normal.

The condition is self-limiting, but in the active stage rest is required. In more severe cases, especially those affecting a number of thoracic segments where kyphosis exceeds 30°, a spinal brace (Milwaukee brace) may be required to prevent gross deformity. An exercise programme to prevent further deformity is essential. This normally involves

strengthening in extension, and patient education to avoid repeated flexion during activities and prolonged flexion in sitting and lying. In addition, increasing the lumbar lordosis and stretching the hamstrings has been recommended (Corrigan and Maitland, 1983).

Exercise therapy for the thoracic spine

As well as restoring fitness components (p. 111) to this body area (such as mobility and strength) following injury, posture is a prime consideration. As was seen on p. 162, one of the common postural faults in this region is an increase in kyphosis. The increased thoracic curve often begins with scapular abduction which moves the centre of gravity of the upper body forwards. In time, the thoracic spine flexes further as a result of the change in equilibrium. The increased curvature has a direct effect on scapulo-humeral rhythm by limiting scapulo-thoracic motion and preventing the final degrees of abduction and extension of the gleno-humeral joint (p. 170). Reversing this trend requires a reduction in thoracic curvature to move the centre of gravity posteriorly, shortening of the shoulder retractors and often restoration of correct shoulder depressor action. Exercises to restore muscle balance for scapulo-humeral rhythm are covered on p. 151. In the following section, examples are given of exercises to correct thoracic curvature by increasing extension. General examples of mobility exercises are also given for use in the restoration phase of injury.

Thoracic extension can be performed in a lying position. The pelvis is posteriorly tilted to flatten and block the lumbar spine, and the arms are lifted to the side and eventually overhead (Fig. 16.5a). Lifting the sternum to extend the thoracic spine without expanding the rib cage (Fig. 16.5b) is also a useful exercise and may be practised in a sitting, high kneeling or standing position. In elbow sup-

Figure 16.5 Exercise therapy for thoracic extension. (a) Overhead reach. (b) Sternal lift. (c) Chest thrust. (d) Thoracic extension.

port prone kneeling (Fig. 16.5c) thoracic extension is performed by pressing (thrusting) the chest towards the floor. Passive extension may be performed by lying over a rolled towel, with the towel positioned at the apex of the thoracic curve (Fig. 16.5d). If the head does not rest on the mat, a thin pillow is used to prevent a protracted head position.

Thoracic mobility to rotation and lateral flexion may be localized to various segmental levels (Fig. 16.6). Mobility to rotation is performed in a sitting position, and may be localized by changing the position of the arms. Leaving the arms at the sides and leading the movement with the head (looking around to the direction of movement) will focus movement to the upper thoracic spine. Holding the elbows horizontally stres-

ses the mid-thoracic spine, which when reaching overhead pulls through the thoracolumbar fascia to stress the lower thoracic spine. Side (lateral) flexion may be mobilized by side-bending against a wall to prevent flexion/extension. With the hands by the sides (reach for the side of the knee) the lower thoracic region is stressed. Placing the hands behind the head and reaching up with the elbow transfers the centre of rotation higher up. Side-lying over a cushion or roll with the upper arm reaching overhead will stretch the muscles of side flexion as well as mobilizing the thoracic spine.

Examples of strength exercises for the thoracic spine musculature include single- or double-handed rowing actions, pull-downs and modified dips (Fig. 16.7).

Figure 16.6 Thoracic mobility exercises. (a) Thoracic rotation, (i) upper, (ii) mid, (iii) lower. (b) Thoracic side flexion, (i) lower region, (ii) upper region, (iii) side flexor stretch.

Figure 16.7 Resistance exercises for the thorax. (a) Lateral pull down. (b) Seated rowing. (c) One arm dumb-bell row. (d) Modified dip.

References

Bailey, P. (1985) Surfer's rib: isolated first rib fracture secondary to indirect trauma. *Annals of Emergency Medicine*, **14**, 346–349

Bourdillon, J.F. (1982) *Spinal Manipulation*, Butterworth-Heinemann, Oxford

Butler, D.S. and Slater, H. (1994) Neural injury in the thoracic spine: a conceptual basis for manual therapy. In *Physical Therapy of the Cervical and Thoracic Spine*, 2nd edn (ed. R. Grant), Churchill Livingstone, Edinburgh

Butler, D.S. (1991) *Mobilization of the Nervous System*, Churchill Livingstone, Edinburgh

Corrigan, B. and Maitland, G.D. (1983) *Practical Orthopaedic Medicine*, Butterworth, London

Cyriax, J. (1982) *Textbook of Orthopaedic Medicine*, Vol. 1, 8th edn, Baillière Tindall, London

Gartland, J.J. (1987) *Fundamentals of Orthopaedics*, 4th edn, W.B. Saunders, Philadelphia

Gilmore, O.J.A. (1995) personnal communication

Greene, T.L., Hensinger, R.N. and Hunter, L.Y. (1985) Back pain and vertebral changes simulating Scheuermann's disease. *Journal of Pediatric Orthopaedics*, **5**, 1–7

Grieve, G.P. (1986) *Modern Manual Therapy of the Vertebral Column*, Churchill Livingstone, London

Gurtler, R., Pavlov, H. and Torg, J.S. (1985) Stress fracture of the ipsilateral first rib in a pitcher. *American Journal of Sports Medicine*, **13**, 277–279

Halbach, J.W. and Tank, R.T. (1990) The shoulder. In *Orthopaedic and Sports Physical Therapy*, 2nd edn (ed. J.A. Gould), C.V. Mosby, St Louis

Kendall, F.P. and McCreary, E.K. (1983) *Muscles Testing and Function*, 3rd edn, Williams and Wilkins, Baltimore

Lacote, M., Chevalier, A.M., Miranda, A., Bleton, J.P. and Stevenin, P. (1987) *Clinical Evaluation of Muscle Function*, Churchill Livingstone, Edinburgh

Lankenner, P.A. and Micheli, L.J. (1985) Stress fracture of the first rib: a case report. *Journal of Bone and Joint Surgery*, **67A**, 159–160

Maitland, G.D. (1986) *Vertebral Manipulation*, 5th edn, Butterworth, London

McGuckin, N (1986) The T4 syndrome. In *Modern Manual Therapy of the Vertebral Column* (ed. G.P. Grieve), Churchill Livingstone, Edinburgh

McKenzie, R.A. (1990) *The Cervical and Thoracic Spine. Mechanical Diagnosis and Therapy*, Spinal Publications, New Zealand

Nachemson, A. (1987) Lumbar intradiscal pressure. In *The Lumbar Spine and Back Pain* (ed. M.I.V. Jayson), Churchill Livingstone, London

Norris, C.M. (1995) *Postural Considerations in Training*, Presentation to the Football Association Medical Committee, Lilleshall, England

Palastanga, N., Field, D. and Soames, R. (1994) *Anatomy and Human Movement*, 2nd edn, Butterworth-Heinemann, Oxford

Slater, H., Butler, D.S. and Shacklock, M.O. (1994) The dynamic central nervous system: examination and assessment using tension tests. In *Grieve's Modern Manual Therapy*, 2nd edn (eds J.D. Boyling and N. Palastanga), Churchill Livingstone, Edinburgh

17

The cervical spine

The cervical spine consists of eight mobile segments generally categorized into two functional units. The first comprises the occiput, C1 and C2 (the sub-occipital region) and the second the segments from C2 to T1 (the lower cervical region).

Within the sub-occipital region, an important distinction is made between the atlanto-occipital and atlanto-axial joints. The atlanto-occipital joint, formed between the occipital condyle and lateral masses of C1 allows no rotation, but free flexion/extension and some lateral flexion. There are three atlanto-axial joints. The median joint is formed between the odontoid peg of the axis and the anterior arch and transverse ligament of the atlas. The lateral two joints are between the lateral articular processes of the atlas and axis. The atlanto-axial joint allows free rotation to about 35°, and only minimal flexion/extension. As rotation occurs, the head is depressed vertically by about 1 mm, causing ligamentous slackening and increasing the available range of motion.

The discs of the lower cervical region are fairly thick, allowing free movement in all planes. Flexion and extension combined has a range of about 110°, with only 25° being flexion, and the least movement occurring between C7 and T1. With flexion, the upper vertebra of a pair slides anteriorly, pulling its inferior facet up and forwards, thus widening the facet joint space posteriorly. With extension the situation is reversed, the upper vertebra tilting and sliding posteriorly, gapping the facet joint anteriorly but narrowing the intervertebral foramen. Lateral flexion has a range of about 40° to each side. This is not a pure movement, but is combined with rotation and slight extension. Rotation occurs in the lower cervical region in either direction to about 50°, and is limited by grinding of the facets and torsion stress on the discs and facet capsules. The functional side of the intervertebral foramen is increased on the opposite side to the rotation, but reduced on the same side. Thus, manual therapy to the cervical spine for unilateral pain often involves contralateral rotation to relieve root pressure.

The lateral edge of each vertebra in the cervical region is lipped to form an uncovertebral joint, lying anteriorly to the intervertebral foramen. Each joint is surrounded by a capsule which blends medially with the disc. The joints help to stabilize the neck and control its movements.

Within the total range of any cervical movement some regions move more than others. The upper cervical segments allow more rotation than the lower, but less lateral flexion. With head retraction the upper segments flex while the lower ones extend. In fact, with this movement a greater range of upper cervical flexion is obtained than with neck flexion itself (McKenzie, 1990). As flexion occurs, the spinal canal lengthens, stretching the cord and nerve roots. Extension reverses this effect relaxing the spinal structures.

Vertebral arteries

One important difference between the cervical and other spinal areas is the presence of the vertebral arteries. These branch from the subclavian artery (Fig. 17.1i) and pass through the foramina transversaria of each cervical vertebra from C6 and above (Fig. 17.1ii). When the artery reaches the atlas, it runs almost horizontally (Fig. 17.1iii) and then enters the foramen magnum to join with its neighbour and form the basilar artery (Fig. 17.1iv). The vertebral arteries supply about 11% of the cerebral blood flow, the carotid system supplying 89% (Grant 1994a).

Variations in the diameter of the vertebral arteries are common, and in some cases the basilar artery is supplied almost entirely by one dominant vertebral artery (Bogduk, 1986). During its course, the artery is in close relation to a number of structures, including the scalenus anterior and longus colli muscles, the uninate processes, the superior surface of the facet joint, and of course the transverse process itself.

Vertebrobasilar insufficiency (VBI) may occur with occlusion, in which case the predominant symptom is dizziness, although other symptoms may be seen (Table 17.1). Occlusion may be either intrinsic or extrinsic. Intrinsic causes include atherosclerosis blocking the artery causing either focal narrowing, or more extensive constriction over the whole length of the artery. Extrinsic causes of occlusion occur by compression to the vessel wall. This is most commonly caused during rotation of the neck if an anomaly of the artery exists. Three such anomalies have been described in the lower part of the artery (Bogduk, 1986). First, an irregularity in the origin of the artery from the subclavian, secondly, bands of deep cervical fascia crossing the artery which tighten on rotation, and thirdly squeezing of the artery within the fascicles of either longus colli or scalenus anterior.

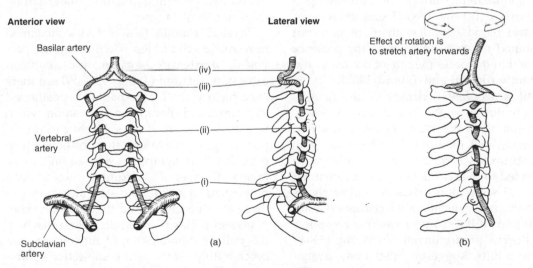

Figure 17.1 Structure of the vertebral artery. (a) Anterior and lateral view. (i) Branch from subclavian artery to C6. (ii) Vertical track through foramen transversaria. (iii) Horizontal section from C1. (iv) Entry to foramen magnum to join neighbour. (b) Effect of rotation is to stretch artery forwards. After Grant (1994a).

Table 17.1 Symptoms of vertebrobasilar insufficiency (VBI)

Dizziness (in over 60% of cases)
Visual disturbances
— spots before the eyes
— blurred vision
— hallucination
— field defects
Diplopia
Ataxia
Drop attacks
Visceral/vasomotor disturbances
— nausea
— faintness
— light-headedness
Tingling around lips (peri-oral dysaesthesia)
Nystagmus
Hemi-anaesthesia
Hemi-plegia

From Grant (1994b).

The major vertical portion of the artery (Fig. 17.1b) is most commonly affected by osteophytes and adhesive scar tissue, with neck rotation compromising the ipsilateral vessel. In the upper region (Fig. 17.1c), the artery may be occluded should the atlas move on the axis, through trauma, rheumatoid arthritis or abnormalities of the odontoid. Passive rotation of the neck can shut the contralateral artery by stretching it (Brown and Tatlow, 1963). Extension reduces cerebral blood flow less than rotation, but combined rotation-extension in the presence of traction increases the rate of occlusion significantly (Brown and Tatlow, 1963).

VBI is a potential danger of any manual therapy to the neck, particularly rotation, with some 60 cases of stroke being reported following neck manipulation (Bogduk, 1986). Twenty six cases, reported in one series, were subjected to X-ray following the incident. Of these, 23 were reported as normal or showing only minor degenerative changes (Grant, 1994b). In addition, major vascular complications occur predominantly in young (35–40 years) adults, suggesting that bony degenerative changes are not responsible for VBI. Trauma following manipulation occurs predominantly in the atlanto-axial component of the artery, which is stretched forwards during rotation. The more mobile neck of a younger adult will allow a greater range of rotatory motion and therefore greater stretch. Mechanical stress to the vertebral artery may lead to spasm (transient or persistent), subintimal tearing, perivascular haemorrhage or embolus formation leading to brain-stem ischaemia. Repeated rotatory manipulation is especially dangerous as it builds on trauma which may already have occurred.

Pre-manipulative testing of the cervical spine

Testing for VBI should be carried out for all patients undergoing cervical manipulation (APA, 1989; Grant, 1994a, 1994b). Aspects of these tests (especially subjective history) will be relevant for all manual therapy procedures. Initially, subjective examination is used to determine the presence of dizziness or other symptoms suggesting VBI. The frequency of these symptoms and aggravating and alleviating factors are noted, especially with relevance to the neck. Any previous treatment (particularly multiple rotatory manipulation or manipulation under strong axial traction) is noted.

Physical examination includes sustained movements (10 s or less if symptoms are provoked) of extension, rotation, and combined extension/rotation (Table 17.2). Where there is no history of VBI, the patient is positioned in a simulated manipulation position which is again sustained. If the subjective examination suggests dizziness, the position which provokes this symptom is used in a sustained fashion. In addition, rapid head movement is used to distinguish between dizziness due to VBI and that due to vestibular origin. This is especially relevant where the patient describes rapid movement as a precipitating factor in the subjective examination. The therapist holds the patient's head (but not covering the ears) and body rotation is performed (for example in a swivel chair,

Table 17.2   Physical examination for vertebrobasilar insufficiency (VBI)

No history of VBI	History of VBI (dizziness)
Sustained extension	Sustained extension
Sustained rotation (left and right)	Sustained rotation (left and right)
Sustained rotation with extension (left and right)	Sustained rotation with extension (left and right)
Simulated manipulation position	Test position or movement which provokes dizziness
	Rapid movement of relevant head position within available range

After Grant (1994b).

or trunk twisting in standing) to both sides and held for 10 seconds. As the head itself is not moving, any symptoms are due to cervical rotation rather than vestibular disturbance.

The production of VBI symptoms is an obvious bar to full range rotation manipulation. However, even if the test is negative, a small risk still remains so the patient should be continually questioned about dizziness throughout any treatment involving rotation techniques.

Nature of cervical injury in sport

The most common mechanism of severe cervical injury is axial loading (Torg et al., 1985). This may be caused as a player hits another by using his head as a battering ram (spearing), or if the athlete falls on to his or her head or runs into an object head first. In this situation, the neck is slightly flexed, flattening the cervical lordosis. Now, the cervical spine absorbs considerably less energy than it would in its normal state as a flexible column. Initially, maximal discal compression occurs, and then the spine rapidly buckles and fails in flexion, resulting in fracture, subluxation or dislocation.

An illustration of the importance of this mechanism and its preventive possibilities is found in American football. The incidence of cervical quadriplegia in this sport dropped dramatically from a peak of 34 cases per year

to 5 since head-first tackling and blocking were forbidden (Torg et al., 1985).

A similar mechanism has been described in rugby football. Cord injuries have occurred in scrum, ruck, and maul situations when a player was attempting to pick the ball up from the ground (Silver and Gill, 1988), and as two forwards engage (Taylor and Coolican, 1987). The vertex of the head is restrained, either against another player or the ground, and the trunk continues to move forwards forcing the cervical spine into flexion and dislocation (McCoy et al., 1984).

In ice hockey, axial loading is again the culprit, when a player hits the boards or an opponent with his helmeted head while the neck is slightly flexed (Tator and Edmonds, 1986).

Where significant axial loading has occurred, permanent abnormalities exist within the cervical spine (Torg et al., 1993). These may include interspace narrowing at C5–C6 with deformity of the C5 end plate due to Schmorl's node formation. In addition, reversal of the cervical spine lordosis with fixation from C2 to C6 may be seen. Where these changes are present, they should preclude an athlete from participation in sports involving collision activities.

In all full-body contact sports such as rugby, American football and ice hockey, it is essential that players are taught that the initial point of contact in a tackle or block should be the shoulders or chest and not the head. In addition, strengthening the neck musculature may reduce the intensity of injury (Torg, 1982).

Less severe trauma may occur to the neck with indirect impact or a sudden mistimed movement. A type of whiplash injury may occur in a rear impact where one player runs into another. Hyperextension of the neck can result with varying degrees of tissue damage.

Diving into a shallow swimming pool or lake is also a common cause of injury, with fracture dislocation occurring as the neck is forced into flexion (or extension in some cases) when the head strikes the pool bottom. The condition may occur if a swimming pool is too shallow, especially if left unsupervised or without depth markings. In addition, this tragic injury is common in lakes and rivers with youngsters under the influence of alcohol or drugs.

In gymnastics the most usual mechanism of injury is flexion of the cervical spine, with injury occurring most commonly at C4 and C7 levels (Silver, Silver and Godfrey, 1986). Again, there is an axial loading, with the gymnast landing on his or her head. Of note is the potential for abuse of the trampette by young athletes. This piece of equipment enables the young athlete to gain both height and speed in an inverted body position—a potentially lethal combination.

Screening examination

The subjective assessment will give the practitioner an indication of the depth of examination required objectively. A great number of tests and procedures exist, but not all will be used with every patient. Following the subjective assessment, a screening examination is used to indicate where further tests, including palpation, should concentrate.

Initial objective examination includes posture and head position in both sitting and standing. Muscle tension and both active and passive motions are examined. Flexion/extension, rotation and lateral flex-

ion are examined for range and end feel. Movements are isolated by eliminating unwanted shoulder elevation or trunk rotation. Resisted movements may be similarly tested, and the shoulder range to abduction and flexion/abduction assessed to determine if there is an associated shoulder or arm pathology. Pain referral and any sensation loss is mapped, and upper limb muscle power and reflexes assessed if the history suggests neurological involvement.

Two further movements and their adaptations are important with reference to mechanical therapy, these are head protrusion (protraction) and retraction. As with other tests, the location and intensity of symptoms is established prior to testing. Head protrusion is performed in a sitting position, with the patient instructed to slide the head forwards horizontally as far as possible by 'poking the chin out'. This is performed singly and to repetition. Head retraction is the opposite action, sliding the head back and 'pulling the chin in'. Again, overpressure may be used to assess end feel and symptoms. Where postural pain is suspected, the movements are performed statically and maintained to load the structures and cause tissue deformation. The capsular pattern of the cervical spine is an equal limitation of all movements except flexion, which is usually of greater range. Asymmetrical limitation of movement suggests a non-capsular lesion such as disc displacement (Cyriax and Cyriax, 1983).

Classification of disc displacement by pain pattern and presence of deformity is similar to that of the lumbar spine (McKenzie, 1990). Derangements one and two give pain travelling as far as the shoulder, three and four give pain referred into the arm but no further than the elbow. Derangements five and six can refer pain down to the wrist. Derangements one, three, and five do not show deformity, whereas derangement two may show cervical kyphosis, and derangements four and six may show torticollis.

Special tests

Further detail in cervical examination is gained by palpation to test accessory movements, and special tests such as the quadrant position and the upper limb tension test (ULTT). These two latter procedures are useful where the clinical picture is not clear, and to confirm or refute involvement of the cervical spine. The quadrant test combines extension, lateral flexion and rotation to the same side. For the lower cervical spine, the neck is taken back into extension and lateral flexion towards the painful side, and then rotated, again towards the pain. Testing the upper cervical spine is performed by extension with pressure to localize the movement to the upper cervical segments. When full extension has been gained, rotation is added towards the pain, and then followed by lateral flexion. Various sequences of combined movements may produce the patient's symptoms, and it is important that the same sequence of movements be used when comparing between both sides, or assessing prior to and following treatment.

The ULTT (Elvey's test) may be thought of as the 'straight leg raise of the upper limb'. It develops tension in the cervical nerve roots and their sheaths and dura, and places greatest stress to the C5 and C6 structures. Four variations are used to place greater or lesser stress on particular nerves (ULTT1, ULTT2a, ULTT2b, ULTT3).

For ULTT1 (Fig. 17.2) the patient is supine with the therapist facing the patient and standing at his or her side. The patient's shoulder girdle is depressed by caudal pressure from the therapist's hand. The forearm is supinated and the wrist and fingers extended, then the shoulder is laterally rotated and the elbow extended. Finally, cervical lateral flexion (but not rotation) is added away from the tested arm. The instruction to 'keep looking at the ceiling but take your ear away' is helpful.

Pain from two-joint muscle stretch over the shoulder is eliminated by altering the head or finger position (which will not affect the shoulder muscles but will alter the nerve tension) to establish if this affects the pain. In normal subjects an ache is usually felt in the cubital fossa, and some sensation on the radial side of the forearm and hand is common. The test is only positive if symptoms other than these, and similar to the patient's complaint are produced.

ULTT2a is used to place bias on the median nerve. The test is performed by depressing the patient's shoulder girdle and extending the elbow. The shoulder is laterally rotated and the wrist, fingers and thumb are then extended. Slight abduction of the shoulder may be added to sensitize the test. ULTT2b places bias on the radial nerve. From the previous position, the shoulder is medially rotated and the forearm pronated. The wrist is then flexed, and ulnar deviation of the wrist further sensitizes the nerve.

ULTT3 is used to test the ulnar nerve. The patient's wrist is extended and forearm supinated, and then the elbow is flexed. The shoulder girdle is depressed, and the glenohumeral joint abducted as though trying to place the patient's hand over his or her ear.

The ULTT is useful in patients with shoulder girdle or upper limb involvement where the origin of the symptoms is unclear, or where other tests do not reproduce the symptoms (Magarey, 1986). For a test to be positive, it must reproduce the patient's symptoms and be different from the uninjured side of the body. Furthermore, the test responses should be altered by movement of the distal body parts (forearm, wrist and fingers).

In sport, traction injury of the brachial plexus can occur, in a position similar to that of the ULTT. With blocking or tackling in rugby or American football, the shoulder may be forcibly depressed while the cervical spine is simultaneously laterally flexed to the contralateral side. The upper trunk of the brachial plexus may suffer a neurapraxia as a result. Nerve function is tem-

Figure 17.2 The upper limb tension test (ULTT). Finishing positions are shown: (a) ULTT 1: Median nerve. Shoulder abduction. (b) ULTT 2a: Median nerve. Shoulder girdle depression and external rotation of the shoulder. (c) ULTT 2b: Radial nerve. Shoulder girdle depression and internal rotation of shoulder. (d) ULTT 3: Ulnar nerve. Shoulder abduction and elbow flexion. From Butler (1991).

porarily disturbed and a burning sensation is felt in the upper limb. The condition is often referred to as a 'stinger' or 'burner' by players, and recovery is usually full in a matter of minutes.

The stinger may also be associated with extension compression, and during this mechanism the athlete with cervical spine stenosis is more at risk. The presence of such stenosis also makes the likelihood of developing a stinger three times greater (Meyer et al., 1994). Decreased canal diameter is associated with a narrow intervertebral foramen, and it is this structure which is likely to cause compression of the nerve root.

Manual therapy for the cervical spine

Joint mobilization

One of the most useful mobilization techniques for the cervical spine in the presence of unilateral symptoms is rotation, usually performed in a direction away from the patient's pain (Maitland, 1986). The patient lies supine on the treatment couch with his or her head extending over the couch end. The therapist grasps the patient's occiput and chin, and rotates the head away from the painful side. The upper cervical (suboccipital) spine is better mobilized with the head and neck in line. With the lower cervical area, the neck is flexed further the lower down the spine the lesion is. Grading for mobilization is described on p. 355.

Where pain is intense, or if the patient is particularly nervous, longitudinal oscillations are useful. The same grip may be used as with rotation movements, and the longitudinal motion is imparted by the therapist pulling through his or her arms. Stronger manual traction is also of use (Cyriax, 1980). This may be applied with the patient's shoulders stabilized by an assistant, couch horns, or body weight with heavier patients. Traction is applied through straight arms by the therapist leaning back. The use of a belt or harness can reduce the strain on the therapist considerably. Rotation mobilizations and manipulations may also be applied during traction. Some authors claim that this procedure makes cervical manipulation safer by ensuring that any displaced fragment will move centrally (Cyriax and Cyriax, 1983). Others dispute this claim, arguing that the mechanics of the vertebral arteries makes injury more likely with this technique (Grieve, 1986; Grant, 1994a).

Accessory intervertebral movements are normally performed with the patient in a prone lying position with his or her hands beneath the forehead. The chin is tucked in slightly to reduce the cervical lordosis. The tips or pads of the therapist's thumbs are used to impart the mobilization. Power for the movement comes from the shoulders and is transmitted through the arms and hands, so that the thumbs deliver rather than create the force.

Postero-anterior central vertebral pressures are performed with the therapist's thumbs in contact with the patient's spinous process. More pressure is required to feel movement in the mid-cervical region than in the sub-occipital or lower cervical areas. The atlas has no spinous process, but rather a posterior tubercle, and pressure here is through the overlying muscles and ligaments. The spinous process of C2 overhangs that of C3, so palpation is aided in this region

by asking the patient to tuck the chin in further and so increase cervical flexion. The oscillation is repeated two or three times each second, and the direction of travel may be angled towards the patient's head or feet depending on comfort. Postero-anterior central pressures are very useful where symptoms are central, or evenly distributed to either side.

Postero-anterior unilateral pressures are similarly performed, but this time the therapist's thumbs are in contact with the patient's articular processes, and angled towards the mid-line. The technique is used for unilateral symptoms over the painful side. Transverse vertebral pressures are given against the side of a single spinous process with one thumb reinforcing the other. This technique is used mostly where there are unilateral symptoms which are well localized to the vertebrae. The movement is usually performed from the painless side pressing towards the pain.

Mechanical therapy

The same rules apply for the assessment of mechanical lesions as for the lumbar spine (p. 351). The postural syndrome is managed largely by correcting sitting posture with the slouch overcorrect exercise. This time, however, the elimination of head protrusion is an important aim.

Extension dysfunction occurs more commonly in the lower cervical spine, making it impossible for the patient to sit correctly. Retraction is performed initially in sitting or standing, followed by extension. Overpressure is most easily given with the patient in a prone lying position. From this position the patient props him or herself on to the elbows, and places the fingers beneath the chin, pushing the head into further extension. Alternatively, a supine lying position may be used with the head over the couch end. The patient allows his or her head to slowly move back into full extension (traction being applied by the weight of the head). Small rotation movements may be used at end range to complete the movement. This latter procedure is really only suitable for younger patients, and even then caution should be exercised with consideration to the vertebral arteries (see p. 385).

Rotation and flexion movements may also be performed with overpressure. The patient gently presses on his or her chin or pulls the back of the head down respectively.

Nags and snags

Nags are mid-range oscillatory mobilizations applied to the facet joints between C2 and T3, in an antero-superior direction (Mulligan, 1989). They are used with the patient seated, placing the cervical spine in a functional weight-bearing position.

Assuming the therapist is using the right hand, he or she stands to the right of the patient, blocking any unwanted shoulder movement with his or her own lower trunk. The patient's head is held in the therapist's cupped right hand, with the little finger hooked below the spinous process at the level to be treated. The therapist's left thenar eminence reinforces the pressure of his or her right little finger. The mobilization is applied through the hand and little finger at an angle of 45° to the cervical spine, and repeated 6–10 times.

Varying degrees of flexion, and traction may be applied until a movement is found which reduces the patient's symptoms. The cradled head position is particularly useful in that it gives confidence to the especially nervous patient.

Snags are sustained motions applied at end range. The therapist places the side of his or her thumb over the level to be treated, and presses upwards along the plane of the facet joint as the patient rotates or laterally flexes his or her head. The thumb follows the motion as the neck moves. Similar snags may be used where flexion or extension is limited, and to C2 in the case of headaches. In this case the direction of movement is horizontal, again in line with the facet joint plane.

Soft tissue techniques

Additional soft tissue techniques involve massage and muscle stretching, which are particularly effective when used in combination with other forms of manual therapy. Stretching of the sternomastoid and upper fibres of trapezius (see also p. 160) is useful where the neck has been held to one side for any time, or if the athlete (usually a child) wakes with an acute torticollis. The technique is used initially as a passive stretch in a supine-lying position and continued as an autostretch technique in a sitting position. In a supine position, the neck is straightened as far as possible. For tightness on the left side, the therapist places his or her left hand against the left side of the patient's head, and the right hand over the antero-lateral aspect of the left shoulder, so that the forearms cross. The movement is left shoulder depression combined with right cervical lateral flexion and rotation where this increases the stretch of tight structures. A gentle continuous pressure is used initially followed by PNF stretching techniques or spray stretch procedures.

The autotherapy stretch is applied with the patient sitting on a dining chair. The head is laterally flexed to the right, and as this occurs, the tight trapezius and sternomastoid will elevate the shoulder. The head position is held by the right hand reaching over the head to grip the left side. The action is an active depression of the left scapula to apply the stretch. It is important that the right hand stabilizes but does not violently pull on the irritable neck structures.

If the pain is initially too intense for stretching, positional traction is used. Here the patient is supine and the head is straightened as far as possible and held in this position with a rolled towel until the pain starts to subside. The neck is then taken to a new end-range position limited by the pain. This procedure is continued over a 30-minute period until full lateral flexion (with or without rotation) to the contralateral side is achieved.

The sub-occipital muscles may be massaged and stretched in the supine-lying position. The therapist places his or her supinated forearms beneath the patient's head, and grips the sub-occipital structures with the pads of his or her flexed fingers. Gently gripping and relaxing the fingers imparts the massage. The muscles are stretched by retracting and flexing the neck, and then applying gentle overpressure. Transverse frictions may be given in prone lying or lean support sitting, using the thumb and forefinger, or forefinger supported by the middle finger.

Stabilization techniques for the cervical spine

Restoration of cervical function using exercise therapy begins with spinal stabilization. This topic was covered for the lumbar spine on pp. 363–366, and the principles are broadly similar for the cervical spine. The stabilizers of the cervical spine are the deep neck flexors. These have a tendency to be poorly recruited following injury, while the superficial neck flexors (sternomastoid and scalenes) tend to be overactive. Retraining cervical stabilization depends on increasing the work of the deep neck flexors while reducing that of the superficial muscles. Imbalance of the cervical region is usefully assessed by a screening test in a supine lying position. The patient is instructed to flex their neck ('look at your toes'). If the deep neck flexors are overpowered by the superficial neck flexors, the chin juts forwards at the beginning of the movement (Fig. 17.3). This leads to hyperextension of the cervical spine in the sub-occipital region, and the head then follows an arc-like movement as flexion continues in the lower cervical region only. This is more apparent when slight resistance is given against the forehead, and sternomastoid is seen to stand out prominently as soon as the movement begins (Janda, 1994).

Figure 17.3 Neck flexion test. (a) Normal: cervical lordosis reverses and neck flexes. (b) Abnormal: cervical lordosis increases as chin juts forwards. Upper cervical spine hyperextends.

Re-education of deep neck flexor activity begins in a supine-lying starting position. The head rests on the couch or small pad so that its weight does not act as a resistance to the movement. A pressure biofeedback unit is used to monitor head/neck movement. The cuff of the unit is folded and placed behind the upper cervical spine. The aim is to achieve sub-occipital rather than lower cervical flexion. The action is a minimal flexion or 'nodding' action of the head alone (dropping the chin to the throat), avoiding forceful actions or lifting the head from the couch. The cuff is inflated sufficiently to fill the space between the cervical spine and couch, which is usually about 20 mmHg. The action is to slowly draw the chin back (chin tuck) to increase the pressure by 6–10 mmHg. If the pressure reduces, the head is being lifted by the sternomastoid and scalenes, so the exercise is re-started. The holding time of the movement is built up until the patient can maintain 10 repetitions each of 10 seconds duration.

Cervical strengthening in sport

Following the restoration of appropriate stabilization and segmental control, many sports require general muscle strengthening. This may be achieved by resisted movements (partner or elastic band) through range and static muscle work in bridging. Several exercise examples are given in Fig. 17.4. In each case it is essential to maintain cervical alignment. Once good alignment is lost the exercise should be stopped.

Figure 17.4   Examples of neck strengthening exercises. (a) Isometric resistance against the hand. (b) Pressing a sponge against a wall. (c) Resistance provided by a partner. (d) Neck bridge on bench. (e) Resistance provided by a weight disc.

References

Australian Physiotherapy Association (APA) (1989) Testing of the cervical spine prior to manipulation. *Physiotherapy Practice*, **5**, 207–211

Bogduk, N. (1986) Cervical causes of headache and dizziness. In *Modern Manual Therapy of the Vertebral Column* (ed. G.P. Grieve), Churchill Livingstone, Edinburgh

Brown, B. St J. and Tatlow, W.F.T. (1963) Radiographic studies of the vertebral arteries in cadavers. *Radiology*, **81**, 80–88

Butler, D.S. (1991) *Mobilisation of the Nervous System*, Churchill Livingstone, Edinburgh

Cyriax, J (1980) *Textbook of Orthopaedic Medicine*, Vol. 2, 10th edn, Treatment by manipulation massage and injection, Baillière Tindall, London

Cyriax, J.H. and Cyriax, P.J. (1983) *Illustrated Manual of Orthopaedic Medicine*, Butterworth, London

Grant, R (1994a) Vertebral artery concerns: premanipulative testing of the cervical spine. In *Physical Therapy of the Cervical and Thoracic Spine*, 2nd edn (ed. R. Grant), Churchill Livingstone, Edinburgh

Grant, R. (1994b) Vertebral artery insufficiency: a clinical protocol for pre-manipulative testing of the cervical spine. In *Grieve's Modern Manual Therapy*, 2nd edn (eds J.D. Boyling and N. Palastanga), Churchill Livingstone, Edinburgh

Grieve, G.P. (1986) *Modern Manual Therapy of the Vertebral Column*, Churchill Livingstone, Edinburgh

Janda, V. (1994) Muscles and motor control in cervicogenic disorders: assessment and management. In *Physical Therapy of the Cervical and Thoracic Spine*, 2nd edn (ed. R. Grant), Churchill Livingstone, Edinburgh

Magarey, M.E. (1986) Examination and assessment in spinal joint dysfunction. In *Modern Manual Therapy of the Vertebral Column* (ed. G.P. Grieve), Churchill Livingstone, Edinburgh

Maitland, G.D. (1986) *Vertebral Manipulation*, 5th edn, Butterworth, London

McCoy, G.F., Piggot, J. and Macafee, A.L. (1984) Injuries of the cervical spine in schoolboy rugby football. *Journal of Bone and Joint Surgery*, **66B**, 500–503

McKenzie, R.A. (1990) *The Cervical and Thoracic Spine. Mechanical Diagnosis and Therapy*, Spinal Publications, New Zealand

Meyer, S.A., Schulte, K.R., Callaghan, J.J. and Albright, J.P. (1994) Cervical spinal stenosis and stingers in collegiate football players. *American Journal of Sports Medicine*, **22**, 158–166

Mulligan, B.R. (1989) *Manual Therapy — Nags, Snags, and PRP's etc*, Plane View Services, New Zealand

Silver, J.R. and Gill, S. (1988) Injuries of the spine sustained during rugby. *Sports Medicine*, **5**, 328–334

Silver, J.R., Silver, D.D. and Godfrey, J.J. (1986) Injuries of the spine sustained during gymnastic activities. *British Medical Journal*, **293**, 861–863

Tator, C.H. and Edmonds, V.E. (1986) Sports and recreation are a rising cause of spinal cord injury. *Physician and Sports Medicine*, **14**, 157–167

Taylor, T.K.F. and Coolican, M.R.J. (1987) Spinal-cord injuries in Australian footballers, 1960–1985. *Medical Journal of Australia*, **147**, 112–118

Torg, J.S. (1982) *Athletic Injuries to the Head, Neck and Face*. Lea and Febiger, Philadelphia

Torg, J.S., Vegso, J.J., Sennett, B. and Das, M. (1985) The national football head and neck injury registry: 14-year report on cervical quadriplegia, 1971 through 1984. *Journal of the American Medical Association*, **254**, 3439–3443

Torg, J.S., Sennett, B., Pavlov, H., Leventhal, M.R. and Glasgow, S.G. (1993) Spear tackler's spine: an entity precluding participation in tackle football and collision activities that expose the cervical spine to axial energy inputs. *American Journal of Sports Medicine*, **21**, 640–649

18

Facial injury

Ocular injury

Eye injuries may arise from collisions in which a finger or elbow goes into the eye. Small balls (especially squash balls) may cause ocular damage, and mud, grit or stone chips can enter the eye. It is interesting to note the speed at which a ball may move. In squash, the ball can travel at 140 mph, in cricket at 110 mph and in football 35–75 mph (Reid, 1992). A small object travelling at these speeds obviously creates considerable force and potential for damage. This is borne out by the sad fact that over 10% of eye injuries in sport result in blindness in that eye (Pashby, 1986).

Where a foreign body is in the eye, quantities of water should be used to irrigate the eye and wash the object out (a squeeze bottle is particularly useful). No attempt should be made to probe the eye as this may cause the object to scratch the cornea. In some instances, particularly if the foreign body is an eyelash, the eyelid may be rolled back on itself. This procedure is carried out by first asking the athlete to look down. The practitioner then grasps the lashes of the upper lid, pulling them down and out, away from the eye. A cotton swab is placed on the outside of the lid level with the lid crease. The lashes are then folded upwards over the swab to reveal the inside of the eyelid, and the foreign body is washed away. The eyelid goes back to its normal position when the athlete looks up and blinks.

A foreign body is one of the most common eye problems on the sports field. The reaction is usually pain and tear production. If the object is not removed, blinking may cause corneal abrasion and extreme pain for about 48 hours.

Contact lenses can cause problems. Hard lenses may break or become scratched or roughened causing corneal damage. Soft lenses are easily torn. When the eye has been injured or infected, a contact lens should never be re-inserted until the eye has healed completely for at least 24 hours.

When contact lenses become dislodged, the wearer, with the aid of a mirror, is often the person most capable of removing them. Hard lenses may be removed with a small suction cup available from an optician, and persistent soft lenses may be dislodged by water from a squeeze bottle, or by gently wiping with a cotton swab.

Following injury, basic vision assessment should be carried out and if any abnormalities are detected the athlete should be referred to an ophthalmologist. A distance chart (placed 6 metres from the subject) and a near vision chart (35 cm from the eyes) should be used. Failure to read the 20/40 line on either chart is a reason for referral (Ellis, 1987). Visual fields are tested in all four quadrants. One eye is covered, and the athlete should look into the examiner's eyes. The examiner moves his or her finger to the edge of the visual field in both horizontal and vertical directions until the athlete loses sight of it. Decreased visual acuity or loss of the visual field in one area warrants referral (Ellis, 1987).

Pupil reaction may be tested with a small pen torch. Pupil size, shape and speed of reaction is noted. Pupil dilation in reaction to illumination requires immediate referral, as does any irregularity in pupil shape and an inability to clear blurring of vision by blinking.

Eye protection

Sports trauma accounts for 25% of all serious ocular injuries (Jones, 1989), an even more tragic statistic when we realize that 90% of sports injuries to the eye could be prevented by wearing eye protection (Pashby, 1989). Prevention of ocular trauma comes from two sources, sports practice and eye protection.

Changes in sports practice include rule modification, and increasing player awareness. For example, rule changes in Canadian ice hockey to prevent high sticking have greatly reduced eye injury. Injury in badminton is more frequent at the net, so teaching young players to cover their face with the racquet when receiving a smash at the net would seem sensible.

Individual athletes should also protect themselves. The eye protectors worn must be capable of dissipating force, but should not restrict the field of vision or the player's comfort. In addition, if they are to be acceptable to a player they must be cosmetically attractive and inexpensive.

Each sport will have its own specific requirements. Where the blow is of great intensity, the eye protector must be incorporated into a helmet, and if there is a danger of irritation (chlorine in a swimming pool) the material used must be chemically resistant.

Goggles for skiing must filter out ultraviolet light, while those for shooting may have to be suitable for low light conditions or capable of screening out glare.

For general protection in racquet sports polycarbonate lenses mounted in plastic rather than wire frames are the choice. The nasal bridge and sides of such a protector should be broad and strong to deflect or absorb force.

Dental injury

The simplest form of tooth injury is a concussion in which the anterior teeth are knocked against something. This may occur from a head butt, a punch, or someone running into a piece of apparatus. There is only minor soft tissue damage and the teeth and mouth are sore. The front teeth may be painful when the athlete eats, so he or she should avoid eating hard foods until the pain subsides.

Tooth subluxation occurs when a tooth becomes mobile after a direct injury, but is not displaced. On examination, the tooth may be loose and tender, and there may be some gum damage. It is usual for the teeth to tighten up and heal within a week, but the athlete should see his or her dentist. A subluxed tooth may have damaged its dental artery or vein. When this happens the venous blood can stagnate in the tooth and the haemoglobin seeps into the dentine turning the tooth dull yellow and eventually grey.

Displacement of a tooth is more common when a gum shield is not worn. The displaced tooth should be washed in tepid water and replaced in the socket, taking care to put the tooth back the right way round. The athlete may hold the tooth in place by biting on a cloth or handkerchief, until specialist advice can be sought. In children, a displaced tooth may be soaked in whole milk (Mackie and Warren, 1988) until help is available. The tooth should be handled by the crown to avoid further damage to the cells at its root. Good results may be expected if re-implantation is carried out within 30 minutes of trauma, but after 2 hours the prognosis is poor.

Examination of the tooth after an impact injury initially is by a pressure test. The biting edge of the tooth is gently pressed inwards towards the tongue and then outwards towards the lips. If the tooth is painless (but not numb) and moves only as much as its neighbours, injury is normally restricted to the gums alone. If the tooth is numb, painful, mobile, or depressed below the level of the other teeth, the athlete requires dental referral.

A number of tooth fractures may occur (Fig. 18.1). A small corner of the tooth may be chipped off, leaving a sharp edge which may cut into the tongue. Larger chips can expose the tooth dentine, causing pain when the athlete sucks air into the mouth, or the tooth pulp, which can be seen by looking up into the mouth. This latter injury is a dental emergency, as are complete tooth fractures of the root apex or at gum level.

Mouth guards

Custom-made mouth guards (gum shields) have been shown to reduce the incidence of dental injuries by as much as 90% (Jennings, 1990). In addition, they stop the teeth from cutting into the lips and cheeks. When the jaw is hit from below, the bottom teeth will

impact into the guard, absorbing some of the impact force. A mouth guard will also modify the transmission of force through the temporo-mandibular joints. The combination of altered force transmission and shock absorption can reduce the likelihood of concussion and mandibular fracture (Chapman, 1990). Any guard must cover the surfaces of the upper teeth, be comfortable to wear, and allow unhindered breathing and speech. Furthermore, they must show good properties of retention in the mouth, and give proper inter-maxillary positioning.

Mouth guards were originally worn in boxing, when they were simply curved pieces of rubber gripped between the teeth. Progress has been made in their design, and nowadays three types are available, custommade, mouth-formed and ready moulded. Most protection is given to the upper front teeth, these being the ones most susceptible to injury.

For custom-made gum shields the first step is to take an impression of the upper teeth using a material such as alginate. Dental stone is poured into the impression to create a positive model of the teeth. Polyvinyl acetate-polyethelene (PVAc-PE) is vacuum formed over the model, and the mouth guard is trimmed and smoothed off (Kerr, 1986).

Self-moulded guards come in two types. The first is soaked in hot water to soften it and moulded over the upper teeth ('boil and

Figure 18.1 Tooth fractures. (a) Small corner fracture involving enamel only. (b) Larger corner fracture with dentine exposure. (c) Nerve root pulp exposed. (d) Fracture close to root apex. (e) Fracture at gum level. From Reid (1992).

bite'). The second type consists of a pre-formed outer shell into which a plasticized acrylic gel or silicone rubber is added. The outer shell and fluid gel are placed over the teeth and pressed into position until the gel sets.

The dentally fitted type of mouth protector is better in terms of both safety and effectiveness. The model made from the impression of the athlete's mouth can be re-used to form a number of mouth shields.

The ready moulded kind are available off the shelf in many sports shops. They do not fit well, and have to be held in place by gritting the teeth. They should not be recommended to athletes as they are easily dislodged and may block the airway.

Auricular injury

Cauliflower ear

Auricular haematoma (cauliflower ear) is normally caused by a direct blow to the ear. Blood and serum accumulate between the perichondrium and external ear cartilage, and secondary infection may arise. First aid treatment involves the use of ice and compression. As soon as possible the haematoma should be aspirated or drained through an incision, and the ear compressed to prevent further fluid accumulation. The injury occurs particularly in contact sports such as wrestling, boxing and rugby, and is very common. Schuller et al. (1989) found 39% of high school and collegiate wrestlers from a group of 537 with one or both of the auricles permanently deformed by injury. Some degree of prevention may be achieved by wearing protective headgear.

Underwater diving injury

Air either side of the tympanic membrane should be at equal pressure. Externally, the air is at atmospheric pressure, and internally the Eustachian tube leads to the nasopharynx. Pressure changes, such as those that occur in an aeroplane, are equalized by swallowing or yawning, through the Eustachian tube mechanism. If the free exchange of air is impaired, barotrauma may occur. If the outside air pressure rises, such as may occur in diving, and the Eustachian tube mechanism is unable to equalize pressure, pain will result, a condition referred to as 'the squeeze'. Small haemorrhages may occur in the middle ear and the tympanic membrane may burst in depths below 3 m (Sperryn, 1985). With a severe cold, the Eustachian tube may be blocked, so an athlete should not dive (or fly if the condition is severe).

Barotrauma to the inner ear secondary to decompression is less common, but considerably more serious. This type of trauma usually occurs at depths below 35 m. Symptoms may be caused by the formation of gas bubbles in the blood vessels supplying the inner ear (Renon et al., 1986).

The reduction in air volume at increasing depths is responsible for another danger with diving and underwater swimming, the phenomenon of 'mask squeeze'. A relative vacuum is created in a diving mask or swimming goggles, as the diver descends. With a mask, this is equalized by breathing out through the nose into the mask, but with swimming goggles this is not possible. A swimming pool may be as deep as 3 or 4 m. Children who dive down for objects at this depth, face the very real danger of conjunctival haemorrhage and oedema (Craig, 1984). As the air space within the goggles is not connected to a body cavity, the air pressure will not be equalized. The pressure within the goggles will drop lower than that inside the body causing the ocular vascular system to over-distend and fluid to accumulate in the tissues covered by the goggles.

Diving with ear plugs in, or with an upper respiratory tract infection, should also be avoided because of danger to the eardrum (tympanic membrane). Water pressure will press an ear plug further in, compressing the air between the plug and eardrum. This can cause severe pain and may even rupture the drum. During any change in air pressure, the pressure inside the eardrum is equalized through the Eustachian tube mechanism when swallowing or yawning. With upper respiratory tract infections, this tube can become blocked, giving severe pain (middle-ear squeeze) as the eardrum is stretched inwards.

Swimming pool ear

Swimming pool ear (otitis externa) is an irritable condition of the outer ear which can occur in athletes who swim regularly (Eichel, 1986). The symptoms are mainly itching, bordering on pain, but in extreme cases discharge may occur and even partial hearing loss. The ear canal produces its own protective layer of cerumen (wax). With prolonged exposure to chlorinated water especially, the wax may degenerate and the skin of the inner ear can become macerated. This leaves the ear open to bacterial or fungal infection, especially as the skin is damaged by vigorous drying (corner of a towel or cotton swabs) or scratching (finger nail).

Prevention is the key to this condition. Ear wax should not be removed, and nothing inserted into the ear. If ear protection is required, a drop of baby oil placed in the ear will form a protective coating. To limit water contact, rather than using ear plugs a close fitting swimming cap can be used. Where itching is present, anti-bacterial eardrops should be used and the athlete should avoid water contact until the symptoms settle.

Maxillofacial injuries

Sport accounts for about 12% of maxillofacial injuries (Handler, 1991), with fractures of the maxilla and zygomatic bones being more common in contact sports. If the upper jaw has been subjected to a blow, injury should be suspected if the teeth are out of alignment or one half of the cheek feels numb. Direct palpation of these fractures is painful, and pain may be elicited as far back as the temporo-mandibular joint if the athlete is asked to bite on a folded cloth. Chewing will be painful and local swelling may be apparent. Bony deformity is often better assessed by looking at both cheekbones from the top of the patient's head.

Mandibular fracture may occur with a direct blow to the chin, with pain being experienced as the mouth is opened or closed, in an area in front of the ear. There is malocclusion and abnormal mobility of the mandible. Most of these fractures extend through the intra-oral mucosa and so bleeding is often noticed from the mouth. The primary aim is to ensure a clear airway. Blood, bone and tooth fragments, and saliva must be cleared from the mouth. The mobile jaw fragment may be temporarily secured with a bandage around the head and chin.

The local application of ice will ease pain, and direct pressure by the athlete himself supports the area until hospitalization is achieved.

Temporo-mandibular joint pain

The temporo-mandibular joint (TMJ) can give rise to facial pain of various types, and although not strictly a sporting injury, will be briefly considered. TMJ pain may be the result of alterations in the way the teeth come together (occlusion), and this in turn is affected by mouth guards used in contact sports.

Structure and function

The TMJ is a synovial condyloid joint found between the mandibular fossa of the temporal bone, and the condyle of the mandible. The two bony surfaces are covered with fibrocartilage, and separated by an articular disc. Movements of the jaw include protraction, retraction, elevation, depression and lateral gliding, all of which are used to some extent when chewing. The three main muscles contributing to TMJ motion are the temporalis, masseter and the pterygoids. The temporalis fans out from the temporal fossa to insert into the coronoid process of the mandible. The masseter has both deep and superficial portions, and attaches from the zygomatic arch and maxillary process to the angle of the mandible. The medial pterygoid is similar in position to the masseter, but the lateral pterygoid arises from the sphenoid bone and inserts into the mandibular condyle and articular disc, playing a large part in stabilization of the TMJ.

In the occluded position, the upper teeth are normally in front of the lower ones. As the mouth is opened, the lower inscisors move downwards and forwards, a movement encompassing forward gliding and rotation at the TMJ. Depression of the mandible is controlled by eccentric action of the temporalis, but if resisted, the geniohyoid, mylohyoid and digastric muscles contract. The jaw is closed powerfully by masseter, temporalis and the medial pterygoid. The lateral pterygoid pulls the mandible forwards (protraction) while the temporalis is the main effector of retraction.

Pathology

Dysfunction of the TMJ may present as local muscle tenderness, limited motion and a general dull ache over the side of the face. Clicking may be present, and patients often protrude the mandible as the jaw is opened, or sublux the joint. When chronic, the condition may show reduced range of motion, with contracture of the masticatory muscles. Pain and muscle spasm are common, with the lateral pterygoids most usually affected (Hertling and Kessler, 1990). Emotional stress which presents as teeth clenching is a common factor, as is an alteration in bite pattern and chewing action.

Trauma to the area is common in contact sports, and soft tissue damage and subluxation/dislocation may occur. Whiplash injuries can also give rise to the condition. As the head tips back rapidly, the jaw flies open stretching the masseter and joint structures. Immediately following this the jaw snaps shut, which may in turn compromise the articular meniscus.

Management

Limited mandibular movement can be corrected by a number of autotherapy techniques. Initially, the patient starts by simply opening and closing the mouth, gradually increasing the range until a yawning motion is used. Prolonged static stretch is used by placing a number of tongue depressors (about ten to begin with) between the teeth. The stretched position is maintained for 5 to 10 minutes until the muscles relax. Ice is useful for cryostretch. As the range of motion increases, the number of tongue depressors is increased. Alteratively, a tapered cork may be used to hold the teeth apart. This is inserted thin side first and gradually moved inwards as movement range increases. Translation movements occur when the mouth is opened further than about 1 cm. From this position the patient is instructed to protrude and retract the chin, and to use lateral gliding movements.

Mobilization procedures include caudal traction, where the therapist presses down on the patient's lower jaw, and medial-lateral gliding and protrusion. In each case the hold is over the chin using the web of the therapist's hand, or over the inner aspect of the lower molars. Direct mobilization may be used with the patient in a side-lying position with the head supported on a pillow. Contact is made with the therapist's thumbs over the posterior surface of the head of the mandible.

In persistent cases referral to a dental practitioner is recommended. Bite patterns may be corrected with the use of a dental appliance, but the precise value of mandibular orthopaedic repositioning appliances (MORA) is still largely uncertain. Some authors (Laskin and Greene, 1972; Gelb, 1977) have used these devices to optimize the positioning of the condyles and fossa of the TMJ to restore neuromotor function to the joint. It has been suggested (Gelb, 1977) that in addition to TMJ pain, cervical and spinal problems may also benefit, and muscle strength may be enhanced in other body parts (Schwartz and Novich, 1980). The use of a MORA has however been criticized. Burkett and Berstein (1982), and McArdle et al. (1984) found no increase in strength with subjects using a MORA, and Kerr (1986) concluded that physiological improvement by the use of a MORA had not been scientifically proven.

In all cases of TMJ pain, the cervical and thoracic spines must be examined and excluded as a cause or contributory factor of the patient's complaint.

Nasal injury

Nasal injuries mainly require treatment for haemorrhage (nose bleed). Direct pressure should be applied to the distal part of the nose with the head held forward. The athlete is able to breathe through his or her mouth. In cases where bleeding is severe a cotton-wool ball or compress may be placed inside the nostril providing the pad is large enough not to be inhaled. If bleeding continues, hospitalization may be required to cauterize the ruptured vessels or apply vessel-constricting agents.

Nasal fracture is one of the most common maxillofacial injuries in sport. Often the nasal bones are obviously deviated to one side or depressed. Gently running the finger down the edge or bridge of the nose may reveal a step deformity, but this can easily be disguised when oedema is excessive (frequently the case). Radiographs are useful, but not definitive as many nasal features cannot be identified on X-ray (Handler, 1991). The nasal septum and orbit must be examined at the same time as the nose, as concurrent injures here can often go unnoticed.

Reduction of a displaced fracture should be performed within 7 days, because, after this , fibrosis makes accurate realignment of the bony fragments difficult.

References

Burkett, L.N. and Berstein, A.K. (1982) Strength testing after jaw repositioning with a mandibular orthopaedic appliance. *Physician and Sports Medicine*, **10**(2), 101–107

Chapman, P.J. (1990) Orofacial injuries and international rugby players' attitudes to mouthguards. *British Journal of Sports Medicine*, **24**, 3

Craig, A.B. (1984) Physics and physiology of swimming goggles. *Physician and Sports Medicine*, **12**(12), 107

Eichel, B.S. (1986) How I manage external otitis in competitive swimmers. *Physician and Sports Medicine*, **14**, 108

Ellis, G.S. (1987) Sports eye injuries: first aid and prevention. In *Sports Ophthalmology* (eds L.D. Pizzarello and B.G. Haik), Charles C. Thomas, Springfield, Illinois

Gelb, H. (1977) *Clinical Management of Head, Neck and Temporomandibular Joint Pain and Dysfunction*, W.B. Saunders, Philadelphia

Handler, S.D. (1991) Diagnosis and management of maxillofacial injuries. In *Athletic Injuries to the Head, Neck, and Face*, 2nd edn (ed. J.S. Torg), Mosby Year Book, St Louis

Hertling, D. and Kessler, R.M. (1990) *Management of Common Musculoskeletal Disorders*, J.B. Lippincott, Philadelphia

Jennings, D.C. (1990) Injuries sustained by users and non-users of gum shields in local rugby union. *British Journal of Sports Medicine*, **24**, 3

Jones, N.P., (1989) Eye injury in sport. *Sports Medicine*, **7**, 163–181

Kerr, I.L. (1986) Mouth guards for the prevention of injuries in contact sports. *Sports Medicine*, **3**, 415–427

Laskin, D.M. and Greene, G.S. (1972) Splint therapy for the myofacial pain dysfunction (MPD) syndrome in a comparative study. *Journal of the American Dental Association*, **84**, 624–628

Mackie, I.C. and Warren V.N. (1988) Dental trauma: 4. Avulsion of immature incisor teeth. *Dental Update*, December, 406–407

McArdle, W.D., Goldstein, L.B., Last, F.C., Spena, R. and Lechtman, S. (1984) Temporomandibular joint repositioning and exercise performance: a double blind study. *Medicine and Science in Sports and Exercise*, **16** (3), 228–233

Pashby, R.C. (1986) Sports injuries to the eye. *Medical Clinics of North America*, **33**, 4672

Pashby, T. (1989) Eye injuries in sports. *Journal of Ophthalmic Nursing and Technology*, **8**(3), 99–101

Reid, D.C. (1992) *Sports Injuries. Assessment and Rehabilitation*, Churchill Livingstone, Edinburgh

Renon, P., Lory, R., Belliato, R. and Casanova, M. (1986) Inner ear trauma caused by decompression accidents following deep sea diving. *Annals of Otolaryngology (Paris)*, **103**, 259–264

Schuller, D.E., Dankle, S.K., Martin, M. and Strauss, R.H. (1989) Auricular injury and the use of headgear in wrestlers. *Archives of Otolaryngology: Head and Neck Surgery*, **115**, 714–717

Schwartz, R. and Novich, M.M. (1980) The athlete's mouthpiece. *American Journal of Sports Medicine*, **8** (5), 357–359

Sperryn, P.N. (1985) *Sport and Medicine*, Butterworth, London

19

The shoulder

Functional anatomy

The upper limb attaches to the trunk via the shoulder (pectoral) girdle. The shoulder complex in total consists of the scapula and clavicle, articulating with the rib cage and sternum to form four joints, all of which require attention in the management of shoulder pain (Fig. 19.1). The clavicle forms a strut for the shoulder, holding the arm away from the side of the body, and allowing a greater range of unincumbered movement. At one end the clavicle joins the sternum through the sternoclavicular joint, while at the other it joins the scapula via the acromioclavicular joint. The scapula rests on the rib cage through muscle tissue alone, an essential point when dealing with stability of the shoulder complex. The gleno-humeral joint is the articulation between the head of the humerus and the shallow glenoid fossa of the scapula.

The glenoid fossa is only one-third the size of the humeral head, but is extended by the glenoid labrum attached to its periphery. This fibrocartilage rim is about 4 mm deep with its inner surface lined by, and continuous with, the joint cartilage. The joint itself is surrounded by a loose capsule with a volume twice as large as the humeral head. The anterior capsule is strengthened by the three gleno-humeral ligaments. The lower portion of the capsule is lax in the anatomical position, and hangs down in folds. It has two openings, one for the passage of the long head of biceps, and the other between the superior and middle gleno-humeral ligaments which communicates with the subscapular bursa (between subscapularis and the joint capsule). The capsule is further strengthened by the rotator cuff muscles which act as 'active ligaments' and blend with the lateral capsule. The 'roof' of the joint is formed by the bony coracoid and acromion processes and the coraco-acromial ligament which runs between them, the three structures together forming an arch.

Most joints have a high degree of passive stability provided by their capsules and ligaments. The shoulder, however, depends more on the active stability provided by its muscles to maintain joint integrity. In the anatomical position, the weight of the arm is largely supported by the coraco-humeral ligament and superior capsule. When the arm moves away from the side of the body, tension in the superior capsule is immediately lost (see p. 167). Now joint stability is provided only by the rotator cuff muscles alone.

The fibres of the joint capsule are angled forwards and slightly medially when the arm is hanging by the side of the body. As abduction progresses, tension within these fibres causes the shoulder to passively externally rotate. This movement prevents the humeral head from being pulled closer to the glenoid

Figure 19.1 Joints of the shoulder complex.
1. Sternoclavicular joint. 2. Acromioclavicular joint.
3. Gleno-humeral joint. 4. Scapulo-thoracic joint.

and facilitates a greater range of movement. Importantly, the external rotation also allows the greater tuberosity to clear the acromion process (see below).

Abduction of the humerus is accomplished by the supraspinatus and deltoid, acting as the prime movers. With the arm dependent, contraction of the deltoid (particularly the middle fibres) merely approximates the joint (upward translation), because the medial muscle fibres run almost parallel with the humerus. Unopposed, this pull would force the head of the humerus into the coraco-acromial arch, resulting in impingement. Contraction of the infraspinatus, subscapularis, and teres minor (Fig. 19.2) causes compression and downward translation to offset the upward translation of deltoid (Culham and Peat, 1993). In an overhead throwing or serving action, the intraspinatus and teres minor stabilize the joint anteriorly when it is abducted and externally rotated (Cain et al., 1987). By 90° abduction, the pull of the deltoid no longer tends to cause impingement, as shear forces are exceeded by compression, and the humeral head is

Figure 19.2 (a) Deltoid pull at 30° and 90° abduction. (b) Muscles counteracting pull of deltoid. (i) Supraspinatus, (ii) infraspinatus and teres minor, (c) subscapularis. Resolution of muscle force: S, shear. C, compression.

stabilized into the glenoid (Perry and Glousman, 1995).

The supraspinatus is better placed to produce a rotatory action and therefore initiates abduction for the first 20°. The line of action of supraspinatus is such that less translation is caused, and its contribution to abduction is to reduce the reliance on deltoid and, as a consequence, reduce translation. After 30° of abduction the scapula starts to rotate to alter the glenoid position (see p. 167).

The biomechanics of throwing

In sport, throwing is to the upper limb what gait is to the lower limb. It is an activity seen in many sports in some form, and there are similarities between all types of throw, and with shots in racquet sports. Throwing can be divided into five stages which form a single continuous motion (Fig. 19.3). In the early stages, up to ball release, the body is accelerating the object. By the later stages, following release, the aim is to decelerate and reduce the effect of stress on the body.

In the wind-up phase (I) the athlete positions himself in the best position for the throw. A right-handed thrower will plant the back foot on the ground and turn the body perpendicular to the direction of throw (left side of the body forward). The thrower then steps towards the target and begins to move his or her arms. During the cocking phase (II), the front leg moves forwards and the throwing arm moves backwards, effectively stretching the body out and building elastic energy. The shoulder is abducted to 90° and taken into extension and external rotation. The elbow is flexed to 45°. In the acceleration phase (III) the body moves forwards leaving the arm behind. The elbow begins to extend and the shoulder internally rotates.

The deceleration phase (IV) sees the release of the object being thrown, and the energy built up to throw the object must now be

Figure 19.3 (a) Stages of throwing: (i) wind-up—athlete positions him or herself for the throw; (ii) cocking—lead leg moves forwards, arm moves backwards, stretching body; (iii) acceleration—body drives forwards, leaving arm behind; (iv) deceleration—object released. Elbow continues to extend and shoulder to internally rotate; (v) follow through—trunk and lead leg show eccentric activity to dissipate energy. (b) Similarity to tennis serve. After Fleisig, Dillman and Andrews (1994).

effectively dissipated to reduce stress on the body tissues. The arm continues to extend at the elbow and internally rotate at the shoulder, bringing the knuckles up. The rotator cuffs (external rotators) decelerate the internal rotation motion, and limit distraction to the gleno-humeral joint. The elbow flexors similarly decelerate extension and limit hyperextension of the elbow joint. In the final phase, the follow through (V), the trunk is flexed eccentrically and the lead leg is extended pushing into the ground eccentrically to absorb energy. The throwing arm continues to move, giving a longer period over which to dissipate energy, and the hand may end up near the knee of the lead leg. Angular displacement for the shoulder and elbow throughout the throwing action is shown in Fig. 19.4.

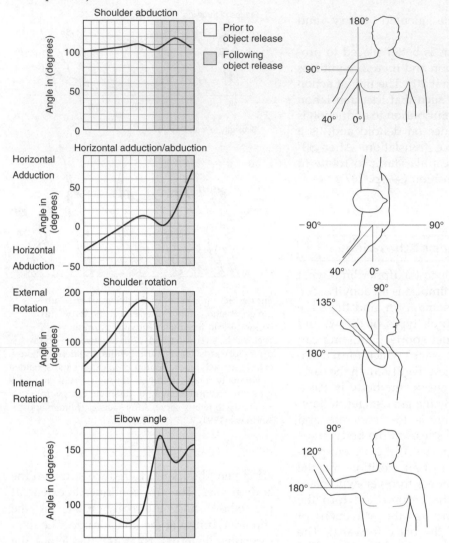

Figure 19.4   Angular displacement of the shoulder during the throwing action. After Fleisig, Dillman and Andrews (1994).

Screening examination of the shoulder complex

After a subjective history has been taken, a screening examination is performed to enable the examiner to focus more closely on the injured area. The patient's posture and actions are noted while undressing, and the area is inspected for swelling, colour and deformity. A combination of active, resisted and passive movements are used to assess the shoulder complex (Cyriax, 1982). The patient is viewed from behind, to note any alteration in scapulo-humeral rhythm. It is helpful to have the patient facing a full length mirror, so the anterior aspect of the shoulder and the patient's facial expression may also be assessed. Active abduction, and flexion-abduction are performed with over-pressure applied at end range, to assess end feel. Positional changes of the scapula, either at rest or during movement, warrant closer inspection. Active gleno-humeral rotation may be performed by asking the patient to place his or her hand behind his or her back (medial rotation) and then behind the head (lateral rotation). Passive lateral rotation is performed with the elbow flexed and upper arm held into the side. This is also the position for resisted lateral and medial rotations. Passive medial rotation is performed with the patient placing his or her hand into the small of the back. The examiner stabilizes the upper arm, and keeps the patient's elbow tucked into the side of the body. He or she then gently pulls the patient's forearm away from the body, increasing medial rotation. Any limitation of movement is noted, and the percentages of limitation relative to each other reveal if a capsular pattern exists. The capsular pattern for the gleno-humeral joint is gross limitation of abduction with some limitation of lateral rotation and little limitation of medial rotation.

Resisted abduction and adduction are performed in mid-range, the examiner stabilizing the patient's pelvis to prevent any lateral trunk flexion occurring at the same time as the shoulder moves. Elbow flexion, extension, and forearm rotation may be assessed at the same time with the elbow flexed and the upper arm held close to the body. The patient's forearm rests on the examiner's when testing the triceps, and resistance is given from above when testing the biceps. Resisted shoulder shrugging tests the trapezius. When a small physiotherapist is examining a large athlete, it is particularly important that resistance is applied from a position which gives maximum mechanical advantage to the therapist.

Referred pain from the neck must always be considered in cases of shoulder pain, and the neck screening examination (see p. 388) is performed to establish whether movement is painful or reproduces the patient's shoulder symptoms. This simple, but methodical, examination should take no more than 2–3 minutes and tells the examiner whether the shoulder is the cause of pain, if a contractile or non-contractile structure is affected, and reveals if a capsular pattern exists to suggest an intracapsular lesion.

Should movement apparently be full and painless at the gleno-humeral joint, two further procedures are useful to reproduce the patient's symptoms. These are the locking test and the quadrant position (Maitland, 1991). Both tests refer to the position of the greater tuberosity relevant to acromial arch and glenoid (Corrigan and Maitland, 1994). The locking position combines internal rotation, extension and abduction of the shoulder with the scapula fixed. In this position the subacromial space is compressed and will give pain should an impingement syndrome be present. The quadrant position stresses the anterior capsule, and combines external rotation, slight flexion and full abduction of the shoulder. Each test should be assessed for pain and end feel, and compared with the uninjured side.

To perform the tests, the patient is in a supine position, and the practitioner stands by the patient's side towards his or her shoulders. To test the locking position, the therapist places the palmar aspect of his or her forearm beneath the patient's shoulder, and grips the trapezius muscle to stop the shoulder shrugging. The therapist holds the patient's elbow, slightly medially rotates the arm, and lifts it into abduction (Fig. 19.4a). The movement is continued into the quadrant position (Fig. 19.5b) by allowing the arm to externally rotate and flex, while the humerus is abducted to full range.

Sternoclavicular joint

The sternoclavicular (SC) joint provides, via the clavicle, the only structural attachment of the scapula to the rest of the body (Norkin and Levangie, 1992). The joint performs functionally as a ball and socket. The medial end of the clavicle articulates with the clavicular

(a)

(b)

Figure 19.5 (a) Locking position; (b) quadrant position.

notch of the sternum, and the adjacent edge of the first costal cartilage. The congruity of the joint is enhanced by the presence of an interarticular fibrocartilage disc, which separates the joint cavity into two. In addition to improving the congruity of the joint, the disc also provides cushioning between the two bone ends. Furthermore, it holds the medial end of the clavicle against the sternum, preventing it moving upwards and medially when pushing actions are performed.

The joint is strengthened by a capsule attached to the articular margins, and four ligaments (anterior SC, posterior SC, interclavicular, and costoclavicular). Three degrees of movement are possible at the joint, elevation-depression, protraction-retraction, and axial rotation. The axis of rotation for the first two movements (not rotation) is lateral to the joint itself, passing through the costoclavicular ligament. Consequently, when the lateral end of the clavicle moves in one direction, its medial end moves in the opposite direction (Fig. 19.6), an important consideration with clavicular joint dislocation.

A total of about 60° of elevation and depression is available, elevation being limited by tension in the costoclavicular ligament, and depression by the interclavicular ligament and articular disc. When the lateral end of the clavicle is protracted, the medial

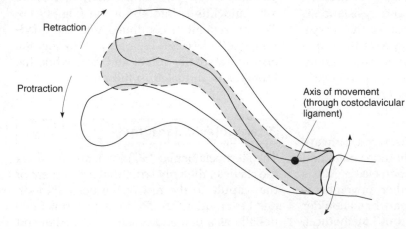

Retraction

Protraction

Axis of movement
(through costoclavicular
ligament)

Figure 19.6 Movement of the clavicle. After Palastanga, Field and Soames (1989).

end moves backwards, the opposite movement occurring with retraction. The total range of motion here is about 35°. Axial rotation is purely a passive action accompanying scapular movements. The range of rotation is small (20–40°), but increases slightly as the lateral end of the clavicle is pulled back.

Injury

Injury to the SC joint is unusual. Normally, the clavicle will fracture or the acromioclavicular joint will give way before the SC joint is seriously injured. However, when damage does occur, it is frequently the result of direct lateral compression of the shoulder, such as occurs when falling onto the side of the body. The injury is more common in horse-riding and cycling where sufficient force is produced, but is seen in rugby and wrestling. The SC joint will dislocate in the opposite direction to the applied force (Fig. 19.7), thus an anterior force (falling onto the back) will dislocate the joint backwards. Several important structures lie in close proximity to the joint including the oesophagus, trachea, lungs, pleurae, brachial plexus and major arteries and veins. Posterior dislocation therefore, if it is severe, may be potentially life threatening. In contrast, anterior dislocation can occur in the absence of trauma, and frequently results only in slight discomfort.

Initial examination (of posterior dislocation) on the field must obviously be aimed at ruling out life-threatening injury. The presence of stridor, dyspnoea, cyanosis, difficulty with speech, pulsating vessels and neurological signs may all necessitate immediate hospitalization.

If these are not present, joint examination may continue. Pain is generally well localized, and may become progressively more limiting over time. Anterior dislocation leaves a visible step deformity, and with posterior dislocation the usual prominence over the medial clavicle is lost. Local swelling is sometimes present, with crepitus and pain to motion, especially horizontal flexion. The shoulder is frequently held protracted.

Radiographic investigation will rule out clavicular fracture, and may enable differentiation between fracture and epiphyseal injury in the young (below 25 years) athlete. Closed reduction is often possible immediately after injury if pain is not too severe and before muscle spasm sets in. Both anterior and posterior dislocations may be reduced by placing a knee between the scapulae of the seated athlete and gently pulling

Figure 19.7 Sternoclavicular dislocation. (a) Anteriorly directed force causes posterior dislocation. (b) Posteriorly directed force causes anterior dislocation. From Garrick and Webb (1990), with permission.

the shoulders back. The joint often reduces with an audible thud. After reduction the joint is immobilized with a figure-of-eight bandage and ice is used to reduce local swelling. Posterior dislocations, even if successfully reduced, will still require hospital referral and observation. Posterior dislocations usually stay reduced, but anterior dislocations are apt to recur. Surgical fixation of anterior dislocation is possible, but the number of complications makes the procedure undesirable. Migration of a Steinmann pin or Kirchner wire into the heart or major vessels has been reported (Garrick and Webb, 1990). Rockwood and Odor (1989) reported excellent results following conservative management of atraumatic anterior displacement 8 years after initial treatment. Patients treated surgically (not by these authors) in the same study had complications including scarring, instability, pain and limitation of activity.

Even though the joint is frequently hypermobile, joint mobilizations may be used to relieve pain (Maitland, 1991). Antero-posterior gliding may be performed with the therapist placing his or her thumbs over the sternal end of the clavicle.

Acromioclavicular joint

This joint is formed between the oval facet on the lateral end of the clavicle and the similarly shaped area on the acromion process. The lateral end of the clavicle overrides the acromion, slightly. The joint capsule is fairly loose and strengthened above by fibres from trapezius, and by capsular thickenings which make up the superior and inferior acromioclavicular (AC) ligaments. As with the SC joint there is an intra-articular disc, but this time it does not divide the cavity into two. The joint is further stabilized by the coracoclavicular ligament, divided into its conoid and trapezoid parts. The conoid ligament is fan-shaped and resists forward movement of

the scapular, while the stronger trapezoid ligament is flat and restricts backward movements. As with the SC joints, the AC joint moves only in association with the scapula. Three types of movement are again present, protraction–retraction, elevation–depression and axial rotation.

Injury

The most common conditions affecting the AC joint are sprains and degeneration. AC joint sprains vary in intensity between minor grade I injuries to grade III ruptures representing complete disruption of the coracoclavicular ligament and AC joint dislocation (sprung shoulder) (Fig. 19.8). The injury may be further classified using weight-lifting radiographs. Here, the anterior deltoid is contracted by having the patient hold a

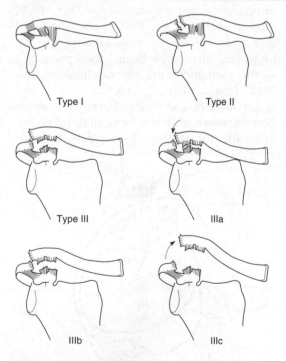

Figure 19.8 Acromioclavicular joint injuries. Type I (sprain), type II (subluxation), type III (dislocation), type IIIa (reduces as weight taken), type IIIb (no change as weight taken), type IIIc (lateral end of clavicle more prominent as weight taken).

weight with the elbow flexed and arm next to the body. If the clavicular attachment of the deltoid is intact, the joint may reduce as weight is taken (IIIa), or there may be no change in the joint appearance (IIIb). However, if the lateral end of the clavicle becomes more prominent, the clavicular attachment of the deltoid may have been stripped off (Dias and Gregg, 1991). Radiographs are also used to differentiate the condition from fractures of the distal clavicle where this is suspected.

Injury is usually the result of a superiorly directed force as occurs with a fall onto the point of the shoulder or being struck from above. The force drives the scapula downwards, an action resisted by the coracoclavicular ligament. Examination reveals local tenderness over the AC joint, sometimes with a noticeable step deformity. The deformity may occur later, if initial muscle spasm reduces acromioclavicular separation.

Initial treatment aims to reduce the symptoms. Ice and a sling support to take the weight of the arm are recommended. The joint is immobilized in the sling for 2–3 weeks, and then gradually mobilized within pain-free limits. With grade I injuries, some relief may be provided by taping.

Acromioclavicular taping

Stress may be taken off the AC joint by a simple taping designed to press the clavicle down and take some of the weight of the arm away from the distal shoulder structures (Austin, Gwynn-Brett and Marshall, 1994; Macdonald, 1994). The athlete is positioned in sitting at the side of the couch with the elbow flexed to 90° and the shoulder abducted to 30°. The shoulder is slightly elevated and the arm rests on a couch. The shoulder and chest on the injured side of the body should be shaved of long hair. Spray adhesive is applied, making sure that the athlete turns their head away from the spray and covers their eyes with their unaffected hand. Also, the nipple area must be protected with a non-adhesive pad.

A felt pad is placed over the acromion to protect it from abrasion. Two anchors of 7.5 cm elastic adhesive tape are applied. The first runs horizontally from the sternum to the paravertebral area on the side of injury. The second is placed around the mid-humerus with light tension, ensuring that the limb is not excessively compressed (Fig. 19.9a). Two stirrups of 7.5 cm elastic adhesive tape are placed (pre-stretched) from the front to the back of the chest anchor, passing over the acromion (Fig. 19.9b). These are then rein-

Figure 19.9 Acromioclavicular joint taping. (a) Anchors. (b) Stirrup applied under tension. (c) Arm stirrups.

forced by two strips of 5 cm zinc-oxide taping. Two further strips of elastic adhesive tape are place (pre-stretched) laterally from the arm anchor across the anterior aspect of the shoulder to join the chest stirrups over the acromion, and laterally from the anchor passing posteriorly over the shoulder to the acromion (Fig. 19.9c). Again, these stirrups are reinforced by 5 cm zinc-oxide taping. If the shoulder stirrups have been applied correctly, their tension will tend to lift the arm into abduction slightly. The chest and arm stirrups are closed by reapplying the chest and arm anchors (7.5 cm elastic adhesive tape) to act as fixing strips. Sensation and pulse should be re-tested after tape application.

In the acute phase of injury, the forearm weight may also be taken by a collar and cuff sling. With time, when pain-free arm motion to 90° is available, the humeral portion of the tape may be dispensed with.

Specific exercise therapy

As inflammation subsides, exercise therapy is commenced to restore function. This is used initially to maintain muscle tone in the absence of joint movement. Isometric contractions of the scapular and gleno-humeral muscles are used, and the athlete maintains general fitness and lower body strength by exercising with the AC joint taped. When pain subsides and movement commences, gentle scapular actions are used, such as shoulder shrugging and bracing within the limits of pain. These may progress to a scapular stabilization programme (p. 150). Range of motion exercises for the gleno-humeral joint are begun, ensuring that correct scapulo-humeral rhythm is maintained.

When full pain-free motion is obtained, the athlete may be seen to have a permanent step deformity, and some joint degeneration may occur in later years. The major problem resulting from this injury is lack of confidence when falling in contact sports. The effects of direct trauma may be limited by placing a felt doughnut pad over the joint. Confidence is built using progressive closed chain exercises (p. 174) and rehearsal of falling actions. These may begin with forward rolls onto the outstretched arm on a mat, initially from a kneeling position, progressing to standing and finally a diving forward roll over a bench. Pressure over the point of the shoulder begins with log rolling on the floor, and builds up to shoulder blows on to a rolled mat or punch bag.

Surgical intervention

There is some controversy concerning the treatment of this condition. Both conservative and surgical approaches restore function to a similar degree (Larsen, Bjerg-Nielsen and Christensen, 1986; Dias et al., 1987; Bannister et al., 1989), and some surgical methods have been shown to give long-term functional detriment. Certainly, removal of the distal end of the clavicle (Gurd, 1941) will disrupt the acromioclavicular ligament, a main stabilizer of the joint (Fukuda et al., 1986). In the literature, the main argument for surgery has been the development of degenerative changes in the joint as a result of non-operative management. However, degeneration does not occur in all patients, and when it does occur, it is not necessarily a limitation (Dias et al., 1987). In addition, surgery is often as effective if done in the acute or chronic condition, so there is normally no advantage to operating immediately. Importantly, surgery carries with it a high risk of complications (Ejeskar, 1974; Lancaster, Horowitz and Alonso, 1987; Taft, Wilson and Oglesby, 1987).

In a literature review of 11 papers detailing the long-term results of both surgical and conservative management of this injury, Dias and Gregg (1991) found poor results to have occurred in 13 out of 247 patients treated conservatively (5.3%), and 22 out of 233 managed surgically (9.4%). These authors argued that as comparable results were obtained regardless of the method used, conservative management was the treatment of choice for most AC injuries. Looking at strength testing following grade III AC injuries treated conservatively (average 4.5 year follow-up), Tibone, Sellers and Tonino (1992) found no subjective complaints in patients, all of whom were able to participate in sport. Full motion occurred in all subjects, and no significant differences were found in muscle strength of injured and non-injured sides in rotation, abduction/adduction or flexion/extension.

AC joint degeneration

Joint degeneration is common in later years following injury, regardless of the grade of damage which occurred, and particularly after repeated trauma. In addition, some sports, such as weight-lifting, have a higher incidence of degenerative changes in the AC joint, even where no incidents of trauma may have occurred. Cahill (1982) reported 46 cases of osteolysis of the distal clavicle, all but one occurring in weight-lifters. He argued that degeneration occurred as a result of sub-chondral stress fractures resulting from repeated microtrauma. The condition presents as pain, usually dull and aching in nature, brought on by activities such as lifting and throwing. To examination there is point tenderness over the joint, with pain and crepitus to passive horizontal flexion.

Where the diagnosis is uncertain, radiographs will frequently reveal degeneration, and injection of local anaesthetic into the joint is helpful to establish if the degeneration is the cause of the patient's symptoms.

Movements which stress the joint (for example, press-ups, weight training or throwing) should be avoided. Initially, immobilization in a sling may be required in the very acute lesion. Later, joint mobilization provides good results. Antero-posterior gliding may be performed with the patient in a sitting position. The therapist grasps the distal end of the clavicle with his or her thumb and forefingers of one hand, and the acromion process in a similar fashion with the other hand. The hands are worked against each other to glide the joint. Injection of corticosteroid may give many months of relief, a technique made easier if the shoulder is laterally rotated to distract the AC joint.

Fractures of the clavicle

The most common mechanism of injury is a fall onto the outstretched arm, and occasionally direct trauma to the shoulder. Although common, these injuries should not be taken too lightly, as it must be remembered that the subclavian vessels and brachial plexus lie in close proximity, as does the upper lobe of the lung. There is usually a cracking sensation at the time of injury, with immediate pain over the fracture sight, and rapid swelling. Signs of injury to vital structures are rare, but include dyspnoea and paraesthesia and obviously warrant immediate hospitalization. Laceration of the subclavian artery presents as a readily expanding pulsating haematoma. Deformity is common, as is crepitus.

Fractures of the proximal and middle thirds of the clavicle make up the largest proportion (80%) of such injuries. If not displaced these should be immobilized with the shoulders retracted in a figure-of-eight bandage for 6 weeks. With young athletes the risk of non-union may make it necessary to curtail activity for up to 3 months after injury. Figure-of-eight bandages must not be applied too tightly as to constrict the blood or nerve supply to the arm. When little displacement is present, support in a sling may be all that is required. Some step deformity usually occurs as complete immobilization of athletes (other than in a cast) is difficult. This type of deformity is usually cosmetic rather than functional.

Distal fractures tend to be displaced by retraction immobilization, and are better wired. Internal fixation of the proximal clavicle carries with it similar complications to that of the sternoclavicular (SC) joint.

Winged scapula

During normal scapulo-humeral rhythm, the scapula slides over the rib cage, and is held in place by the serratus anterior. If weakness or paralysis of the serratus anterior occurs, the scapula will stand prominent from the rib cage when the arm is protracted against resistance. In addition to muscular weakness, there are a number of causes including damage to the long thoracic nerve, brachial plexus injury, conditions affecting the fifth, sixth and seventh cervical nerve roots, and certain types of muscular dystrophy (Apley and Solomon, 1989).

Where weakness is due to nerve palsy, spontaneous recovery is to be expected. Re-education of scapulo-humeral movement is required as habitual alteration of scapulo-humeral rhythm is often seen. Strengthening the shoulder musculature in general, and especially serratus anterior, is also useful.

Occasionally, a congenitally undescended scapula (Sprengel's shoulder) is seen, sometimes associated with marked thoracic kyphosis. Normally, the scapulae descend completely by the third month of fetal life. However, if undescended, the scapula appears slightly smaller, higher, and more prominent. Scapulo-humeral rhythm is affected and abduction is limited as a consequence. Minor cases respond to rehabilitation although marked deformity may require surgery.

Apparent winging may occur when the scapulae abduct through lengthening of the scapular retractors and tightening of the protractors (see p. 150). As the scapulae move away from the mid-line, they roll around the rib cage, lifting their medial border. This is not true winging however, because the condition is present at rest and during muscle contraction.

Impingement syndrome

The sub-acromial space (Fig. 19.10) lies beneath the coraco-acromial arch formed by the coroco-acromial ligament together with the coracoid and acromion, the so-called 'roof of the joint'. The coraco-acromial arch is covered by the deltoid, and inferiorly its fascia is continuous with that of the supraspinatus. The arch prevents upward dislocation of the gleno-humeral joint. The supraspinatus passes beneath the arch being separated from it by the sub-acromial bursa. The sub-acromial distance (space between the inferior acromion and the head of the humerus) is normally about 1 cm (Petersson and Redlund-Johnell, 1984). If the supraspinatus tendon has ruptured, or the muscle is no longer active, this space will reduce by as much as 50% due to the unopposed pull of the deltoid. During elevation and internal rotation the greater tuberosity, with the supraspinatus riding on top, may press against the anterior edge of the underside of the acromion (or a spur from a degenerating AC joint) causing impingement pain. During flexion, impingement may also involve the long head of biceps (Peat and Culham, 1994).

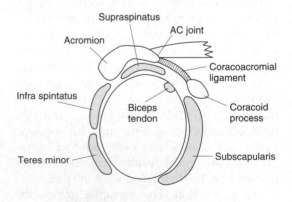

Figure 19.10 Impingement and the rotator cuff.

The action of abduction involves a complex series of movements as described on p. 167. At the point where the greater tuberosity comes close to the acromion (70–120° abduction), a number of structures may be pinched between the involved bones or the tuberosity and the coraco-clavicular ligament. Normally, the structures affected are the suprasinatus tendon, the long head of biceps, and the sub-acromial bursa.

Following the screening examination described on p. 406, two further tests are useful. In test one (Fig. 19.11a) the arm is fully abducted and overpressure is put onto the internally rotated (thumb forwards) shoulder. For the second test (Fig. 19.11b), the gleno-humeral joint is flexed and internally rotated (Hawkins test). Overpressure is then added to internal rotation and abduction or horizontal flexion. Resisting flexion by placing pressure over the elbow may

also bring on the athlete's pain (Hawkins and Hobeika, 1983; Reid, 1992).

In addition to a purely mechanical impingement, changes in the microvascular supply to the area have been noted. Pressure exerted by the humeral head on the supraspinatus tendon, has the effect of 'wringing out' the tendon vessels and creating an avascular zone (Rathbun and Macnab, 1970). This area, known as the critical zone (Fig. 19.12), is an anastomosis between the osseous vessels and the tendinous vessels (Moseley and Goldie, 1963). Furthermore, repeated microtrauma results in local oedema within the tendon and an increase in tissue volume. This in turn makes the structures more susceptible to impingement by reducing the sub-acromial space and so perpetuates the problem.

A reduction in the sub-acromial space may be the result of individual variation in the

(a)

(b)

Figure 19.11 Impingement tests. (a) Full abduction with overpressure to the internally rotated shoulder. (b) Hawkin's sign. Flexion and internal rotation. Overpressure to internal rotation and abduction or horizontal flexion.

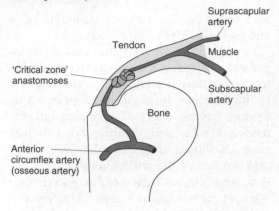

Figure 19.12 Vascularity of the critical zone. From Keirns (1994).

anatomical architecture of this region, with some individuals more prone to impingement than others (Ticker and Bigliani, 1994). Cadaveric studies of 140 specimens have identified three types of acromion associated with full thickness tears of the rotator cuff (Bigliani, Morrison and April, 1986). The flat (type I) acromion occurred in 17% of subjects, the curved (type II) acromion was seen in 43%, and the hooked (type III) type in 39% (Fig. 19.13). The hooked acromion was present in 70% of rotator cuff tears whereas the flat type was only seen in 3%. By assessing the supraspinatus outlet view X-ray, Morrison and Bigliani (1987) showed 80% of those with positive arthrograms to have a hooked acromion. The same authors showed that 66% of patients who underwent open sub-acromial decompression had a hooked acromion.

Impingement is not simply the result of a lack of sub-acromial space, however. Weakness in the rotator cuff (or pain inhibition) can cause instability (see below) and allow the humeral head to ride up through deltoid contraction, making examination of rotator cuff strength, and order of muscle contraction, vital with this condition. The interaction between biomechanics, physiology and pathology creates a painful progressive condition which ultimately may cause mechanical failure as detailed in Fig. 19.14.

Figure 19.13 Acromion types. (a) Type I, flat; (b) type II, curved; (c) type III, hooked. After Ticker and Bigliani (1994).

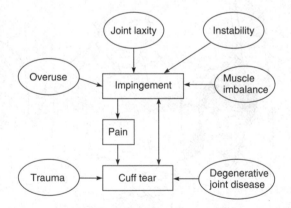

Figure 19.14 Interrelation between pain, impingement and cuff tear. After Reid (1992).

Three stages of impingement have been described (Neer, 1972). Stage I is a self-limiting overuse syndrome. It presents as a dull ache occurring after repeated overhead activity. The most significant sign is a painful arc of movement. Here, as abduction is commenced, no pain is felt. As the tuberosity moves closer to the glenoid, structures are compressed and pain occurs between 70–120°. As abduction goes further, the tuberosity moves away from the acromion and pain subsides as the arm is taken overhead (Fig. 19.15). In addition to a painful arc, palpable pain may be found over the anterior edge of the acromion in some cases. Resisted movements may or may not be painful depending on whether a contractile structure is impinged. If the supraspinatus is affected, the painful arc exists in combination with pain to resisted lateral rotation and initiation of abduction. However, the situation is far from being clear cut because pain is frequently caused when a resisted movement approximates the joint, pulling the humerus onto the acromion. In addition, pain in this condition may be so acute that resisted actions appear weak. The weakness, how-

ever, is due to the pain itself rather than neurological involvement. Involvement of the biceps tendon gives pain along the intertubercular sulcus with resisted shoulder and elbow flexion in combination with resisted forearm supination.

The stage I lesion is basically inflammatory in nature and so reversible. Treatment aims to reduce pain and swelling, and to remove the cause of impingement by resting the impinged structures through training modification. If modalities are used, the position of the athlete for treatment must be considered. The standard resting position of adduction and neutral rotation causes the blood vessels within the region to be tractioned and compressed (McNab, 1973). A better resting position during treatment is to have the athlete sit at the side of the couch with the arm abducted to 30–70° and the forearm supported (Lovinger, Mangus and Ingersoll, 1991). There should be neutral rotation of the gleno-humeral joint and slight extension.

Stage II lesions involve the development of thickening and fibrosis. They generally give more intense pain, at night as well as with activity, and are not so readily reversed. Movement becomes increasingly limited as fibrosis and scarring occur in the sub-acromial space. Pain relief and reduction of inflammation are as for a stage I condition, but now stretching exercises become more important to limit loss of range through fibrosis. The stage III lesion involves chronic bony changes and is more usually seen in the older athlete (Thein, 1989). Prolonged mechanical impingement gives rise to sclerosis and osteophyte formation of the acromion and tuberosity, and occasionally calcification of the supraspinatus tendon. Active movements are more limited than passive, with weakness and rotator cuff atrophy being commonly seen. Treatment aims are essentially to restore limited function, and frequently require surgical intervention. Both decompression and anterior acromioplasty are used.

Internal rotation of the shoulder is one biomechanical factor which predisposes to

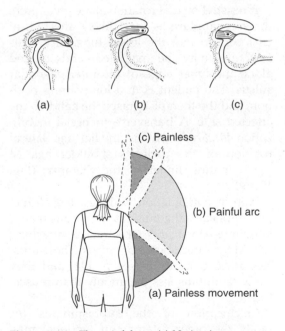

Figure 19.15 The painful arc. (a) No impingement, painless. (b) Tuberosity pinches painful structure. (c) Tuberosity moves beneath acromion, pain disappears.

impingement (Halbach and Tank, 1990), and should be limited in patients with this condition. While external rotation helps the greater tuberosity clear the acromion, internal rotation has the reverse effect, compressing the two structures. Exercise therapy aims to redevelop scapular stability and to restore the normal internal/external rotation, ratio of the gleno-humeral joint to 3:2 (Baechle, 1994). As the supraspinatus is affected, external rotation range and strength is normally greatly reduced in these athletes. External rotation exercises, beginning with the arm held to the side and eventually in 90° abduction are therefore used. Combinations of abduction, extension and external rotation may be performed on a pulley or with elastic tubing, within the pain-free range.

The structures affected by impingement may also be injured in isolation. So, either the supraspinatus or biceps tendons may be subjected to tendinitis, and the sub-acromial bursa inflamed without muscular involvement.

Tendon injuries

Rotator cuff

Tendonitis of the rotator cuff muscles is common both as a result of overuse and through trauma. Common examples of overuse include excessive repetitions on a single weight-training exercise, while trauma may result from an ill-timed 'wrenching' action which combines rotation with abduction.

The most commonly affected tendon in the shoulder is that of the supraspinatus. Pain is elicited with resisted external rotation and initiation of abduction. More specifically, pain occurs with the arms abducted to 90°, brought forwards into 30° flexion and internally rotated so that the thumbs point towards the floor (Reid, 1992).

Palpation to the muscle insertion is performed with the injured arm medially rotated (hand behind the back) to bring the greater tuberosity forwards and make the tendon more superficial (Fig. 19.16a). This is also the most convenient position for transverse frictions, the area of scarring being found by palpating about one finger's width below the anterior tip of the acromion. The musculotendinous junction is more conveniently palpated with the injured arm abducted to 90° and supported (Cyriax and Cyriax, 1983). The palpating finger is directed at the space between the posterior aspect of the lateral clavicle and the scapular spine. Again, this is the most convenient starting position for transverse frictional massage (Fig. 19.16b).

Pain on resisted lateral rotation but not abduction implicates the infraspinatus. Local pain may be found by palpation to the posterior aspect of the greater tuberosity with the patient's shoulder flexed, slightly adducted and laterally rotated. The most convenient position for this is elbow support in a prone-lying position, with the patient leaning forwards and outward over the injured shoulder (Fig. 19.16c).

If resisted medial rotation alone gives pain, the subscapularis is most likely affected, at its insertion into the lesser tuberosity. This structure may be palpated and treated along the inner edge of the intertubercular sulcus. The patient is in a long sitting position, and the therapist grasps the hand on the affected side. A transverse frictional mobilization is carried out by medial and lateral rotation of the patient's shoulder against the palpating finger of the therapist (Fig. 19.16d).

Pain in combination with resisted adduction implicates the muscles (pectoralis major, latissimus dorsi and teres major) attaching within the intertubercular sulcus. These muscles are usually tight (see p. 144) and they show tendonitis less commonly than muscle tearing.

Calcification of the supraspinatus (or rarely the other rotator cuff tendons) may develop following chronic tendonitis within the critical zone (Moseley and Goldie, 1963),

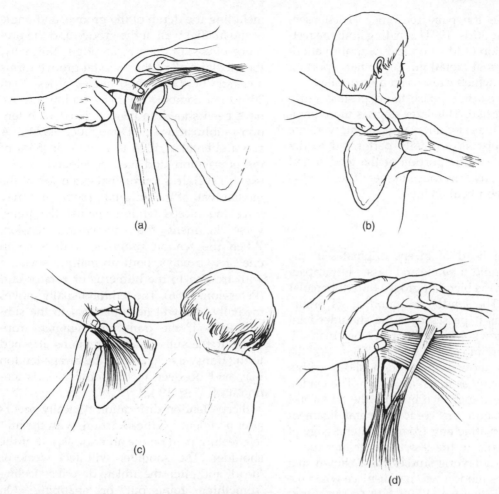

Figure 19.16 Palpation and treatment of rotator cuff tendon injury. (a) Supraspinatus: tendon. (b) Supraspinatus: musculotendinous junction. (c) Infraspinatus. (d) Subscapularis. After Cyriax and Cyriax (1983).

an area susceptible to injury due to reduced vascularity (Rothman and Parkes, 1965). This area, near the attachment of the supraspinatus (see Fig. 19.12), tends to be wrung out when the arm is held in its resting position of adduction and neutral rotation. Compression of the tendon vessels and microtrauma leads to repetitive hypoxia, and is especially common in activities which involve repeated internal rotation at 90° shoulder abduction. Fibrocytes within the tendon are transformed to chondrocytes, and collagen disintegration, coupled with the accumulation of mucopolysaccharides,

begins. Hydroxyapatite mineral deposit deposition is then initiated (Lemak, 1994).

During the acute and sub-acute phase the deposit is of toothpaste-like consistency (and will escape into the sub-acromial bursa if punctured during an injection procedure). Conservative management is usually successful if the condition is caught early enough. Active rest and exercise are called for. The repetitive forces causing hypoxia must be removed by correcting impingement. Exercise therapy is then used to enhance the blood supply of the tendon, and healing is good. High repetitions are performed in the pain-free range (Torstensen, Meen and Stiris, 1994) avoiding both the resting position (adduction and neutral rotation) and internal rotation. All other sporting activities which cause pain are curtailed.

In the chronic phase the deposit is gritty and sand-like. This later stage is more painful and may require surgical intervention. Arthroscopy is normally performed to debride the calcific portion of the tendon and remove any necrotic tissue. The tendon should then heal well.

Biceps

The long head of biceps originates at the supraglenoid tubercle and passes intracapsularly into the bicipital groove (intertubercular sulcus). The tendon is round at its origin, flattens as it passes over the shoulder joint and narrows within the intertubercular sulcus (Mariani and Cofield, 1988). As the humerus moves, the tendon slides within its groove by as much as 3–4 cm. The tendon is held in the groove by both the transverse ligament and the coraco-humeral ligament (the latter attaching from the lateral edge of the coracoid to the lesser and greater tuberosities). Cadaveric studies have shown that the biceps tendon will not displace when the transverse ligament is cut, if the coraco-humeral ligament remains intact (Slatis and Alato, 1979). The tendency for subluxation or dislocation of the tendon from the bicipital groove is dependent on a number of factors

including the depth of the groove, and angle of the medial wall of the groove and the presence of a supratubercular ridge. Normally, the medial wall of the bicipital groove forms an angle of 60–70°, and angles of less than 30° when combined with a shallow groove have been shown to be associated with tendon subluxation (O'Donoghue, 1973). A supratubercular ridge is present in 55% of the population, and well developed in 18% (Reid, 1992). It is a proximal extension of the medial wall of the bicipital groove, and may force the biceps tendon against the transverse ligament thus increasing tension. When the tendon subluxes, it does so in one of two ways, both normally associated with trauma to the humerus or rotator cuff (Petersson, 1986). The tendon usually moves medially and will lie superficial to the subscapularis if the transverse ligament ruptures. If the subscapularis remains attached to the transverse ligament, the biceps tendon may end up deep to the subscapularis tendon itself (Fig. 19.17).

Biceps tendon dislocation typically occurs after a violent overhead action, with the athlete feeling pain on the anterior aspect of the shoulder. The shoulder will feel weak or 'dead' and often the athlete describes feeling 'something going out' or 'snapping'. On examination there is tenderness to palpation over the tendon, and medial and lateral rotation may elicit a palpable click. This may be further investigated using Yergason's sign

Figure 19.17 Biceps tendon subluxation. (a) Normal alignment. (b) Transverse ligament tears, biceps tendon rides over subscapularis. (c) Transverse ligament intact, biceps tendon slides beneath subscapularis. After Reid (1992).

(Yergason, 1931) or Speed's test. For Yergason's test the patient attempts to supinate the flexed elbow while externally rotating the shoulder. Speed's test involves shoulder flexion from a position of extension with the forearm supinated. Management of the condition is usually surgical followed by intensive rehabilitation to restore correct scapulo-thoracic and gleno-humeral function.

Tendonitis of the long head of biceps presents as pain to resisted shoulder and elbow flexion and resisted forearm supination. Yergason's sign and Speed's test may again be used. The teno-osseous junction of the muscle at the supraglenoid tubercle and adjacent glenoid labrum is difficult to palpate directly, but the tendon itself within the intertubercular sulcus is easier. A painful arc is only present with these conditions if the inflamed area of tendon is within a pinchable position in mid-range abduction, in which case impingement tests will be positive.

Overuse is the predominant causal factor with alteration in the biomechanics of overhead actions often being present. The synovial sheath of the tendon may become swollen and inflamed, with thickening and haemorrhaging frequently seen. Adhesions are often present. If the locking position and quadrant test reproduce pain, postero-anterior (PA) gliding should be assessed. If limited, PA pressures against the humeral head (see below) should be used.

Rupture of the biceps brachii occurs more commonly at the insertion of the long head into the supraglenoid tubercle, but tears to the short head, distal attachment or belly may occur. The rupture more frequently follows sub-acromial impingement and tendon degeneration (Reid, 1992). The mechanism of injury for proximal tendon injuries is normally a forced extension while the muscle is contracting. This can result from an arm tackle or block, where the arm is held abducted and then pushed back behind trunk level. Distal tendon injuries may

occur as a result of heavy lifting with the elbow flexed to $90°$.

On examination, pain is elicited to resisted elbow flexion and supination (which may be combined with shoulder flexion), and passive end-range extension. A visible defect may be noted in the muscle, with retraction of the tendon. In the case of the long head, the tendon may no longer be palpable in the intertubercular sulcus, and as the muscle is contracted the belly of the long head is seen to bunch up into a ball-shaped mass. Local swelling and bruising are noted, and lead to an increased arm girth measurement.

Both surgical and conservative management have been recommended in the literature (Friedman, 1963; Morrey et al., 1985; Bandy, Lovelace-Chandler and Holt, 1991). Surgical management is normally favoured (in the young especially) because conservative treatment has been said to give a loss of supination power (Baker and Bierwagen, 1985; Morrey et al., 1985). However, the reason for this deficit may be the lack of adequate rehabilitation following conservative management (Bandy, Lovelace-Chandler and Holt, 1991).

Conservative management consists of the RICE protocol to minimize inflammation, with gentle mobility exercises to the elbow within the pain-free range. Exercise therapy is used to maintain shoulder function. Multi-angle isometric training begins as soon as possible to reduce muscle atrophy, the deciding factor for starting this being pain. As pain to resisted movement reduces, dynamic exercise is begun against manual, and later isokinetic, resistance. PNF techniques combining shoulder flexion/adduction/medial rotation with elbow flexion/supination are used, as well as static stretching to elbow and shoulder extension. The resistance training programme is progressed with power actions, and functional sporting activities are introduced. The long-term prognosis is good, in terms of restoration of function, but a palpable defect will usually remain in the muscle.

Surgery for distal tendon injuries includes re-inserting the tendon into the radial tuberosity, or the use of a fascia lata graft, where surgery has been delayed and the tendon has retracted. The long head may be re-inserted into the supraglenoid tubercle in the case of an avulsion or, in some instances, to the wall of the bicipital groove.

Pectoralis major

Rupture of the pectoralis major is unusual, but when it does occur, the muscle is usually already under tension when further force is imposed on it. The most common example of this scenario is the bench press exercise in weight-training. The injury normally occurs during the eccentric phase of the exercise as the bar is being lowered. During the last 30° of humeral extension of this action the inferior fibres of the muscle have been shown to lengthen disproportionately (Wolfe, Wickiewicz and Cavanaugh, 1992). In addition, with fatigue, the athlete may move his or her whole body in an attempt to lift the weight, and so bring accessory muscle groups into action enabling him or her to exceed his or her safe limit. When lowering this excessive weight, he or she loses control and the injury occurs.

A tearing sensation is felt, and a large haematoma is apparent over the anterior axilla. Weakness and pain to resisted adduction and medial rotation is noted to manual muscle testing. No defect may be seen at rest, but if the muscle is contracted isometrically by asking the athlete to press his or her hands together as if clapping, a defect may be apparent. Following injury, the muscle does not retract very far, perhaps due to its varied fibre direction and wide origin. The insertion into the humerus (just lateral to the intertubercular sulcus) of the non-dominant arm is more normally affected (Kretzler and Richardson, 1989).

Non-surgical treatment can be successful for partial tears (Roi, Respizzi and Dworzak, 1990), and in the non-athletic individual (Delport and Piper, 1982). However, surgical management is more generally recommended (Kretzler and Richardson, 1989; Reut, Bach and Johnson, 1991). At operation the deltoid is retracted and the tendon is re-attached either via drill holes in the humerus or by suturing the tendon to the remnant of tissue insertion.

The arm is immobilized in a sling and isometric contractions started as soon as the pain stabilizes. Assisted movements are begun 1 week after surgery, and thereafter the rehabilitation programme aims to restore strength, mobility and function. As strength training progresses, eccentric movements must be used to prepare the muscle for its action of decelerating the bar in the bench press exercise. In addition, pectoral muscle stretches and retraction work must be used to avoid a protracted shoulder posture.

Triceps

In addition to the more common elbow site for triceps injury (p. 450), occasionally the muscle may avulse from its glenoid attachment (O'Donoghue, 1976), especially in throwing athletes. Pain occurs to triceps stretching, often palpable at the inferior rim of the glenoid. With rest, a fibrous union will normally fix the fragment back in place, but surgery to remove the avulsed fragment and re-suture the tendon may be required where the injury recurs. When the muscle belly itself is injured, it is usually the medial head which is involved and the treatment of choice is conservative (Kunichi and Torisu, 1984).

It is important to note that the normal tendon is capable of sustaining considerable force before it will rupture, making avulsion fracture the more usual injury. Where tendon rupture occurs, an underlying pathology may be present. High dosage oral steroids may weaken the tendons (Hunter, Shybut and Nuber, 1986), a situation especially important with athletes using heavy resistance exercise, or power movements.

Conditions such as rheumatoid arthritis, systemic lupus erythematosus and hormone disorders may also predispose to tendon rupture (Reid and Kushner, 1989).

Bursitis

Gray's anatomy (1973) lists some eight bursae around the shoulder joint, but the one most commonly affected in sport is the sub-acromial (sub-deltoid) bursa. This lies between the deltoid and the joint capsule and stretches beneath the acromion process and coraco-acromial ligament. The bursa extends over the supraspinatus tendon, and does not usually communicate with the joint capsule except in the case of a supraspinatus tear, where the bursa may be damaged as well.

Acute sub-acromial bursitis is unusual and occurs with sudden onset. The whole bursa is inflamed, and this severely limits abduction, but not in the capsular pattern. Pain is acute and often referred as far down as the wrist in extreme cases. Resisted movements are largely painless, and a painful arc only appears in a sub-acute case as initially no abduction at all is possible. Treatment in this acute stage is aimed at reducing the intense pain. The arm is supported in a sling to limit all gleno-humeral movement, and anti-inflammatory modalities used.

Chronic sub-acromial bursitis occurs when the bursal sac becomes thickened and adherent, but in one part only. The condition is not a progression of acute bursitis, but a separate clinical entity (Cyriax, 1982). The onset is gradual and a painful arc is present, but movements are largely of full range. Injecting the bursa with a local anaesthetic to inflate it is surprisingly effective, and may act mechanically by simply pushing the walls of the bursal sac apart.

In all cases of bursitis, shoulder mechanics should be closely examined to detect any abnormality which may give rise to microtrauma. Typically, postural changes around the chest and shoulder can alter the mechanics of gleno-humeral movement. This may predispose the athlete to impingement leading eventually to bursitis.

Shoulder instability

The stability of the gleno-humeral joint lies very much on a continuum. At one end there is the stable, fully functional joint, and at the other the dislocated joint requiring surgery. In many cases, there is a progression which begins with a reduction of stability through alteration in static, dynamic or proprioceptive factors (see p. 364, Fig. 15.20 for joint stability model). Individual differences in bony or soft tissue configuration can give some athletes a greater risk of instability, and training activities can alter the subtle muscle balance that exists around the joint. Trauma will cause both mechanical changes to stabilizing structures and alteration in proprioception. Any or all of these factors may co-exist to push the athlete from a position of stability to instability of some degree. The progression from minor instability to major instability may then occur with time, unless there is treatment intervention of some type.

Instability may be classified using the TUBS/AMBRI acronyms (Matsen, Harryman and Sidles, 1991). These acronyms represent two ends of the spectrum (Table 19.1) from instability through trauma to instability through congenital factors. The patient with a TUBS lesion will have suffered trauma instability in one direction only (unidirectional). The glenoid labrum will have been detached from the anterior rim of the glenoid (Bankart lesion) and they will probably require surgery, although rehabilitation should be tried first as this can be successful with minor degrees of injury. The AMBRI patient has an atraumatic etiology causing multidirectional instability in both shoulders (bilateral). Usually this patient responds well to intensive rehabilitation, but if they do

Table 19.1   Classification of shoulder instability

TUBS Born loose ←————————————————————→	AMBRI Torn loose
T— Traumatic aetiology U—Unidirectional instability B—Bankart lesion S—Surgical repair	A—Atraumatic aetiology M—Multidirectional instability B—Bilateral condition R—Rehabilitation normally successful I—Inferior capsular shift if rehabilitation fails

require surgery, an inferior capsular shift is normally the treatment of choice.

Shoulder stability is supplied by both static and dynamic factors. Static stability is provided by the glenoid labrum, joint capsule and ligaments, while dynamic stability comes from muscle action (Table 19.2). As the arm hangs by the side of the body, the pull of gravity is resisted by the superior capsule and the coraco-humeral ligament. If the arm is loaded, when carrying a bag for example, the greater force is resisted by the supraspinatus which shares a common distal attachment with the two previous structures and has a line of action which is virtually identical to them (Norkin and Levangie, 1992).

The middle gleno-humeral ligament lies directly under the tendon of subscapularis and is attached to it (Fig. 19.18). The ligament varies tremendously between subjects. In some it may be 2 cm wide, while in others it may be completely absent (Peat and Culham, 1994). Both the subscapularis and middle gleno-humeral ligament limit external rotation, and are important anterior stabilizers in the lower and middle ranges of abduction.

The inferior gleno-humeral ligament (the thickest position of the gleno-humeral ligament in total) is the most important stabilizing structure in overhead actions. The ligament is divided into three bands with the inferior portion forming the axillary pouch. The anterior band wraps around the humeral head at 90° abduction with external rotation and prevents anterior head migration (O'Brian et al., 1990). It is, therefore, the anterior band of the inferior gleno-humeral ligament which is most significant in stabiliz-

Table 19.2   Stability of the gleno-humeral joint

Dependent position	Coraco-humeral ligament Superior gleno-humeral ligament Supraspinatus muscle
Elevation Lower range (0–45°)	Anterior capsule Superior gleno-humeral ligament Coraco-humeral ligament Middle gleno-humeral ligament Subscapularis, infraspinatus, and teres minor muscles
Middle range (45–75°)	Middle gleno-humeral ligament Supscapularis muscle (decreasing importance) Infraspinatus and teres minor muscles Inferior gleno-humeral ligament (superior band)
Upper range (>75°) Throughout elevation	Inferior gleno-humeral ligament (axillary pouch) Dynamic activity of rotator cuff

From Peat and Culham (1994).

Figure 19.18   Anterior ligaments of the gleno-humeral joint.

ing the arm in overhead throwing sports. As this ligament tightens, abduction is limited and the humerus must laterally rotate and move towards the scapular plane.

The gleno-humeral and coraco-humeral ligaments form a 'Z' shape on the anterior aspect of the shoulder, with the middle gleno-humeral ligament providing the crossbar of the 'Z'. Above and below the crossbar are spaces which create areas of potential weakness. Superiorly (foramen of Weitbrecht) the opening allows the subscapularis bursa to communicate with the joint cavity. Inferiorly, a smaller bursa is sometimes present (Ferrari, 1990). In some subjects, if the 'Z' crossbar (middle gleno-humeral ligament) is missing, the anterior defect formed may contribute to anterior instability.

Active stability is provided by the rotator cuff muscles (Fig. 19.19). As previously stated (p. 404), the pull of the deltoid is almost vertical and it tends to cause upward translation of the humeral head. This is counteracted by the rotator cuff muscles, which tend to downwardly translate the head. The combination of the two sets of muscle translation forces stabilize the head of the humerus in the glenoid. These compressor forces are at their maximum between 60–80° and are minimal after 120° (Comtet, Herberg and Naasan, 1989).

Assessing instability

Static instability may be assessed clinically by a number of drawer and apprehension tests. Anterior and posterior instability is initially tested with the athlete in a sitting position. The therapist grasps the athlete's upper arm over the humeral head and applies forward and backward pressure while stabilizing the scapula (Fig. 19.20a). The injured and uninjured sides are compared for range and end feel. Excessive anterior glide leaves a posterior hollow, and the movement can be graded as mild (less than one-third of the head coming off the glenoid), moderate (head riding on the edge of the glenoid) or severe (complete dislocation of the head). Posterior subluxation is considered abnormal when more than 50% of the humeral head comes off the glenoid.

The apprehension test is again performed in a sitting position. The athlete's arm is taken into 90° abduction and externally rotated. At the same time an anterior pressure is exerted on the proximal humerus (Fig. 19.20b). The test is positive in the presence of spasm or a feeling of impending (or actual) subluxation. A more rigorous procedure is to position the athlete in a supine-lying position, with the injured shoulder over the table edge. The arm is abducted to 90° and externally rotated. From this position the examiner applies an anteriorly directed pressure to increase pain and a posteriorly directed pressure to reduce pain (Fig. 19.20c).

Exercise therapy

In an overhead motion the arm externally rotates, causing the humeral head to move superiorly. In this position the subscapularis is not able to control the humeral head any longer and the tendency to anterior translation is therefore increased. The joint must depend on the inferior gleno-humeral ligament for passive stability, the only effective active control coming from the infraspinatus.

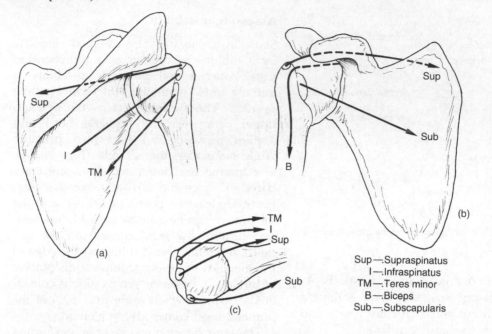

Sup —.Supraspinatus
I —.Infraspinatus
TM —.Teres minor
B —.Biceps
Sub —.Subscapularis

Figure 19.19   Active stabilizers of the gleno-humeral joint. (a) Posterior, (b) anterior, (c) superior.

Figure 19.20   Assessing static instability of the gleno-humeral joint. (a) Antero-posterior gliding. (b) Apprehension test—pain/apprehension increases as an anteriorly directed force is applied. (c) Modified apprehension test—pain reduces with posterior pressure.

If the ligamentous control is failing, enhancement of infraspinatus action can effectively control the humeral head (Reid, 1992).

As with all shoulder rehabilitation, the cornerstone of exercise therapy is scapular stabilization. Proximal stability must be obtained before distal mobility and function are attempted. In cases of anterior instability of the gleno-humeral joint, single channel sEMG is an extremely useful rehabilitation tool. The sEMG electrode is placed over the bulk of the infraspinatus below the scapular spine avoiding the posterior deltoid. The shoulder is flexed to activate the sEMG signal and the athlete is instructed to maintain the audible or visual signal from the machine by tightening the rotator cuff muscles. Isometric rotator cuff tightening is performed for multiple repetitions (10 sets of 10 repetitions), and then holding time is built (up to a 10 second hold) before active gleno-humeral movements are commenced. Short lever shoulder flexion (in neutral rotation) is performed between 70–90° as the patient tries to push the sEMG signal up as high as possible. If pain or apprehension occur, the exercise is regressed to isometric holding alone. As sEMG signals can be maintained with active shoulder flexion, further exercises are added in a progression (Table 19.3). When painless and confident full-range motion has been obtained, general shoulder rehabilitation is begun (see p. 434).

Although anterior instability is by far the most common type, posterior or inferior instability is seen. Rehabilitation follows similar guidelines building scapular stability and then emphasizing general rotator cuff control, while avoiding movements which stress the pathological joint.

Table 19.3 Use of surface EMG in rehabilitation of anterior instability of ther shoulder

1	Forward flexion with a straight elbow
2	Forward flexion with increasing external rotation
3	Abduction with flexion, progressing to elbow extension
4	Abduction with elbow extension with increasing external rotation
5	Abduction from flexion
6	Abduction from flexion with increasing external rotation
7	Reaching for objects behind the back or overhead

From Reid (1992).

Taping and mobilization with movement

When assessing static alignment of the gleno-humeral joint (p. 162) no more than one-third of the head of the humerus should lie anterior to the acromion. In cases where the head of the humerus lies further forward (normally with impingement or instability symptoms), mobilization with movement and taping may be of help. Mobilization with movement (MWM) is a technique where a sustained mobilization is applied to a joint, normally at 90° to the plane of movement, to correct joint tracking (Mulligan, 1989).

The mobilization is applied at the same time as the patient performs a painful action with the affected joint. In the case of the shoulder, the painful action is abduction. The therapist stands behind the patient with one hand cupped over the anterior aspect of the shoulder, and the other braced against the scapula. A posterior gliding force is applied over the head of the humerus as the patient performs a previously painful abduction movement. The aim of the MWM is to allow the patient to perform the action painlessly to repetition. Eventually, the posterior glide is released, and the patient should still be able to perform the action with less (or no) pain.

If this technique is successful, a proprioceptive taping, which gives the patient the feeling of posterior glide and scapular depression, is often helpful (McConnell, 1992). The taping consists of the strips of 5 cm zinc-oxide taping placed over adhesive net tape (Fig. 19.21). The first strip passes from the anterior aspect of the shoulder around the lateral aspect of the joint and down to the inferior angle of the scapula. The second strip passes from the anterior aspect of the shoulder, over the middle fibres of trapezius and again down to the inferior angle of the scapula. The adhesive net tape is placed on the shoulder in a relaxed state, but the zinc-oxide tape pulls the skin to give the patient the sensation of posterior gliding

(a)   (b)

Figure 19.21 Proprioception taping of the shoulder. (a) Strip one passes from the anterior shoulder to the inferior angle of the scapula. Strip two passes over the middle trapezius. (b) Gap between the two strips corresponds to the humeral sulcus at 90° abduction.

(strip one) and scapula depression (strip two). The gap between the two pieces of tape should correspond to the sulcus which appears at the tip of the acromion at 90° abduction. As with the MWM the taping should reduce the pain of abduction to re-test.

Gleno-humeral dislocation

Dislocation (often a progression of instability) is a commonly seen shoulder injury, with anterior displacement being encountered more often than posterior. Forced movements involving rotation and abduction are common mechanisms, and a fall onto the outstretched arm is also a frequent aetiology. Acute anterior dislocation gives considerable pain. The arm is usually held slightly abducted and externally rotated, and the normal rounded contour of the shoulder is lost. Close inspection shows the acromion process to be more prominent than

usual, and a hollow is visible below it. The displaced humeral· head can usually be felt on the anterior aspect of the shoulder.

The question of whether to reduce an acute injury is one of debate. On the positive side, early reduction of an uncomplicated injury may be achieved without anaesthetic and little discomfort. If left, muscle spasm sets in, making reduction under anaesthetic necessary. The main problem is the likelihood of further injury by reduction without X-ray by inexperienced staff. Fracture of the head or neck of the humerus may have occurred at the time of injury and epiphyseal displacement is seen with adolescents. Displaced bone fragments may easily be pulled onto the circumflex or radial nerves causing injury, and vascular damage may also occur. For these reasons, an acute injury occurring for the first time is better referred to an orthopaedic consultant.

Recurrent anterior dislocation may be reduced more easily. The forces required to dislocate the shoulder in the first place are considerably less than with the acute injury, and so the chance of associated fracture is minimal. Spontaneous reduction may occur, and frequently the athlete has learnt to reduce the dislocation him or herself, and the joint is fairly lax. For assisted reduction, the patient is in a supine position, on the ground, with the therapist sitting on the patient's injured side. The therapist places his stockinged foot just below the ipsilateral axilla, while holding the patient's arm. He or she then simply leans back to provide traction, and may gently rotate the arm to facilitate reduction. The simplest self-reduction procedure is for the athlete to bend his or her ipsilateral leg and grasp the knee with both hands, keeping the arms locked straight. Slowly leaning back produces in-line traction which usually allows the shoulder to reduce. It must be emphasized that these procedures should only be performed in the absence of pain and spasm. The traction is applied gently, brute force or 'yanking' the arm by another athlete being an obvious contraindication. If the recurrently dislocated shoulder does not reduce readily, referral is still necessary.

Acute posterior dislocation is not as obvious as anterior. Pain is still intense, with the arm held adducted and internally rotated. Any attempt to move the arm is resisted by intense muscle spasm. In thin individuals the coracoid process is more visible than usual, and fullness is often apparent posteriorly. Heavy musculature in an athlete will however obscure these signs. Posterior dislocations require referral and reduction under sedation. Gentle in-line traction is applied to the adducted/internally rotated arm with gentle pressure over the humeral head.

Rehabilitation following anterior dislocation

Following reduction, rest and ice are used to limit inflammation. The arm is immobilized, and the initial period of immobilization is an important determinant of recurrence. Normally the recurrence rate for young (20–30 years) athletes may be as high as 85% (Halbach and Tank, 1990). However, this may be reduced considerably, with one study of 50 individuals showing a recurrence rate of 20% after 6 weeks immobilization (Reid, 1992). Exercise therapy is divided into four phases (Table 19.4).

In phase one (0–3 weeks), isometric exercises are used. These are performed twice daily with only minimal active abduction allowed to facilitate axillary hygiene. Limited flexion and extension are allowed, but external rotation is avoided. Gentle pendular swinging actions are used in transverse and sagittal planes. In phase two (3–6 weeks), active resisted internal rotation is used, and external rotation to neutral using elastic tubing. Abduction is limited to 45° and exercise for the rest of the body is progressed. Strengthening concentrates on medial rotation, to strengthen the subscapularis and support the anterior joint, and limited range adduction to work latissimus dorsi, teres major, the pectorals and coraco-brachialis to resist abduction forces.

After 6–8 weeks (phase three), abduction increases to 90° and limited external rotation is used to reduce stiffness. Only when strength has increased to 75% of the uninjured shoulder should full-range motion be attempted. To reduce stiffness, self-stretches such as 'finger walking' along a table top or up a wall, and limited joint distractions are useful (Fig. 19.22). Autotherapy distractions may be performed in a prone kneeling position, holding the couch end.

Slow velocity (< 90°/s) isokinetics may be used, with the velocity gradually increasing to functional sporting levels as the athlete is able to control the movement. Pool exercises are used to incorporate faster actions against the resistance of a paddle, and range of motion exercise using floatation to take the weight of the arm. PNF techniques involving extension/adduction/medial rotation are used initially against manual resistance and subsequently with a weight and pulley system. Later, flexion/abduction/lateral rotation is used with caution. Restoration of kinaesthetic awareness is important after anterior dislocation (Smith and Brunolli, 1989) and is described on p. 434.

Figure 19.22 Self-stretching procedures for the shoulder.

Table 19.4   Guidelines for rehabilitation following anterior gleno-humeral dislocation

Initial post-reduction period
Rest and ice
Immobilization

0–3 weeks
Isometrics twice daily
Minimal abduction for axillary hygiene only
Limited flexion and extension
Avoid external rotation
Gentle pendular swinging in transverse and sagittal planes
Scapular stability work

3–6 weeks
Resisted internal rotation
External rotation to neutral only
Abduction limited to 45°
Re-education of scapulo-humeral rhythm
Extension/adduction/medial rotation pattern on pulley
Limited range resisted adduction
Pendular swinging giving way to automobilization techniques
Proprioceptive work including static joint repositioning

6–8 weeks
Abduction increased to 90°
External rotation gradually increased
Flexion/abduction/lateral rotation pattern on pulley
Full resistance training below shoulder height
Introduce fast throwing and catching below head height
Closed chain work on balance board and trampette (two hands)

Final rehabilitation
Full range motion resisted
Ensure muscle balance (internal rotation:external rotation ratio)
Closed chain work (single arm)
Push up with clap
Fast reaction work—throwing/catching/blocking
Re-education of falling—forward roll/handstand/fall back

Frozen shoulder

Frozen shoulder or 'adhesive capsulitis' is an increasingly common pathology found in sport. As the number of elderly people involved in sport continues to rise, this condition is likely to be seen even more frequently. The problem is more common in females, and presents as a gradual loss of shoulder movement, with or without pain. The initial loss of movement may go unnoticed until function is limited. Patients complain that activities of everyday living become increasingly difficult. Combing the hair at the back of the head and fastening a bra strap are frequent sources of complaint. Active sports persons frequently notice the onset of the condition earlier than sedentary individuals. Elderly athletes often complain that their golf swing is affected, or overhead badminton shots are painful for example.

The term 'frozen shoulder' (Codman, 1934) is not an accurate diagnosis, but rather a description of the major symptom, which is lack of movement. 'Adhesive capsulitis' (Neviaser, 1945) describes the finding of capsular thickening, contraction and adhesions. The condition may be associated with a number of other soft tissue and medical pathologies including rotator cuff injuries, impingement syndrome, traumatic arthritis, osteoarthritis, shoulder joint immobilization, autoimmune disease, diabetes and thyroid dysfunction (Boissonnault and Janos, 1989; Hertling and Kessler, 1990; Ott, Clancy and Wills, 1994).

The joint capsule seems to be a major source of movement limitation in this condition. The capsule is thickened and may adhere to the humeral head, with the axillary pouch frequently being obliterated. A reduction in joint volume has been noted on arthrogram (Reeves, 1966), and a loss of bone mineral content can be seen on X-ray (Lundberg and Nilsson, 1968). An increase in vascularity and thickening has been noted in the sub-acromial bursa and rotator cuff (Simmonds, 1949), and a contracture of the coraco-humeral ligament (Ozaki et al., 1989). Many studies, subsequent to Neviaser, have noted an absence of adhesions and degenerative changes (Ha'eri and Maitland, 1981; Uitvlugt, Detrisac and Johnson 1988). Changes to the subscapular bursa, rotator cuff, and biceps tendon (Uitvlugt, Detrisac and Johnson, 1988; Wiley, 1991) indicate that these structures may be key factors in the initiation of the condition. On examination, movement is usually limited in a capsular pattern (sub-acute) or by muscle guarding (acute), but resisted movements are normally pain free. Accessory movements are limited, particularly inferior and anterior gliding, and the quadrant position is limited and painful when compared to the uninvolved side. Three stages of the condition have been described (Maitland, 1991). In stage I, pain is the dominant feature, which almost completely prevents movement. With stage II conditions, painful limitation is again a feature. This time, however, some movement is present, and when the joint is stretched the pain increases. Stage III lesions have restricted range but very little pain.

The frozen shoulder responds well to joint mobilization techniques. The condition is sometimes self-limiting within a year, but with mobilization may resolve in a matter of months. Pain may be greatly reduced by postero-anterior (PA) oscillations (Maitland, 1991), and scapulo-thoracic mobilization, and these are the manual treatments of choice for the stage I lesion. For PA mobilization the patient lies in a supine position with the arm supported in a pain-free position. The elbow is flexed with a folded towel placed under the arm. The patient's forearm rests on his or her trunk. This position limits adduction, extension and excessive medial rotation. The therapist kneels on the floor and directs his or her thumbs to the posterior aspect of the humeral head. The oscillations are produced by the therapist's arms rather than the finger flexors. For scapulo-thoracic mobilization the patient lies on his or her side with the injured arm uppermost. The arm should be in a pain-free position supported by towels. The therapist grasps the medial edge of the scapula with his or her finger tips in an attempt to release the scapula from the rib cage first, and secondly to abduct it, easing it away from the spine.

With the stage II condition, the pain is limited first, and then stiffness is addressed. As pain is reduced, the starting position is changed to use the patient's upper arm as a lever. The therapist grips the patient's upper arm in his or her cupped hands, high into the axilla. Initially, the arm is by the patient's side (Fig. 19.23a). From this position the slack is taken up in the joint by lifting it anteriorly, and then the arm is lifted and lowered to perform the PA glide. As pain lessens and movement returns, the same action is performed with the arm held abducted to 45° (Fig. 19.23b), and then in full flexion overhead (Fig. 19.23c).

Inferior gliding, if limited, may be regained with the patient's shoulder flexed to 90° and his or her hand on the trapezius (central fibres). The therapist stabilizes the patient's elbow against his or her own shoulder and grips the upper arm in his or her cupped hands. The gliding motion pulls the humeral head inferiorly. As pain reduces, a similar movement may be performed with

Figure 19.23 Postero-anterior gleno-humeral joint movement. (a) Patient's arm by his or her side. (b) 45° abduction. (c) Maximal flexion-abduction.

the patient's arm abducted and supported. The therapist pushes down on the humeral head with the web of his or her free hand (Fig. 19.24).

The final range of movement may be regained using the quadrant position (see above) as a mobilization to stretch the anterior capsule. This is only used when pain is minimal and stiffness is the predominant symptom (late stage II and stage III lesions). The therapist stands at the head of the couch with his or her knee resting on the couch top (Fig. 19.25a). The arm is then oscillated through approximately 30° to facilitate a grade II mobilization. A grade IV movement

Figure 19.24 Inferior gliding gleno-humeral joint. Patient in (a) supine, or (b) sitting position. The arm is grasped near the elbow to stabilize it in 90° abduction. The web of the other hand contacts the head of the humerus. The head of the humerus is then depressed inferiorly.

may be used by placing the therapist's near-side arm under the patient's upper rib angles, a small 5° oscillation is all that is required (Fig. 19.25b).

Following each treatment the patient is shown exercise and autotherapy techniques to maintain the new range of motion. Such movements include pendular swinging in the early stages and later, overhead reaching into flexion. Cord and pulley exercises are used if abduction is not painful, and rotation movements, placing the hand behind the head or the small of the back, are begun. Strength development and movement re-education must parallel the restoration of joint mobility.

Snapping scapulae

This unusual condition occurs especially in adolescent females just after skeletal maturity, and in both sexes following surgery. Patients experience a snapping sensation, which is sometimes audible, near the vertebral border of the scapula. Pain is often localized to the rhomboids and levator scapulae over the medial scapular border or the trapezius over the medial aspect of the scapular spine. It appears to be from tendonitis to these muscles. This occurs through micro-trauma from excessive shearing forces beneath the scapular due to abnormal scapulo-thoracic rhythm. Management relies on the restoration of a more normal scapulo-thoracic rhythm (Percy, Birbrager and Pitt, 1988).

Nerve entrapment syndromes

Two relatively uncommon nerve entrapments are seen around the shoulder, quadrilateral space syndrome and entrapment of the suprascapular nerve.

The quadrilateral (quadrangular) space lies between the teres minor and the subscapularis above and the teres major below. The long head of triceps forms its medial wall and the surgical neck of the humerus lies laterally (Fig. 19.26a). Entrapment by tethering can occur to both the axillary nerve and circumflex humeral artery (Cahill and Palmer, 1983). The patient, frequently a throwing athlete, is usually young (22–35

(a)

(b)

Figure 19.25 Gleno-humeral mobilizations in the quadrant position to regain final degrees of movement.

years) and complains of shoulder pain of insidious onset. Muscle fatigue and loss of abduction power are apparent and tenderness may be elicited to palpation over the involved quadrilateral space. Arteriograph frequently shows posterior circumflex artery occlusion. Most patients respond to alteration of throwing technique but some may go on to surgical decompression.

The suprascapular nerve (Fig. 19.26b) may be trapped as it passes through the suprascapular notch beneath the suprascapular ligament, or as it winds around the lateral edge of the scapular spine. Direct blows in contact sports are one cause as the nerve is superficial, and occult ganglions pressing on the shoulder have been described (Fritz et al., 1992; Gerscovich and Greenspan, 1993). Entrapment can affect the motor response of both the supraspinatus and infraspinatus, either together or in isolation (Black and Lombardo, 1990). The patient presents with visible muscular atrophy and weakness is often noticed to backhand shots or in serving. Vague pain occurs deep in the posterior aspect of the shoulder. Treatment involves decompression of the nerve at the suprascapular notch and scapular nerve block.

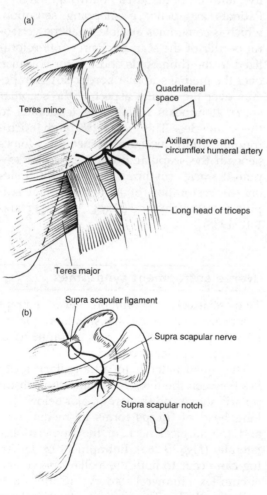

Figure 19.26 Entrapment neuropathy in the shoulder. (a) Quadrilateral space; (b) Suprascapula notch.

Shoulder rehabilitation

Shoulder rehabilitation begins with an assessment of scapulo-humeral rhythm and then localized scapula stability exercises as detailed in Chapter 7. It is essential that provision of a stable base is made before further shoulder work is begun. Rehabilitation must start at the base of the kinetic chain and progress outward into the extremity (Kibler, 1991).

Gleno-humeral stability

The gleno-humeral joint must then be restored and a balanced action of all the rotator cuff muscles obtained. Gleno-humeral stability has been described as a circle concept (Dempster, 1965; Wilk and Arrigo, 1993). Translational movement of the humeral head is related to laxity of both the anterior and posterior structures. For example, anterior translation may be caused by tightness in the anterior structures, but will only be noticeable if the posterior structures are lax. Active stability is achieved through cocontraction of the rotator cuff muscles compressing the humeral head into the glenoid. Rehabilitation must involve work for the entire rotator cuff, rather than simply the supraspinatus, which has a contributory role only (Wilk and Arrigo, 1993).

A differentiation must be made between joint laxity and functional instability (see also p. 364). Shoulder laxity is present when the humeral head can be passively translated on the glenoid. Functional instability, on the other hand, exists when unwanted humeral head motion compromises the comfort and function of a movement (Matsen, Harryman and Sidles, 1991). The difference is the patient's ability to control the translational motion of the humeral head. Three interrelating systems exist to contribute to gleno-humeral stability. The first is an increase in joint compression brought about by a force couple between the deltoid and rotator cuff. Secondly, dynamic stability is provided by the rotator cuff tendons with the shoulder capsule. Muscular contraction directly tensions the joint ligaments, therefore creating 'dynamic ligament tension' (Cleland, 1866). The third method of stabilization is via neuromuscular control. Proprioceptive rehabilitation (movement awareness drills) has been shown to reduce muscle reaction speed in a number of joints and has been used successfully for shoulder rehabilitation (Smith and Brunolli, 1989; Lephart et al., 1994).

Exercises begin in starting positions which place minimal stress on the shoulder joint capsule. Initially, the arm is held by the side with the elbow flexed to 90°. The patient is instructed to hold the arm inactive against alternating manual pressure (medial and lateral rotation) from the therapist to apply rhythmic stabilization. The movement then progresses to 45° and finally 90° of shoulder abduction.

A variety of weight-training exercises may be performed to re-strengthen the shoulder musculature as a whole, and four exercises (Fig. 19.27) in particular have been shown using intramuscular EMG synchronized with cinematography to be maximally challenging to the gleno-humeral muscles (Jobe et al., 1991).

In overhead motions, the cocking phase provides an eccentric pre-stretch to the muscles (adductors and internal rotators) closely followed by an explosive acceleration phase. Concentric–eccentric coupling of this type requires plyometric rehabilitation. Plyometrics involve a pre-stretch (eccentric) and short amortization phase where the movement direction is reversed, and finally a rapid facilitated concentric action. Activities include overhead soccer throws, basketball chest passes, single arm tennis ball throws, use of exercise tubing in PNF patterns and use of small medicine balls (Wilk et al., 1993).

Figure 19.27 Gleno-humeral exercises from EMG analysis. (a) Elevation in the sagittal plane. (b) Elevation in the scapular plane. (c) Horizontal abduction in lateral rotation. (d) Sitting press-up. From Jobe et al. (1991).

Closed kinetic chain activities

The concept of kinetic chain activity was introduced on p. 174. Essentially, closed kinetic chain activity involves movement of the proximal body segment on a fixed distal segment. This is common in the lower limb during the stance phase of gait for example. In the upper limb the majority of daily actions occur in open chain format, with the distal segment (arm) moving on a fixed proximal base (thorax). However, the upper limb must be able to work in a closed kinetic chain pattern for 'fall' and 'push' actions. In many sports, the athlete is likely to fall onto the hand or elbow, and in some sports, such as gymnastics, complex closed kinetic chain actions are involved (handstand/vault). During a closed chain action, such as falling onto the outstretched arm, gravity assists in closing the chain of movement, approximating the joint surfaces. The muscle action is primarily eccentric to control the deceleration of movement and provide a protective role. As concentric action begins to accelerate the body segment, the joint surfaces are still approximated (push-up) whereas during open chain actions, the joint surfaces are under traction (throwing).

Traditional closed chain exercises include body weight (push-ups, dips) resistance and weights (bench and shoulder presses). Additional movements include the push-up with-a-press, and the sitting push-up. Hand walking activities are useful and may be performed on a wall, floor, treadmill, stepper, static cycling or on steps, either from a kneeling or prone falling position. Use of a rocker board for double-handed activities, and a balance board for single handed activities, is also useful for closed kinetic chain rehabilitation and is challenging to proprioception. The same would apply to activities on the Swiss ball and slide trainer.

References

Akeson, W.H., Amiel, D. and Woo, S. (1980) Immobility effects of synovial joints: the pathomechanics of joint contracture. *Biorheology*, **17**, 95

Apley, A.G. and Solomon, L. (1989) *Concise System of Orthopaedics and Fractures*, Butterworth, London

Austin, K.A., Gwynn-Brett, K.A. and Marshall, S.C. (1994) *Illustrated Guide to Taping Techniques*, C.V. Mosby, St Louis

Baechle, T.R. (1994) *Essentials of Strength Training and Conditioning*, Human Kinetics, Champaign, Illinois

Baker, B.E. and Bierwagen, D. (1985) Rupture of the distal tendon of the biceps brachii: operative versus non-operative treatment. *Journal of Bone and Joint Surgery*, **67A**, 414–417

Bandy, W.D., Lovelace-Chandler, V. and Holt, A. (1991) Rehabilitation of the ruptured biceps brachii muscle of an athlete. *Journal of Orthopaedic and Sports Physical Therapy*, **13**(4), 184–190

Bannister, G.C., Wallace, W.A., Stableforth, P.G. and Hutson, M.A. (1989) The management of acute acromioclavicular dislocation: a randomised prospective controlled trial. *Journal of Bone and Joint Surgery*, **71B**, 848–850

Bigliani, L.U., Morrison, D.S. and April, E.W. (1986) The morphology of the acromion and its relationship to rotator cuff tears. *Orthopaedic Transactions*, **10**, 228

Black, K. and Lombardo, J. (1990) Suprascapular nerve injuries with isolated paralysis of the infraspinatus. *American Journal of Sports Medicine*, **18**(3), 225–228

Boissonnault, W.G. and Janos, S.C. (1989) Dysfunction, evaluation, and treatment of the shoulder. In *Orthopaedic Physical Therapy* (eds R. Donatelli and M.J. Wooden), Churchill Livingstone, Edinburgh

Cahill, B.R. (1982) Osteolysis of distal part of clavicle in male athletes. *Journal of Bone and Joint Surgery*, **64A**, 1053–1058

Cahill, B.R. and Palmer, R.E. (1983) Quadrilateral space syndrome. *Journal of Hand Surgery*, **8**, 65

Cleland, J. (1866) On the actions of muscles passing over more than one joint. *Journal of Anatomy and Physiology*, **1**, 85–93

Codman, E.A. (1934) *The Shoulder*, Thomas Todd, Boston

Comtet, J.J., Herberg, G. and Naasan, I.A. (1989) Biomechanical basis of transfers for shoulder paralysis. *Hand Clinics*, **5**, 1

Corrigan, B. and Maitland, G.D. (1994) *Musculoskeletal and Sports Injuries*, Butterworth-Heinemann, Oxford

Cyriax, J. (1982) *Textbook of Orthopaedic Medicine*, Vol. 1, 8th edn, Baillière Tindall, London

Cyriax, J.H. and Cyriax, P.J. (1983) *Illustrated Manual of Orthopaedic Medicine*, Butterworth, London

Delport, H.P. and Piper, M.S. (1982) Pectoralis major rupture in athletes. *Archives of Orthopaedic and Traumatic Surgery*, **100**, 135–137

Dempster, W.T. (1965) Mechanisms of shoulder movement. *Archives of Physics in Medicine and Rehabilitation*, **46**, 49–70

Dias, J.J. and Gregg, P.J. (1991) Acromioclavicular joint injuries in sport. *Sports Medicine*, **11**, 125–132

Dias, J.J., Steingold, R.F., Richardson, R.A., Tesfayohannes, B. and Gregg, P.J. (1987) The conservative treatment of acromioclavicular dislocation: review after five years. *Journal of Bone and Joint Surgery*, **69B**, 719–722

Ejeskar, A. (1974) Coracoclavicular wiring for acromioclavicular joint dislocation: a ten year follow-up study. *Acta Orthopaedica Scandinavica*, **45**, 652–661

Ferrari, D.A. (1990) Capsular ligaments of the shoulder: anatomical and functional study of the anterior superior capsule. *American Journal of Sports Medicine*, **18**, 20

Freidman, E. (1963) Rupture of the distal biceps tendon. Report on 13 cases. *Journal of the American Medical Association*, **184**, 60–63

Fritz, R.C., Helms, C.A., Steinbach, L.S. and Genant, H.K. (1992) Suprascapular nerve entrapment: evaluation with MR imaging. *Radiology*, **182**, 437–444

Fukuda, K., Craig, E.V., An, K., Cofield, R.H. and Chao, E.Y.S. (1986) Biomechanical study of the ligamentous system of the acromioclavicular joint. *Journal of Bone and Joint Surgery*, **68A**, 434–439

Garrick, J.G. and Webb, D.R (1990) *Sports Injuries: Diagnosis and Management*, W.B. Saunders, Philadelphia

Gerscovich, E.O. and Greenspan, A. (1993) Magnetic resonance imaging in the diagnosis of suprascapular nerve syndrome. *Canadian Association of Radiologists Journal*, **44**, 307–309

Gurd, F.B. (1941) The treatment of complete dislocation of the outer end of the clavicle—a hitherto undescribed operation. *Annals of Surgery*, **113**, 1041

Ha'eri, G.B. and Maitland, A. (1981) Arthroscopic findings in the frozen shoulder. *Journal of Rheumatology*, **8**, 149

Halbach, J.W. and Tank, R.T. (1990) The shoulder. In *Orthopaedic and Sports Physical Therapy*, 2nd edn (ed. J.A. Gould), C.V. Mosby, St Louis

Hawkins, R.J. and Hobeika, P.E. (1983) Impingement syndrome in the athletic shoulder. *Clinics in Sports Medicine*, **2**, 391

Hertling, D. and Kessler, R.M. (1990) *Management of Common Musculoskeletal Disorders*, J.B. Lippincott, Philadelphia

Hunter, M.B., Shybut, G.T. and Nuber, G. (1986) The effect of anabolic steroid hormones on the mechanical properties of tendons and ligaments. *Transactions of the Orthopaedic Research Society*, **11**, 240

Keirns, M.A. (1994) Conservative management of shoulder impingement. In *The Athletes Shoulder* (eds J.R. Andrews and K.E. Wilk). Churchill Livingstone, New York

Kibler, W.B. (1991) Role of the scapula in the overhead throwing motion. *Contemporary Orthopaedics*, **22**, 525–532

Kretzler, H.H. and Richardson, A.B. (1989) Rupture of the pectoralis major muscle. *American Journal of Sports Medicine*, **17**, 453–458

Kunichi, A. and Torisu, T. (1984) Muscle belly tear of the triceps. *American Journal of Sports Medicine*, **12**(6), 485

Lancaster, S., Horowitz, M. and Alonso, J. (1987) Complete acromioclavicular separations: a comparison of operative methods. *Clinical Orthopaedics and Related Research*, **216**, 80–88

Larsen, E., Bjerg-Nielsen, A. and Christensen, P. (1986) Conservative or surgical treatment of acromioclavicular dislocation: a prospective controlled randomised study. *Journal of Bone and Joint Surgery*, **68A**, 552–555

Lemak, L.J. (1994) Calcifying tendonitis. In *The Athlete's Shoulder* (eds J.R. Andrews and K.E. Wilk), Churchill Livingstone, Edinburgh

Lephart, S.M., Warner, J.P., Borsa, P.A. and Fu, F.H. (1994) Proprioception of the shoulder in normal, unstable, and surgical individuals. *Journal of Shoulder and Elbow Surgery*, **3**, (4) 116–119

Lovinger, A., Mangus, B.C. and Ingersoll, C.D. (1991) Shoulder positioning for optimal treatment effects. *Athletic Training, Journal of the National Athletic Training Association*, **26**, 81–82

Lundberg, B.J. and Nilsson, B.E. (1968) Osteopenia in the frozen shoulder. *Clinical Orthopaedics and Related Research*, **60**, 187

Macdonald, R. (1994) *Taping Techniques. Principles and Practice*, Butterworth-Heinemann, Oxford

Maitland, G.D. (1991) *Peripheral Manipulation*, 3rd edn, Butterworth-Heinemann, Oxford

Mariani, E.M. and Cofield, R.H. (1988) The tendon of the long head of biceps brachii: instability, tendinitis, and rupture. *Advances in Orthopaedic Surgery*, **11**, 262

Matsen, F.A., Harryman, D.T. and Sidles, J.A. (1991) Mechanics of glenohumeral instability. *Clinical Sports Medicine*, **10**(4), 783–788

McConnell, J. (1992) *The Challenge of the Problem Shoulder*, Course notes, London

McNab, I. (1973) Rotator cuff tendinitis. *Annals of the Royal College of Surgeons of England*, **53**, 271

Morrey, B.F., Askew, L.J., An, K.N. and Dobyns, J.H. (1985) Rupture of the distal tendon of the biceps brachii: a biomechanical study. *Journal of Bone and Joint Surgery*, **67A**, 418–421

Morrison, D.S. and Bigliani, L.U. (1987) The clinical significance of variations in acromial morphology. *Orthopaedic Transactions*, **11**, 234

Moseley, H.F. and Goldie, I. (1963) The arterial pattern of the rotator cuff of the shoulder. *Journal of Bone and Joint Surgery*, **45B**, 780

Mulligan, B.R. (1989) *Manual Therapy*, Plane View Services, Wellington, New Zealand

Neer, C. (1972) Anterior acromioplasty for the chronic impingement syndrome in the shoulder. *Journal of Bone and Joint Surgery*, **54A**, 41–50

Neviaser, J.S. (1945) Adhesive capsulitis of the shoulder. *Journal of Bone and Joint Surgery*, **27**, 211

Norkin, C.C. and Levangie, P.K. (1992) *Joint Structure and Function*, 2nd edn, F.A. Davis, Philadelphia

O'Brian, S.J., Neves, M.C., Arnoczky, S.P. et al. (1990) The anatomy and histology of the inferior gleno-humeral ligament complex of the shoulder. *American Journal of Sports Medicine*, **18**, 451

O'Donoghue, D.H. (1973) Subluxing biceps tendon in the athlete. *Journal of Sports Medicine*, **1**, 20

O'Donoghue, D.H. (1976) *Treatment of Injuries to Athletes*, W.B. Saunders, Philadelphia

Ott, J.W., Clancy, W.G. and Wilk, K.E. (1994) Soft tissue injuries of the shoulder. In *The Athlete's Shoulder* (eds J.R. Andrews and K.E. Wilk), Churchill Livingstone, Edinburgh

Ozaki, J., Nakagawa, Y., Sakurai, G. and Tamia, S. (1989) Recalcitrant chronic adhesive capsulitis of the shoulder. *Journal of Bone and Joint Surgery*, **71A**, 1511

Palastanga, N., Field, D. and Soames, R. (1989) *Anatomy and Human Movement*, Heinemann Medical, Oxford

Peat, M. and Culham, E. (1994) Functional anatomy of the shoulder complex. In *The Athlete's Shoulder* (eds J.R. Andrews and K.E. Wilk), Churchill Livingstone, Edinburgh

Percy, E.C., Birbrager, D. and Pitt, M.J. (1988) Snapping scapula: a review of the literature and presentation of 14 patients. *Canadian Journal of Surgery*, **31**, 248–250

Perry, J. and Glousman, R.E. (1995) Biomechanics of throwing. In *The Upper Extremity in Sports Medicine*, 2nd edn (eds. J.A. Nicholas and E.B. Hershman), C.V. Mosby, St Louis

Petersson, C.J. (1986) Spontaneous medial dislocation of the tendon of the long biceps brachii: an anatomic study of prevalence and pathomechanics. *Clinical Orthopaedica and Related Research*, **211**, 244

Petersson, C.J. and Redlund-Johnell, I. (1984) The sub-acromial space in normal shoulder radiographs. *Acta Orthopaedics Scandinavica*, **55**, 57

Rathbun, J. and Macnab, I. (1970) The microvascular pattern of the rotator cuff. *Journal of Bone and Joint Surgery*, **52B**, 540–553

Reeves, B. (1966) Arthrographic changes in frozen shoulder and post traumatic stiff shoulders. *Proceedings of the Royal Society of Medicine*, **59**, 827

Reid, D.C. (1992) *Sports Injury Assessment and Rehabilitation*, Churchill Livingstone, Edinburgh

Reid, D.C. and Kushner, S. (1989) The elbow region. In *Orthopaedic Physical Therapy* (eds R. Donatelli and M.J. Wooden), Churchill Livingstone, Edinburgh

Reut, R.C., Bach, B.R. and Johnson, C. (1991) Pectoralis major rupture: diagnosing and treating a weight-training injury. *Physician and Sports Medicine*, **19**(3), 89–96

Rockwood, C.A. and Odor, J.M. (1989) Spontaneous atraumatic subluxation of the sternoclavicular joint. *Journal of Bone and Joint Surgery*, **71A**, 1280–1288

Roi, G.S., Respizzi, S. and Dworzak, F. (1990) Partial rupture of the pectoralis major muscle in athletes. *International Journal of Sports Medicine*, **11**, (1) 85–87

Rothman, R.H. and Parkes, W.W. (1965) The vascular anatomy of the rotator cuff. *Clinical Orthopaedics and Related Research*, **41**, 176

Simmonds, F.A. (1949) Shoulder pain with particular reference to the frozen shoulder. *Journal of Bone and Joint Surgery*, **31B**, 426

Slatis, P. and Alato, K. (1979) Medial dislocation of the tendon of the long head of biceps brachii. *Acta Orthopaedica Scandinavica*, **50**, 73

Smith, R.L. and Brunolli, J. (1989). Shoulder kinesthesia after anterior glenohumeral joint dislocation. *Physical Theapy*, **69**, 106–112

Taft, T.N., Wilson, F.C. and Oglesby, J.W. (1987) Dislocation of the acromioclavicular joint: an end-result study. *Journal of Bone and Joint Surgery*, **69A**, 1045–1051

Thein, L.A. (1989) Impingement syndrome and its con-servative management. *Journal of Orthopaedic and Sports Physical Therapy*, **11**(5), 183–191

Tibone, J., Sellers, R. and Tonino, P. (1992) Strength test-ing after third degree acromioclavicular dislocations. *American Journal of Sports Medicine*, **20**, 328–331

Ticker, J.B. and Bigliani, L.U. (1994) Impingement pathology of the rotator cuff. In *The Athlete's Shoulder* (eds J.R. Andrews and K.E. Wilk), Churchill Livingstone, Edinburgh

Torstensen, T.A., Meen, H.D. and Stiris, M. (1994) The effect of medical exercise therapy on a patient with chronic supraspinatus tendinitis. Diagnostic ultra-sound—tissue regeneration: a case study. *Journal of Orthopaedic and Sports Physical Therapy*, **20**, 319–327

Uitvlugt, G., Detrisac, D.A. and Johnson, L.L. (1988) The pathology of the frozen shoulder: an arthroscopic perspective. *Arthroscopy*, **4**, 137

Wiley, A.M. (1991) Arthroscopic appearance of frozen shoulder. *Arthroscopy*, **7** 138

Wilk, K.E. and Arrigo, C. (1993) Current concepts in the rehabilitation of the athletic shoulder. *Journal of Orthopaedic and Sports Physical Therapy*, **18**(1), 365–378

Wilk, K.E., Voight, M.L., Keirns, M.A., Gambetta, V., Andrews, J.R. and Dillman, C.J. (1993) Stretch short-ening drills for the upper extremities: theory and clinical application. *Journal of Orthopaedic and Sports Physical Therapy*, **17**(5), 225–239

Wolfe, S.W., Wickiewicz, T.L. and Cavanaugh, J.T. (1992) Ruptures of the pectoralis major muscle: an anatomic and clinical analysis. *American Journal of Sports Medicine*, **20**, 587–593

Yergason, R.M. (1931) Supination sign. *Journal of Bone and Joint Surgery*, **13A**, 160

20

The elbow

The primary purpose of the shoulder is often described as positioning the arm to facilitate hand action. The elbow, in turn, functions to shorten or lengthen the arm, largely to allow the hand to be brought to the mouth. The elbow complex consists of the humero-ulnar and humero-radial articulations and the superior radio-ulnar joint, all of which share the same capsule.

When viewed from the side, the distal end of the humerus is larger anteriorly and inferiorly, and sits at an angle of 45° to the longitudinal axis of the bone. Similarly, the trochlear notch of the ulna bulges, making a comparable angle to its axis. This structure postpones contact between the humerus and ulna on flexion, and allows more space between the bones to accommodate soft tissues. The 'nutcracker effect' is therefore reduced, as the bones come together.

Viewed from the front, the radius and ulna are slanted laterally to the shaft of the humerus, the angulation forming the carrying angle (Fig. 20.1a). This is approximately 10–15° for men, increasing to 20–25° for women. This bony alignment means that normally, as the arm is flexed the hand moves towards the shoulder, and the radius and ulna end up in line with the humerus (Fig. 20.1c). Variations in carrying angle between individuals, mainly due to altered configuration of the trochlear groove, may occur and will alter the resting position of

the radius and ulnar at full flexion (Fig. 20.1b,d). Changes in bony alignment may also occur after injury—an important factor in rehabilitation following elbow fractures.

The contact area between the joint surfaces of the elbow complex increases throughout flexion. In full extension the lower medial part of the trochlear notch of the ulna is used, with no contact occurring between the radius and ulna. At 90° the contact area is a diagonal (lower medial to upper lateral) across the trochlear surface, with only slight pressure between the humerus and radial head. In full flexion definite contact occurs between the radius and ulna, and the trochlear contact areas increase (Fig. 20.2). Full flexion is thus required to ensure adequate nutrition of the whole articular cartilage, a situation sometimes not possible in obese or heavily muscled individuals due to the approximation of the flexor soft tissues.

As occurs in the knee, the collateral ligaments of the elbow become taut at different degrees of flexion. The anterior fibres of both the medial and lateral collateral ligaments are taut in extension, whereas the posterior fibres are taut in flexion. Protection is provided against valgus and varus strains throughout the whole range of joint movement as a result.

Flexion is limited by muscle contact and impingement of the radial head on to the radial fossa. In addition, tension occurs in

Figure 20.1 (a) Carrying angle. (b) Lateral orientation. (c) Most common configuration of trochlear groove. (d) Medial orientation. After Norkin and Levangie (1992).

Figure 20.2 Contact areas at different elbow positions. (a) The trochlear notch. (b) The head of the radius. From Palastanga, Field and Soames (1989).

the triceps and posterior joint capsule, and finally in lean individuals the shafts of the radius and humerus themselves come into contact (Fig. 20.3a)

In extension, when the muscles are relaxed, valgus stability is provided by the medial collateral ligament, anterior capsule and bony configuration. As the elbow flexes, the anterior capsule relaxes, and its role is taken on by the medial collateral ligament, which provides 31% of joint stability in extension and 54% at 90° flexion (Table 20.1). In contrast, varus stress is resisted in the main by bone contact supplemented by the anterior capsule. The lateral collateral ligament only contributes 14% of the total stability of the joint with the elbow in full extension, and 9% with it flexed to 90° (Morrey and Kai-Nan, 1983). With joint distraction, the main limiting factor in extension is the joint capsule, and with the joint flexed to 90°, the medial collateral ligament. End range is limited by a combination of the olecranon impinging into the olecranon fossa, and tension in the anterior capsule and biceps (Fig. 20.3b).

Pronation and supination of the forearm involve not just the superior and inferior radio-ulnar joints, but also the ulno-humeral, radio-humeral and radio-carpal joints. With

Table 20.1 Percentage contribution of elbow structures to stability of the joint

Limiting structure	Valgus %		Varus %		Distraction %	
	0°	90°	0°	90°	0°	90°
Medial collateral ligament	31	54	–	–	6	78
Lateral collateral ligament	–	–	14	9	5	10
Joint capsule	38	10	31	13	85	8
Bone contact	31	33	55	75	–	–

After Morrey and Kai-Nan (1983).

Range 150-160° flexion

Range 0-10° flexion

Constraints to flexion

1 Muscle contact
2 Radial head impingement
3 Posterior capsule tension
4 Triceps tension
5 Radius-humerus contact

(a)

Constraints to extension

1 Olecranon impingement
2 Anterior capsule tension
3 Biceps tension

(b)

Figure 20.3 Constraints to flexion (a) and extension (b). From Reid (1992).

pronation, the head of the radius twists on the capitulum and swings on the radial notch of the ulna, tightening the quadrate ligament. The radial head tilts, and is pulled into the capitulotrochlear groove, and the ulna moves into slight extension and abduction at the ulno-humeral joint (Lee, 1986). Consequent to this, at the inferior radio-ulnar joint the ulnar notch of the radius swings medially over the ulnar head. A traumatic injury to the elbow is therefore likely to affect the wrist, and clinical examination should include both joints to be complete.

Screening examination

Following inspection, objective examination begins with flexion and extension, each performed to full range, noting the joint end feel. The normal end feel to extension is hard while that to flexion is soft. Pronation and supination are performed with the elbow held to the side of the body and arm flexed to 90°. The end feel should be springy. Further differentiation may be obtained by combining flexion and extension with abduction and adduction (valgus/varus) stresses, and by assessing gliding motions of the individual component joints of the elbow complex. The capsular pattern is of flexion more limited than extension, and rotations relatively free.

The inferior radio-ulnar joint is stressed by pronation and supination, and may require further examination if pain is produced. Screening examinations of the neck and shoulder are performed if referred pain is suspected, and full neurological examination may be required. The front of the elbow lies within the C5 and C6 dermatomes, while the back of the elbow is in the C7 dermatome. Pain may therefore be referred to the elbow from the cervical nerve roots or the shoulder region.

The contractile structures are examined by resisted movements, performed firstly with the elbow flexed to 90°. One of the therapist's hands supports the elbow to restrict shoulder movement and the other applies resistance to flexion and extension. For pronation and supination, the lower forearm (not the hand) is gripped. The grip must be tight and positioned over the radial styloid to avoid a friction burn to the patient's skin. Resisted wrist flexion and extension are performed with the elbow locked.

Lateral pain

The term tennis elbow is often used colloquially as a blanket description for any soft tissue pain between the shoulder and wrist, and there has been little agreement in the past as to the exact site of the lesion. The condition was first documented in the late 1800s when it was described as 'lawn tennis arm'. Cyriax (1936) described 26 different lesions to which the condition had been attributed, while Lee (1986) cited 12 more general causes as shown in Table 20.2. The terms lateral and medial tennis elbow have been used (Nirschl, 1986), but in this book the name tennis elbow is used to describe lateral epicondylitis while 'golfer's elbow' refers to medial epicondylitis. The ratio of lateral to medial epicondylitis encountered

Table 20.2   General causes of tennis elbow

Radio-humeral bursitis
Periostitis of the common extensor tendon
Tendinitis: extensor carpi radialis brevis, supinator
Microtendinous tears of the common extensor tendon with sub-tendinous granulation and fibrosis
Myofasciitis
Radial head fibrillation/chondromalacia
Calcification
Radial nerve entrapment and subsequent fibrosis
Stenosis of the orbicular ligament
Hyperaemic synovial fringe
Inflammation of the annular ligament
Cervical radiculopathy

From Lee (1986).

clinically has been shown to be 7:1 (Leach and Miller, 1987).

Tennis elbow is a lesion to the common extensor origin (CEO), with the primary site being the tendon of extensor carpi radialis brevis. Less frequently, the extensor carpi radialis longus is affected at its attachment to the supracondylar ridge, and in some cases the anterior portion of the extensor digitorum. Most commonly, the injury is at the tenoperiosteal junction but scar tissue may form onto the tendon itself, or the musculotendinous junction. Repeated activity causes microtrauma, with subsequent granulation tissue formation on the underside of the tendon unit and at the tenoperiosteal junction. The granulation tissue formed appears to contain large numbers of free nerve endings, hence the pain of the condition. The major problem is that the granulation tissue does not progress quickly to a mature form, and so healing fails to take place, almost a type of tendinous 'non-union' (Goldie, 1964; Bernhang, 1977).

Clinical presentation

Tennis elbow usually presents as pain over the region of the lateral epicondyle, extending distally. The pain may build up slowly (overuse) or be the result of a single incident (trauma). Pain is usually increased with resisted wrist extension. Depending on the site of the lesion, pain can be made worse by adding forearm supination (but see radial tunnel syndrome below), and radial deviation of the wrist (Halle, Franklin and Karalfa, 1986). Performing resisted wrist extension with the elbow fully extended will usually elicit pain even in mild cases.

The condition is most common with athletes over 30 years of age, and occurs normally when repeated wrist extension is combined with forearm supination. Racquet sports involve this action, but several occupational stresses can also be causal factors. Hammering, painting and using heavy spanners will all exacerbate the problem, so any training modification which is prescribed must also take into account an athlete's job. Pain usually increases when small objects are gripped, as this hand position places additional stretch on the forearm extensors.

As with most overuse syndromes, the ache may initially subside when the stressful activity is discontinued, but as the condition progresses, pain even occurs at rest. Patients complain of a weak grip, and wasting of the affected muscles may be seen in long-standing cases. Close inspection will often reveal slight swelling over the affected area, but this is rarely obvious to the patient.

Treatment

Treatment aims initially to reduce pain and swelling. The RICE protocol is used, and several authors have reported good results by using ultrasound, alone or with hydrocortisone gel (Griffen and Touchstone, 1963; Klienkort and Wood, 1975; Halle, Franklin and Karalfa, 1986). Reducing the stress applied to the tendon is important. Rest from exacerbating activities, and the use of counterforce bracing is effective. The counterforce brace consists of a tight strap which is placed around the upper forearm, to create a lateral pressure when an object is gripped. The aim is to redirect and disperse overload to healthy tissue or to the band itself, and in so doing reduce painful inhibition and permit a more forceful contraction. Using this technique, grip strength has been shown to improve (Burton, 1985; Wadsworth et al., 1989), and a positive effect has been shown using biomechanical analysis and technique correction of tennis serves and backhand strokes (Groppel and Nirschl, 1986).

As the local swelling adheres and shrinks, inelastic scar tissue is formed. Stretching exercises are therefore of particular value. A useful forearm extensor stretch may be performed with the athlete facing a wall (Fig. 20.4a). The dorsum of the hand is placed flat onto the wall, and the elbow remains

Figure 20.4 Exercise therapy for tennis elbow. (a) Forearm extensor stretch against wall. (b) Combined flexion-pronation of wrist. (c) Resisted forearm extension (dumb-bell). (d) Resisted extension (band).

locked. By leaning forwards the wrist is forced into 90° flexion, stretching the posterior forearm tissues. Wrist flexion may be combined with a pronation stretch (Fig. 20.4b). Keeping the elbow locked, the forearm is maximally pronated and the wrist flexed. Overpressure is applied with the other hand and a static stretch performed. The scar tissue is more pliable when warm and so the athlete is advised to practise stretching after a hot bath or shower.

Resistance exercises (weight or powerband) are used to re-strengthen the forearm extensors. Wrist extension may be performed holding a small (2 kg) dumb-bell. The forearm is supported on a block or over the couch side and full range movement is attempted (Fig. 20.4c). Powerband extension is performed with the athlete sitting. One end of the band is placed beneath the foot and the other end gripped. The forearm is supported along the athlete's thigh (Fig. 20.4c). Initially, eccentric contractions are likely to be less painful than concentric, and the use of ice massage to produce a temporary anaesthesia before exercise is applied (cryokinetics) is often used.

One word of caution, negative transfer effects (see p. 116), have been described by Nirschl (1988) when using high weight low repetition training following tennis elbow. To avoid this they recommended the use of high speed skill training as part of the total rehabilitation programme.

Manual therapy, including local massage to reduce swelling and produce hyperaemia, and transverse frictions to form a mobile scar, are both of use. It is important to locate the exact site of injury for transverse frictions to be effective. The forearm should be pronated

and supinated while the area is palpated to find the exact site of the CEO. The lateral epicondyle should be identified as should the supracondylar ridge, and each considered as a possible source of pain. The teno-osseous junction is best frictioned with the forearm in mid-position to let the CEO relax slightly and allow the palpating finger to get right on to the bony surface. The tendon itself is treated on stretch with the elbow and wrist flexed, and forearm pronated (Fig. 20.5a).

Mills manipulation (Mills, 1928), although originally designed to stress the annular ligament, can be performed to stretch the CEO. The patient's arm is held in extension at the shoulder, with the elbow comfortably flexed, and wrist and forearm fully flexed and pronated (Fig. 20.5b). A high velocity low ampli-

Figure 20.5 Manual therapy for tennis elbow. (a) Deep transverse friction to the common extensor origin. (b) Mills manipulation. (c) Mobilization with movement using belt.

tude thrust is applied to the elbow to fully extend it. Cyriax and Cyriax (1983) claimed this procedure would pull apart the tissue surfaces joined by a painful scar, the fresh tear being replaced by new fibrous tissue under no tension.

Mobilization with movement has been shown to be an effective treatment for this condition (Vicenzino and Wright, 1995). In this technique, a sustained mobilization is applied to a joint, normally at 90° to the plane of movement, to correct joint tracking (Mulligan, 1989). The mobilization is applied at the same time as the patient performs a painful action with the affected joint. In the case of tennis elbow, this action is normally extension of the wrist or fingers (especially the third finger).

With the patient in a supine position, the therapist wraps a belt around his or her hips and the athlete's forearm. The proximal edge of the belt is level with the elbow joint. The humerus and forearm are stabilized by the therapist's hands. The mobilization (lateral glide of the ulna) is carried out by the therapist gently leaning back (Fig. 20.5c). The aim is to reduce the pain of the finger extension action, initially while the mobilization is applied and eventually during free movement.

Biomechanics

The extensor carpi radialis brevis is under maximum tension when it contracts in a position of forearm pronation, wrist flexion and ulna deviation (Briggs and Elliott, 1985). This is a typical position for a backhand shot in racquet sports, and elements of this anatomical alignment are seen in many repetitive actions in sport. Repeated practice will cause hypertrophy of this muscle and often a resultant loss of flexibility. In addition, an imbalance frequently exists between the forearm flexors and extensors. Normally, the wrist extensors should be at least 50% of the flexors, but in many recreational sports an individual may have considerably weaker wrist extensors in proportion to flexors. The combination of weaker and less flexible wrist extensors, placed in a demanding situation of the backhand stroke (or similar occupational action), exceeds the adaptability of the tissues. One action an athlete may take as part of a preventive programme for this condition, therefore, is to maintain the flexibility of the wrist musculature, and build up the strength of the wrist extensors to as much as 75% of the flexor strength (Reid, 1992).

Ergonomics plays an important part in the management of this condition. Enlarging the grip of any object being held, be it a racquet or a spanner, is important in most cases. The correct grip size can be calculated by measuring from the tip of the ring finger to the bottom lateral crease of the palm, directly below (Fig. 20.6). The figure obtained represents the circumference of the racquet handle. Placing a thick piece of sponge around a handle is also useful to enlarge the grip and reduce shock travelling from the handle to the hand. In some cases a grip which is too large may also be a problem, so to assess if grip size is a relevant feature, ask the patient to grip a thin object (a pencil) and a large one

Figure 20.6 Hand size measurement to determine proper grip handle size. The distance from the proximal palmar crease to the tip of the middle finger determines the proper size. From Nirschl (1988), with permission.

(a bottle) and find which gives less pain. In general terms, when prolonged grip is applied, the therapist should be able to place one finger between the tips of the athlete's fingers and thumb.

In tennis, higher impact and torsion forces are produced by a wet, heavy, ball or a racquet which is too tightly strung. The closer the ball is to the centre of percussion (the mathematical point on the racquet face where no torsion will occur on impact) the less strain on the elbow tissues.

Oversize racquets, by increasing the likelihood of keeping the ball away from the frame may reduce torsion and in turn overload stress on the elbow. In addition, leverage forces may be reduced in these racquets by moving the centre of percussion closer to the racquet handle (Nirschl, 1988). A heavier racquet will have more momentum, and will place a greater strain on the forearm. Nirschl (1988) recommended a mid-sized (90–100 square inch) graphite composite light-weight racquet to give the best protection, and Bullard (1982) recommended fibreglass or graphite as the best materials to absorb vibration.

Osteochondrosis

The most common site for osteochondrosis in the elbow is the anterolateral surface of the capitulum (Panner's disease). The aetiology is generally either traumatic or vascular, although some familial tendency may be present. The condition is most commonly related to throwing or racquet sports. In throwing, the angular velocity experienced at the joint may exceed $300°/s$ (Jobe and Nuber, 1986). This, coupled with a valgus force and an extension stress, causes the radial head to impinge against the capitulum. Ultimately, a breakdown can occur in the capitulum surface and the radial head may hypertrophy.

The vascular supply to the area can be disrupted by this repeated trauma. Up until the age of 5 years the capitulum has a good blood supply, but later the nucleus of the capitulum receives only one or two vessels. These pass into the area posteriorly through soft, compressible cartilage—a possible site of damage.

The typical patient is an athlete in early adolescence (usually male) who shows limitation of elbow extension with local swelling. Onset is often insidious and the patient may report that he or she has been experiencing difficulties over a protracted period. If the osteochondrotic fragment is free within the joint, locking or catching may be experienced with certain movements. Radiographs may show blunting of the capitulum with enlargement of the radial head. Often an island of bone is seen surrounded by an area of rarefaction. Premature epiphyseal closure may also be noted to either the humerus or proximal radius.

In the initial stages of the condition with a young athlete, rest is all that is required, splinting being indicated if the patient fails to heed this advice. If stress has been allowed to continue and bony degeneration has occurred, drilling or grafting of the attached fragment may be required. In late stage conditions loose bodies may need to be removed, and unfortunately the prognosis is sometimes poor.

Medial pain

Lesions to the medial side of the joint occur most often with throwing actions. Although different sports demand different throwing techniques, similarities still exist (p. 405). Initially, the shoulder is abducted and taken into extreme external rotation and extension, while the elbow remains flexed (cocking phase). Then, the shoulder and trunk rapidly move forward leaving the arm behind (acceleration phase). This action imposes a valgus stress on the joint and stretches the ulnar collateral ligament in particular. The shoulder flexors and internal rotators contract powerfully, flinging the arm forward resulting in stress to the olecranon as the arm extends rapidly to full range (deceleration phase and follow through).

The throwing action imposes a number of stresses on the elbow (Fig. 20.7). The lateral joint line is subjected to compression forces, in the olecranon fossa there are shearing forces, while the medial joint line experiences tensile forces (Jobe and Nuber, 1986). These forces, if repeated, can give rise to specific injuries and general degeneration reflecting the stress imposed on the elbow structures (Table 20.3).

Medial epicondylitis

This is a lesion of the common flexor origin (CFO) on the medial epicondyle, and is commonly called golfer's elbow. The primary site is the origin of pronator teres and flexor carpi radialis on the medial epicondyle. The flexor carpi ulnaris may occasionally be affected. Golfer's elbow is less common than tennis elbow, occurring at a ratio of about 1:15 (Coorad and Hooper, 1973). The injury can be complicated by ulnar nerve involvement, the nerve being compressed at a point distal to the medial epicondyle. Sensory symptoms are often present and Tinel's sign (tapping the

Table 20.3   Throwing injuries to the elbow

Medial tension
Muscular overuse
Ligamentous injury
Capsular injury
Ulnar traction spur
Medial epicondylitis

Lateral compression
Osteochondrosis
Fractured capitulum
Lateral epicondylitis

Posterior shear
Muscular strain
Impingement
Olecranon fracture
Bony hypertrophy
Loose bodies

ulnar nerve at the elbow to produce pain or tingling in the ulnar portion of the hand) is positive (Nirschl, 1986). Chronic conditions may see calcium deposits developing within the tendon itself (Leach and Miller, 1987).

Pain is felt more locally than with tennis elbow, and is increased on resisted wrist flexion and sometimes forearm pronation. The condition may be differentiated from chronic medial ligament sprain by applying the valgus stress test which should not give pain or laxity in epicondylitis.

The treatment is for the most part like that for tennis elbow, including soft tissue manipulation and biomechanical changes. Transverse frictions are now performed with the elbow and wrist in extension, with the forearm supinated. Counterforce bracing is again used, but this time the brace extends up to the medial epicondyle to avoid interfering with elbow flexion.

Figure 20.7   Forces on the elbow during throwing. 1. Hypertension—olecranon shear. 2. Valgus—compresses laterally, radial head damage. 3. Valgus—distracts medially, collateral ligament damage.

Medial collateral ligament (Thrower's elbow)

Repetitive stresses to this ligament are common in throwing athletes, particularly in events such as the javelin. Pain is generally quite localized over the medial joint line, and exacerbated by applying an elbow abduction stress test, forcing a valgus strain on the joint in 20° flexion. With severe injuries, gapping of the joint may be apparent.

Initial treatment is to remove the causal stress and rest from throwing. Operative repair of a ruptured medial collateral ligament is often recommended for athletes and those involved in heavy manual labour. The theory is that instability may produce problems later in life. However, Kuroda and Sakamaki (1986) reported surgical repair in ten patients and conservative management in three others. Before surgery valgus instability averaged 14.9°. Those treated surgically later showed average laxity of 5.1° while those managed conservatively had average values of 8.0°. With figures for instability which are so similar, it may be questionable whether surgery offers substantial advantage over conservative management in many cases.

Posterior elbow pain

Pain at the back of the elbow is common in sports which rapidly extend or hyperextend the joint. These include the throwing sports, punching in martial arts, and pressing actions in weight training. Structures involved, either individually or in combination, include the insertion of the triceps, the olecranon bursa, and the olecranon itself.

Olecranon bursitis

The olecranon bursa is placed at the bony point of the elbow, over the olecranon process subcutaneously. A deeper bursa is sometimes present between the capsule and triceps. When the elbow is extended, the margins of the olecranon bursa cause a circular ridge of skin about 1.5–2 cm in diameter to be pulled up on the posterior aspect of the elbow.

The bursa can become inflamed by leaning on the elbow for a prolonged period (student's elbow), or from a direct fall onto the point of the elbow. This latter case may induce haemorrhage into the bursal sac itself. Examination of the joint reveals no abnormality, but pain and thickening occur to direct palpation over the bursa. Treatment is to remove the cause, pad the point of the elbow, and aspirate the fluid.

Triceps insertion

Triceps tendinitis may occur in throwing athletes (especially javelin) and weight-lifters. Inflammation and microtrauma are usually limited to the olecranon insertion of the muscle. Damage is usually to the musculotendinous or teno-osseous junctions, and cessation of activity and correction of technique, coupled with modalities to reduce local inflammation and pain are usually curative. Unusually, the medial head of the triceps may sublux over the medial epicondyle during flexion causing a snapping sensation ('snapping elbow syndrome', Dreyfuss and Kessler, 1978). This must be distinguished from subluxation of the ulnar nerve from its groove, which is common in 16% of the population (Reid, 1992). This is normally due to laxity of the ulnar collateral ligament and/ or a shallow ulnar groove.

Rupture of the triceps tendon, either partial or complete, is unusual, and the muscle belly itself is even less frequently injured. When rupture does occur, there is usually a palpable defect in the musculotendinous junction of the muscle, with scarring in the chronic injury. Active extension is lost, and a large haematoma, later developing into bruising, is noted locally. The majority of patients are in their 30s or 40s, and the injury almost always occurs either following a fall onto the outstretched hand or a 'chopping' action. In either case, the stress is one of deceleration imposed on an already contracting muscle.

A small fragment of the olecranon may be avulsed and show up on a lateral radiograph of the elbow, and occasionally radial head fractures are associated with the condition. Conservative management is reserved for partial ruptures (Bach, Warren and Wickiewicz, 1987) distinguished by an ability to partially extend the arm against gravity. Surgical management for avulsion injuries involves drilling the olecranon and suturing the muscle. Post-operatively, the patient is immobilized for 3–4 weeks in a cast or splint at 30°–45° elbow flexion.

Posterior impingement

Posterior impingement of the olecranon into its fossa is common in sports where the elbow is 'snapped back'. This is especially the case with rapid weight (circuit) training, and martial arts, where athletes 'punch the air' while performing forms. Throwing events will tend to cause impingement of the medial aspect of the olecranon on the follow through movement.

Examination usually reveals point tenderness over the posterior or posteromedial aspect of the olecranon. This is made worse by forced extension, and extension/abduction. Chronic injuries may show osteophyte formation posteromedially. Cortical thickening is also usually seen on radiograph, but this is thought to represent adaptation of the bone to repetitive stress (Garrick and Webb, 1990).

Treatment is initially to limit extension and valgus stress by strapping, or if this fails, to rest the elbow completely. The elbow flexors are strengthened (especially eccentrically) to enhance their action as decelerators of elbow extension, and to shorten them and therefore limit hyperextension.

Stress fracture of the olecranon is a rare but often overlooked outcome of posterior impingement, and has been described in javelin throwers (Hulkko, Orava and Nikula, 1968) and baseball pitchers (Nuber and Diment, 1992). Pain usually follows the pattern typical of a stress fracture (p. 294) eventually limiting performance. Many lesions will respond to rest and splinting, but some require surgery including excision of the olecranon tip and inlaid bone block graft (Torg, 1993).

Muscular injury

The biceps, triceps, and brachialis may all be injured in sport. The most common injury for the biceps is to its long head (see p. 420), but its lower insertion may also be injured occasionally. Pain is reproduced to resisted elbow flexion and supination, and passive pronation, resisted shoulder flexion may also be added. If resisted flexion is painful but supination is not, the brachialis is indicated. The site of pain is the centre of the front of the arm, often radiating as far as the wrist in severe cases.

The usual site for injury to the triceps is the musculotendinous junction, but the belly may be injured. Pain on resisted elbow (and shoulder) extension is the clinical sign, but when this test gives pain in the upper arm felt nearer to the shoulder, referred pain from impingement of a shoulder structure should be considered. In this case the triceps contraction pulls the humerus up into the acromion approximating the joint.

Myositis ossificans traumatica

Injury to the brachialis should always be treated with caution, because this muscle shares with the quadriceps the potential for myositis development (see p. 53).

The history is usually that of a direct blow, for example from a knee or head in rugby or a foot in martial arts. Most commonly, a second blow has been experienced to the same area. The typical findings are tenderness persisting for 2–3 weeks after injury, and difficulty in regaining full range motion. On examination, a fibrous mass is often palpable within the muscle over the anterior aspect of the arm. Where these findings are present, X-ray is required. Often heterotrophic bone formation is seen, showing a diffuse fluffy callous. As the callus matures it will shrink and its margins become better defined. Bone scan will reveal whether the condition is still active.

Management aims initially to minimize the damage. Local swelling is reduced where possible, and activity limited. Mobility exercise is begun with caution when radiographic evidence shows that the condition is no longer active. Resisted work is the last exercise to be started, and when sport is resumed, the area is protected with padding.

Elbow dislocations

Posterior or posterolateral dislocation of the elbow is seen following a fall onto the outstretched arm, sometimes associated with a fracture to the olecranon or coronoid process. This is common when falling from a horse or bicycle, and from gymnastic accidents. Rollerskating and skateboarding are also prime causes, as the athlete usually falls backwards onto an abducted straight arm. There is often a snap or crack at the time of injury with immediate swelling. On examination, the arm is held flexed, and a gross deformity is apparent on the posterior aspect of the elbow. The normal triangular alignment of the olecranon and two epicondyles is lost. Radiographic examination is required to assess bony damage, and on no account should reduction on the field be attempted because of the risk of neural complications. Reduction is achieved by downward pressure on the forearm initially to disengage the coronoid from the olecranon fossa and then the forearm is brought forwards. As with the shoulder, reduction, unless immediate, will usually require analgesia. Operative intervention has often been recommended where reduction is unstable due to ligament

avulsion. However, Josefsson et al. (1987) compared the results of patients treated by primary surgical repair to those treated by closed reduction. Although the surgery group included those with complete collateral ligament ruptures or avulsions (all patients) and muscle origin tears from the humeral epicondyles (half the patients) the results from the two groups were the same.

If the arm is immobilized for more than a week, the resting position should be in as much extension as possible (Garrick and Webb, 1990). This is important because reduced flexion is far easier to regain during rehabilitation than is extension. With an uncomplicated injury, gentle isometric exercise is begun as pain and swelling settles. After 2–3 days, active mobility exercise is started with caution in the pain-free range, the athlete remaining in a sling between exercise periods for protection.

Early mobilization of this injury is essential. Mehlhoff et al. (1988) described 52 adults with elbow dislocation. Those immobilized for less than 18 days showed significantly better results than those inactive for longer periods, and patients immobilized for more than 4 weeks all showed only fair or poor results. None of the patients redislocated.

Following this injury, there is normally a slight loss of extension. If the elbow had previously hyperextended, this is not usually a problem. However, where the arm remains slightly flexed, weight-bearing activities, such as handstands and cartwheels will tend to push the arm into flexion. To stabilize the arm and obtain some degree of functional locking, the triceps must be built up extensively.

Radial head

Compression fracture of the radial head may occur with a vertical fall onto the outstretched arm, but more commonly the injury which affects the radial head is a dislocation. This is usually seen in children, where the radial head is pulled through the annular ligament, limiting extension. The peak incidence of injury occurs between the ages of 2 and 3 years, this being the age when the annular ligament is thinner and more easily disrupted. The injury is twice as common in girls as in boys (Quan and Marcuse, 1985), and the left elbow is affected more often than the right (Corrigan and Maitland, 1994). The mechanism of injury is a sudden traction applied to an extended and pronated arm as an adult lifts the child while gripping his or her hand.

Reduction, if carried out before muscle spasm sets in, may be performed by holding the elbow flexed to 90° and lightly rotating the forearm. The therapist holds the child's elbow in his or her cupped hand and places the thumb over the radial head. The other hand holds the child's hand, and the manipulation is produced with a high velocity supination of the patient's forearm while maintaining thumb pressure over the radial head. At the same time, the radius and humerus are gently pulled together and the radial head is felt to click back beneath the annular ligament on full supination. Often this condition reduces spontaneously.

Nerve involvement

Ulnar nerve

The ulnar nerve may be involved with medial collateral ligament injuries of the elbow, as outlined above. Friction against this nerve or its sheath may give rise to symptoms, described by Wadsworth and Williams (1973) as the cubital tunnel syndrome.

Since the sensory fibres of the ulnar nerve are more superficial than the motor fibres, sensory symptoms are more prevalent, with paraesthesia occurring in the fourth and fifth fingers.

The nerve passes through the groove behind the medial epicondyle and is covered by a fibrous sheath, forming the cubital tunnel (Fig. 20.8). The roof of the tunnel is the aponeurosis of the two heads of flexor carpi ulnaris. This is taut at 90° flexion, constricting the tunnel, and slack on extension. The floor of the cubital tunnel is formed from the tip of the trochlea and the medial collateral ligament. The ligament bulges with elbow flexion, an additional factor leading to nerve compression, especially with prolonged periods of end range flexion.

Dislocation of the nerve from the ulnar groove can also occur following fracture and is accompanied by a persistent tingling sensation with certain elbow actions. If motor symptoms are present, wasting may be seen in the hypothenar eminence and the first dorsal interosseous space. Tinel's sign (see pp. 292 and 461) and the elbow flexion test may be positive. This latter test involves maximal flexion of the elbow for 5 minutes to compress the cubital tunnel. Symptoms produced, including pain, altered sensation and numbness constitute a positive test.

Management depends very much on the severity of the symptoms. Often rest, and elbow padding to avoid irritation in contact sports may be all that is required for frictional neuritis. Corticosteroid injection along the cubital tunnel may be useful

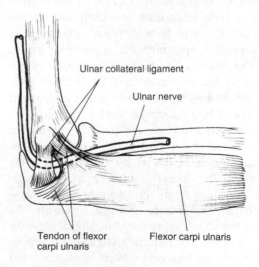

Ulnar collateral ligament

Ulnar nerve

Tendon of flexor carpi ulnaris

Flexor carpi ulnaris

Figure 20.8 The cubital tunnel.

(Corrigan and Maitland, 1994). Surgery, if performed early, can be successful. Nerve transposition combined with excision of a portion of the medial epicondyle and division of the tendinous origin of the flexor carpi ulnaris has been described (Hirsch and Thanki, 1985).

Radial nerve

The radial nerve can be injured in the elbow region. The nerve travels in front of the lateral condyle of the humerus to divide into deep (posterior interosseous) and superficial branches. The superficial branch may be exposed to direct trauma, sometimes being damaged as a complication of fractures to the radial head or neck.

Radial tunnel syndrome (Roles and Maudsley, 1972) occurs when the deep branch of the radial nerve is compressed as it passes under the origin of the extensor carpi radialis brevis and along the fibrous edge of the supinator muscle (arcade of Frohse). Pain is produced when the arm is fully pronated with the wrist flexed.

Differential diagnosis of radial tunnel syndrome is made by eliciting pain by palpation of the radial head, and pain on resisted supination. True tennis elbow will give pain over the lateral epicondyle (not the radial head), with pain on resisted wrist extension but not supination alone (Lee, 1986). The condition is seen following repeated contraction of the wrist extensors and forearm supinators against resistance, as in racquet sports in a novice sportsperson (Cailliet, 1983).

Treatment by local injection and surgery have both been described (Moss and Switzer, 1983).

Testing the elbow following injury

A sportsperson must be able to perform actions relevant to his or her sport and to his or her competitive role within that sport (Wright, 1981). Maximal functional work of the biceps may be performed by the subject chinning a bar, and for the triceps, dipping between two chairs, or performing a push-up with the feet on a chair, both of these actions should be slow and controlled until confidence is built. Faster, more demanding actions include press-ups with a clap in between each repetition, and walking hand to hand while hanging at arms length from a horizontal ladder.

Racquet sportspeople should mimic their stroke action with a weighted racquet or heavy club, and can assess their resilience to jarring strains by hitting a club or bat against a firm surface (a medicine ball is ideal). The elbow must be able to take repeated traction and approximation strains, and be pain-free when the arm is locked while holding a weight at arms length.

References

Bach, B.R., Warren, R.F. and Wickiewicz, T.L. (1987) Triceps rupture. A case report and literature review. *American Journal of Sports Medicine*, **15**(3), 285–289

Bernhang, A.M. (1979) The many causes of tennis elbow. *New York State Journal of Medicine*, 1363–1366

Briggs, C.A. and Elliott, B.G. (1985) Lateral epicondylitis: a review of structures associated with tennis elbow. *Anat Clin*, **7**, 149

Bullard, J.A.A (1982) Tennis elbow. *Canadian Family Physician*, **28**, 961-963

Burton, A.K. (1985) Grip strength and forearm straps in tennis elbow. *British Journal of Sports Medicine*, **19**, 37–38

Cailliet, R. (1983) *Soft Tissue Pain and Disability*, F.A. Davis, Philadelphia

Coorad, R.W. and Hooper, W.R., (1973) Tennis elbow: course, natural history, conservative and surgical management. *Journal of Bone and Joint Surgery*, **55A**, 1177

Corrigan, B. and Maitland, G.D. (1994) *Musculoskeletal and Sports Injuries*, Butterworth-Heinemann, Oxford

Cyriax, J. (1936) Pathology and treatment of tennis elbow. *Journal of Bone and Joint Surgery*, **18A**, 921

Cyriax, J.H. and Cyriax, P.J. (1983) *Illustrated Manual of Orthopaedic Medicine*, Butterworth, London

Dreyfuss, U. and Kessler, I. (1978) Snapping elbow due to dislocation of the medial head of triceps. *Journal of Bone and Joint Surgery*, **60B**, 56

Garrick, J.G. and Webb, D.R. (1990) *Sports Injuries: Diagnosis and Management*, W.B. Saunders, Philadelphia

Goldie, I. (1964) Epicondylitis lateralis humeri: a pathological study. *Acta Chirugica Scandinavica* (suppl.), **34**, 339

Griffen, J.E. and Touchstone J.C., (1963) Ultrasonic movement of cortisol into pig tissues. (I). Movement into skeletal muscle. *American Journal of Physical Medicine*, **43**, 77

Groppel, J.L. and Nirschl, R.P. (1986) A mechanical and electromyographical analysis of the effects of various joint counterforce braces on the tennis player. *American Journal of Sports Medicine*, **14**, 195–200

Halle, J.S., Franklin, R.J. and Karalfa, B.L. (1986) Comparison of four treatment approaches for lateral epicondylitis of the elbow. *Journal of Orthopaedic and Sports Physical Therapy*, **8**(2), 62–69

Hirsch, L.F. and Thanki, A. (1985) Ulnar nerve entrapment at the elbow. Tailoring the treatment to the cause. *Postgraduate Medicine*, **77**, 211–215

Hulkko, A., Orava, S. and Nikula, P. (1968) Stress fractures of the olecranon in javelin throwers. *International Journal of Sports Medicine*, **7**, 210

Jobe, F.W. and Nuber, G. (1986) Throwing injuries of the elbow. *Sports Medicine*, **5**(4), 621–635

Josefsson, P.O., Gentz, C., Johnell, O. and Wendeberg, B. (1987) Surgical versus non-surgical treatment of ligamentous injuries following dislocation of the elbow joint: a prospective randomized study. *Journal of Bone and Joint Surgery*, **69A**, 605–608

Kleinkort, J.B. and Wood, F. (1975) Phonophoresis with 1% versus 10% hydrocortisone. *Physical Therapy*, **55**, 1320

Kuroda, S. and Sakamaki, K. (1986) Ulnar collateral ligament tears of the elbow joint. *Clinical Orthopaedics and Related Research*, **208**, 266–271

Leach, R.E. and Miller, J.K. (1987) Lateral and medial epicondylitis of the elbow. *Clinics in Sports Medicine*, **6**(2), 259–272

Lee, D.G. (1986) Tennis elbow: a manual therapist's perspective. *Journal of Orthopaedic and Sports Physical Therapy*

Mehlhoff, T.L., Noble, P.C., Bennett, J.B. and Tullos, H.S. (1988) Simple dislocation of the elbow in the adult: results after closed treatment. *Journal of Bone and Joint Surgery*, **70A**, 244–249

Mills, G.P. (1928) Treatment of tennis elbow. *British Medical Journal*, **1**, (12)

Morrey, B.F. and Kai-Nan, A. (1983) Articular and ligamentous contributions to the stability of the elbow joint. *American Journal of Sports Medicine*, **11**, 315–318

Moss, S.H. and Switzer, H.E. (1983) Radial tunnel syndrome: a spectrum of clinical presentations. *Journal of Hand Surgery*, **8**, 414–420

Mulligan, B.R. (1989) *Manual Therapy*, Plane View Services, Wellington, New Zealand

Nirschl, R.P. (1986) Soft tissue injuries about the elbow. *Clinics in Sports Medicine*, **5**(4), 637–652

Nirschl, R.P. (1988) Prevention and treatment of elbow and shoulder injuries in the tennis player. *Clinics in Sports Medicine*, **7**(2), 289–309

Norkin, C.C. and Levangie, P.K. (1992) *Joint Structure and Function. A Comprehensive Analysis*, 2nd edn, F.A. Davis, Philadelphia

Nuber, G.W. and Diment, M.T. (1992) Olecranon stress fractures in throwers: a report of two cases and a review of the literature. *Clinical Orthopaedics and Related Research*, **278**, 58–61

Quan, L. and Marcuse, E.K. (1985) The epidemiology and treatment of radial head subluxation. *American Journal of Diseases of Children*, **139**, 1194–1197

Reid, D.C. (1992) Sports injury assessment and rehabilitation. Churchill Livingstone, Edinburgh

Roles, N.C. and Maudsley, R.H. (1972) Radial tunnel syndrome. Resistant tennis elbow as a nerve entrapment. *Journal of Bone and Joint Surgery*, **54B**, 499–508

Torg, J.S. (1993) Comment. *Yearbook of Sports Medicine*, C.V. Mosby, St Louis, pp. 72

Vicenzino, B. and Wright, A. (1995) Effects of a novel manipulative physiotherapy technique on tennis elbow: a single case study. *Manual Therapy*, **1**, 30–35

Wadsworth, C.T., Nielsen, D.H., Burns, L.T., Krull, J.D. and Thompson, C.G. (1989) Effect of the counterforce armband on wrist extension and grip strength and pain in subjects with tennis elbow. *Journal of Orthopaedic and Sports Physical Therapy*, **11**, 192–197

Wadsworth, T.G. and Williams, J.R. (1973) Cubital tunnel external compression syndrome. *British Medical Journal*, **1**, 662

Wright, D. (1981) Fitness testing after injury. In *Sports Fitness and Sports Injuries* (ed. T. Reilly), Faber and Faber, London

21

The wrist and hand

The wrist area has a series of articulations between the distal end of the radius and the carpal bones (radiocarpal joint), and between the individual carpals themselves (intercarpal joints). The radiocarpal joint is formed between the distal end of the radius and the scaphoid, lunate and triquetral. The end of the radius being covered by a concave articular disc. The eight carpal bones are arranged in two rows, the junction between the rows forming the mid-carpal joint. This joint is convex laterally and concave medially, giving it an 'S' shape (Fig. 21.1).

The wrist is strengthened by collateral, palmar and dorsal ligaments. The ulnar collateral ligament is a rounded cord stretching from the ulnar styloid to the triquetral and pisiform. The radial collateral ligament passes from the radial styloid to the scaphoid and then to the trapezium. The dorsal radiocarpal ligament runs from the lower aspect of the radius to the scaphoid, lunate and triquetral. On the palmar surface, the radiocarpal and ulnocarpal ligaments attach from the lower ends of the radius and ulna to the proximal carpal bones (Fig. 21.2).

The available range of movement at the wrist is a combination of radiocarpal and mid-carpal movement. Flexion occurs more at the mid-carpal joint while extension is greater at the radiocarpal joint, but the combined movement is about 85° in each direction. Abduction occurs mostly at the mid-carpal joint and has a range of about 15°, whereas adduction involves more movement of the radiocarpal joint and has a range of 45° (Palastanga, Field and Soames, 1989). The difference in range occurs because the radial styloid comes down further than the ulnar styloid, and so is more limiting to abduction.

The carpal bones form a transverse arch, concave on their palmar aspect (Fig. 21.3). This arch is maintained by the flexor retinaculum, which attaches medially to the pisiform and the hook of hamate. Laterally, the retinaculum binds to the scaphoid tubercle and to the groove of trapezium, through which runs the tendon of flexor carpi radialis. The space formed beneath the retinaculum is called the 'carpal tunnel', and the tendons of flexor pollicis longus, flexor digitorum profundus, flexor digitorum superficialis and the median nerve pass through it.

On the posterior aspect of the wrist the extensor retinaculum stretches from the radius to the hamate and pisiform bones and extends inferiorly to form six longitudinal compartments for the passage of the extensor tendons.

Grip

Prehension is an advanced skill in humans, resulting largely from the ability of the thumb to oppose the fingers. Two types of

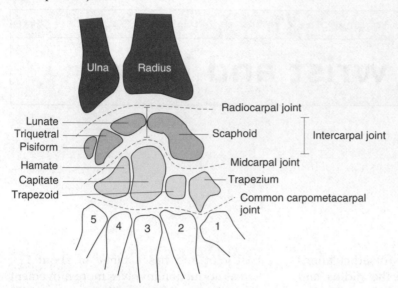

Figure 21.1   The joints of the wrist.

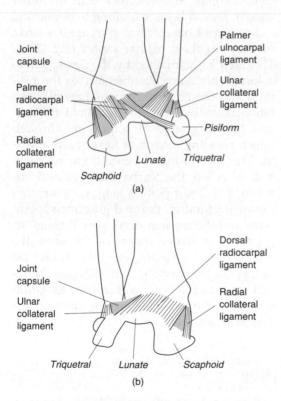

Figure 21.2   The capsular and collateral ligaments of the radiocarpal joint. (a) Anterior. (b) Posterior. After Palastanga et al. (1994).

Figure 21.3   Transverse arch of the wrist.

grip may be described, 'precision' involving the thumb and fingers and 'power', involving the whole hand.

With precision grip, the object is usually small and light. The grip is applied with the nails or fingertips (terminal opposition), pads of the fingers (subterminal opposition), or the pad and side of another finger (subterminal-lateralopposition). This action involves rotation of both the carpometacarpal joints of the thumb and fingers involved in the gripping action. The small finger muscles work in combination with the flexor digitorum profundus and superficialis as well as the flexor pollicis longus.

In power grips the long flexors and extensors work to lock the wrist and grip the object. In the palmar grip, the whole hand surrounds the object, and the thumb works against the fingers. The shape taken up by the hand is largely determined by the size of the object, but the grip is strongest when the thumb can still touch the index finger. This is the type of grip used when holding a racquet or javelin. When the fingers are closed firmly, the fourth and fifth metacarpals move over the hamate bone to further tighten the grip and prevent a smooth object from slipping out of the hand. The hook grip is used when lifting something with a handle, such as a suitcase. Now, the object is held between the flexed fingers and palm, the thumb not being used. Although the grip is quite powerful, the power is in one direction only.

Screening examination

Initial examination of the wrist utilizes a number of movements to cover all the joints involved in wrist articulation. The superior and inferior radioulnar joints are stressed by passive pronation and supination. The wrist itself is assessed by flexion, extension, abduction and adduction performed both passively and against resistance. At the same time as the wrist is examined, the fingers are also assessed as the two areas are intimately linked. Passive and resisted movements are performed at the thumb and finger joints. Again, flexion, extension, abduction and adduction are used. The capsular pattern for the wrist joint is an equal limitation to passive flexion and extension. Painful resisted movement at the wrist indicates that the lesion is not local, but higher up in the muscle bellies, whereas pain to resisted finger movements may give local pain. In

addition to pain, crepitus to active movements is an important sign for the long finger tendons.

This examination, described by Cyriax (1982), provides the examiner with enough information to establish whether a lesion is intracapsular or not, and whether contractile tissue is affected. For the physiotherapist, further assessment is usually required to assess and record range of motion and accessory movements. Movements of the individual carpel bones gives more detail about the exact site of the lesion, and the sequence for testing is shown in Table 21.1. In addition, specific tests are used once the initial examination has focused the therapist's attention onto a specific area or series of tissues.

Table 21.1   Assessing motion of individual carpal joints

Movements around the capitate
Fixate capitate and move:
1 trapezoid
2 scaphoid
3 lunate
Fixate capitate and move:
4 Hamate
Movements on the radial side
Fixate scaphoid and move:
5 the two trapezii
Movements of the radiocarpal joint
Fixate radius and move:
6 scaphoid
7 lunate
Fixate ulna (including the disc) and move:
8 triquetrum (triquetral)
Movements on the ulnar side
Fixate triquetrum and move:
9 hamate
10 pisiform (position the patient's hand in palmar flexion)

From Kaltenborn (1989).

Scaphoid fracture

The important feature of this fracture is not the frequency with which it occurs, but the number of times it is missed, with pain so often being put down to 'just a sprain'. The usual history is of a fall onto the outstretched arm with the wrist fully extended. When the hand is locked into extension, the athlete is more likely to sustain a scaphoid fracture, this can occur with a vertical fall from gymnastic apparatus for example. When the hand is more relaxed, and the force has some horizontal component, as with a fall when running, the distal radius will usually break (Colles' fracture). The scaphoid fracture is common in the young athlete while the Colles' fracture is seen more frequently in the elderly. This is partially due to the weakness of the radius with the onset of osteoporosis in the aged.

A further cause of injury to the scaphoid is striking an object with the heel of the hand, a mechanism seen in contact sports, such as the martial arts or in a collision with another player. In addition, scaphoid fracture can be seen as a punching injury. Horii (1994) described a series of 125 patients with fractured scaphoid, 14% of whom had acquired the injury through punching. Normally it is a bending force within the scaphoid which creates the fracture line when falling onto the outstretched hand. With a punching scaphoid fracture however, stress force creates the fracture making displacement and delayed union more likely.

The major symptom of scaphoid fracture is one of well-localized pain to the base of the thumb, within the 'anatomical snuffbox'. The athlete's hand is pronated and gently stressed into ulnar deviation, as the snuffbox is palpated. In addition, pain is exacerbated by longitudinal compression of the first metacarpal against the scaphoid by pressing the thumb proximally. Radiographic examination is helpful, but a negative X-ray does not rule out fracture (Garrick and Webb, 1990). Non-displaced fractures are often normal to begin with and only become positive when some bone reabsorption has occurred, the fracture line beginning to show up 2–4 weeks after injury.

The blood supply to the scaphoid is confined to its distal pole in 30% of subjects. The fracture, which usually travels transversely through the neck of the bone, can cut off the blood supply to the proximal fragment making non-union or mal-union more likely. Scaphoid fracture requires prolonged immobilization of the wrist and thumb. The cast usually extends to the interphalangeal (IP) joint of the thumb to just below the elbow. In some cases an above elbow splint is used to limit pronation and supination. Uncomplicated fractures of the scaphoid tubercle may heal in as little as 4 weeks, but fracture to the proximal part of the bone may take as much as 20 weeks.

Complications to scaphoid fracture have a poor prognosis. Avascular necrosis may require excision of the avascular fragment, or prosthetic replacement of the whole bone. Non-union usually demands bone graft or screw fixation, but the failure rate can be high. Successful union has however been shown in 90% of patients treated with a Herbert differential pitch screw (which is completely buried in the bone) combined with bone grafting (Bunker, McNamee and Scott, 1987). This type of fixation significantly reduces the time to return to active sport. With fixation, return in some athletes is immediate, but on average 4.3 weeks. Athletes treated non-operatively with a playing cast return on average in 11 weeks (Rettig, Weidenbener and Gloyeske, 1994).

Wrist pain

Sprains

A 'sprained wrist' is a common 'diagnosis', but really only indicates the area of pain, and the fact than soft tissue is the likely structure affected. The most common tissues affected are the intercarpal ligaments, with or without subluxation of a carpal bone. Pain is reproduced to passive wrist flexion and is generally well-localized to the particular tissue injured. Common ligaments affected include the lunate-capitate (Cyriax, 1982) and scapho-lunate (Wilkes, 1989). Transverse frictions to the ligament with the wrist flexed is effective, but manipulation to rupture adhesive scarring is not (Cyriax, 1982).

Sprain to the ulnar or radial collateral ligaments is rare, but if present gives pain to end-range passive abduction and adduction.

Carpal dislocation

Subluxation or dislocation of a carpal bone, rather than a scaphoid fracture, may occur from a fall onto the outstretched hand. The bone most commonly affected is the lunate, although the capitate may also sublux (Cyriax and Cyriax, 1983). Movement is generally limited in one direction only (contrast the capsular pattern). Pain is localized by palpating in a line along the third finger to reach the third metacarpal. In the normal hand the capitate lies in a hollow just proximal to the base of the third metacarpal and the lunate is felt proximal to this, and slightly towards the ulna.

When the capitate subluxes, the wrist is held in flexion, and a prominent bump is seen over the dorsum of the wrist as the capitate stands proud of its neighbours. Reduction of a minor subluxation is often spontaneous, but if not, may be achieved during traction by a repeated anterior and posterior glide, with the wrist positioned over the edge of the treatment couch. The wrist is immobilized in a splint until the acute pain subsides, when rehabilitation is begun.

Full dislocation of the lunate may occur with a fall onto the extended wrist. The shape and position of the lunate lying between the lower radius and capitate make it prone to dislocation. On forced wrist extension, the wedged-shaped lunate is squeezed out from between the two bones to lie on the palmar surface of the carpal region (Fig. 21.4) as an apparent 'swelling'. The scaphoid-lunate ligament usually ruptures and the lunate rotates. Radiographs taken with the forearm fully supinated show a separation of the scaphoid-lunate joint of more than 2 mm (Corrigan and Maitland, 1983). The dislocated lunate may impinge on the median nerve, and the flexor tendons may be compressed within the carpal tunnel.

Reduction under anaesthesia is possible if the condition is diagnosed early, with the wrist being immobilized in some degree of flexion initially, and then protected from forced extension when sport is resumed. If left, damage to the median nerve is more likely and open reduction is usually required.

Occasionally, the lunate may stay in place against the radius, and the carpal bones surrounding it dislocate posteriorly to give a perilunar dislocation. This normally occurs

Figure 21.4 Lunate dislocation. (a) The injury occurs when the radius forces the lunate in a palmar direction, resulting in dislocation (b). From Hertling and Kessler (1990), with permission.

in association with a scaphoid fracture, part of the fractured bone remaining with the radius and lunate (O'Donoghue, 1976; Williams and Sperryn, 1976).

Wrist pain in gymnasts

Repetitive forced extension causes compression and impaction forces on the wrist. This type of movement is common in gymnastics, and in exercises such as the 'press-up with clap'. In addition, heavy bench press exercises used in training or powerlifting force extension at the wrist. When this occurs, the athlete may experience pain over the dorsum of the wrist, and end-range flexion and extension are painfully limited. The main fault initially may be an impingement of the dorsal wrist structures, resulting in capsular inflammation (Aronen, 1985). If impact forces continue, however, carpal subluxation or fracture may occur in the adult, and epiphyseal damage in the adolescent.

The distal end of the ulna has a fibrocartilage disc which separates it from the lunate. The disc prevents ulnocarpal abutment by cushioning forces between the ulna and lunate. Trauma may cause thinning of the articular disc, and a reduction in shock-absorbing capacity. Cadaver studies have shown that the radius takes 60% of axial loading to the wrist when the articular disc is intact, but this is increased to 95% when the disc is excised (Palmer and Werner, 1981).

Forced extension is of particular concern in the child. Normally, closure of the distal ulnar growth plate should precede that of the radius. However, the structure and function of the distal radial growth plate can be altered by repetitive loading from gymnastics or other sports, and may fuse prematurely giving radial shortening with respect to the normal ulna (Albanese et al., 1989). On posterior-anterior radiographs, the position of the ulna may be compared to that of the radius. If the ulnar is longer, positive ulnar variance exists, if shorter, negative variance is present. As the radial growth plate closes after that of the ulna, negative ulnar variance is the norm. However, gymnasts have been shown to have significant positive ulnar variance when compared to controls (Mandelbaum et al., 1989).

With positive variance, in addition to bone changes, the articular disc between the ulna and lunate may be thinner, and less stable. The combination of reduced shock absorption and stability may lead to a chronic degenerative condition.

In the adolescent, rest from activities involving extension and loading of the wrist is essential. Carter et al. (1988) have demonstrated significant healing of this condition within 3 months following cessation of gymnastics.

Kienbock's disease

This is an aseptic necrosis (osteochondritis) of the lunate. The condition may result from direct trauma, such as a compression fracture (Cetti, Christensen and Reuther, 1982), or following repeated microtrauma from impact stresses. Industrial stresses, such as hammering, and impact forces in sports, such as tennis, karate, volleyball and golf, have been identified as factors (Nakamura et al., 1991). Although the progress of the condition is similar in both sporting and non-sporting populations, athletes develop symptoms more quickly.

The condition is seen from adolescence up to the mid-30s. The lunate atrophies, becomes sclerosed, and later decalcifies, showing flattening and fragmentation on X-ray. The main symptom is wrist pain, with range of motion and grip strength reducing.

Marked deformity of the bone occurs, unless the condition is identified early enough, when pressure on the wrist during sport should be eliminated. If the condition is too advanced to respond to conservative management, surgery is required. As the patients are young, and remodelling of the lunate can be expected, osteotomy is frequently performed rather than carpectomy (Nakamura et al., 1991).

Wrist mobilization

Mobilization of the various joints of the wrist is useful both for pain reduction and movement enhancement. The inferior radioulnar joint is mobilized by gripping the lower ends of the radius and ulna and working the hands forwards and backwards against each other (Fig. 21.5a). The radiocarpal joint may be mobilized by gripping the athlete's wrist in one hand and his or her hand in the other. The edge of the therapist's hands are aligned with the radiocarpal joint line. Again, the hands are worked against each other to perform transverse mobilizations and antero-posterior movements. Greater purchase may be gained by supporting the athlete's forearm on a low block or on the couch edge (Fig. 21.5b). Pronation and supination at the radiocarpal joint is performed using a 'wringing' action (Fig. 21.5c), and intercarpal movements (see Table 21.1) are performed using the thumb pads (Fig. 21.5d).

Compression neuropathies

Carpal tunnel syndrome

Carpal tunnel syndrome is a compression neuropathy of the median nerve as it passes beneath the transverse carpal ligament. It is more common in women than men, and occurs typically later in life (40–60 years), although it is seen in younger individuals secondary to trauma. Paraesthesia (numbness, burning, tingling) is felt over the first three fingers and the radial half of the fourth. Pain is made worse with repeated movements, and prolonged (1 minute) wrist flexion can reproduce the symptoms (Phalen's test). Percussion of the medial nerve (Tinel's

Figure 21.5 Examples of wrist joint mobilization. From Corrigan and Maitland (1994).

sign) within the centre of the carpal tunnel with the wrist extended may also be positive.

A number of factors may contribute to the condition, and these generally fall into one of two categories. First, factors which increase the size of the structures within the carpal tunnel. This could be through swelling of the flexor tendon sheaths (tenosynovitis) as a result of repeated or sustained flexor activity (gymnasts, cyclists, weight-lifters). Secondly, factors which reduce the size of the carpal tunnel itself, such as arthritic changes secondary to a Colles' fracture, fluid retention during pregnancy, and obesity. The condition must be differentiated from vascular insufficiency which usually gives a glove-like distribution of symptoms, and entrapment of the C6/C7 nerve root, which does not give increased pain to repeated wrist movements.

Management of the condition is initially to rest the wrist in a splint (day and night), as in the neutral position there is less pressure within the carpal tunnel (Hertling and Kessler, 1990). In addition, the flexor retinaculum may be stretched by separating the pisiform and hamate from the trapezium and scaphoid (Maitland, 1991). It is interesting to note that vitamin B6 may facilitate healing in this condition (Diamond, 1989).

Ulnar nerve compression

Ulnar nerve compression (cyclist's palsy) is an unusual condition. The nerve passes into the hand through a shallow trough (canal of Guyan) between the pisiform and the hook of hamate, to emerge and divide into two. During cycling, the nerve is stretched by hyperextension and ulnar deviation of the wrist. Stresses taken by the hand in cycling can be greater than the athlete's body weight (Haloua, Collin and Coudeyre, 1987), and altered conduction velocity of the distal ulnar nerve has been shown in long-distance cyclists (Wilmarth and Nelson, 1988).

Motor and sensory symptoms may be caused, affecting the fourth and fifth fingers. Weakness and clumsiness of fine finger movements may be seen with a reduction in pinch grip strength. The latter is tested by asking the athlete to pinch a piece of paper between the thumb and radial side of the second finger.

Initial management is by ensuring a correct cycle frame size to prevent the athlete overstretching. Extra padding on the handlebars or in cycling gloves will reduce compression stress, but if symptoms persist, the athlete should refrain from cycling for as long as 4 months to allow recovery of motor function.

Thumb

Ulnar collateral ligament rupture

Injury to the ulnar collateral ligament (UCL) of the metacarpophalangeal (MCP) joint of the thumb is common in any sport where the thumb is forced into excessive abduction. This may occur in alpine skiing, where the strap of the ski pole pulls the thumb. It has been estimated that around 10% of all alpine skiing injuries involve this ligament, giving a total of 50 000–200 000 injuries per year (Peterson and Renstrom, 1986). The injury also occurs less commonly in contact sports when the thumb becomes trapped as a player falls.

Chronic insufficiency of the ligament (gamekeeper's thumb) is distinct from complete rupture (skier's thumb). Complete rupture usually occurs from the distal attachment at the base of the proximal phalanx, and in about 30% of cases an avulsion fracture occurs. The UCL lies beneath the adductor pollicis, and with complete rupture the aponeurosis of this muscle may be trapped between the pieces of torn ligament—a so-called 'Stener lesion' (Stener, 1962). When the ligament is completely ruptured, contraction of the adductor pollicis will tend to sublux the joint rather than give true adduction, and so grip is weakened.

Symptoms are reproduced by passive extension and abduction of the thumb, and the pain is usually well-localized to the ulnar side of the joint. A valgus strain to the MCP joint will stretch the ligament and again gives pain. In complete rupture, the end feel of the joint is limp, and a dorsal haematoma may be visible over the thumb interphalangeal joint, indicating that blood has diffused along the extensor pollicis longus (Moutet et al., 1989). Treatment of a grade I injury is initially by rest and ice in the acute phase and then the joint is actively mobilized as pain and swelling settle. Grade II injuries require immobilization for as much as 4 weeks in a strapping or splint to limit abduction, and in severe cases a cast may be required. Complete ligamentous ruptures generally require surgery, and about a quarter may be expected to have displaced bone fragments (Moutet et al., 1989) which will require fixation by Kirschner wires.

Following surgical repair the thumb is immobilized in a cast for 4–6 weeks, and later a full rehabilitation programme is begun.

De Quervain's tenovaginitis

This is an inflammation and thickening of the synovial lining of the common sheath of the abductor pollicis longus and extensor pollicis brevis tendons. The thickening occurs particularly at the point where the tendons pass over the distal aspect of the radius. The history is usually of overuse, and the condition represents a common occupational injury, but is also seen in rock climbers. There is pain to resisted thumb extension and abduction. In addition, pain is caused by passively ulnar deviating the wrist while keeping the thumb fully flexed, a movement which stretches the tendon and sheath. Local tenderness is found to palpation, again with the tendon on stretch. Crepitus is often present to repeated movements. The condition must be differentiated from arthritis of the carpometacarpal joint of the thumb which will not give pain on resisted movements, or tendon stretch, but will give pain in roughly the same area.

De Quervain's tenovaginitis responds well to frictional massage with the tendon on stretch, and immobilization of the thumb in a splint. Corticosteroid injection into the tendon sheath is reserved for persistent cases.

Importantly, the stressor causing this injury must be identified and removed. Often, the type of grip and repetition of movement are the two deciding factors. Experimenting with alternative grip types and size of grip is useful to increase the variety of stress imposed on the affected tissues.

Arthrosis

The capsular pattern at the carpometacarpal joint is a limitation of abduction only. By far the most common intra-articular lesion is osteoarthrosis. The condition is more usual in women and is frequently bilateral, but can also occur secondary to Bennett's fracture. The typical patient seen by the sports physiotherapist is a mature female who plays casual racquet sports. The pain is made worse with increasing frequency of play, particularly with a sustained grip. Pain is well localized to the base of the thumb and must be distinguished from tenovaginitis (see above). Sudden shooting pains may often cause the patient to drop an object in extreme cases, and accessory movements are limited and painful, particularly axial rotations. Pinch grip power is reduced.

Splinting the joint may allow the acute inflammation to subside. Joint mobilization, including longitudinal oscillations, and abduction/adduction while stabilizing the trapezium are effective for pain relief or increasing motion.

Fracture

The base of the first metacarpal is often fractured from a longitudinally applied force, as occurs from a punch in sports such as boxing and karate. Transverse or oblique fracture lines may occur, and if the fracture line affects the joint surface (Bennett's fracture), secondary osteoarthritis may occur in later years. Oblique fractures are often displaced, with the abductor pollicis longus pulling the shaft of the metacarpal proximally (Fig. 21.6). These injuries require manipulation under anaesthetic to reduce them. Maintenance of reduction is by casting the thumb, wrist and forearm, keeping the first metacarpal in extension. Fixation may be required where

Figure 21.6 Bennett's fracture displaced proximally by the pull of the abductor pollicis longus. From Reid (1992).

Figure 21.7 Hyperextension injury of the finger. Hyperextension injury (ball hitting finger) may damage the joint capsule and palmar ligament. Greater force creates a dislocation.

the joint surface is involved to improve the alignment of the bone fragments.

Immobilization is usually for a period of about 3 weeks. Active mobility exercises are begun immediately the cast is removed, as stiffness is a severe impairment to normal hand function.

The fingers

The fingers are commonly injured in sport by being 'pulled back' when hit by a ball or opponent (Fig. 21.7). In addition, sports which place great strain on the fingers themselves, such as rock climbing and certain martial arts techniques may also give problems.

Dislocation

Dislocations of the proximal interphalangeal (PIP) joints, especially that of the fifth finger, are the most commonly seen types. These result from a hyperextension force, with posterior dislocation being more common. Radiographic appearance is of the middle

phalanx overriding the proximal, a condition which is often associated with detachment of the palmar ligament (volar plate) from the base of the middle phalanx. Once reduced, these injuries should be protected in a splint which prevents hyperextension, but allows early flexion.

Where the force is less severe, dislocation may be avoided, but the palmar ligament and joint capsule may still be disrupted. The anterior aspect of the joint is tender to palpation, and the joint is splinted as for a dislocation.

Fracture dislocation can result when an axially directed force is imposed on a semi-flexed finger. The middle phalanx shears and hits onto the condyle of the proximal phalanx, dislodging a bony fragment. When the fragment involves less than one-third of the articular line (Fig. 21.8) the collateral ligament usually remains intact and ensures joint stability. Closed reduction is used, with splinting to prevent the last 15% of extension. Where the joint surface is fragmented the collateral ligament will usually be disrupted, and repeated sub-

Figure 21.8   Dislocations of the proximal interphalangeal joint. (a) Reducible dislocation. (b) Fracture-dislocation involving less than one third of the articular base. (c) Articular fragmentation involving more than one third of the articular base. (d) Anterior (volar) dislocation.

tion. Close examination is needed, and longitudinal traction should be gently applied. The joint may reduce easily, but this should be checked by X-ray (Rimmer, 1981).

Collateral ligament injuries

The MCP and IP joints have loose capsules which are lax in extension. Each joint has obliquely placed collateral ligaments which become increasingly tight with flexion. In addition, the palmar ligaments are fibrocartilage structures attached loosely to the metacarpals but firmly to the bases of the proximal phalanges. Proximally, the palmar ligament thins out to become membranous. During flexion, this thin portion folds like a bellows, but with hyperextension it is stretched and provides the support lacking from the joint capsule (Fig. 21.9). The fibrous flexor sheaths (containing the tendons of

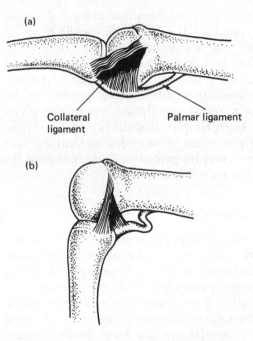

Figure 21.9   Interphalangeal joint of the finger. (a) Extension—collateral ligament lax, palmar ligament tight. (b) Flexion—collateral ligament tight, palmar ligament lax. From Hertling and Kessler (1990), with permission.

luxation is likely to occur. Open reduction with internal fixation is therefore required (Isani, 1990).

It is often tempting to reduce finger dislocations straight away, and this is certainly easier than when muscle spasm has set in. As the joint capsule is intact the procedure is usually quite successful. However, the danger of fracture dislocation or the imposition of soft tissue between the bone ends makes it necessary to err on the side of cauflexor digitorum superficialis and flexor digitorum profundus) in turn attach to the palmar ligaments.

Valgus and varus forces directed against the PIP joints will usually result in partial tearing of the collateral ligaments but leave the joint stable. The injuries respond to strapping to the adjacent finger (buddy splinting) to protect the joint and at the same time facilitate early mobility.

Complete ligamentous disruption may warrant surgical intervention, especially where the radial collateral ligament of the index or little finger is affected, as these are subjected to greater stress in normal gripping activities (Isani, 1990). The ligament normally ruptures at the level of the joint line, possibly with avulsion. After suture repair the finger is maintained in 60° flexion for 3 weeks (Rimmer, 1981).

Muscles

The muscles most commonly injured within the hand are the interossei, usually by overstretching the fingers. Pain is highly localized, and increased to abduction (dorsal interossei) or adduction (plantar interossei). As the muscle fibres travel parallel to the finger, transverse friction massage is given by the therapist placing his or her finger between those of the athlete and using a rotation action by pronating and supinating his or her own forearm.

Tendon injury

Prolonged gripping with the tips of the fingers, such as may occur in rock climbing, can cause injury to the flexor tendons. The distal IP joint is extended, while the proximal IP is flexed, stressing flexor digitorum profundus. Long-term exposure to this type of stress may also damage the flexor sheath, increasing the bowstringing effect to resisted finger flexion (Bollen, 1988).

Hyperflexion may disrupt the extensor tendon, and avulse it from the base of the distal phalanx (mallet finger) or cause the middle section of the tendon to rupture (Boutonniere or 'buttonhole' deformity) (Fig. 21.10). This can occur when the end of the terminal phalanx is struck by a ball for example. When the extensor mechanism is disrupted in this way, the athlete can flex the finger, and while elastic recoil enables the joint to extend slightly, normal extension is impossible. With mallet finger, tenderness occurs at a point between the nail and the distal IP joint, and the fingertip is held slightly flexed when resting. In a buttonhole deformity, tenderness is more proximal, and the finger is hyperextended at the distal interphalangeal joint. Radiographs reveal the avulsed fragment. Treatment is by immobilization in a splint which maintains hyperextension of the distal IP joint, or occasionally surgical intervention.

Inflammation of the extensor tendons (tendonitis), or tendon sheaths (tenosynovitis) may occur with repetitive finger movements. Although more common as an occupational injury (keyboard operators), the condition can occur through excessive training activities. Pain and crepitus occur to repeated movements, with pain localized to the extensor tendon sheaths. Treatment is to remove the stressor and reduce the inflammation with ice and modalities.

Figure 21.10 Results of injury to the extensor tendon mechanism. (a) Mallet deformity. (b) Buttonhole deformity. From Reilly (1981), with permission.

Rehabilitation of wrist and hand injuries

There is often a tendency for athletes to play down wrist and finger injuries. Because they can run, and because they largely look normal, athletes may often be found some years later to still have a lack of movement or strength when compared to the uninjured side. This, of course, leads to faults in sports technique in those areas where the hand is used extensively, and lays the foundation for arthritis in later years. Hand rehabilitation is no less important than that of, say, a hamstring or injured collateral ligament of the knee, and this must be stressed over and over again.

For soft tissue injuries, especially those affecting the fingers, mobility following injury is the all-important factor. Where splinting is required, this should be in the 'protective position', which prevents capsular and ligamentous contracture while protecting the joint from further injury. The IP joints are immobilized in extension, the MCP joints in flexion, and the thumb in abduction (Isani, 1990). Movement must be begun as soon as possible after injury. Gentle isometrics and mobility exercise within the pain-free range can usually be begun 1 or 2 days after injury. Following this, exercise progresses as hand function returns. For convenience, wrist and finger exercises will be dealt with separately, although many of the exercises will be used together.

Wrist exercise

Three exercises can be used to form a basis for regaining wrist mobility. The first two are performed with the hand flat on a table top. Initially, the hand is placed palm down on the table surface, with the wrist crease at the table edge. The contralateral hand is placed on top of the injured one, and the elbow is moved up and down to produce flexion and extension of the wrist. The leverage of the forearm and body weight may be used to

actively assist movement at end range (Fig. 21.11a). The hand is then moved into the centre of the table, so that the whole forearm is supported, again, the contralateral hand holds the injured one flat against the table surface, stopping it moving. The elbow on the injured side is moved from side to side, sliding over the table surface to perform abduction and adduction of the injured wrist (Fig. 21.11b). Finally, the arm is held at 90° flexion with the elbow held close into the side of the body, the injured forearm supported by the cupped contralateral hand. A stick is held in the hand, and pronation and supination performed, aiming to move the stick into a horizontal position (Fig. 21.11c). Range of motion is measured regularly and realistic targets are set for the athlete to achieve.

Strength of the wrist is regained by performing movements against the resistance of a powerband or small weight. Flexion/extension may be performed holding a light dumb-bell, with the forearm supported. The other movements are performed with one

Figure 21.11 Autotherapy wrist mobilizations. (a) Flexion/extension of the wrist. (b) Abduction/adduction. (c) Pronation/supination with broom handle.

weight of the dumb-bell removed (hammer-bell), or using a hammer. The forearm is positioned with the side supported, and the hand holds the free end of the dumb-bell. Abduction is performed with the dumb-bell weight above the hand, and adduction with it below, in each case a 'chopping' action is used (Fig. 21.12). Pronation and supination are again executed using the hammerbell. The forearm is supported, and pronated and supinated to perform an arc with the hammerbell weight.

In addition to mobility and strength, compression, distraction and combined movements using functional activities are important. The ability of the wrist to take weight (press-up, bench press), to lock (straight arm actions holding a dumb-bell), and to take tension (chinning a bar) must be redeveloped. Rapid actions such as punching, catching, and throwing all form part of the late stage rehabilitation programme.

Finger exercise

Many finger exercises may be begun using simple pinch grip and power grip actions. Grip and release movements, holding, and

lifting may be performed using small objects with two fingers (pinch) or larger objects and all the fingers (power). Mobility may be performed by isolating the movement to the affected joint and simply teaching the athlete to perform autotherapy activities with the other hand. These are easier when the joint is warm and any tight skin is made more flexible, so hot soaking and the use of oil or cream is encouraged.

Isolation exercises for strength may be accomplished using therapeutic putty, rubber bands of varying sizes, and small weights. Again, functional activities, the ability to push, pull, and lock, and rapid grip and release actions are important. Simple actions such as screwing and unscrewing varying sized nuts and bolts improve dexterity. Pushing with the finger straight into a thick piece of foam rubber, and pulling using pinch, ring, power, and key grips help to restore tension and compression ability. Rapid throwing and catching actions with objects of varying sizes and weight rehabilitate grip and release.

Figure 21.12 Wrist abduction/adduction using a modified dumb-bell.

References

Albanese, S.A., Palmer, A.K., Kerr, D.R., Carpenter, C.W., Lisi, D. and Levinsohn, E.M. (1989) Wrist pain and distal growth plate closure of the radius in gymnasts. *Journal of Pediatric Orthopaedics*, **9**, 23–28

Aronen, J.G. (1985) Problems of the upper extremity in gymnasts. *Clinics in Sports Medicine*, **4**(1), 61–71

Bollen, S.R. (1988) Soft tissue injury in extreme rock climbers. *British Journal of Sports Medicine*, **22**(4), 145–147

Bunker, T.D., McNamee, P.B. and Scott, T.D. (1987) The Herbert screw for scaphoid fractures: a multicentre study. *Journal of Bone and Joint Surgery*, **69B**, 631–634

Carter, S.R., Aldridge, M.J., Fitzgerald, R. and Davies, A.M. (1988) Stress changes of the wrist in adolescent gymnasts. *British Journal of Radiology*, **61**, 109–112

Cetti, R., Christensen, S.E. and Reuther, K. (1982) Fracture of the lunate bone. *Hand*, **14**, 80–84

Corrigan, B. and Maitland, G.D. (1983) *Practical Orthopaedic Medicine*, Butterworth, London

Corrigan, B. and Maitland, G.D. (1994) *Musculoskeletal and Sports Injuries*, Butterworth-Heinemann, Oxford

Cyriax, J. (1982) *Textbook of Orthopaedic Medicine*, Vol. 1, 8th edn, Baillière Tindall, London

Cyriax, J.H. and Cyriax, P.J. (1983) *Illustrated Manual of Orthopaedic Medicine*, Butterworth, London

Diamond, M.R. (1989) Carpal tunnel syndrome: a review. *Chiropractic Sports Medicine*, 3(2), 46–53

Garrick, J.G. and Webb, D.R. (1990) *Sports Injuries: Diagnosis and Management*, W.B. Saunders, London

Haloua, J.P., Collin, J.P. and Coudeyre, L. (1987) Paralysis of the ulnar nerve in cyclists. *Annales de Chirurgie de la Main*, 6, 282–287

Hertling, D. and Kessler, R.M. (1990) *Management of Common Musculoskeletal Disorders*, J.B. Lippincott, Philadelphia

Horii, E., Nakamura, R., Watanabe, K. and Tsunoda, K. (1994) Scaphoid fracture as a 'Puncher's fracture'. *Journal of Orthopaedic Trauma*, 8, 107–110

Isani, A. (1990) Prevention and treatment of ligamentous sports injuries to the hand. *Sports Medicine*, 9(1), 48–61

Maitland, G.D. (1991) *Peripheral Manipulation*, 3rd edn, Butterworth-Heinemann, London

Mandelbaum B.R., Bartolozzi, A.R., Davis, C.A., Teurlings, L. and Bragonier, B. (1989) Wrist pain syndrome in the gymnast: pathogenetic, diagnostic and therapeutic considerations. *American Journal of Sports Medicine*, 17(3), 305–317

Moutet, F., Guinard, D., Lebrun, C., Bello-Champel, P. and Massart, P. (1989) Metacarpo-phalangeal thumb sprains: based on experience with more than 1000 cases. *Annales de Chirurgie de la Main*, 8, 99–109

Nakamura, R., Imaeda, T., Suzuki, K. and Miura, T. (1991) Sports-related Kienbock's disease. *American Journal of Sports Medicine*, 19(1), 88–91

O'Donoghue, D.H. (1976) *Treatment of Injuries to Athletes*, W.B. Saunders, Philadelphia

Palastanga, N., Field, D. and Soames, R. (1989) *Anatomy and Human Movement*, Heinemann Medical, Oxford

Palastanga, N., Field, D. and Soames, R. (1994) *Anatomy and Human Movement*, 2nd edn, Butterworth-Heinemann, Oxford

Palmer, A.K. and Werner, F.W. (1981) The triangular fibrocartilage complex of the wrist—anatomy and function. *Journal of Hand Surgery*, 6, 153–162

Peterson, L. and Renstrom, P. (1986) *Sports Injuries*, Martin Dunitz, London

Reid, D.C. (1992) *Sports Injury Assessment and Rehabilitation*, Churchill Livingstone, Edinburgh

Reilly, T. (1981) The concept, measurement and development of flexibility. In *Sports Fitness and Sports Injuries* (ed. T. Reilly), Faber and Faber, London

Rettig, A.C., Weidenbener, E.J. and Gloyeske, R. (1994) Alternative management of midthird scaphoid fractures in the athlete. *American Journal of Sports Medicine*, 22, 711–714

Rimmer, J.N. (1981) Injuries to the hand in sports. In *Sports Fitness and Sports Injuries* (ed. T. Reilly), Faber and Faber, London

Stener, B. (1962) Displacement of the ruptured ulnar collateral ligament of the metacarpophalangeal joint of the thumb: a clinical and anatomical study. *Journal of Bone and Joint Surgery*, **44B**, 869

Wilkes, J.S. (1989) Reconstructive surgery of the wrist and hand. In *Orthopaedic Physical Therapy* (eds R. Donatelli and M.J. Wooden), Churchill Livingstone, Edinburgh

Williams, J.G.P. and Sperryn, P.N. (1976) *Sports Medicine*, Edward Arnold, London

Wilmarth, M.A. and Nelson, S.G. (1988) Distal sensory latencies of the ulnar nerve in long distance bicyclists: pilot study. *Journal of Orthopaedic and Sports Physical Therapy*, 9, 370–374

Appendix

Manual muscle tests

The upper extremity

The following tests draw largely on the work of Kendall, McCreary and Provance (1993) and Clarkson and Gilewich (1989) to which the reader is referred for further information.

Serratus anterior

The serratus anterior is a scapular abductor and lateral rotator, which works in opposition to the rhomboids. As a screening test, the wall push-up or full push-up is performed and any scapular winging is noted. In both cases winging is more noticeable on eccentric activity. A similar, but less powerful, movement is obtained in a supine-lying position by performing a 'punch with a plus'. Again, weakness is apparent with scapular winging, but it should be noted that pectoralis minor can partially perform the punching action from this starting position by causing the coronoid to pull the scapular into subtle tilt. Resisted shoulder flexion (120°) in sitting is a more accurate test (Fig. A.1). If serratus anterior is weak, the rhomboids are usually found to be tight, due to an inability to abduct the scapulae fully. The rhomboids may be stretched by pulling on the vertebral border of the scapula, or by abducting the scapulae and crossing the arms fully.

Trapezius

The upper trapezius, levator scapulae and the rhomboids all elevate the scapulae. However, the upper trapezius upwardly rotates the scapula while the rhomboids and levator scapulae downwardly rotate it. These latter two muscles may be differentiated through the action of levator scapulae on the cervical spine. Elevation is tested in a sitting position, resisting both elevation of the shoulder and lateral flexion of the cervical spine (Fig. A.2).

The middle fibres of trapezius are tested with the athlete in a prone-lying position with the arm hanging over the couch side initially, and then abducted to 90° (Fig. A.3). The athlete adducts the scapula towards the mid-line. The rhomboids are differentiated from the middle trapezius by their action on scapular rotation. Laterally rotating the humerus, by pointing the thumb to the ceiling, tractions the teres major (a medial rotator of the gleno-humeral joint) causing it to pull on the axillary border of the scapular sufficiently to draw the scapula into upward rotation. As scapular adduction is begun, movement of the scapula into downward rotation shows the

Figure A.1 Serratus anterior.

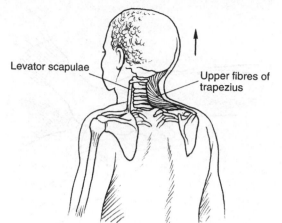

Figure A.2 Levator scapulae and upper trapezius.

(a)

(b)

Figure A.3 (a) Middle trapezius, (b) rhomboids.

rhomboids to be working with or without the middle trapezius. Medially rotating the humerus (thumb to floor) emphasizes the rhomboids and is an alternative test.

The lower trapezius is again assessed in a prone-lying position. Initially, the scapula is passively depressed and adducted into an optimal position (see p. 162). The arm is held by the side, slightly off the couch and the test assesses the athlete's ability to maintain scapular stabilization against the weight

of the arm. Progression is made by lengthening the arm lever while maintaining an optimal scapular position. The final test position is with the arm held diagonally overhead in line with the lower trapezius fibres (Fig. A.4)

The rhomboids

The rhomboids are tested with the athlete in a prone position (Fig. A.5). The athlete places the dorsum of his or her hand over the but-

Figure A.4 Lower fibres of trapezius.

Figure A.6 Anterior deltoid.

Figure A.5 Rhomboids.

tock on the non-test side, and attempts to raise the arm away from the back. Resistance is applied over the scapula, not the humerus. Differentiation from the middle trapezius relies on scapular rotation as described above.

Deltoid

Each of the three sets of deltoid fibres are assessed in a sitting position (Fig. A.6). For the anterior fibres, the athlete flexes the shoulder joint to 90° (in slight medial rotation). Where coracobrachialis is tested, the

anterior deltoid is placed at a disadvantage by maintaining an externally rotated position. Flexion adduction is used (Fig. A.7). The medial deltoid and supraspinatus are tested with the arm abducted to 90°. Supraspinatus may not be distinguished from the medial deltoid in initiation of abduction, as both muscles are active. However, palpation of supraspinatus and use of surface EMG will indicate if the muscle is contracting. As the muscle is covered by the middle and upper trapezius, the trapezius must remain as relaxed as possible throughout the action. The posterior fibres of the deltoid are assessed using horizontal

Figure A.7 Coracobrachialis.

abduction combined with slight lateral rotation (Fig. A.8).

Latissimus dorsi

The latissimus dorsi and teres major are tested in a prone-lying position with the arm by the athlete's side. The action is to extend the arm while maintaining adduction (Fig. A.9).

Figure A.8 Posterior deltoid.

Pectoralis major

The pectoralis major is assessed in a supine-lying position. Initially, the whole muscle is tested using horizontal adduction. Any excessive activity in the anterior deltoid is noted. The clavicular and sternal heads of the muscle may be differentiated by aligning the direction of pull with the appropriate muscle fibres. Both sets of fibres are tested using adduction and slight medial rotation. The clavicular (upper) head is tested from a 70° abducted position, aiming the pull to the sternal end of the clavicle. The sternal head is tested from 135° abduction, pulling towards the opposite iliac crest (Fig. A.10). Pectoralis minor is tested again in supine lying, but the action is a forward thrust with the shoulder region, with no direct movement of the humerus (Fig. A.11). This muscle is commonly short, and an important factor in altered mechanics of the gleno-humeral joint (see p. 164).

Internal and external rotation

Rotation is assessed either in a prone-lying position with the shoulder abducted to 90° (upper arm supported) and the elbow flexed, or in a sitting position with the upper arm

Latissimus dorsi   Teres major

Figure A.9 Latissimus dorsi and teres major.

Figure A.10 Pectoralis major.

Figure A.11 Pectoralis minor.

Figure A.13 External rotation of infraspinatus and teres minor.

tucked into the side. Internal rotation tests the subscapularis with teres major, pectoralis major, latissimus dorsi, and the anterior deltoid acting as assistant movers (Fig. A.12). External rotation tests the infraspinatus and teres minor with the posterior deltoid acting as an assistant (Fig. A.13).

Elbow flexors

Biceps, brachialis and brachioradialis are all assessed in supine lying with the shoulder adducted. The athlete performs resisted elbow flexion with the forearm supinated for biceps (Fig. A.14), pronated for brachialis and in mid-position for brachioradialis. The

Figure A.14 Biceps brachii.

effect of biceps on gleno-humeral flexion, and radio-humeral supination must also be tested, with the athlete in a sitting position.

Triceps

The athlete may be tested in supine lying, with the shoulder internally rotated and flexed to 90°. Elbow extension is resisted (Fig. A.15). In prone lying, with the shoulder abducted to 90°, elbow extension may be combined with shoulder extension.

Pronation and supination

Both movements are tested with the athlete in a sitting position, with the arm positioned in mid-position (Fig. A.16).

Figure A.12 Internal rotation of subscapularis.

Figure A.15   Triceps.

Figure A.17   Iliopsoas.

Figure A.16   Supinator.

The lower extremity

Iliopsoas

Iliopsoas is tested in a sitting position, with resisted hip flexion, and the knee remaining flexed (Fig. A.17). The muscle is differentiated from rectus femoris by the action of rectus over the knee.

Sartorius

The starting position is supine lying, and hip flexion, abduction and external rotation (FABER) are combined with knee flexion (Fig. A.18).

Figure A.18   Sartorius.

Gluteus maximus

The athlete is positioned in prone lying, and inner range hip extension is performed with the knee remaining flexed to reduce the activity of the hamstrings. Through range, activity is assessed from four point kneeling, with the athlete's abdomen supported over a stool (Fig. A.19) The movement must be pure extension with no abduction.

Hip abductors

The starting position is side lying. The gluteus minimus and gluteus medius are both tested in side lying (Fig. A.20). Emphasis is placed on the posterior fibres of gluteus medius (postural portion of the muscle) by combining hip abduction with external rotation

Figure A.19   Gluteus maximus.

Figure A.21   Tensor fascia lata.

Hip adductors

A side-lying starting position is chosen with the tested leg down (Fig. A.22). Adduction is resisted to test the whole adductor group. Flexing the knee will shorten gracilis and place it at a mechanical disadvantage, thus

Figure A.20   Gluteus medius.

(see p. 150). Tensor fascia lata is again tested in side lying. It is differentiated from gluteus minimus by the action of tensor fascia lata on hip flexion, knee extension and in tightening the ilio-tibial band (Fig. A.21)

Figure A.22   Adductors.

emphasizing the short adductors. Gracilis should also be tested with the hamstrings by resited knee flexion. It is differentiated from the hamstrings by its inability to extend the hip. Adductor longus and brevis, together with pectineus, aid in hip flexion, so a tendency for the leg to drift into flexion is an indication that these adductors are dominant and/or that the hip extensors are failing to neutralize the flexion movement.

Hip rotators

A prone-lying starting position may be used with the pelvis stabilized by the therapist. The hip and knee are flexed to 90°, and resisted internal rotation (foot out) and external rotation (foot in) are performed (Fig. A.23).

Hamstrings

The starting position is prone lying with the pelvis stabilized. Resisted knee flexion is performed with internal rotation (semi-membranosus and semi-tendinosus) or external rotation (biceps femoris) (Fig. A.24). The action of the hamstrings and gluteus maximus in extending the hip is an important

Figure A.24 Hamstrings.

factor to muscle imbalance assessment in this region (see p. 150)

Quadriceps

The quadriceps are tested in a sitting position. Resisted knee extension is performed to assess the vasti, and resisted knee extension and hip flexion are combined to test the rectus femoris (Fig. A.25).

Figure A.23 Hip rotation.

Figure A.25 The quadriceps.

Popliteus

The athlete is tested in a sitting position, and the action is resisted medial rotation of the tibia on the fixed femur. In cases where the lateral hamstrings are dominant over the medial, active medial rotation may be extremely weak. During the test tibial rotation must be differentiated from foot inversion (Fig. A.26).

References

Clarkson, H.M. and Gilewich, G.B. (1989) *Musculoskeletal Assessment*, Williams and Wilkins, Baltimore

Kendall, F.P., McCreary, E. and Provance, P.G. (1993) *Muscles. Testing and Function*, Williams and Wilkins, Baltimore

Figure A.26   Popliteus.

Index